Cancer
SOURCEBOOK

Eighth Edition

Health Reference Series

Eighth Edition

Cancer
SOURCEBOOK

Basic Consumer Health Information about Major Forms and Stages of Cancer, Featuring Facts about Head and Neck Cancers, Lung Cancers, Gastrointestinal Cancers, Genitourinary Cancers, Lymphomas, Blood Cell Cancers, Endocrine Cancers, Skin Cancers, Bone Cancers, Metastatic Cancers, and More

Along with Facts about Cancer Treatments, Cancer Risks and Prevention, a Glossary of Related Terms, Statistical Data, and a Directory of Resources for Additional Information

OMNIGRAPHICS

615 Griswold, Ste. 901, Detroit, MI 48226

* * *

OMNIGRAPHICS
Angela L. Williams, *Managing Editor*

***

ISBN 978-0-7808-1622-0
E-ISBN 978-0-7808-1623-7

Library of Congress Cataloging-in-Publication Data

Names: Omnigraphics, Inc.

Title: Cancer sourcebook: basic consumer health information about major forms and stages of cancer, featuring facts about head and neck cancers, lung cancers, gastrointestinal cancers, genitourinary cancers, lymphomas, blood cell cancers, endocrine cancers, skin cancers, bone cancers, metastatic cancers, and more; along with facts about cancer treatments, cancer risks and prevention, a glossary of related terms, statistical data, and a directory of resources for additional information.

Description: Eighth edition. | Detroit, MI: Omnigraphics, [2018] | Series: Health reference series | Includes bibliographical references and index.

Identifiers: LCCN 2018002745 (print) | LCCN 2018004155 (ebook) | ISBN 9780780816237 (eBook) | ISBN 9780780816220 (hardcover: alk. paper)

Subjects: LCSH: Cancer--Popular works. | Cancer--Handbooks, manuals, etc.

Classification: LCC RC263 (ebook) | LCC RC263.C294 2018 (print) | DDC 616.99/4--dc23

LC record available at https://lccn.loc.gov/2018002745

Printed in the United States

Table of Contents

Part II: Common Types of Cancer

Cancers Affecting the Brain and Central Nervous System

Cancers Affecting the Endocrine System

Cancers Affecting the Eyes, Mouth, and Neck

Cancers Affecting the Breasts and Reproductive Organs

Cancers Affecting the Blood Cells and Immune System

Cancers Affecting the Skin and Bones

Cancers Affecting Other or Multiple Body Systems

Part III: Cancer-Related Tests and Treatments

Part IV: Recurrent and Advanced Cancer

Part V: Clinical Trials and Cancer Research

Part VI: Additional Help and Information

Preface

About This Book

Every year, nearly 1.6 million Americans receive a diagnosis of cancer. Cancer is not a single disease, however. It is many different diseases that all share one common characteristic: Some of the body's cells do not die when they should. Instead they continue to grow and divide. Through this process, cancer cells can damage the body's tissues and organs, leading to a broad array of symptoms and even death. The cellular changes that lead to the development of cancer are sometimes inherited but they may also result from environmental or lifestyle factors. Although the survival rates for many types of cancer have improved in recent years and innovative treatment protocols are being developed, cancer remains one of the leading causes of death in the United States.

Cancer Sourcebook, Eighth Edition provides updated information about common types of cancer affecting the head, neck, central nervous system, endocrine system, lungs, digestive and urinary tracts, blood cells, immune system, skin, bones, and other body systems. It explains how people can reduce their risk of cancer by adopting a healthy life-style, addressing issues related to cancer risk, and taking advantage of screening exams. Various treatment choices—including surgery, chemotherapy, radiation therapy, bone marrow transplantation, and biological therapies—are discussed, and facts are provided about cancer clinical trials and other ongoing research. The book concludes with a glossary of related terms, a directory of national cancer organizations, and suggestions for finding community-based resources.

How to Use This Book

This book is divided into parts and chapters. Parts focus on broad areas of interest. Chapters are devoted to single topics within a part.

Part I: Cancer Risk Factors and Cancer Prevention introduces cancer and discusses hereditary, lifestyle, and environmental factors that can sometimes set the stage for the growth of cancer. It explains which factors can be prevented and which factors are unavoidable. Statistical information about cancer prevalence, mortality, and survival is also provided, along with facts about specific population groups that suffer disproportionately from cancer. It concludes with myths and misconceptions regarding cancer.

Part II: Common Types of Cancer includes a head-to-toe list of the most frequently occurring types of cancer. Individual chapters describe the development, identification, and treatment of cancers that affect the various components of the body, including the brain and central nervous system, endocrine system, respiratory system, blood and immune system, digestive and urinary tracts, and reproductive organs, as well as the bones and skin.

Part III: Cancer-Related Tests and Treatments describes the screening methods used to find cancers at their earliest stages and the procedures most commonly used in cancer diagnosis and treatment. It also provides information on how to find healthcare services. These include medical imaging tests, surgical procedures, chemotherapy, radiation therapy, precision medicine, stem cell transplantation, and various complementary and alternative medicine (CAM) practices used in cancer care.

Part IV: Recurrent and Advanced Cancer explains the factors that cause cancer to spread to distant parts of the body and to come back again after a time of remission. It also describes end-of-life care, decisions to be taken by cancer patients and their families, and offers suggestions regarding ways to make wishes known.

Part V: Clinical Trials and Cancer Research discusses cancer treatment trials and various researches related to cancer. Emerging therapies, including gene therapy, oncolytic virus therapy, and liquid biopsy, for cancer treatment and prevention are also described.

Part VI: Additional Help and Information includes a glossary of terms, a directory of national cancer organizations, and suggestions for finding local resources. A chapter offering cautionary guidance about cancer-related health fraud, especially on the Internet, is also provided.

Bibliographic Note

This volume contains documents and excerpts from publications issued by the following U.S. government agencies: Centers for Disease Control and Prevention (CDC); Genetic and Rare Diseases Information Center (GARD); National Cancer Institute (NCI); National Institute of Environmental Health Sciences (NIEHS); National Institutes of Health (NIH); *NIH News in Health*; Office on Women's Health (OWH); U.S. Environmental Protection Agency (EPA); and U.S. Food and Drug Administration (FDA).

It may also contain original material produced by Omnigraphics and reviewed by medical consultants.

About the Health Reference Series

The *Health Reference Series* is designed to provide basic medical information for patients, families, caregivers, and the general public. Each volume takes a particular topic and provides comprehensive coverage. This is especially important for people who may be dealing with a newly diagnosed disease or a chronic disorder in themselves or in a family member. People looking for preventive guidance, information about disease warning signs, medical statistics, and risk factors for health problems will also find answers to their questions in the *Health Reference Series*. The *Series*, however, is not intended to serve as a tool for diagnosing illness, in prescribing treatments, or as a substitute for the physician/patient relationship. All people concerned about medical symptoms or the possibility of disease are encouraged to seek professional care from an appropriate healthcare provider.

A Note about Spelling and Style

Health Reference Series editors use *Stedman's Medical Dictionary* as an authority for questions related to the spelling of medical terms and the *Chicago Manual of Style* for questions related to grammatical structures, punctuation, and other editorial concerns. Consistent adherence is not always possible, however, because the individual volumes within the *Series* include many documents from a wide variety of different producers, and the editor's primary goal is to present material from each source as accurately as is possible. This sometimes means that information in different chapters or sections may follow other guidelines and alternate spelling authorities. For example, occasionally a copyright holder may require that eponymous terms be shown in possessive forms (Crohn's disease vs. Crohn disease) or that British spelling norms be retained (leukaemia vs. leukemia).

Medical Review

Omnigraphics contracts with a team of qualified, senior medical professionals who serve as medical consultants for the *Health Reference Series*. As necessary, medical consultants review reprinted and originally written material for currency and accuracy. Citations including the phrase, "Reviewed (month, year)" indicate material reviewed by this team. Medical consultation services are provided to the *Health Reference Series* editors by:

Dr. Vijayalakshmi, MBBS, DGO, MD
Dr. Senthil Selvan, MBBS, DCH, MD
Dr. K. Sivanandham, MBBS, DCH, MS (Research), PhD

Our Advisory Board

We would like to thank the following board members for providing initial guidance on the development of this series:

- Dr. Lynda Baker, Associate Professor of Library and Information Science, Wayne State University, Detroit, MI
- Nancy Bulgarelli, William Beaumont Hospital Library, Royal Oak, MI
- Karen Imarisio, Bloomfield Township Public Library, Bloomfield Township, MI
- Karen Morgan, Mardigian Library, University of Michigan-Dearborn, Dearborn, MI
- Rosemary Orlando, St. Clair Shores Public Library, St. Clair Shores, MI

Health Reference Series *Update Policy*

The inaugural book in the *Health Reference Series* was the first edition of *Cancer Sourcebook* published in 1989. Since then, the *Series* has been enthusiastically received by librarians and in the medical community. In order to maintain the standard of providing high-quality health information for the layperson the editorial staff at Omnigraphics felt it was necessary to implement a policy of updating volumes when warranted.

Medical researchers have been making tremendous strides, and it is the purpose of the *Health Reference Series* to stay current with the most recent advances. Each decision to update a volume is made on an individual basis. Some of the considerations include how much new information is available and the feedback we receive from people who use the books. If there is a topic you would like to see added to the update list, or an area of medical concern you feel has not been adequately addressed, please write to:

Managing Editor
Health Reference Series
Omnigraphics
615 Griswold, Ste. 901
Detroit, MI 48226

Part One

Cancer Risk Factors and Cancer Prevention

Chapter 1

What Is Cancer?

Cancer is the name given to a collection of related diseases. In all types of cancer, some of the body's cells begin to divide without stopping and spread into surrounding tissues. Cancer can start almost anywhere in the human body, which is made up of trillions of cells. Normally, human cells grow and divide to form new cells as the body needs them. When cells grow old or become damaged, they die, and new cells take their place.

When cancer develops, however, this orderly process breaks down. As cells become more and more abnormal, old or damaged cells survive when they should die, and new cells form when they are not needed. These extra cells can divide without stopping and may form growths called tumors. Many cancers form solid tumors, which are masses of tissue. Cancers of the blood, such as leukemias, generally do not form solid tumors.

Cancerous tumors are malignant, which means they can spread into, or invade, nearby tissues. In addition, as these tumors grow, some cancer cells can break off and travel to distant places in the body through the blood or the lymph system and form new tumors far from the original tumor. Unlike malignant tumors, benign tumors do not spread into, or invade, nearby tissues. Benign tumors can sometimes be quite large, however. When removed, they usually don't grow back, whereas malignant tumors sometimes do. Unlike most benign tumors elsewhere in the body, benign brain tumors can be life threatening.

This chapter includes text excerpted from "What Is Cancer?" National Cancer Institute (NCI), February 9, 2015.

Differences between Cancer Cells and Normal Cells

Cancer cells differ from normal cells in many ways that allow them to grow out of control and become invasive. One important difference is that cancer cells are less specialized than normal cells. That is, whereas normal cells mature into very distinct cell types with specific functions, cancer cells do not. This is one reason that, unlike normal cells, cancer cells continue to divide without stopping.

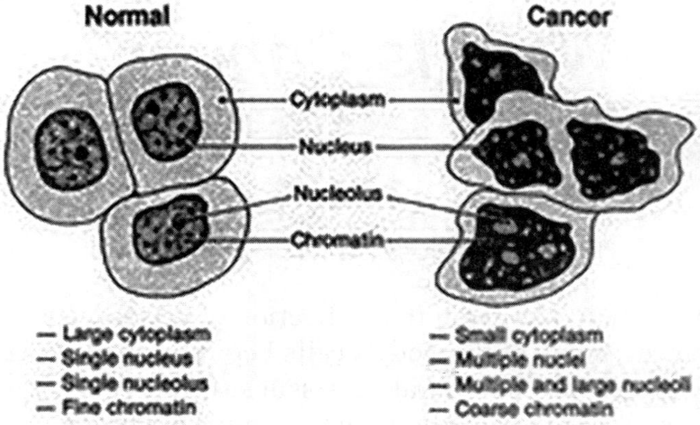

Figure 1.1. *Normal Cell versus Cancer Cell* (Source: "Normal and Cancer Cells Structure," National Cancer Institute (NCI).)

In addition, cancer cells are able to ignore signals that normally tell cells to stop dividing or that begin a process known as programmed cell death, or apoptosis, which the body uses to get rid of unneeded cells. Cancer cells may be able to influence the normal cells, molecules, and blood vessels that surround and feed a tumor—an area known as the microenvironment. For instance, cancer cells can induce nearby normal cells to form blood vessels that supply tumors with oxygen and nutrients, which they need to grow. These blood vessels also remove waste products from tumors.

Cancer cells are also often able to evade the immune system, a network of organs, tissues, and specialized cells that protects the body from infections and other conditions. Although the immune system normally removes damaged or abnormal cells from the body, some cancer cells are able to "hide" from the immune system.

Tumors can also use the immune system to stay alive and grow. For example, with the help of certain immune system cells that normally prevent a runaway immune response, cancer cells can actually keep the immune system from killing cancer cells.

How Cancer Arises

Cancer is a genetic disease—that is, it is caused by changes to genes that control the way our cells function, especially how they grow and divide.

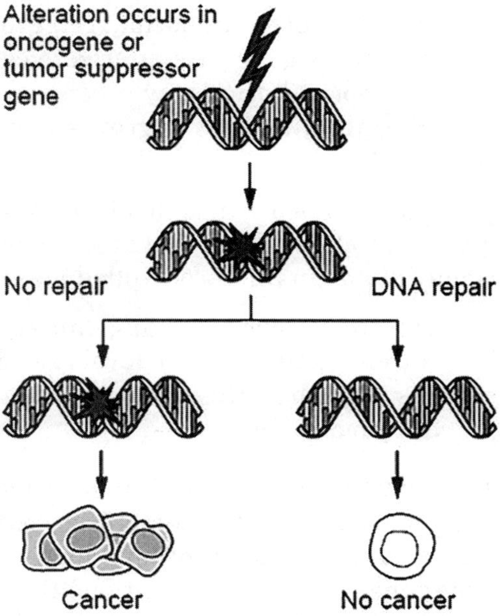

Figure 1.2. *How Cancer Arises* (Source: "Cancer and the Environment," National Institute of Environmental Health Sciences (NIEHS).)

Genetic changes that cause cancer can be inherited from our parents. They can also arise during a person's lifetime as a result of errors that occur as cells divide or because of damage to deoxyribonucleic acid (DNA) caused by certain environmental exposures. Cancer-causing environmental exposures include substances, such as the chemicals in tobacco smoke, and radiation, such as ultraviolet rays from the sun.

Each person's cancer has a unique combination of genetic changes. As the cancer continues to grow, additional changes will occur. Even within the same tumor, different cells may have different genetic changes. In general, cancer cells have more genetic changes, such as mutations in DNA, than normal cells. Some of these changes may have nothing to do with the cancer; they may be the result of the cancer, rather than its cause.

"Drivers" of Cancer

The genetic changes that contribute to cancer tend to affect three main types of genes—proto-oncogenes, tumor suppressor genes, and DNA repair genes. These changes are sometimes called "drivers" of cancer.

- **Proto-oncogenes** are involved in normal cell growth and division. However, when these genes are altered in certain ways or are more active than normal, they may become cancer-causing genes (or oncogenes), allowing cells to grow and survive when they should not.
- **Tumor suppressor genes** are also involved in controlling cell growth and division. Cells with certain alterations in tumor suppressor genes may divide in an uncontrolled manner.
- **DNA repair genes** are involved in fixing damaged DNA. Cells with mutations in these genes tend to develop additional mutations in other genes. Together, these mutations may cause the cells to become cancerous.

As scientists have learned more about the molecular changes that lead to cancer, they have found that certain mutations commonly occur in many types of cancer. Because of this, cancers are sometimes characterized by the types of genetic alterations that are believed to be driving them, not just by where they develop in the body and how the cancer cells look under the microscope.

When Cancer Spreads

A cancer that has spread from the place where it first started to another place in the body is called metastatic cancer. The process by which cancer cells spread to other parts of the body is called metastasis. Metastatic cancer has the same name and the same type of cancer cells as the original, or primary, cancer. For example, breast cancer that spreads to and forms a metastatic tumor in the lung is metastatic breast cancer, not lung cancer.

Under a microscope, metastatic cancer cells generally look the same as cells of the original cancer. Moreover, metastatic cancer cells and cells of the original cancer usually have some molecular features in common, such as the presence of specific chromosome changes. Treatment may help prolong the lives of some people with metastatic cancer. In general, though, the primary goal of treatments for metastatic cancer is to control the growth of the cancer or to relieve symptoms caused by it. Metastatic tumors can cause severe damage to how the body functions, and most people who die of cancer die of metastatic disease.

Tissue Changes That Are Not Cancer

Not every change in the body's tissues is cancer. Some tissue changes may develop into cancer if they are not treated, however. Here are some examples of tissue changes that are not cancer but, in some cases, are monitored:

- **Hyperplasia** occurs when cells within a tissue divide faster than normal and extra cells build up, or proliferate. However, the cells and the way the tissue is organized look normal under a microscope. Hyperplasia can be caused by several factors or conditions, including chronic irritation.
- **Dysplasia** is a more serious condition than hyperplasia. In dysplasia, there is also a buildup of extra cells. But the cells look abnormal and there are changes in how the tissue is organized. In general, the more abnormal the cells and tissue look, the greater the chance that cancer will form. Some types of dysplasia may need to be monitored or treated. An example of dysplasia is an abnormal mole (called a dysplastic nevus) that forms on the skin. A dysplastic nevus can turn into melanoma, although most do not.

An even more serious condition is carcinoma in situ. Although it is sometimes called cancer, carcinoma in situ is not cancer because the abnormal cells do not spread beyond the original tissue. That is, they do not invade nearby tissue the way that cancer cells do. But, because some carcinomas in situ may become cancer, they are usually treated.

Types of Cancer

There are more than 100 types of cancer. Types of cancer are usually named for the organs or tissues where the cancers form. For example, lung cancer starts in cells of the lung, and brain cancer starts in cells of the brain. Cancers also may be described by the type of cell that formed them, such as an epithelial cell or a squamous cell.

Here are some categories of cancers that begin in specific types of cells:

Carcinoma

Carcinomas are the most common type of cancer. They are formed by epithelial cells, which are the cells that cover the inside and outside surfaces of the body. There are many types of epithelial cells, which often have a column-like shape when viewed under a microscope.

Carcinomas that begin in different epithelial cell types have specific names:

- **Adenocarcinoma** is a cancer that forms in epithelial cells that produce fluids or mucus. Tissues with this type of epithelial cell are sometimes called glandular tissues. Most cancers of the breast, colon, and prostate are adenocarcinomas.
- **Basal cell carcinoma** is a cancer that begins in the lower or basal (base) layer of the epidermis, which is a person's outer layer of skin.
- **Squamous cell carcinoma** is a cancer that forms in squamous cells, which are epithelial cells that lie just beneath the outer surface of the skin. Squamous cells also line many other organs, including the stomach, intestines, lungs, bladder, and kidneys. Squamous cells look flat, like fish scales, when viewed under a microscope. Squamous cell carcinomas are sometimes called epidermoid carcinomas.
- **Transitional cell carcinoma** is a cancer that forms in a type of epithelial tissue called transitional epithelium, or urothelium. This tissue, which is made up of many layers of epithelial cells that can get bigger and smaller, is found in the linings of the bladder, ureters, and part of the kidneys (renal pelvis), and a few other organs. Some cancers of the bladder, ureters, and kidneys are transitional cell carcinomas.

Sarcoma

Sarcomas are cancers that form in bone and soft tissues, including muscle, fat, blood vessels, lymph vessels, and fibrous tissue (such as tendons and ligaments).

Osteosarcoma is the most common cancer of bone. The most common types of soft tissue sarcoma are leiomyosarcoma, Kaposi sarcoma, malignant fibrous histiocytoma, liposarcoma, and dermatofibrosarcoma protuberans.

Leukemia

Cancers that begin in the blood-forming tissue of the bone marrow are called leukemias. These cancers do not form solid tumors. Instead, large numbers of abnormal white blood cells (leukemia cells and leukemic blast cells) buildup in the blood and bone marrow, crowding out normal blood cells. The low level of normal blood cells can make it harder for the body to get oxygen to its tissues, control bleeding, or fight infections.

There are four common types of leukemia, which are grouped based on how quickly the disease gets worse (acute or chronic) and on the type of blood cell the cancer starts in (lymphoblastic or myeloid).

Lymphoma

Lymphoma is cancer that begins in lymphocytes (T cells or B cells). These are disease-fighting white blood cells that are part of the immune system. In lymphoma, abnormal lymphocytes build up in lymph nodes and lymph vessels, as well as in other organs of the body.

There are two main types of lymphoma:

- **Hodgkin lymphoma**—People with this disease have abnormal lymphocytes that are called Reed-Sternberg cells. These cells usually form from B cells.
- **Non-Hodgkin lymphoma**—This is a large group of cancers that start in lymphocytes. The cancers can grow quickly or slowly and can form from B cells or T cells.

Multiple Myeloma

Multiple myeloma is cancer that begins in plasma cells, another type of immune cell. The abnormal plasma cells, called myeloma cells, buildup in the bone marrow and form tumors in bones all through the body. Multiple myeloma is also called plasma cell myeloma and Kahler disease.

Melanoma

Melanoma is cancer that begins in cells that become melanocytes, which are specialized cells that make melanin (the pigment that gives skin its color). Most melanomas form on the skin, but melanomas can also form in other pigmented tissues, such as the eye.

Brain and Spinal Cord Tumors

There are different types of brain and spinal cord tumors. These tumors are named based on the type of cell in which they formed and where the tumor first formed in the central nervous system. For example, an astrocytic tumor begins in star-shaped brain cells called astrocytes, which help keep nerve cells healthy. Brain tumors can be benign (not cancer) or malignant (cancer).

Other Types of Tumors

Germ Cell Tumors

Germ cell tumors are a type of tumor that begins in the cells that give rise to sperm or eggs. These tumors can occur almost anywhere in the body and can be either benign or malignant.

Neuroendocrine Tumors

Neuroendocrine tumors form from cells that release hormones into the blood in response to a signal from the nervous system. These tumors, which may make higher-than-normal amounts of hormones, can cause many different symptoms. Neuroendocrine tumors may be benign or malignant.

Carcinoid Tumors

Carcinoid tumors are a type of neuroendocrine tumor. They are slow-growing tumors that are usually found in the gastrointestinal system (most often in the rectum and small intestine). Carcinoid tumors may spread to the liver or other sites in the body, and they may secrete substances such as serotonin or prostaglandins, causing carcinoid syndrome.

Chapter 2

Cancer Statistics

Chapter Contents

Section 2.1

Understanding Statistics on Incidence, Prevalence, and Mortality

This section includes text excerpted from "Cancer Statistics," National Cancer Institute (NCI), March 22, 2017.

Cancer has a major impact on society in the United States and across the world. Cancer statistics describe what happens in large groups of people and provide a picture in time of the burden of cancer on society. Statistics tell us things such as how many people are diagnosed with and die from cancer each year, the number of people who are currently living after a cancer diagnosis, the average age at diagnosis, and the numbers of people who are still alive at a given time after diagnosis. They also tell us about differences among groups defined by age, sex, racial/ethnic group, geographic location, and other categories. Although statistical trends are usually not directly applicable to individual patients, they are essential for governments, policy makers, health professionals, and researchers to understand the impact of cancer on the population and to develop strategies to address the challenges that cancer poses to the society at large. Statistical trends are also important for measuring the success of efforts to control and manage cancer.

Statistics at a Glance: The Burden of Cancer in the United States

- In 2016, an estimated 1,685,210 new cases of cancer will be diagnosed in the United States and 595,690 people will die from the disease
- The most common cancers in 2016 are projected to be breast cancer, lung and bronchus cancer, prostate cancer, colon and rectum cancer, bladder cancer, melanoma of the skin, non-Hodgkin lymphoma, thyroid cancer, kidney and renal pelvis cancer, leukemia, endometrial cancer, and pancreatic cancer

- The number of new cases of cancer (cancer incidence) is 454.8 per 100,000 men and women per year (based on 2008–2012 cases)
- The number of cancer deaths (cancer mortality) is 171.2 per 100,000 men and women per year (based on 2008–2012 deaths)
- Cancer mortality is higher among men than women (207.9 per 100,000 men and 145.4 per 100,000 women). It is highest in African American men (261.5 per 100,000) and lowest in Asian/Pacific Islander women (91.2 per 100,000). (Based on 2008–2012 deaths)
- The number of people living beyond a cancer diagnosis reached nearly 14.5 million in 2014 and is expected to rise to almost 19 million by 2024
- Approximately 39.6 percent of men and women will be diagnosed with cancer at some point during their lifetimes (based on 2010–2012 data)
- In 2014, an estimated 15,780 children and adolescents ages 0–19 were diagnosed with cancer and 1,960 died of the disease
- National expenditures for cancer care in the United States totaled nearly $125 billion in 2010 and could reach $156 billion in 2020

Statistics at a Glance: The Burden of Cancer Worldwide

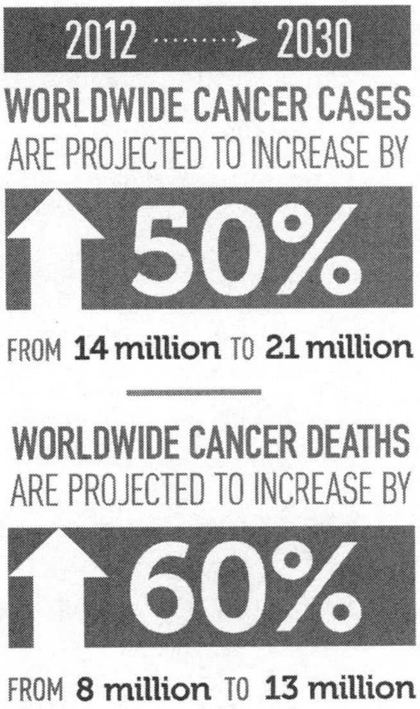

Figure 2.1. *Worldwide Cancer Cases*

- Cancer is among the leading causes of death worldwide. In 2012, there were 14 million new cases and 8.2 million cancer-related deaths worldwide
- The number of new cancer cases will rise to 22 million within the next two decades
- More than 60 percent of the world's new cancer cases occur in Africa, Asia, and Central and South America; 70 percent of the world's cancer deaths also occur in these regions

U.S. Cancer Mortality Trends

The best indicator of progress against cancer is a change in age-adjusted mortality (death) rates, although other measures, such as quality of life, are also important. Incidence is also important, but it is not always straightforward to interpret changes in incidence. For example, if a new screening test detects many cancer cases that would never have caused a problem during someone's life (called overdiagnosis), the incidence of that cancer would appear to increase even though the death rates do not change. But a rise in incidence can also reflect a real increase in disease, as is the case when an increase in exposure to a risk factor causes more cases of cancer. In this scenario the increased incidence would likely lead to a rise in mortality from the cancer.

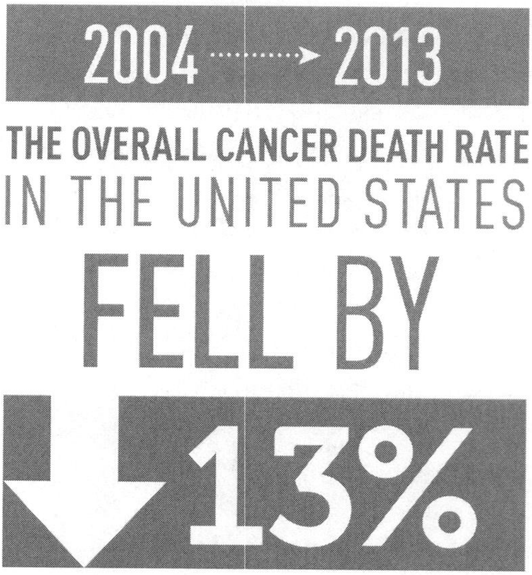

Figure 2.2. *U.S. Cancer Death Rates*

In the United States, the overall cancer death rate has declined since the early 1990s. The most recent Surveillance, Epidemiology, and End Results Program (SEER) Cancer Statistics Review, updated in September 2016, shows that cancer death rates decreased by:

- 1.8 percent per year among men from 2004–2013
- 1.4 percent per year among women from 2004–2013
- 1.4 percent per year among children ages 0–19 from 2009–2013

Although death rates for many individual cancer types have also declined, rates for a few cancers have stabilized or even increased. As the overall cancer death rate has declined, the number of cancer survivors has increased. These trends show that progress is being made against the disease, but much work remains. Although rates of smoking, a major cause of cancer, have declined, the U.S. population is aging, and cancer rates increase with age. Obesity, another risk factor for cancer, is also increasing.

Section 2.2

Statistics for Different Kinds of Cancer

This section includes text excerpted from "Cancer Prevention and Control—Statistics for Different Kinds of Cancer," Centers for Disease Control and Prevention (CDC), August 16, 2016.

Every year, cancer claims the lives of more than half a million Americans. Cancer is the second leading cause of death in the United States, exceeded only by heart disease. One of every four deaths in the United States is due to cancer. According to the *United States Cancer Statistics: 1999–2014 Incidence and Mortality Web-based Report,* 591,686 people died of cancer in the United States in 2014, the latest year for which statistics are available. The following statistics are for some of the most common kinds of cancer in the United States, based on data from the *United States Cancer Statistics: 1999–2014 Incidence and Mortality Web-based Report.*

Statistics for Specific Cancer Types

Bladder Cancer Statistics

In the United States in 2014 (the most recent year for which numbers are available):

- 72,462 people (55,014 men and 17,448 women) got bladder cancer
- 15,775 people (11,291 men and 4,484 women) died from bladder cancer
- Men were about three times as likely as women to get bladder cancer, and white people had higher rates of bladder cancer than people of other races and ethnicities
- Among men, white men had the highest rates of getting bladder cancer (36.4 per 100,000 men), followed by black men (19.0), Hispanic men (18.6), American Indian/Alaska Native men (14.8), and Asian/Pacific Islander men (14.0)
- Among women, white women had the highest rates of getting bladder cancer (9.0 per 100,000 women), followed by black women (6.4), Hispanic women (4.8), Asian/Pacific Islander women (3.7), and American Indian/Alaska Native women (3.4)

Breast Cancer Statistics

Not counting some kinds of skin cancer, breast cancer in the United States is:

- The most common cancer in women, no matter your race or ethnicity
- The most common cause of death from cancer among Hispanic women
- The second most common cause of death from cancer among white, black, Asian/Pacific Islander, and American Indian/Alaska Native women

In 2014 (the most recent year numbers are available):

- 236,968 women and 2,141 men in the United States were diagnosed with breast cancer
- 41,211 women and 465 men in the United States died from breast cancer

Cervical Cancer Statistics

Cervical cancer used to be the leading cause of cancer death for women in the United States. However, in the past 40 years, the number of cases of cervical cancer and the number of deaths from cervical cancer have decreased significantly. This decline largely is the result of many women getting regular Pap tests, which can find cervical precancer before it turns into cancer.

In 2014 (the most recent year numbers are available):

- 12,578 women in the United States were diagnosed with cervical cancer
- 4,115 women in the United States died from cervical cancer

Colorectal Cancer Statistics

Of cancers that affect both men and women, colorectal cancer is the second leading cause of cancer-related deaths in the United States. It is the third most common cancer in men and in women.

In 2014 (the most recent year numbers are available):

- 139,992 people in the United States were diagnosed with colorectal cancer, including 73,396 men and 66,596 women
- 51,651 people in the United States died from colorectal cancer, including 27,134 men and 24,517 women

Head and Neck Cancers Statistics

The following statistics apply to cancers of the oral cavity and pharynx, which includes cancers of the lip, tongue, mouth, pharynx, and tonsils.

In the United States in 2014 (the most recent year for which numbers are available):

- 43,371 people (30,883 men and 12,488 women) got cancers of the oral cavity and pharynx
- 9,404 people (6,768 men and 2,636 women) died from cancers of the oral cavity and pharynx
- Among men, white men had the highest rate of getting cancers of the oral cavity and pharynx (18.0 per 100,000 men), followed by black men (13.9), Asian/Pacific Islander men (11.1), American Indian/Alaska Native men (10.5), and Hispanic men (10.0)

- Among women, white women had the highest rate of getting cancers of the oral cavity and pharynx (6.5 per 100,000 women), followed by black women (4.9), Asian/Pacific Islander women (4.7), Hispanic women (4.4), and American Indian/Alaska Native women (3.8)

Kidney Cancer Statistics

In the United States in 2014 (the most recent year for which numbers are available):

- 59,395 people (37,531 men and 21,864 women) got kidney and renal pelvis cancers
- 13,917 people (9,203 men and 4,714 women) died from kidney and renal pelvis cancers
- Among men, black men are the most like to get kidney and renal pelvis cancers (24.7 per 100,000 men), followed by white men (22.0), Hispanic men (20.6), American Indian/Alaska Native men (19.5), and Asian/Pacific Islander men (10.4)
- Among women, black women are the most like to get kidney and renal pelvis cancers (12.4 per 100,000 women), followed by Hispanic women (11.9), white women (11.4), American Indian/Alaska Native women (10.8), and Asian/Pacific Islander women (4.9)

Leukemia Statistics

In the United States in 2014 (the most recent year for which numbers are available):

- 47,135 people (27,489 men and 19,646 women) were diagnosed with leukemia, and 23,564 people (13,542 men and 10,022 women) died from it
- Among men, white men had the highest rate of developing leukemia (17.5 per 100,000 men), followed by black men (13.0), Hispanic men (12.3), Asian/Pacific Islander men (9.4), and American Indian/Alaska Native men (9.2)
- Among women, white women had the highest rate of developing leukemia (10.6 per 100,000 women), followed by Hispanic

women (8.9), black women (8.4), Asian/Pacific Islander women (6.2), and American Indian/Alaska Native women (5.3)

Liver Cancer Statistics

In the United States in 2014 (the most recent year numbers are available):

- 31,411 people (22,472 men and 8,939 women) were diagnosed with liver cancer
- 24,598 people (16,623 men and 8,075 women) died from liver cancer
- Among men, Hispanic men had the highest rates of getting liver cancer (20.1 per 100,000 men), followed by Asian/Pacific Islander men (18.4), black men (17.0), American Indian/Alaska Native men (15.7), and white men (11.2)
- Among women, Hispanic women had the highest rates of getting liver cancer (7.7 per 100,000 women), followed by Asian/Pacific Islander women (7.6), American Indian/Alaska Native women (6.8), black women (5.0), and white women (4.0)
- Among Asian/Pacific Islander men, liver cancer was the fourth most common cancer and the second most common cause of cancer death
- Among Asian/Pacific Islander women, liver cancer was the ninth most common cancer and the fifth most common cause of cancer death

Lung Cancer Statistics

More people in the United States die from lung cancer than any other type of cancer. This is true for both men and women.

In 2014 (the most recent year numbers are available):

- 215,951 people in the United States were diagnosed with lung cancer, including 113,326 men and 102,625 women*
- 155,526 people in the United States died from lung cancer, including 84,859 men and 70,667 women*

**Incidence counts cover about 99 percent of the U.S. population; death counts cover about 100 percent of the U.S. population. Use caution when comparing incidence and death counts.*

Lymphoma Statistics

In the United States in 2014 (the most recent year for which numbers are available):

- 8,581 people (4,780 men and 3,801 women) were diagnosed with Hodgkin lymphoma, and 1,077 people (633 men and 444 women) died from it
- 66,769 people (36,728 men and 30,041 women) were diagnosed with non-Hodgkin lymphoma, and 20,387 people (11,285 men and 9,102 women) died from it

Among men:

- White men had the highest rate of getting Hodgkin lymphoma (3.1), followed by black men (3.0), Hispanic men (2.7), Asian/Pacific Islander men (1.5), and American Indian/Alaska Native men (1.3)
- White men had the highest rate of getting non-Hodgkin lymphoma (23.0), followed by Hispanic men (19.0), black men (16.7), Asian/Pacific Islander men (15.2), and American Indian/Alaska Native men (10.6)

Among women:

- White women had the highest rate of getting Hodgkin lymphoma (2.4), followed by Hispanic women (2.3), black women (2.2), and Asian/Pacific Islander women (1.0), Rates for American Indian/Alaska Native women could not be presented
- White women had the highest rate of getting non-Hodgkin lymphoma (15.7), followed by Hispanic women (15.1), black women (11.8), Asian/Pacific Islander women (10.8), and American Indian/Alaska Native women (9.3)

Myeloma Statistics

In the United States in 2014 (the most recent year for which numbers are available):

- 23,555 people (13,190 men and 10,365 women) were diagnosed with myeloma
- 12,112 people (6,589 men and 5,523 women) died from myeloma
- Among men, black men had the highest rate of getting myeloma (15.0 per 100,000 men), followed by Hispanic men (7.5), white

men (7.2), American Indian/Alaska Native men (6.1), and Asian/Pacific Islander men (4.6)

- Among women, black women had the highest rate of getting myeloma (10.5 per 100,000 women), followed by Hispanic women (5.2), white women (4.5), American Indian/Alaska Native women (4.2), and Asian/Pacific Islander women (3.1)

Ovarian Cancer Statistics

Each year, about 20,000 women in the United States get ovarian cancer. Among women in the United States, ovarian cancer is the tenth most common cancer and the fifth leading cause of cancer death, after lung and bronchus, breast, colorectal, and pancreatic cancers. Ovarian cancer causes more deaths than any other cancer of the female reproductive system, but it accounts for only about 3 percent of all cancers in women. When ovarian cancer is found in its early stages, treatment works best.

In 2014 (the most recent year numbers are available):

- 21,161 women in the United States were diagnosed with ovarian cancer
- 14,195 women in the United States died from ovarian cancer

Prostate Cancer Statistics

Aside from nonmelanoma skin cancer, prostate cancer is the most common cancer among men in the United States. It is also one of the leading causes of cancer death among men of all races and Hispanic origin populations.

In 2014 (the most recent year for which numbers are available):

- 172,258 men in the United States were diagnosed with prostate cancer
- 28,343 men in the United States died from prostate cancer

Skin Cancer Statistics

Skin cancer is the most common form of cancer in the United States. The following statistics refer to melanomas of the skin. Nonepithelial skin cancers, which are not reflected below, represent 7 percent of skin cancers that are tracked by central cancer registries. These statistics also do not include data for basal cell and squamous cell carcinomas, which are not tracked by central cancer registries.

In 2014 (the most recent year numbers are available:

- 76,665 people in the United States were diagnosed with melanomas of the skin, including 45,402 men and 31,263 women
- 9,324 people in the United States died from melanomas of the skin, including 6,161 men and 3,163 women

Thyroid Cancer Statistics

In the United States in 2014 (the most recent year for which numbers are available):

- 48,288 people (12,198 men and 36,090 women) got thyroid cancer
- 1,832 people (796 men and 1,036 women) died from thyroid cancer
- Women are almost three times as likely as men to get thyroid cancer, and white people have higher rates of thyroid cancer than people of other races and ethnicities
- Among men, white men have the highest rates of getting thyroid cancer (7.7 per 100,000 men), followed by Asian/Pacific Islander men (7.2), Hispanic men (5.8), and black and American Indian/Alaska Native men (4.0)
- Among women, white women have the highest rates of getting thyroid cancer (22.2 per 100,000 women), followed by Asian/Pacific Islander women (21.6), Hispanic women (20.9), black women (13.9), and American Indian/Alaska Native women (11.8)

Uterine Cancer Statistics

Uterine cancer is the fourth most common cancer in women in the United States and the most commonly diagnosed gynecologic cancer.

In the United States in 2014 (the most recent year for which numbers are available):

- 53,028 women in the United States were diagnosed with uterine cancer
- 9,727 women in the United States died from uterine cancer

Vaginal and Vulvar Cancers Statistics

Vaginal and vulvar cancers are very rare. While all women are at risk for these cancers, very few will get them. Together, they account for 6–7 percent of all gynecologic cancers diagnosed in the United States.

In 2014 (the most recent year numbers are available):

- 1,312 women in the United States were diagnosed with vaginal cancer
- 430 women in the United States died from vaginal cancer
- 5,133 women in the United States were diagnosed with vulvar cancer
- 1,085 women in the United States died from vulvar cancer

Chapter 3

Cancer Health Disparities

Chapter Contents

Section 3.1

Overview of Cancer Health Disparities

This section includes text excerpted from "Cancer Disparities," National Cancer Institute (NCI), October 21, 2016.

Cancer affects all population groups in the United States. But certain groups may bear a disproportionate burden of cancer compared with other groups. Cancer disparities (sometimes called cancer health disparities) are differences in cancer measures such as:

- incidence (new cases)
- prevalence (all existing cases)
- mortality (deaths)
- morbidity (cancer-related health complications)
- survivorship, including quality of life after cancer treatment
- burden of cancer or related health conditions
- screening rates
- stage at diagnosis

Cancer disparities can also be seen when outcomes are improving overall but the improvements are delayed in some groups relative to other groups. Although disparities are often considered in the context of race/ethnicity, other population groups may experience cancer disparities. These include groups defined by disability, gender/sexual identity, geographic location, income, education, and other characteristics.

Contributing Factors

Cancer disparities are thought to reflect the interplay of socioeconomic factors, culture, diet, stress, the environment, and biology.

Members of minority racial/ethnic groups in the United States are more likely to be poor and medically underserved (that is, to have little or no access to effective healthcare) than whites, and limited access to

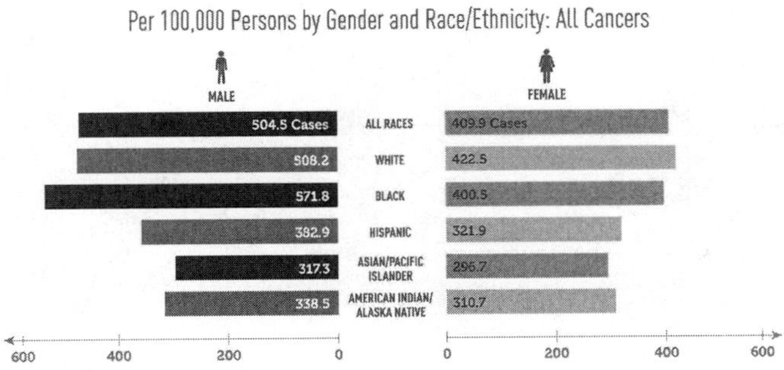

Figure 3.1. *Number of New Cancer Cases Each Year*

quality healthcare is a major contributor to disparities. For example, regardless of their racial/ethnic background, the poor and medically underserved are less likely to have recommended cancer screening tests than those who are medically well served. They are also more likely to be diagnosed with late-stage cancer that might have been treated more effectively if diagnosed earlier.

The higher cancer burden in poor and medically underserved individuals may also reflect different rates of behavioral risk factors for cancer, such as higher rates of tobacco smoking, physical inactivity, obesity, and excessive alcohol intake, and lower rates of breastfeeding. In addition, individuals who live in poverty may experience higher rates of exposure to environmental risk factors, such as cancer-causing substances in motor vehicle exhaust in dense urban neighborhoods.

Even among people of higher socioeconomic status, certain racial/ethnic minority groups may experience cancer disparities. These differences may reflect cultural differences such as mistrust of the healthcare system, fatalistic attitudes about cancer, or apprehension or embarrassment about having certain kinds of medical procedures. They may also reflect geographic or other differences in access to quality care.

Cancer disparities may also reflect differences in clinical trial participation. Clinical trials often have low participation by racial/ethnic minorities, which raises the possibility that the results may not be fully applicable to them. Biological differences also appear to play a role in some cancer disparities. Advances in genomics and other molecular technologies are improving our understanding of how biological differences among population groups contribute to health disparities and how biological factors interact with other potentially relevant factors, such as diet and the environment.

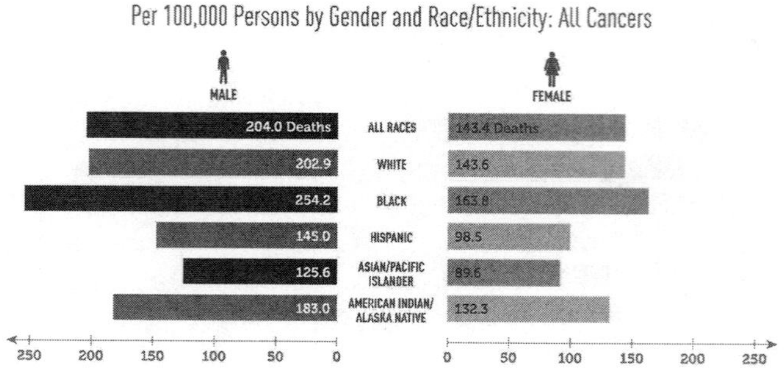

Figure 3.2. *Number of Deaths Each Year*

For example, some evidence suggests that there are genetic or other biological differences between the triple-negative breast, colorectal, and prostate cancers that arise in African Americans and those that arise in people of other racial/ethnic groups and that these differences may explain differences in incidence or aggressiveness of these cancers.

Examples of Cancer Disparities

Although cancer incidence and mortality overall are declining in all racial/ethnic groups in the United States, certain groups continue to be at increased risk of developing or dying from particular cancers.

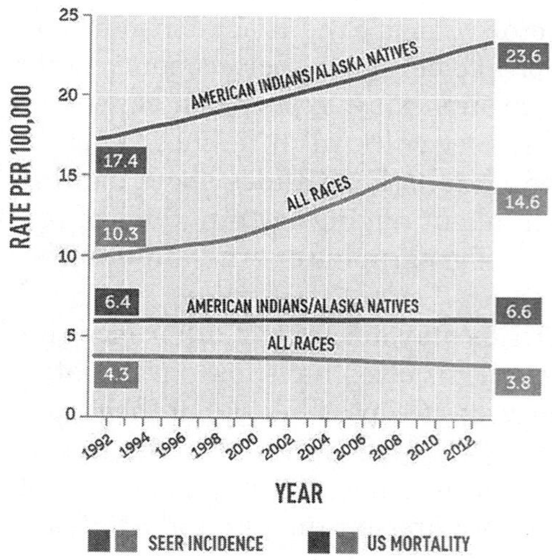

Figure 3.3. *American Indian/Alaska Native Kidney and Renal Pelvis Cancer Incidence and Mortality Rates*

Some key cancer incidence and mortality disparities among U.S. racial/ethnic groups include:

- African Americans have higher death rates than all other groups for many, although not all, cancer types
- African American women are much more likely than white women to die of breast cancer. The mortality gap is widening as the incidence rate in African American women, which in the past had been lower than that in white women, has caught up to that in white women.
- African Americans are more than twice as likely as whites to die of prostate cancer and nearly twice as likely to die of stomach cancer
- Colorectal cancer incidence is higher in African Americans than in whites. Incidence in all groups is declining, but the difference between the groups remains

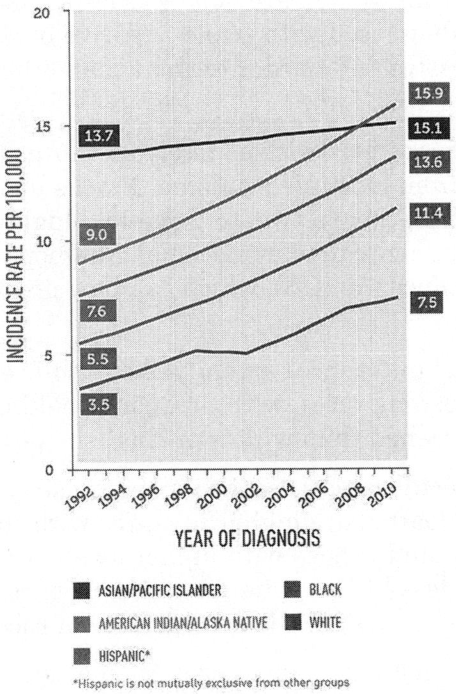

Figure 3.4. *Trends in Liver and Intrahepatic Bile Duct Cancer Incidence*

- Hispanic and African American women have higher rates of cervical cancer than women of other racial/ethnic groups; African American women have the highest rates of death from the disease
- American Indians/Alaska Natives and Asian Pacific Islanders have the highest rates of liver and intrahepatic bile duct cancer, followed by Hispanics.
- American Indians/Alaska Natives have higher death rates from kidney cancer than people of other racial/ethnic groups
- Both the incidence of lung cancer and death rates from the disease are higher in African American men than in men of other racial/ethnic groups

Other notable examples of disparities include:

- The incidence rates of colorectal, lung, and cervical cancers are much higher in the Appalachian region of Ohio than in wealthier and more populated areas of the state
- African American women are nearly twice as likely as white women to be diagnosed with triple-negative breast cancer, which is more aggressive and harder to treat than other subtypes of breast cancer
- African Americans are twice as likely as whites to be diagnosed with and die from multiple myeloma. Blacks in the United States and Africa have a two- to three-fold higher incidence than whites of a disorder called monoclonal gammopathy of undetermined significance (MGUS), which can be a precursor to multiple myeloma
- There are large differences among racial/ethnic groups in colorectal cancer screening rates, with Spanish-speaking Hispanics less likely to be screened than whites or English-speaking Hispanics
- Rates of colorectal cancer deaths among those younger than 65 ("premature" deaths) are higher in states with the lowest education levels than in those with higher levels. People with more education are less likely to die prematurely of colorectal cancer than those with less education, regardless of race or ethnicity
- Behaviors that increase cancer risk, such as smoking and drinking alcohol, may be more prevalent among lesbian, gay, and bisexual youths than among heterosexual youths

Addressing Cancer Disparities

Because many different factors can cause cancer disparities—in particular, poverty and a resultant lack of quality medical care—addressing them is not simple or straightforward. Nevertheless, researchers are identifying ways to address the most critical factors in specific disparities and are already meeting with some success.

One approach is to specifically address access to care. For example, in 2002, seeking to address disparities in colorectal cancer among African Americans, Delaware created a statewide colorectal cancer screening program that paid for screening and treatment and made patient navigators available to coordinate screening and cancer care. By 2009, this program had eliminated disparities in screening rates, cut the percentage of African Americans diagnosed with cancer that had already spread, and almost completely abolished racial/ethnic differences in colorectal cancer incidence and mortality. Similar efforts are under way to address cancer disparities among rural populations.

Researchers are also addressing biological differences in cancers across racial/ethnic groups. For example, they are identifying genetic variants that may explain the higher risk of prostate cancer among African American men compared with white men. Researchers are also looking at other molecular differences that may explain why African American men tend to get more aggressive prostate cancers than white men. Studies of this type may eventually help identify ways to reduce risk among African American men.

Section 3.2

Health Disparities among Different Cancer Types

This section includes text excerpted from "Health Disparities in Cancer," Centers for Disease Control and Prevention (CDC), April 12, 2017.

Health disparities refer to differences in health between groups of people. These differences in health may be seen among people of various races and ethnicities, residents of rural areas, women, men, children and adolescents, the elderly, people with disabilities, and the uninsured. According to Centers for Disease Control and Prevention (CDC) Office of Minority Health and Health Equity (OMHHE), life expectancy and overall health have improved for most Americans in recent years, but not all Americans have benefited equally. Centers for Disease Control and Prevention (CDC) and its partners track trends in cancer incidence (new cancer cases), deaths, and survival (life after a cancer diagnosis) to learn which groups are affected negatively more than others. Health disparities in cancer can be reduced by expanding access to cancer screening tests, high-quality treatment, and better follow-up after treatment, and by increasing awareness about healthy lifestyle choices that can lower the risk of getting cancer or having cancer come back after it has been treated. Also, social and economic factors which affect health, such as poorer housing and education and lack of transportation, can affect health disparities in cancer.

Breast Cancer

Breast cancer is the second leading cause of cancer deaths among women in the United States. Breast cancer deaths are going down the fastest among white women compared to women of other races and ethnicities. African American women have the highest death rate of all racial and ethnic groups and are 40 percent more likely to die of breast cancer than white women. The reasons for this difference result from many factors, including finding the cancer after it has spread, having more aggressive cancers, treatments that don't work well, and fewer social and economic resources. To reduce this disparity in deaths, African American women need to be screened as recommended, and get better follow-up care for a mammogram that is not normal.

BRCA1 and *BRCA2* are two genes that are important to fighting cancer. Sometimes a change occurs in the *BRCA* genes that prevents them from working normally. This change, or mutation, can raise a person's risk for breast, ovarian, and other cancers. Some groups are at a higher risk for a *BRCA* gene mutation than others, including women with Ashkenazi Jewish heritage. The screening test for breast cancer is a mammogram. Learn about mammography screening recommendations.

Cervical Cancer

Hispanic and African American women have the highest rates of getting and dying from cervical cancer. Getting screened as recommended, starting at age 21, can help prevent cervical cancer or find it early. Getting children vaccinated against human papillomavirus (HPV), the main cause of cervical cancer, can help prevent them from getting cervical cancer later in life.

Colorectal Cancer

Colorectal cancer is the second leading cause of cancer death among cancers that affect men and women. African Americans have the highest rates of getting and dying from colorectal cancer when compared to people of other races and ethnicities. Colorectal cancers typically grow slowly, but a person's risk for colorectal cancer is affected by family and personal health history. It is important to know the signs and symptoms of colorectal cancer. People with average risk for colorectal cancer should begin screening at age 50. There are several options for screening. Talk to your doctor about screening options and ways to reduce your risk of colorectal cancer.

Liver Cancer

New liver cancer cases and deaths are on the rise in the United States. Americans who are Asian, Pacific Islander, or Hispanic have the highest rates of getting and dying from liver cancer. Many liver cancer cases are related to the hepatitis B virus or hepatitis C virus. To lower your risk of getting liver cancer, get vaccinated against hepatitis B, get tested for hepatitis C, and avoid drinking too much alcohol.

Lung Cancer

African-American men have the highest rates of lung cancer in the United States. Cigarette smoking is the number one risk factor for lung cancer and other tobacco-related cancers. Using other tobacco products such as cigars or pipes, as well as smoke from other people's cigarettes, pipes, or cigars (secondhand smoke) also increases the risk for lung cancer. The most important thing you can do to lower your lung cancer risk is to quit smoking and avoid secondhand smoke. For help quitting, call 800-QUIT-NOW (800-784-8669), or text "QUIT" to 47848 from your cell phone. Not all people who get lung cancer have a history of smoking. It is important to discuss your health history and any symptoms with your doctor to find out if you should be screened.

Prostate Cancer

Prostate cancer is more common in African American men and men of African descent. It tends to start at younger ages and grow faster than in other racial or ethnic groups, but medical experts do not know why. Prostate cancers usually grow slowly. Most men diagnosed with prostate cancer are older than 65 years and do not die from the disease. Finding and treating prostate cancer before symptoms occur may not improve your health or help you live longer. A prostate-specific antigen (PSA) test may find prostate cancer at an earlier stage than if you don't get screened, but many medical groups don't recommend screening with the PSA test. Learn about prostate cancer and talk to your doctor before you decide to get tested or treated for prostate cancer.

Chapter 4

Lifestyle Issues and Cancer Risk

Chapter Contents

Section 4.1

Tobacco Use and Cancer Risk

This section includes text excerpted from "Cancer Prevention and Control—Tobacco and Cancer," Centers for Disease Control and Prevention (CDC), November 9, 2016.

If you were asked to describe the relationship between "tobacco smoking" and "cancer," you might immediately think of lung cancer. It's true that smoking tobacco products (including cigarettes and cigars) causes almost nine of every ten cases of lung cancer, but smoking can cause cancer almost anywhere in your body, including in the:

- Bladder
- Blood (acute myeloid leukemia)
- Cervix
- Colon and rectum
- Esophagus
- Kidney and renal pelvis
- Liver
- Lungs, bronchi, and trachea
- Mouth and throat
- Pancreas
- Stomach
- Voice box (larynx)

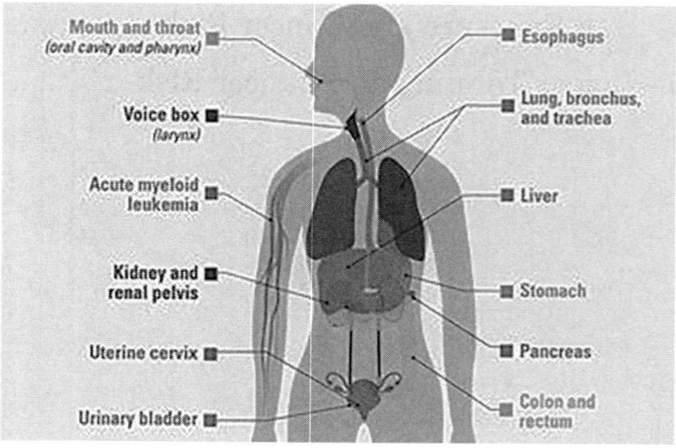

Figure 4.1. *Cancer and Tobacco.*

Tobacco use causes cancer throughout the body.

Health Advice for People Who Use Tobacco or Are Thinking of Using Tobacco

The most important things you can do to avoid health risks from cancer are:

- If you don't smoke or use tobacco—don't start!
- If you do smoke or use tobacco—quit!

No matter how long you have smoked, quitting can reduce your risk for cancer and other chronic diseases. Quitting smoking can be hard for many people, but there is a lot of help out there.

How Tobacco Products Cause Cancer

Tobacco smoke has at least 70 chemicals that cause cancer, also known as carcinogens. Every time you breathe in that smoke, those chemicals get into your bloodstream, which carries the chemicals to all parts of your body. Many of these chemicals can damage your deoxyribonucleic acid (DNA), which controls how your body makes new cells and directs each kind of cell to do what it is made for. Damaged DNA can make cells grow differently from how they are supposed to. These unusual cells can turn into cancer.

Secondhand Smoke

Smokers are not the only people who can get cancer from tobacco smoke. People around them—their kids, partners, friends, coworkers, and others—breathe in that smoke, too. Every year, more than 7,300 nonsmokers die of lung cancer from secondhand smoke.

Other Tobacco Products

Smokeless tobacco products, such as dipping and chewing tobacco, can cause cancer, too, including cancers of the esophagus, mouth and throat, and pancreas. Smoking tobacco in a pipe causes lung cancer and increases the risk of cancers of the mouth, throat, larynx, and esophagus, even though pipe smokers don't inhale the smoke into their lungs.

Health Disparities

Differences between groups of people in their level of health, quality of healthcare, how many have a particular health problem, and so on, are called health disparities. The groups of people might differ by age, race, income, or some other characteristic. People who are poorer, less educated, or part of certain racial or ethnic groups are more likely to smoke.

Section 4.2

Alcohol Use and Cancer Risk

This section contains text excerpted from the following sources: Text in this section begins with excerpts from "Alcohol and Public Health—Fact Sheets—Alcohol Use and Your Health," Centers for Disease Control and Prevention (CDC), January 3, 2018; Text beginning with the heading "What Is the Evidence That Alcohol Drinking Is a Cause of Cancer?" is excerpted from "Alcohol and Cancer Risk," National Cancer Institute (NCI), June 24, 2013. Reviewed March 2018.

Drinking too much alcohol can harm your health. Excessive alcohol use led to approximately 88,000 deaths each year in the United States from 2006–2010, shortening the lives of those who died by an average of 30 years. Further, excessive drinking was responsible for 1 in 10 deaths among working-age adults aged 20–64 years. The economic costs of excessive alcohol consumption in 2010 were estimated at $249 billion, or $2.05 a drink.

Short-Term Health Risks

- Injuries, such as motor vehicle crashes, falls, drownings, and burns.
- Violence, including homicide, suicide, sexual assault, and intimate partner violence.
- Alcohol poisoning, a medical emergency that results from high blood alcohol levels.
- Risky sexual behaviors, including unprotected sex or sex with multiple partners. These behaviors can result in unintended

pregnancy or sexually transmitted diseases (STD), including human immunodeficiency virus (HIV).

- Miscarriage and stillbirth or fetal alcohol spectrum disorders (FASDs) among pregnant women.

Long-Term Health Risks

Over time, excessive alcohol use can lead to the development of chronic diseases and other serious problems including:

- High blood pressure, heart disease, stroke, liver disease, and digestive problems.
- Cancer of the breast, mouth, throat, esophagus, liver, and colon.
- Learning and memory problems, including dementia and poor school performance.
- Mental health problems, including depression and anxiety.
- Social problems, including lost productivity, family problems, and unemployment.
- Alcohol dependence, or alcoholism.

By not drinking too much, you can reduce the risk of these short- and long-term health risks.

What Is the Evidence That Alcohol Drinking Is a Cause of Cancer?

Based on extensive reviews of research studies, there is a strong scientific consensus of an association between alcohol drinking and several types of cancer. In its Report on Carcinogens, the National Toxicology Program (NTP) of the U.S. Department of Health and Human Services (HHS) lists consumption of alcoholic beverages as a known human carcinogen. The research evidence indicates that the more alcohol a person drinks—particularly the more alcohol a person drinks regularly over time—the higher his or her risk of developing an alcohol-associated cancer. Based on data from 2009, an estimated 3.5 percent of all cancer deaths in the United States (about 19,500 deaths) were alcohol related. Clear patterns have emerged between alcohol consumption and the development of the following types of cancer:

- **Head and neck cancer.** Alcohol consumption is a major risk factor for certain head and neck cancers, particularly cancers of the oral cavity (excluding the lips), pharynx (throat), and larynx (voice box). People who consume 50 or more grams of alcohol per day (approximately 3.5 or more drinks per day) have at least a 2–3 times greater risk of developing these cancers than nondrinkers. Moreover, the risks of these cancers are substantially higher among persons who consume this amount of alcohol and also use tobacco.

- **Esophageal cancer.** Alcohol consumption is a major risk factor for a particular type of esophageal cancer called esophageal squamous cell carcinoma. In addition, people who inherit a deficiency in an enzyme that metabolizes alcohol have been found to have substantially increased risks of alcohol-related esophageal squamous cell carcinoma.
- **Liver cancer.** Alcohol consumption is an independent risk factor for, and a primary cause of, liver cancer (hepatocellular carcinoma). (Chronic infection with hepatitis B virus and hepatitis C virus are the other major causes of liver cancer.)
- **Breast cancer.** More than 100 epidemiologic studies have looked at the association between alcohol consumption and the risk of breast cancer in women. These studies have consistently found an increased risk of breast cancer associated with increasing alcohol intake. A meta-analysis of 53 of these studies (which included a total of 58,000 women with breast cancer) showed that women who drank more than 45 grams of alcohol per day (approximately three drinks) had 1.5 times the risk of developing breast cancer as nondrinkers (a modestly increased risk). The risk of breast cancer was higher across all levels of alcohol intake: for every 10 grams of alcohol consumed per day (slightly less than one drink), researchers observed a small (7%) increase in the risk of breast cancer.

The Million Women Study in the United Kingdom (which included more than 28,000 women with breast cancer) provided a more recent, and slightly higher, estimate of breast cancer risk at low to moderate levels of alcohol consumption: every 10 grams of alcohol consumed per day was associated with a 12 percent increase in the risk of breast cancer.

- **Colorectal cancer.** Alcohol consumption is associated with a modestly increased risk of cancers of the colon and rectum. A meta-analysis of 57 cohort and case-control studies that examined the association between alcohol consumption and colorectal cancer risk showed that people who regularly drank 50 or more grams of alcohol per day (approximately 3.5 drinks) had 1.5 times the risk of developing colorectal cancer as nondrinkers or occasional drinkers. For every 10 grams of alcohol consumed per day, there was a small (7%) increase in the risk of colorectal cancer.

Research on Alcohol Consumption and Other Cancers

Numerous studies have examined the association between alcohol consumption and the risk of other cancers, including cancers of the pancreas, ovary, prostate, stomach, uterus, and bladder. For these cancers, either no association with alcohol use has been found or the evidence for an association is inconsistent. However, for two cancers—renal cell (kidney) cancer and non-Hodgkin lymphoma (NHL)—multiple studies have shown that increased alcohol consumption is associated with a decreased risk of cancer. A meta-analysis of the NHL studies (which included 18,759 people with NHL) found a 15 percent lower risk of NHL among alcohol drinkers compared with nondrinkers. The mechanisms by which alcohol consumption would decrease the risks of either renal cell cancer or NHL are not understood.

How Does Alcohol Increase the Risk of Cancer?

Researchers have identified multiple ways that alcohol may increase the risk of cancer, including:

- metabolizing (breaking down) ethanol in alcoholic drinks to acetaldehyde, which is a toxic chemical and a probable human carcinogen; acetaldehyde can damage both deoxyribonucleic acid (DNA)—the genetic material that makes up genes, and proteins
- generating reactive oxygen species (chemically reactive molecules that contain oxygen), which can damage DNA, proteins, and lipids (fats) through a process called oxidation
- impairing the body's ability to break down and absorb a variety of nutrients that may be associated with cancer risk, including vitamin A; nutrients in the vitamin B complex, such as folate; vitamin C; vitamin D; vitamin E; and carotenoids
- increasing blood levels of estrogen, a sex hormone linked to the risk of breast cancer

Alcoholic beverages may also contain a variety of carcinogenic contaminants that are introduced during fermentation and production, such as nitrosamines, asbestos fibers, phenols, and hydrocarbons.

Can a Person's Genes Affect Their Risk of Alcohol-Related Cancers?

A person's risk of alcohol-related cancers is influenced by their genes, specifically the genes that encode enzymes involved in metabolizing (breaking down) alcohol.

For example, one way the body metabolizes alcohol is through the activity of an enzyme called alcohol dehydrogenase, or ADH. Many individuals of Chinese, Korean, and especially Japanese descent carry a version of the gene for ADH that codes for a "superactive" form of the enzyme. This superactive ADH enzyme speeds the conversion of alcohol (ethanol) to toxic acetaldehyde. As a result, when people who have the superactive enzyme drink alcohol, acetaldehyde builds up. Among people of Japanese descent, those who have this superactive ADH have a higher risk of pancreatic cancer than those with the more common form of ADH.

Another enzyme, called aldehyde dehydrogenase 2 (ALDH2), metabolizes toxic acetaldehyde to nontoxic substances. Some people, particularly those of East Asian descent, carry a variant of the gene for ALDH2 that codes for a defective form of the enzyme. In people who have the defective enzyme, acetaldehyde builds up when they drink alcohol. The accumulation of acetaldehyde has such unpleasant effects (including facial flushing and heart palpitations) that most people who have inherited the ALDH2 variant are unable to consume large amounts of alcohol. Therefore, most people with the defective form of ALDH2 have a low risk of developing alcohol-related cancers.

However, some individuals with the defective form of ALDH2 can become tolerant to the unpleasant effects of acetaldehyde and consume large amounts of alcohol. Epidemiologic studies have shown that such individuals have a higher risk of alcohol-related esophageal cancer, as well as of head and neck cancers, than individuals with the fully active enzyme who drink comparable amounts of alcohol. These increased risks are seen only among people who carry the ALDH2 variant and drink alcohol—they are not observed in people who carry the variant but do not drink alcohol.

Section 4.3

Obesity and Cancer Risk

This section includes text excerpted from "Obesity and Cancer," National Cancer Institute (NCI), January 17, 2017.

What Is Obesity?

Obesity is a condition in which a person has an unhealthy amount and/or distribution of body fat. To measure obesity, researchers commonly use a scale known as the body mass index (BMI). BMI is calculated by dividing a person's weight (in kilograms) by their height (in meters) squared (commonly expressed as kg/m^2). BMI provides a more accurate measure of obesity than weight alone, and for most people it is a fairly good (although indirect) indicator of body fatness. Other measurements that reflect the distribution of body fat—that is, whether more fat is carried around the hips or the abdomen—are increasingly being used along with BMI as indicators of obesity and disease risks. These measurements include waist circumference and the waist-to-hip ratio (WHR) (the waist circumference divided by the hip circumference). The standard weight categories based on BMI for adults age 20 years or older are

Table 4.1. BMI for Adults (20 Years or Older of Age)

BMI in kg/m^2	Weight Category
Below 18.5	Underweight
18.5–24.9	Normal
25.0–29.9	Overweight
30.0–39.9	Obese
40.0 or higher	Severely obese

Compared with people of normal weight, those who are overweight or obese are at greater risk for many diseases, including diabetes, high blood pressure, cardiovascular disease, stroke, and many cancers. Extreme or severe obesity is also associated with an increased death

Table 4.2. BMI for Children and Adolescents (Younger than 20 Years of Age)

BMI	Weight Category
BMI-for-age at or above sex-specific 85th percentile, but less than 95th percentile	Overweight
BMI-for-age at or above sex-specific 95th percentile	Obese

rate; heart disease, cancer, and diabetes are responsible for most of the excess deaths.

How Common Is Overweight or Obesity?

Results from the National Health and Nutrition Examination Survey (NHANES) showed that in 2011–2014, nearly 70 percent of U.S. adults age 20 years or older were overweight or obese and more than one-third (36.5%) were obese. In 1988–1994, by contrast, only 56 percent of adults aged 20 years or older were overweight or obese.

The percentage of children and adolescents who are overweight or obese has also increased. In 2011–2014, an estimated 9 percent of 2–5 year-olds, 17 percent of 6–11 year-olds, and 20 percent of 12–19 year-olds were overweight or obese. In 1988–1994, those figures were only 7 percent, 11 percent, and 10 percent, respectively. In 2011–2014, about 17 percent of U.S. youth ages 2–19 years old were obese. In 1988–1994, by contrast, only about 10 percent of 2–19 year-olds were obese.

According to the Centers for Disease Control and Prevention (CDC), the prevalence of obesity in the United States differs among racial/ethnic groups. For example, in 2011–2012 among adults, non-Hispanic blacks had the highest prevalence of obesity (47.8%) followed by Hispanics (42%), non-Hispanic whites (33.4%), and non-Hispanic Asians (10.9%). Among children and adolescents ages 2–19 years, the prevalence of obesity in 2011–2012 was 21.9 percent among Hispanics, 19.5 percent among non-Hispanic blacks, 14.7 percent among non-Hispanic whites, and 8.6 percent among non-Hispanic Asians.

What Is Known about the Relationship between Obesity and Cancer?

Nearly all of the evidence linking obesity to cancer risk comes from large cohort studies, a type of observational study. However, data from observational studies can be difficult to interpret and cannot definitively establish that obesity causes cancer. That is because obese or overweight people may differ from lean people in ways other than their body fat, and it is possible that these other differences—rather than their body fat—are what explains their different cancer risk. Despite the limitations of the study designs, there is consistent evidence that higher amounts of body fat are associated with increased risks of a number of cancers, including:

- **Endometrial cancer.** Obese and overweight women are two to about four times as likely as normal-weight women to develop endometrial cancer (cancer of the lining of the uterus), and extremely obese women are about seven times as likely to develop the more common of the two main types of this cancer. The risk of endometrial cancer increases with increasing weight gain in adulthood, particularly among women who have never used menopausal hormone therapy (MHT).
- **Esophageal adenocarcinoma.** People who are overweight or obese are about twice as likely as normal-weight people to develop a type of esophageal cancer called esophageal adenocarcinoma, and people who are extremely obese are more than four times as likely.
- **Gastric cardia cancer.** People who are obese are nearly twice as likely as normal-weight people to develop cancer in the upper part of the stomach, that is, the part that is closest to the esophagus.
- **Liver cancer.** People who are overweight or obese are up to twice as likely as normal-weight people to develop liver cancer. The association between overweight/obesity and liver cancer is stronger in men than women.
- **Kidney cancer.** People who are overweight or obese are nearly twice as likely as normal-weight people to develop renal cell cancer, the most common form of kidney cancer. The association of renal cell cancer with obesity is independent of its association with high blood pressure, a known risk factor for kidney cancer.
- **Multiple myeloma.** Compared with normal-weight individuals, overweight and obese individuals have a slight (10–20%) increase in the risk of developing multiple myeloma.
- **Meningioma.** The risk of this slow-growing brain tumor that arises in the membranes surrounding the brain and the spinal

cord is increased by about 50 percent in people who are obese and about 20 percent in people who are overweight.

- **Pancreatic cancer.** People who are overweight or obese are about 1.5 times as likely to develop pancreatic cancer as normal-weight people.
- **Colorectal cancer.** People who are obese are slightly (about 30%) more likely to develop colorectal cancer than normal-weight people.

A higher BMI is associated with increased risks of colon and rectal cancers in both men and in women, but the increases are higher in men than in women.

- **Gallbladder cancer.** Compared with normal-weight people, people who are overweight have a slight (about 20%) increase in risk of gallbladder cancer, and people who are obese have a 60 percent increase in risk of gallbladder cancer. The risk increase is greater in women than men.
- **Breast cancer.** Many studies have shown that, in postmenopausal women, a higher body mass index (BMI) is associated with a modest increase in risk of breast cancer. For example, a 5-unit increase in BMI is associated with a 12 percent increase in risk. Among postmenopausal women, those who are obese have a 20–40 percent increase in risk of developing breast cancer compared with normal-weight women. The higher risks are seen mainly in women who have never used menopausal hormone therapy and for tumors that express hormone receptors. Obesity is also a risk factor for breast cancer in men.

In premenopausal women, by contrast, overweight and obesity have been found to be associated with a 20 percent decreased risk of breast tumors that express hormone receptors.

- **Ovarian cancer.** Higher BMI is associated with a slight increase in the risk of ovarian cancer, particularly in women who have never used menopausal hormone therapy. For example, a 5-unit increase in BMI is associated with a 10 percent increase in risk among women who have never used menopausal hormone therapy.
- **Thyroid cancer.** Higher BMI (specifically, a 5-unit increase in BMI) is associated with a slight (10%) increase in the risk of thyroid cancer.

How Might Obesity Increase the Risk of Cancer?

Several possible mechanisms have been suggested to explain how obesity might increase the risks of some cancers.

- Obese people often have chronic low-level inflammation, which can, over time, cause deoxyribonucleic acid (DNA) damage that leads to cancer. Overweight and obese individuals are more likely than normal-weight individuals to have conditions or disorders that are linked to or that cause chronic local inflammation and that are risk factors for certain cancers. For example, chronic local inflammation induced by gastroesophageal reflux disease or Barrett esophagus is a likely cause of esophageal adenocarcinoma. Obesity is a risk factor for gallstones, a condition characterized by chronic gallbladder inflammation, and a history of gallstones is a strong risk factor for gallbladder cancer. Chronic ulcerative colitis (a chronic inflammatory condition) and hepatitis (a disease of the liver causing inflammation) are risk factors for different types of liver cancer.
- Fat tissue (also called adipose tissue) produces excess amounts of estrogen, high levels of which have been associated with increased risks of breast, endometrial, ovarian, and some other cancers.
- Obese people often have increased blood levels of insulin and insulin-like growth factor-1 (IGF-1). (This condition, known as hyperinsulinemia or insulin resistance, precedes the development of type 2 diabetes.) High levels of insulin and IGF-1 may promote the development of colon, kidney, prostate, and endometrial cancers.
- Fat cells produce adipokines, hormones that may stimulate or inhibit cell growth. For example, the level of an adipokine called leptin, which seems to promote cell proliferation, in the blood increases with increasing body fat. And another adipokine, adiponectin—which is less abundant in obese people than in those of normal weight—may have antiproliferative effects.
- Fat cells may also have direct and indirect effects on other cell growth regulators, including mammalian target of rapamycin (mTOR) and AMP-activated protein kinase.

Other possible mechanisms by which obesity could affect cancer risk include changes in the mechanical properties of the scaffolding that surrounds breast cells and altered immune responses, effects on the nuclear factor kappa beta system, and oxidative stress.

How Many Cancer Cases May Be Due to Obesity?

A population-based study using BMI and cancer incidence data from the GLOBOCAN project estimated that, in 2012 in the United States, about 28,000 new cases of cancer in men (3.5%) and 72,000 in women (9.5%) were due to overweight or obesity. The percentage of cases attributed to overweight or obesity varied widely for different cancer types but was as high as 54 percent for gallbladder cancer in women and 44 percent for esophageal adenocarcinoma in men. A 2016 study summarizing worldwide estimates of the fractions of different cancers attributable to overweight/obesity reported that, compared with other countries, the United States had the highest fractions attributable to overweight/obesity for colorectal cancer, pancreatic cancer, and postmenopausal breast cancer.

Does Avoiding Weight Gain or Losing Weight Decrease the Risk of Cancer?

Most of the data about whether avoiding weight gain or losing weight reduces cancer risk comes from cohort and case-control studies. As with observational studies of obesity and cancer risk, these studies can be difficult to interpret because people who lose weight or avoid weight gain may differ in other ways from people who do not.

Nevertheless, when the evidence from multiple observational studies is consistent, the association is more likely to be real. Many observational studies have provided consistent evidence that people who have lower weight gain during adulthood have lower risks of colon cancer, kidney cancer, and—for postmenopausal women—breast, endometrial, and ovarian cancers.

Fewer studies have examined possible associations between weight loss and cancer risk. Some of these have found decreased risks of breast, endometrial, colon, and prostate cancers among people who have lost weight. However, most of these studies were not able to evaluate whether the weight loss was intentional or unintentional (and possibly related to underlying health problems).

Stronger evidence for a relationship between weight loss and cancer risk comes from studies of people who have undergone bariatric surgery (surgery performed on the stomach or intestines to induce weight loss). Obese people who have bariatric surgery appear to have lower risks of obesity-related cancers than obese people who do not have bariatric surgery.

Nevertheless, the follow-up study of weight and breast cancer in the Women's Health Initiative (WHI) found that for women who were already overweight or obese at baseline, weight change (either gain or loss) was not associated with breast cancer risk during follow-up. However, for women who were of normal weight at baseline, gaining more than 5 percent of body weight was associated with increased breast cancer risk.

How Does Obesity Affect Cancer Survivorship?

Most of the evidence about obesity in cancer survivors comes from people who were diagnosed with breast, prostate, or colorectal cancer. Research indicates that obesity may worsen several aspects of cancer survivorship, including quality of life, cancer recurrence, cancer progression, and prognosis (survival). For example, obesity is associated with increased risks of treatment-related lymphedema in breast cancer survivors and incontinence in prostate cancer survivors treated with radical prostatectomy. In a large clinical trial of patients with stage II and stage III rectal cancer, those with a higher baseline BMI (particularly men) had an increased risk of local recurrence. Death from multiple myeloma is 50 percent more likely for people at the highest levels of obesity compared with people at normal weight.

Several randomized clinical trials in breast cancer survivors have reported weight loss interventions that resulted in both weight loss and beneficial changes in biomarkers that have been linked to the association between obesity and prognosis. However, there is little evidence about whether weight loss improves cancer recurrence or prognosis. The National Cancer Institute (NCI)-sponsored Breast Cancer WEight Loss (BWEL) Study, a randomized phase III trial, will compare recurrence rate in overweight and obese women who take part in a weight loss program after breast cancer diagnosis with that in women who do not take part in the weight loss program.

Section 4.4

The Role of Physical Activity in Reducing Cancer Risk

This section includes text excerpted from "Physical Activity and Cancer," National Cancer Institute (NCI), January 27, 2017.

What Is Physical Activity?

Physical activity is defined as any movement that uses skeletal muscles and requires more energy than does resting. Physical activity can include working, exercising, performing household chores, and leisure-time activities such as walking, tennis, hiking, bicycling, and swimming. Physical activity is essential for people to maintain a balance between the number of calories consumed and the number of calories used. Consistently expending fewer calories than are consumed leads to obesity, which scientists have convincingly linked to increased risks of 13 different cancers. Additionally, evidence indicates that physical activity may reduce the risks of several cancers through other mechanisms, independent of its effect on obesity.

What Is Known about the Relationship between Physical Activity and Cancer Risk?

There is substantial evidence that higher levels of physical activity are linked to lower risks of several cancers.

- **Colon cancer.** Colon cancer is one of the most extensively studied cancers in relation to physical activity. A meta-analysis of 52 epidemiologic studies that examined the association between physical activity and colon cancer risk found that the most physically active individuals had a 24 percent lower risk of colon cancer than those who were the least physically active. A pooled analysis of data on leisure-time physical activity (activities done at an individual's discretion generally to improve or maintain fitness or health) from 12 prospective U.S. and European cohort studies reported a risk reduction of 16 percent, when comparing individuals who were most active to those where least active. Incidence of both distal colon and proximal colon cancers is lower in people who are more physically active than in those who are less physically active. Physical activity is also associated with a decreased risk of colon adenomas (polyps), a type of colon polyp that may develop into colon cancer. However, it is less clear whether physical activity is associated with lower risks that polyps that have been removed will come back.

- **Breast cancer.** Many studies show that physically active women have a lower risk of breast cancer than inactive women; in a 2013 meta-analysis of 31 prospective studies, the average breast cancer risk reduction associated with physical activity was 12 percent. Physical activity has been associated with a reduced risk of breast cancer in both premenopausal and postmenopausal women; however, the evidence for an association is stronger for postmenopausal breast cancer. Women who increase their physical activity after menopause may also have a lower risk of breast cancer than women who do not.
- **Endometrial cancer.** Many studies have examined the relationship between physical activity and the risk of endometrial cancer (cancer of the lining of the uterus). In a meta-analysis of 33 studies, the average endometrial cancer risk reduction associated with high versus low physical activity was 20 percent. There is some evidence that the association between physical activity and endometrial cancer risk may reflect the effect of physical activity on obesity, a known risk factor for endometrial cancer.

For a number of other cancers, there is more limited evidence of a relationship with physical activity. In a study of over 1 million individuals, leisure-time physical activity was linked to reduced risks of esophageal adenocarcinoma, liver cancer, gastric cardia cancer (a type of stomach cancer), kidney cancer, myeloid leukemia, myeloma, and cancers of the head and neck, rectum, and bladder. These results are generally corroborated by large cohort studies or meta-analyses.

Nearly all of the evidence linking physical activity to cancer risk comes from observational studies, in which individuals report on their physical activity and are followed for years for diagnoses of cancer. Data from observational studies can give researchers clues about the relationship between physical activity and cancer risk, but such studies cannot definitively establish that being physically inactive causes cancer (or that being physically active protects against cancer). That is because people who are not physically active may differ from active people in ways other than their level of physical activity. These other differences, rather than the differences in physical activity, could explain their different cancer risk. For example, if someone does not feel well, they may not exercise much, and sometimes people do not feel well because they have undiagnosed cancer.

How Might Physical Activity Be Linked to Reduced Risks of Cancer?

Exercise has a number of biological effects on the body, some of which have been proposed to explain associations with specific cancers, including:

- Lowering the levels of hormones, such as insulin and estrogen, and of certain growth factors that have been associated with cancer development and progression
- Helping to prevent obesity and decreasing the harmful effects of obesity, particularly the development of insulin resistance (failure of the body's cells to respond to insulin)
- Reducing inflammation
- Improving immune system function
- Altering the metabolism of bile acids, resulting in decreased exposure of the gastrointestinal tract to these suspected carcinogens
- Reducing the amount of time it takes for food to travel through the digestive system, which decreases gastrointestinal tract exposure to possible carcinogens

Is Being Sedentary Linked to Health Risks?

Yes. Sedentary behavior, such as prolonged periods of television viewing, sitting, and lying down, is a risk factor for developing chronic conditions, including cancer, cardiovascular disease, and type 2 diabetes, and for premature death. In some studies, the association of sedentary behavior with these outcomes is independent of physical activity—that is, the increased risks of disease associated with being sedentary are not lessened by physical activity. However, in one large meta-analysis an increase in cancer mortality was seen only in those sedentary people with the least physical activity.

How Much Physical Activity Is Recommended for General Health Benefits?

The U.S. Department of Health and Human Services (HHS) *Physical Activity Guidelines for Americans* recommends that, for substantial health benefits, adults engage in at least 150 minutes (2 hours and 30 minutes) of moderate-intensity aerobic physical activity, 75 minutes (1 hour and 15 minutes) of vigorous-intensity aerobic physical activity, or an equivalent combination of moderate- and vigorous-intensity activity, every week. Aerobic physical activity should be performed in episodes of at least 10 minutes, preferably spread throughout the week.

For children and adolescents, the guidelines recommend at least 60 minutes (1 hour) of physical activity daily. Most of the 60 or more minutes a day should be either moderate- or vigorous-intensity aerobic physical activity, and should include vigorous-intensity physical activity at least 3 days a week. As part of their 60 or more minutes of daily physical activity, children and adolescents should include muscle-strengthening physical activity on at least 3 days of the week and bone-strengthening physical activity on at least 3 days of the week.

Is Physical Activity Beneficial for Cancer Survivors?

Research indicates that physical activity may have beneficial effects for several aspects of cancer survivorship—specifically, weight gain, quality of life, cancer recurrence or progression, and prognosis (likelihood of survival). Most of the evidence for the potential benefits of physical activity in cancer survivors comes from people diagnosed with breast, prostate, or colorectal cancer.

- **Weight gain.** Both reduced physical activity and the side effects of cancer treatment can contribute to weight gain after a cancer diagnosis. In a cohort study (a type of epidemiologic study), weight gain after breast cancer diagnosis was linked to worse survival. In a 2012 meta-analysis of randomized controlled clinical trials examining physical activity in cancer survivors, physical activity was found to reduce both body mass index and body weight.

- **Quality of life.** A 2012 Cochrane Collaboration systematic review of controlled clinical trials of exercise interventions in cancer survivors indicated that physical activity may have beneficial effects on overall health-related quality of life and on specific quality-of-life issues, including body image/self-esteem, emotional well-being, sexuality, sleep disturbance, social functioning, anxiety, fatigue, and pain. In a 2012 meta-analysis of randomized controlled trials examining physical activity in cancer survivors, physical activity was found to reduce fatigue and depression and to improve physical functioning, social functioning, and mental health.
- **Recurrence, progression, and survival.** Being physically active after a cancer diagnosis is linked to better cancer-specific outcomes for several cancer types.
    - **Breast cancer.** Consistent evidence from epidemiologic studies links physical activity after diagnosis with better breast cancer outcomes. For example, a large cohort study found that women who exercised moderately (the equivalent of walking 3–5 hours per week at an average pace) after a breast cancer diagnosis had approximately 40–50 percent lower risks of breast cancer recurrence, death from breast cancer, and death from any cause compared with more sedentary women. The potential physical activity benefit with regard to death from breast cancer was most apparent in women with hormone receptor–positive tumors.

Another prospective cohort study found that women who had breast cancer and who engaged in recreational physical activity roughly equivalent to walking at an average pace of 2–2.9 miles per hour (mph) for 1 hour per week had a 35–49 percent lower risk of death from breast cancer compared with women who engaged in less physical activity.

- **Colorectal cancer.** Evidence from multiple epidemiologic studies suggests that physical activity after a colorectal cancer diagnosis is associated with reduced risks of dying from colorectal cancer. In a large prospective cohort of patients with colorectal cancer, those who engaged in leisure-time physical activity had a 31 percent lower risk of death than those who did not, independent of their leisure-time physical activity before diagnosis.

- **Prostate cancer.** Limited evidence from a few epidemiologic studies has suggested a possible link between physical activity and better outcomes among men diagnosed with prostate cancer. In one study, men with nonmetastatic prostate cancer who engaged in vigorous activity for at least 3 hours per week had a 61 percent lower risk of death from prostate cancer compared with men who engaged in vigorous activity for less than 1 hour per week. Another study of men with localized prostate cancer found that higher levels of physical activity were associated with reduced overall and prostate cancer–specific mortality.

Findings from epidemiologic studies cannot completely exclude reverse causation as a possible explanation of the link between physical activity and better cancer outcomes. That is, people who feel good are more likely to exercise and be physically active than people who do not feel good.

Section 4.5

Sun Exposure and Cancer Risk

This section includes text excerpted from "Sunlight," National Cancer Institute (NCI), April 26, 2017.

The sun, sunlamps, and tanning booths all give off ultraviolet (UV) radiation. Exposure to UV radiation causes early aging of the skin and skin damage that can lead to skin cancer. People of all ages and skin tones should limit the amount of time they spend in the sun, especially between mid-morning and late afternoon, and avoid other sources of UV radiation, such as tanning beds. It is important to keep in mind that UV radiation is reflected by sand, water, snow, and ice and can go through windshields and windows. Even though skin cancer is more common among people with a light skin tone, people of all skin tones can develop skin cancer, including those with dark skin.

Tips to Protect Your Skin from Sunlight

Follow these tips to protect your skin from sunlight:

- Wear a hat with a wide brim all around that shades your face, neck, and ears. Baseball caps and some sun visors protect only parts of your skin.
- Wear sunglasses that block UV radiation to protect the skin around your eyes.
- Wear long sleeves and long pants. Tightly woven, dark fabrics are best. Some fabrics are rated with an ultraviolet protection factor (UPF). The higher the rating, the greater the protection from sunlight.
- Use sunscreen products with a sun protection factor (SPF) of at least 15. (Some doctors suggest using a product with an SPF of at least 30.) Apply the product's recommended amount to uncovered skin 30 minutes before going outside, and apply again every two hours or after swimming or sweating.

Keep in mind that the sun's rays:

- are strongest between 10 a.m. and 4 p.m.
- can go through light clothing, windshields, windows, and clouds
- are reflected by sand, water, snow, ice, and pavement

Section 4.6

Indoor Tanning and Cancer Risk

This section contains text excerpted from the following sources: Text beginning with the heading "Indoor Tanning" is excerpted from "Skin Cancer—Indoor Tanning Is Not Safe," Centers for Disease Control and Prevention (CDC), April 26, 2017; Text beginning with the heading "Preventing Overexposure to Ultraviolet (UV) Rays" is excerpted from "Skin Cancer—Are There Benefits to Spending Time Outdoors?" Centers for Disease Control and Prevention (CDC), April 25, 2017.

Indoor Tanning

Using a tanning bed, booth, or sunlamp to get tan is called indoor tanning. Exposure to ultraviolet (UV) rays while indoor tanning can cause skin cancers including melanoma (the deadliest type of skin cancer), basal cell carcinoma, and squamous cell carcinoma. UV exposure also can cause cataracts and cancers of the eye (ocular melanoma). UV exposure from the sun and from indoor tanning is classified as a *human carcinogen* (causes cancer in humans) by the International Agency for Research on Cancer (IARC) (part of the World Health Organization (WHO)) and by the U.S. Department of Health and Human Services (HHS).

Facts about Indoor Tanning

Tanning Indoors Is Not Safer than Tanning in the Sun

Indoor tanning and tanning outside are both dangerous. Although indoor tanning devices operate on a timer, the exposure to UV rays can vary based on the age and type of light bulbs. Indoor tanning is designed to give you high levels of UV radiation in a short time. You can get a burn from tanning indoors, and even a tan indicates damage to your skin.

A Base Tan Is Not a Safe Tan

A tan is the body's response to injury from UV rays. A base tan does little to protect you from future damage to your skin caused by

UV exposure. In fact, people who indoor tan are more likely to report getting sunburned.

The best way to protect your skin from the sun is by using these tips for skin cancer prevention.

Indoor Tanning Is Not a Safe Way to Get Vitamin D

Although it is important to get enough vitamin D, the safest way to do so is through what you eat. Tanning harms your skin, and the amount of UV exposure you need to get enough vitamin D is hard to measure because it is different for every person and also varies with the weather, latitude, altitude, and more.

Dangers of Indoor Tanning

Indoor tanning exposes users to two types of UV rays, UVA and UVB, which damage the skin and can lead to cancer. Indoor tanning is particularly dangerous for younger users; people who begin indoor tanning during adolescence or early adulthood have a higher risk of getting melanoma. This may be due to greater use of indoor tanning among those who begin tanning at earlier ages.

Every time you tan you increase your risk of getting skin cancer, including melanoma. Indoor tanning also:

- Causes premature skin aging, like wrinkles and age spots.
- Changes your skin texture.
- Increases the risk of potentially blinding eye diseases, if eye protection is not used.

Preventing Overexposure to Ultraviolet (UV) Rays

Spending time outdoors can improve overall health and wellness. The outdoors offers many opportunities to be physically active. Time outdoors may also promote mental health and stress reduction. While enjoying the benefits of being outdoors, people can decrease skin cancer risk from too much UV exposure by using sun protection. Protect yourself by staying in the shade, wearing protective clothing, and applying and reapplying a broad spectrum sunscreen with a sun protection factor (SPF) of 15 or higher.

UV rays from the sun can stimulate production of vitamin D in the skin. Having little or no sun exposure may put a person at risk for low levels of vitamin D, but too much UV exposure from the sun or artificial sources can increase risk of skin cancers and eye disease. The amount of vitamin D a person's skin makes when they are in the sun depends on many factors, including skin tone, geographic location, weather conditions, time of year, and time of day.

The skin can produce only a limited amount of vitamin D at one time. Once the body has reached this limit, spending more time in the sun will not continue to increase vitamin D levels. However, continued time in the sun will increase your skin cancer risk. There is no known level of UV exposure that would increase vitamin D levels without also increasing skin cancer risk. Vitamin D can be obtained safely through food and dietary supplements without the risks associated with overexposure to UV.

Sun Safety

The sun's UV rays can damage your skin in as little as 15 minutes. Follow these recommendations to help protect yourself and your family.

Shade

You can reduce your risk of skin damage and skin cancer by seeking shade under an umbrella, tree, or other shelter before you need relief from the sun. Your best bet to protect your skin is to use sunscreen or wear protective clothing when you're outside—even when you're in the shade.

Clothing

When possible, long-sleeved shirts and long pants and skirts can provide protection from UV rays. Clothes made from tightly woven fabric offer the best protection. A wet T-shirt offers much less UV protection than a dry one, and darker colors may offer more protection than lighter colors. Some clothing certified under international standards comes with information on its ultraviolet protection factor.

If wearing this type of clothing isn't practical, at least try to wear a T-shirt or a beach cover-up. Keep in mind that a typical T-shirt has an SPF rating lower than 15, so use other types of protection as well.

Hat

For the most protection, wear a hat with a brim all the way around that shades your face, ears, and the back of your neck. A tightly woven fabric, such as canvas, works best to protect your skin from UV rays. Avoid straw hats with holes that let sunlight through. A darker hat may offer more UV protection.

If you wear a baseball cap, you should also protect your ears and the back of your neck by wearing clothing that covers those areas, using a broad spectrum sunscreen with at least SPF 15, or by staying in the shade.

Sunglasses

Sunglasses protect your eyes from UV rays and reduce the risk of cataracts. They also protect the tender skin around your eyes from sun exposure.

Sunglasses that block both UVA and UVB rays offer the best protection. Most sunglasses sold in the United States, regardless of cost, meet this standard. Wrap-around sunglasses work best because they block UV rays from sneaking in from the side.

Sunscreen

Put on broad spectrum sunscreen with at least SPF 15 before you go outside, even on slightly cloudy or cool days. Don't forget to put a thick layer on all parts of exposed skin. Get help for hard-to-reach places like your back. And remember, sunscreen works best when combined with other options to prevent UV damage.

How sunscreen works. Most sunscreen products work by absorbing, reflecting, or scattering sunlight. They contain chemicals that interact with the skin to protect it from UV rays. All products do not have the same ingredients; if your skin reacts badly to one product, try another one or call a doctor.

SPF. Sunscreens are assigned a SPF number that rates their effectiveness in blocking UV rays. Higher numbers indicate more protection. You should use a broad spectrum sunscreen with at least SPF 15.

Reapplication. Sunscreen wears off. Put it on again if you stay out in the sun for more than two hours and after swimming, sweating, or toweling off.

Expiration date. Check the sunscreen's expiration date. Sunscreen without an expiration date has a shelf life of no more than three years, but its shelf life is shorter if it has been exposed to high temperatures.

Cosmetics. Some makeup and lip balms contain some of the same chemicals used in sunscreens. If they do not have at least SPF 15, don't use them by themselves.

Chapter 5

Hereditary Cancer Risks

Genetic Changes and Cancer

Cancer is a genetic disease—that is, cancer is caused by certain changes to genes that control the way our cells function, especially how they grow and divide.

Genes carry the instructions to make proteins, which do much of the work in our cells. Certain gene changes can cause cells to evade normal growth controls and become cancer. For example, some cancer-causing gene changes increase production of a protein that makes cells grow. Others result in the production of a misshapen, and therefore non-functional, form of a protein that normally repairs cellular damage.

Genetic changes that promote cancer can be inherited from our parents if the changes are present in germ cells, which are the reproductive cells of the body (eggs and sperm). Such changes, called germline changes, are found in every cell of the offspring. Cancer-causing genetic changes can also be acquired during one's lifetime, as the result of errors that occur as cells divide or from exposure to carcinogenic substances that damage deoxyribonucleic acid (DNA), such as certain chemicals in tobacco smoke, and radiation, such as ultraviolet rays

This chapter contains text excerpted from the following sources: Text beginning with the heading "Genetic Changes and Cancer" is excerpted from "The Genetics of Cancer," National Cancer Institute (NCI), October 12, 2017; Text under the heading "Hereditary Breast and Ovarian Cancer" is excerpted from "Hereditary Breast and Ovarian Cancer," Centers for Disease Control and Prevention (CDC), November 14, 2017.

from the sun. Genetic changes that occur after conception are called somatic (or acquired) changes.

There are many different kinds of DNA changes. Some changes affect just one unit of DNA, called a nucleotide. One nucleotide may be replaced by another, or it may be missing entirely. Other changes involve larger stretches of DNA and may include rearrangements, deletions, or duplications of long stretches of DNA.

Sometimes the changes are not in the actual sequence of DNA. For example, the addition or removal of chemical marks, called epigenetic modifications, on DNA can influence whether the gene is "expressed"—that is, whether and how much messenger ribonucleic acid (RNA) is produced. (Messenger RNA in turn is translated to produce the proteins encoded by the DNA.) In general, cancer cells have more genetic changes than normal cells. But each person's cancer has a unique combination of genetic alterations. Some of these changes may be the result of cancer, rather than the cause. As the cancer continues to grow, additional changes will occur. Even within the same tumor, cancer cells may have different genetic changes.

Hereditary Cancer Syndromes

Inherited genetic mutations play a major role in about 5–10 percent of all cancers. Researchers have associated mutations in specific genes with more than 50 hereditary cancer syndromes, which are disorders that may predispose individuals to developing certain cancers. Genetic tests for hereditary cancer syndromes can tell whether a person from a family that shows signs of such a syndrome has one of these mutations. These tests can also show whether family members without obvious disease have inherited the same mutation as a family member who carries a cancer-associated mutation.

Many experts recommend that genetic testing for cancer risk be considered when someone has a personal or family history that suggests an inherited cancer risk condition, as long as the test results can be adequately interpreted (that is, they can clearly tell whether a specific genetic change is present or absent) and when the results provide information that will help guide a person's future medical care.

Cancers that are not caused by inherited genetic mutations can sometimes appear to "run in families." For example, a shared environment or lifestyle, such as tobacco use, can cause similar cancers to develop among family members. However, certain patterns in a family—such as the types of cancer that develop, other noncancer conditions that are seen, and the ages at which cancer develops—may suggest the presence of a hereditary cancer syndrome.

Even if a cancer-predisposing mutation is present in a family, not everyone who inherits the mutation will necessarily develop cancer. Several factors influence the outcome in a given person with the mutation, including the pattern of inheritance of the cancer syndrome.

Here are examples of genes that can play a role in hereditary cancer syndromes.

- The most commonly mutated gene in all cancers is *TP53*, which produces a protein that suppresses the growth of tumors. In addition, germline mutations in this gene can cause Li-Fraumeni syndrome, a rare, inherited disorder that leads to a higher risk of developing certain cancers.
- Inherited mutations in the *BRCA1* and *BRCA2* genes are associated with hereditary breast and ovarian cancer syndrome, which is a disorder marked by an increased lifetime risk of breast and ovarian cancers in women. Several other cancers have been associated with this syndrome, including pancreatic and prostate cancers, as well as male breast cancer.
- Another gene that produces a protein that suppresses the growth of tumors is *PTEN*. Mutations in this gene are associated with Cowden syndrome, an inherited disorder that increases the risk of breast, thyroid, endometrial, and other types of cancer.

Genetic Tests for Hereditary Cancer Syndromes

Genetic tests for mutations that cause hereditary cancer syndromes are usually requested by a person's doctor or other healthcare provider. Genetic counseling can help people consider the risks, benefits, and limitations of genetic testing in their particular situations. A genetic counselor, doctor, or other healthcare professional trained in genetics can help an individual or family understand their test results and explain the possible implications of test results for other family members.

People considering genetic testing should understand that their results may become known to other people or organizations that have legitimate, legal access to their medical records, such as their insurance company or employer, if their employer provides the patient's health insurance as a benefit. Legal protections are in place to prevent genetic discrimination, including the Genetic Information Nondiscrimination

Act (GINA) of 2008 and the Privacy Rule of the Health Information Portability and Accountability Act (HIPAA) of 1996.

Identifying Genetic Changes in Cancer

Lab tests called DNA sequencing tests can "read" DNA. By comparing the sequence of DNA in cancer cells with that in normal cells, such as blood or saliva, scientists can identify genetic changes in cancer cells that may be driving the growth of an individual's cancer. This information may help doctors sort out which therapies might work best against a particular tumor.

Tumor DNA sequencing can also reveal the presence of inherited mutations. Indeed, in some cases, the genetic testing of tumors has shown that a patient's cancer could be associated with a hereditary cancer syndrome that the family was not aware of. As with testing for specific mutations in hereditary cancer syndromes, clinical DNA sequencing has implications that patients need to consider. For example, they may learn incidentally about the presence of inherited mutations that may cause other diseases, in them or in their family members.

Hereditary Breast and Ovarian Cancer

Each year, over 200,000 women in the United States learn that they have breast cancer and more than 20,000 find out that they have ovarian cancer. While most of these cancers happen by chance, some are hereditary, meaning that they are caused by genetic changes (called mutations) which are passed down in families.

Effective medical options are available for women at risk for hereditary breast and ovarian cancer that can make them less likely to get these cancers. Because of this, all women should learn about their family health history of breast and ovarian cancer to know if they could be at risk for hereditary breast and ovarian cancer.

The first step to find out if you are at risk is to collect your family health history of breast and ovarian cancer and share this information with your doctor. If your family health history shows that you could be at risk for hereditary breast and ovarian cancer, your doctor may refer you for genetic counseling and genetic testing.

BRCA1 and *BRCA2* Genes

The genes most commonly affected in hereditary breast and ovarian cancer are the breast cancer 1 (*BRCA1*) and breast cancer 2 (*BRCA2*) genes. About 3 percent of breast cancers (about 6,000 women per year) and 10 percent of ovarian cancers (about 2,000 women per year) result from inherited mutations in the *BRCA1* and *BRCA2* genes.

Normally, the *BRCA1* and *BRCA2* genes protect you from getting certain cancers. But some mutations in the *BRCA1* and *BRCA2* genes prevent them from working properly, so that if you inherit one of these mutations, you are more likely to get breast, ovarian, and other cancers. However, not everyone who inherits a *BRCA1* or *BRCA2* mutation will get breast or ovarian cancer.

Everyone has two copies of the *BRCA1* and *BRCA2* genes, one copy inherited from their mother and one from their father. Even if a person inherits a *BRCA1* or *BRCA2* mutation from one parent, they still have the normal copy of the *BRCA1* or *BRCA2* gene from the other parent. Cancer occurs when a second mutation happens that affects the normal copy of the gene, so that the person no longer has a *BRCA1* or *BRCA2* gene that works properly. Unlike the inherited *BRCA1* or *BRCA2* mutation, the second mutation would not be present throughout the person's body, but would only be present in the cancer tissue.

Breast and ovarian cancer can also be caused by inherited mutations in genes other than *BRCA1* and *BRCA2*. This means that in some families with a history of breast and ovarian cancer, family members will not have mutations in *BRCA1* or *BRCA2*, but can have mutations in one of these other genes. These mutations might be identified through genetic testing using multigene panels, which look for mutations in several different genes at the same time.

You and your family members are more likely to have a *BRCA1* or *BRCA2* mutation if your family has a strong history of breast or ovarian cancer. Family members who inherit *BRCA1* and *BRCA2* mutations usually share the same mutation. If one of your family members has a known *BRCA1* or *BRCA2* mutation, other family members who get genetic testing should be checked for that mutation.

If you are concerned that you could have a *BRCA1*, *BRCA2*, or other mutation related to breast and ovarian cancer, the first step is to collect your family health history of breast and ovarian cancer and share this information with your doctor.

Chapter 6

Infectious Diseases and Cancer Risk

Chapter Contents

Section 6.1

Human Papillomaviruses (HPV) and Cancer

This section includes text excerpted from "HPV and Cancer," National Cancer Institute (NCI), February 19, 2015.

What Are Human Papillomaviruses?

Human papillomaviruses (HPVs) are a group of more than 200 related viruses. More than 40 HPV types can be easily spread through direct sexual contact, from the skin and mucous membranes of infected people to the skin and mucous membranes of their partners. They can be spread by vaginal, anal, and oral sex. Other HPV types are responsible for nongenital warts, which are not sexually transmitted.

Sexually transmitted HPV types fall into two categories:

- Low-risk HPVs, which do not cause cancer but can cause skin warts (technically known as condylomata acuminata) on or around the genitals and anus. For example, HPV types 6 and 11 cause 90 percent of all genital warts. HPV types 6 and 11 also cause recurrent respiratory papillomatosis, a less common disease in which benign tumors grow in the air passages leading from the nose and mouth into the lungs.
- High-risk HPVs, which can cause cancer. About a dozen high-risk HPV types have been identified. Two of these, HPV types 16 and 18, are responsible for most HPV-caused cancers.

HPV infections are the most common sexually transmitted infections in the United States. About 14 million new genital HPV infections occur each year. In fact, the Centers for Disease Control and Prevention (CDC) estimates that more than 90 percent and 80 percent, respectively, of sexually active men and women will be infected with at least one type of HPV at some point in their lives. Around one-half of these infections are with a high-risk HPV type. Most high-risk HPV infections occur without any symptoms, go away within 1–2 years, and do not cause cancer. Some HPV infections, however, can persist for many years. Persistent infections with high-risk HPV types can lead to cell changes that, if untreated, may progress to cancer.

Which Cancers Are Caused by HPV?

High-risk HPVs cause several types of cancer.

- **Cervical cancer.** Virtually all cases of cervical cancer are caused by HPV, and just two HPV types, 16 and 18, are responsible for about 70 percent of all cases.
- **Anal cancer.** About 95 percent of anal cancers are caused by HPV. Most of these are caused by HPV type 16.
- **Oropharyngeal cancers** (cancers of the middle part of the throat, including the soft palate, the base of the tongue, and the tonsils). About 70 percent of oropharyngeal cancers are caused by HPV. In the United States, more than half of cancers diagnosed in the oropharynx are linked to HPV type 16.
- **Rarer cancers.** HPV causes about 65 percent of vaginal cancers, 50 percent of vulvar cancers, and 35 percent of penile cancers. Most of these are caused by HPV type 16.

High-risk HPV types cause approximately 5 percent of all cancers worldwide. In the United States, high-risk HPV types cause approximately 3 percent of all cancer cases among women and 2 percent of all cancer cases among men.

Who Gets HPV Infections?

Anyone who has ever been sexually active (that is, engaged in skin-to-skin sexual conduct, including vaginal, anal, or oral sex) can get HPV. HPV is easily passed between partners through sexual contact. HPV infections are more likely in those who have many sex partners or have sex with someone who has had many partners. Because the infection is so common, most people get HPV infections shortly after becoming sexually active for the first time. A person who has had only one partner can get HPV. Someone can have an HPV infection even if they have no symptoms and their only sexual contact with an HPV-infected person happened many years ago.

Can HPV Infections Be Prevented?

People who are not sexually active almost never develop genital HPV infections. In addition, HPV vaccination before sexual activity can reduce the risk of infection by the HPV types targeted by the vaccine. The U.S. Food and Drug Administration (FDA) has approved three vaccines to prevent HPV infection: Gardasil®, Gardasil®9, and

Cervarix®. These vaccines provide strong protection against new HPV infections, but they are not effective at treating established HPV infections or disease caused by HPV. Correct and consistent condom use is associated with reduced HPV transmission between sexual partners, but less frequent condom use is not. However, because areas not covered by a condom can be infected by the virus, condoms are unlikely to provide complete protection against the infection.

Can HPV Infections Be Detected?

HPV infections can be detected by testing a sample of cells to see if they contain viral deoxyribonucleic acid (DNA) or ribonucleic acid (RNA).

Several HPV tests are currently approved by the FDA for three cervical screening indications: for follow-up testing of women who seem to have abnormal Pap test results, for cervical cancer screening in combination with a Pap test among women over age 30, and for use alone as a first-line primary cervical cancer screening test for women ages 25 and older.

The most common HPV test detects DNA from several high-risk HPV types in a group, but it cannot identify the specific type(s) that are present. Other tests do tell in addition whether there is DNA or RNA from HPV types 16 and 18, the two types that cause most HPV-associated cancers. These tests can detect HPV infections before abnormal cell changes are evident, and before any treatment for cell changes is needed. There are no FDA-approved tests to detect HPV infections in men. There are also no currently recommended screening methods similar to a Pap test for detecting cell changes caused by HPV infection in anal, vulvar, vaginal, penile, or oropharyngeal tissues. However, this is an area of ongoing research.

What Are Treatment Options for HPV-Infected Individuals?

There is currently no medical treatment for persistent HPV infections that are not associated with abnormal cell changes. However, the genital warts, benign respiratory tract tumors, precancerous changes at the cervix, and cancers resulting from HPV infections can be treated.

Methods commonly used to treat precancerous cervical changes include cryosurgery (freezing that destroys tissue), LEEP (loop electrosurgical excision procedure, or the removal of cervical tissue using a hot wire loop), surgical conization (surgery with a scalpel, a laser, or both to remove a cone-shaped piece of tissue from the cervix and cervical canal), and laser vaporization conization (use of a laser to destroy cervical tissue).

Treatments for other types of benign respiratory tract tumors and precancerous changes caused by HPV (vaginal, vulvar, penile, and anal lesions) and genital warts include topical chemicals or drugs, excisional surgery, cryosurgery, electrosurgery, and laser surgery. Treatment approaches are being tested in clinical trials, including a randomized controlled trial that will determine whether treating anal precancerous lesions will reduce the risk of anal cancer in people who are infected with human immunodeficiency virus (HIV).

HPV-infected individuals who develop cancer generally receive the same treatment as patients whose tumors do not harbor HPV infections, according to the type and stage of their tumors. However, people who are diagnosed with HPV-positive oropharyngeal cancer may be treated differently than people with oropharyngeal cancers that are HPV-negative. Research has shown that patients with HPV-positive oropharyngeal tumors have a better prognosis and may do just as well on less intense treatment. Ongoing clinical trials are investigating this question.

How Does High-Risk HPV Cause Cancer?

HPV infects epithelial cells. These cells, which are organized in layers, cover the inside and outside surfaces of the body, including the skin, the throat, the genital tract, and the anus. Once HPV enters an epithelial cell, the virus begins to make the proteins it encodes. Two of the proteins made by high-risk HPVs (E6 and E7) interfere with cell functions that normally prevent excessive growth, helping the cell to grow in an uncontrolled manner and to avoid cell death.

Many times these infected cells are recognized by the immune system and eliminated. Sometimes, however, these infected cells are not destroyed, and a persistent infection results. As the persistently infected cells continue to grow, they may develop mutations in cellular genes that promote even more abnormal cell growth, leading to the formation of an area of precancerous cells and, ultimately, a cancerous tumor.

Other factors may increase the risk that an infection with a high-risk HPV type will persist and possibly develop into cancer. These include:

- Smoking or chewing tobacco (for increased risk of oropharyngeal cancer)

- Having a weakened immune system
- Having many children (for increased risk of cervical cancer)
- Long-term oral contraceptive use (for increased risk of cervical cancer)
- Poor oral hygiene (for increased risk of oropharyngeal cancer)
- Chronic inflammation

Researchers believe that it can take between 10 and 30 years from the time of an initial HPV infection until a tumor forms. However, even when severely abnormal cells are seen on the cervix (a condition called cervical intraepithelial neoplasia 3, or CIN3), these do not always lead to cancer. The percentage of CIN3 lesions that progress to invasive cervical cancer has been estimated to be 50 percent or less.

Section 6.2

Human Immunodeficiency Virus (HIV) Infection and Cancer Risk

This section contains text excerpted from the following sources: Text under the heading "What Is HIV?" is excerpted from "HIV Basics—About HIV/AIDS," Centers for Disease Control and Prevention (CDC), May 30, 2017; Text beginning with the heading "Do People Infected with Human Immunodeficiency Virus (HIV) Have an Increased Risk of Cancer?" is excerpted from "HIV Infection and Cancer Risk," National Cancer Institute (NCI), September 14, 2017.

What Is HIV?

HIV stands for human immunodeficiency virus. It is the virus that can lead to acquired immunodeficiency syndrome or AIDS if not treated. Unlike some other viruses, the human body can't get rid of HIV completely, even with treatment. So once you get HIV, you have it for life.

HIV attacks the body's immune system, specifically the CD4 cells (T cells), which help the immune system fight off infections. Untreated, HIV reduces the number of CD4 cells (T cells) in the body, making the person more likely to get other infections or infection-related cancers. Over time, HIV can destroy so many of these cells that the body can't fight off infections and disease. These opportunistic infections or cancers take advantage of a very weak immune system and signal that the person has AIDS, the last stage of HIV infection.

No effective cure currently exists, but with proper medical care, HIV can be controlled. The medicine used to treat HIV is called antiretroviral therapy or ART. If taken the right way, every day, this medicine can dramatically prolong the lives of many people infected with HIV, keep them healthy, and greatly lower their chance of infecting others. Before the introduction of ART in the mid-1990s, people with HIV could progress to AIDS in just a few years. Today, someone diagnosed with HIV and treated before the disease is far advanced can live nearly as long as someone who does not have HIV.

Do People Infected with Human Immunodeficiency Virus (HIV) Have an Increased Risk of Cancer?

Yes. People infected with human immunodeficiency virus (HIV) have a substantially higher risk of some types of cancer compared with uninfected people of the same age. The general term for these cancers is "HIV-associated cancers." Three of these cancers are known as "acquired immunodeficiency syndrome (AIDS)-defining cancers" or "AIDS-defining malignancies": Kaposi sarcoma, aggressive B-cell non-Hodgkin lymphoma (NHL), and cervical cancer. A diagnosis of any of these cancers in someone infected with HIV confirms a diagnosis of AIDS.

Compared with the general population, people infected with HIV are currently about 500 times more likely to be diagnosed with Kaposi sarcoma, 12 times more likely to be diagnosed with non-Hodgkin lymphoma, and, among women, 3 times more likely to be diagnosed with cervical cancer. In addition, people infected with HIV are at higher risk of several other types of cancer (collectively called "non-AIDS-defining cancers"). These other malignancies include cancers of the anus, liver, oral cavity/pharynx, and lung, and Hodgkin lymphoma. People infected with HIV are 19 times more likely to be diagnosed with anal cancer, 3 times as likely to be diagnosed with liver cancer, 2 times as likely to be diagnosed with lung cancer, about 2 times as likely to be diagnosed with oral cavity/pharynx cancer, and about 8 times more likely to be diagnosed with Hodgkin lymphoma compared with the general population. In addition to being linked to an increased risk of cancer, HIV infection is associated with an increased risk of dying from cancer. HIV-infected people with a range of cancer types are more likely to die of their cancer than HIV-uninfected people with these cancers.

Why Might People Infected with HIV Have a Higher Risk of Some Types of Cancer?

Infection with HIV weakens the immune system and reduces the body's ability to fight viral infections that may lead to cancer. The viruses that are most likely to cause cancer in people with HIV are:

- Kaposi sarcoma-associated herpesvirus (KSHV), also known as human herpesvirus 8 (HHV-8), which causes Kaposi sarcoma and some subtypes of lymphoma
- Epstein-Barr virus (EBV), which causes some subtypes of non-Hodgkin and Hodgkin lymphoma
- Human papillomaviruses (HPV), high-risk types of which cause cervical cancer, most anal cancers, and oropharyngeal, penile, vaginal, and vulvar cancer
- Hepatitis B virus (HBV) and hepatitis C virus (HCV), which both cause liver cancer

HIV-infected persons are more likely to be infected with these viruses than people in the general population. In addition, the prevalence of some traditional risk factors for cancer, especially smoking (a known cause of lung and other cancers) and heavy alcohol use (which can increase the risk of liver cancer), is higher among people infected with HIV. Also, because people infected with HIV have compromised immune systems, both immunosuppression and inflammation may have direct or indirect roles in the development of some cancers that are elevated in people infected with HIV. The poorer cancer survival of HIV-infected people may result, at least in part, from the weakened immune system in such individuals. The increased risk of death could also result from the cancer being more advanced at diagnosis, delays in cancer treatment, or poorer access to appropriate cancer treatment.

Has the Introduction of Antiretroviral Therapy Changed the Cancer Risk of People Infected with HIV?

The introduction of highly active antiretroviral therapy (HAART), also called combination antiretroviral therapy (cART), starting in the mid-1990s greatly reduced the incidence of certain cancers in HIV-infected patients, especially Kaposi sarcoma and non-Hodgkin lymphoma. The likely explanation for this reduced incidence is that cART lowers the amount of HIV circulating in the blood, thereby allowing partial restoration of immune system function to fight the viruses that cause many of these cancers.

Although the risk of these AIDS-defining cancers among people infected with HIV is lower than in the past, it is still much higher than among people in the general population. This persistently high risk may reflect the fact that cART does not completely restore immune system functioning. Also, many people infected with HIV are not aware they are infected, have had difficulty in accessing medical care, or for other reasons are not receiving adequate antiretroviral therapy.

The introduction of cART has not reduced the incidence of all HIV-related cancers, and in fact there has been an increase in non-AIDS-defining cancers. For example, the incidence of liver and anal cancer may be increasing among HIV-infected individuals.

An important factor contributing to the increase in non-AIDS-defining cancers is that as cART has reduced the number of deaths from AIDS, the HIV-infected population has grown in size and become older. The fastest growing proportion of HIV-infected individuals is the over-40 age group. These individuals are now developing cancers common in older age and also have an increased cumulative risk of developing HIV-associated cancers.

What Can People Infected with HIV Do to Reduce Their Risk of Cancer or to Find Cancer Early?

Taking cART as indicated based on current HIV treatment guidelines lowers the risk of Kaposi sarcoma and non-Hodgkin lymphoma and increases overall survival.

The risk of lung, oral, and other cancers can be reduced by quitting smoking. Because HIV-infected people have a higher risk of lung cancer, it is especially important that they do not smoke. Help with quitting smoking is available through the National Cancer Institute's (NCI) smoking quitline at 877-44U-QUIT (877-448-7848).

The higher incidence of liver cancer among HIV-infected people appears to be related to more frequent infection with hepatitis virus (particularly HCV in the United States) than among HIV-uninfected people. Therefore, HIV-infected individuals should know their hepatitis status.

In addition, if HIV-infected people currently have viral hepatitis, they should discuss with their healthcare provider whether antiviral treatment is an option for them. Some drugs may be used for both HBV-suppressing therapy and cART.

Because HIV-infected women have a higher risk of cervical cancer, it is important that they be screened regularly for this disease. In addition, the Centers for Disease Control and Prevention (CDC) recommends vaccination against human papillomavirus (HPV) for women and men with HIV infection up to age 26 years. Cervical cancer screening guidelines that incorporate results of a Pap test and an HPV deoxyribonucleic acid (DNA) test are evolving, and women should discuss screening options with their healthcare provider.

Some researchers recommend anal Pap test screening to detect and treat early lesions before they progress to anal cancer. However, it is not clear if this type of screening benefits all HIV-infected people or if treating such lesions prevents anal cancer. These questions are being addressed in an NCI-funded trial called the Anal Cancer/HSIL Outcomes Research (ANCHOR) Study. This study is currently enrolling men and women with HIV to undergo anal Pap testing and then be randomly assigned to receive either treatment or observation (no treatment). The goal is to determine whether treatment of anal lesions prevents anal cancer in HIV-infected people with anal lesions. KSHV is secreted in saliva, and transmission of this virus may occur through deep kissing, through the use of saliva as a lubricant in sex, or through oral–anal sex. Reducing contact through these routes may reduce the chance of being infected with KSHV.

Section 6.3

Kaposi Sarcoma-Associated Herpesvirus

This section includes text excerpted from "Cancer-Causing Viruses," National Institute of Environmental Health Sciences (NIEHS), November 3, 2016.

What Is Kaposi Sarcoma-Associated Herpesvirus (KSHV) and How Are People Exposed to It?

KSHV is a herpes virus transmitted from person to person, primarily through saliva. It can be transmitted from an infected mother to a child, and by contact with other infected family members. In adults, it can be transmitted through sexual contact, primarily among men who have sex with men, and nonsexual routes, such as blood and organ transplants. Healthy individuals can be infected with the virus and show no signs or symptoms.

What Evidence Is There That KSHV Causes Cancer?

There is sufficient human evidence linking KSHV to several cancers, including Kaposi sarcoma, a blood vessel cancer, and two rare lymphomas—primary effusion lymphoma, and a plasmablastic variant of multicentric Castleman disease. KSHV is part of the criteria for diagnosing all three of these cancers. Kaposi sarcoma is a blood vessel cancer that mainly affects the skin, mouth, and lymph nodes. There are four types of Kaposi sarcoma. Approximately 90 percent of Kaposi sarcoma patients are infected with KSHV. More than 100 human studies have demonstrated a link between KSHV infection and all four types of Kaposi sarcoma.

Consistent human findings, coupled with information from tumor tissues, show that KSHV is also associated with primary effusion lymphoma. Additionally, studies of tumor tissue from KSHV-infected patients provide evidence for an association between KSHV infection and a plasmablastic variant of multicentric Castleman disease (CD).

How Does KSHV Lead to Cancer?

KSHV can cause cancer, especially in people with weakened immune systems, or immunosuppression, by transforming normal cells into cancer cells. Kaposi sarcoma is more likely to occur when an infected person becomes immunosuppressed, which can occur in transplant patients and patients receiving chemotherapy, and can be a major problem for persons with acquired immunodeficiency syndrome (AIDS). Nevertheless, KSHV can also cause cancer in people not known to have impaired immune systems, suggesting that immunosuppression may not be required for cancer development.

What Are Some Things I Can Do to Prevent Transmission of the Virus and, If Infected, Prevent My Risk for Cancer?

- Practice safe sex (use condoms and reduce sexual partners).
- Patients diagnosed with Kaposi sarcoma should discuss treatment options with their physician.

Section 6.4

Hepatitis Viruses and Cancer Risk

This section includes text excerpted from "Viral Hepatitis and Liver Cancer," Centers for Disease Control and Prevention (CDC), May 10, 2017.

In the United States, an estimated 3.5 million people are living with hepatitis C and up to 2.2 million people are living with hepatitis B. Hepatitis B and hepatitis C, the most common types of viral hepatitis in the United States, can cause serious health problems, including liver failure and liver cancer. Unfortunately, new liver cancer cases and deaths are on the rise in the United States. Many of these liver cancer cases are related to infection with hepatitis B or hepatitis C.

Unfortunately, many people are unaware they are infected with hepatitis B and hepatitis C, and most people do not have symptoms or feel sick. To find out if you should be tested or vaccinated for viral hepatitis, Centers for Disease Control and Prevention (CDC) developed an online Hepatitis Risk Assessment. The assessment, which takes only five minutes, will provide personalized testing and vaccination recommendations for hepatitis A, hepatitis B, and hepatitis C.

Hepatitis A

Hepatitis A is a short-term disease that is caused by infection with the hepatitis A virus. Hepatitis A was once very common in the United States, but the number of cases that occur each year is less than 3,000. Hepatitis A does not lead to liver cancer and most people who get infected recover over time with no lasting effects. Hepatitis A is easily prevented with a safe and effective vaccine, which is believed to have caused the dramatic decline in new cases in recent years. The vaccine is recommended for all children at one year of age and for adults who may be at risk, including travelers to certain international countries.

Hepatitis B

Hepatitis B is a liver disease that results from infection with the hepatitis B virus. Hepatitis B is common in many parts of the world, including Asia, the Pacific Islands and Africa. Hepatitis B is also preventable with a vaccine. The hepatitis B virus can be passed from an infected woman to her baby at birth, if her baby does not receive the hepatitis B vaccine. As a result, the hepatitis B vaccine is recommended for all infants at birth. Unfortunately, many people got infected before the hepatitis B vaccine was widely available. That's why CDC recommends anyone born in areas where hepatitis B is common, or whose parents were born in these regions, get tested for hepatitis B. Treatments are available that can delay or reduce the risk of developing liver cancer by 50–80 percent.

Hepatitis C

Hepatitis C is a liver disease that results from infection with the hepatitis C virus. For reasons that are not entirely understood, people born from 1945–1965 are five times more likely to have hepatitis C than other age groups. In the past, hepatitis C was spread through blood transfusions and organ transplants. However, widespread screening of the blood supply began in 1990 and the hepatitis C virus was virtually eliminated from the blood supply by 1992. Today, most people become infected with hepatitis C by sharing needles, syringes, or any other equipment to inject drugs. In fact, rates of new infections have been on the rise in young people who inject drugs.

There is currently no vaccine to prevent hepatitis C. Fortunately, new treatments offer a cure for most people. Once diagnosed, most persons with hepatitis C can be cured in just 8–12 weeks, reducing liver cancer risk by 75 percent.

Section 6.5

Human T-Cell Lymphotropic Virus Type 1 (HTLV1) and Cancer Risk

This section includes text excerpted from "Cancer-Causing Viruses," National Institute of Environmental Health Sciences (NIEHS), November 3, 2016.

What Is Human T-Cell Lymphotropic Virus Type 1 (HTLV1) and How Are People Exposed to It?

HTLV-1 is a virus that people are exposed to through contact with contaminated cells or biological tissues, such as breastfeeding, sharing of needles or syringes with infected individuals, organ transplants, or unprotected sexual activity. It is not transmitted by casual contact. Approximately 90,000 people in the United States are infected with HTLV-1, but only a very small number of infected people develop cancer or other diseases related to this virus. This virus is most prevalent in Japan, the Caribbean, and the Middle East, with an estimated 5- to 10-million people infected worldwide. Most HTLV1-infected individuals have the virus in their bodies throughout their lifetime, but do not have any symptoms.

What Evidence Is There That HTLV-1 Causes Cancer?

Human epidemiological studies and molecular studies show that HTLV-1 causes adult T-cell leukemia-lymphoma (ATLL). ATLL is a rare cancer that infects the body's T cells, specifically white blood cells known as CD4 T cells that help fight off infection.

How Does HTLV-1 Lead to Cancer?

A key HTLV-1 protein, called Tax, can initiate and promote cancer, especially in people who have a weakened immune system.

What Are Some Things I Can Do to Prevent Transmission of the Virus and, If Infected, Prevent My Risk for Cancer?

- Practice safe sex (use condoms and reduce sexual partners).
- If infected, women should refrain from breastfeeding.
- Periodic medical evaluations by a physician knowledgeable about this virus is recommended.

Section 6.6

Epstein-Barr Virus and Cancer Risk

This section includes text excerpted from "Cancer-Causing Viruses," National Institute of Environmental Health Sciences (NIEHS), November 3, 2016.

What Is Epstein-Barr Virus (EBV) and How Are People Exposed to It?

Epstein-Barr Virus (EBV) is a herpes virus, transmitted primarily through saliva. It may also be spread through contact with other types of bodily fluids, such as infected blood, genital fluids, and breast milk. It is a common virus, infecting more than 90 percent of adults worldwide. Most people infected with EBV remain healthy and without symptoms. In some cases, EBV can cause infectious mononucleosis, also called mono. EBV was the first human virus ever linked to cancer, about 52 years ago.

What Evidence Is There That EBV Causes Cancer?

Human epidemiological studies, clinical studies, and molecular studies show that EBV can lead to four types of lymphoma—Burkitt, Hodgkin, immune-suppression-related non-Hodgkin, and nasal type extranodal NK/T-cell lymphoma—and two types of epithelial cancer—nasopharyngeal cancer and some types of stomach cancer.

How Does EBV Lead to Cancer?

The way in which EBV leads to various EBV-related cancers is complex and continues to be researched. EBV is held in check by the immune system. For most EBV-related cancers, a weakened immune system can lead to the production of cancer-causing viral proteins. In addition, infectious agents, regional differences in diet, and an individual's genetic susceptibility and make-up can all potentially play a role in the development of some EBV related cancers.

What Are Some Things I Can Do to Prevent Transmission of the Virus and, If Infected, Prevent My Risk for Cancer?

- Don't kiss people who have EBV infection.
- Don't share drinks, food, or personal items, like toothbrushes, with people who have EBV infection.

Section 6.7

Helicobacter pylori and Cancer Risk

This section includes text excerpted from "*Helicobacter Pylori* and Cancer," National Cancer Institute (NCI), September 5, 2013. Reviewed March 2018.

What Is *Helicobacter pylori*?

Helicobacter pylori, or *H. pylori*, is a spiral-shaped bacterium that grows in the mucus layer that coats the inside of the human stomach.

To survive in the harsh, acidic environment of the stomach, *H. pylori* secretes an enzyme called urease, which converts the chemical urea to ammonia. The production of ammonia around *H. pylori* neutralizes the acidity of the stomach, making it more hospitable for the bacterium. In addition, the helical shape of *H. pylori* allows it to burrow into the mucus layer, which is less acidic than the inside space, or lumen, of the stomach. *H. pylori* can also attach to the cells that line the inner surface of the stomach.

Although immune cells that normally recognize and attack invading bacteria accumulate near sites of *H. pylori* infection, they are unable to reach the stomach lining. In addition, *H. pylori* has developed ways of interfering with local immune responses, making them ineffective in eliminating this bacterium.

H. pylori has coexisted with humans for many thousands of years, and infection with this bacterium is common. The Centers for Disease Control and Prevention (CDC) estimates that approximately two-thirds of the world's population harbors the bacterium, with infection rates much higher in developing countries than in developed nations.

Although *H. pylori* infection does not cause illness in most infected people, it is a major risk factor for peptic ulcer disease and is responsible for the majority of ulcers of the stomach and upper small intestine.

In 1994, the International Agency for Research on Cancer (IARC) classified *H. pylori* as a carcinogen, or cancer-causing agent, in humans, despite conflicting results at the time. Since then, it has been increasingly accepted that colonization of the stomach with *H. pylori* is an important cause of gastric cancer and of gastric mucosa-associated lymphoid tissue (MALT) lymphoma. Infection with *H. pylori* is also associated with a reduced risk of esophageal adenocarcinoma. *H. pylori* is thought to spread through contaminated food and water and through direct mouth-to-mouth contact. In most populations, the bacterium is first acquired during childhood. Infection is more likely in children living in poverty, in crowded conditions, and in areas with poor sanitation.

What Is Gastric Cancer?

Gastric cancer, or cancer of the stomach, was once considered a single entity. Now, scientists divide this cancer into two main classes: gastric cardia cancer (cancer of the top inch of the stomach, where it meets the esophagus) and noncardia gastric cancer (cancer in all other areas of the stomach).

Gastric cancer is the second most common cause of cancer-related deaths in the world, killing approximately 738,000 people in 2008. Gastric cancer is less common in the United States and other Western countries than in countries in Asia and South America.

Overall gastric cancer incidence is decreasing. However, this decline is mainly in the rates of noncardia gastric cancer. Gastric cardia cancer, which was once very uncommon, has risen in incidence in recent decades.

Infection with *H. pylori* is the primary identified cause of gastric cancer. Other risk factors for gastric cancer include chronic gastritis; older age; male sex; a diet high in salted, smoked, or poorly preserved foods and low in fruits and vegetables; tobacco smoking; pernicious anemia; a history of stomach surgery for benign conditions; and a family history of stomach cancer. *H. pylori* has different associations with the two main classes of gastric cancer. Whereas people infected with *H. pylori* have an increased risk of noncardia gastric cancer, their risk of gastric cardia cancer is not increased and may even be decreased.

What Evidence Shows That H. pylori *Infection Causes Noncardia Gastric Cancer?*

Epidemiologic studies have shown that individuals infected with *H. pylori* have an increased risk of gastric adenocarcinoma. The risk increase appears to be restricted to noncardia gastric cancer. For example, a combined analysis of 12 case–control studies of *H. pylori* and gastric cancer estimated that the risk of noncardia gastric cancer was nearly six times higher for *H. pylori*-infected people than for uninfected people.

Additional evidence for an association between *H. pylori* infection and the risk of noncardia gastric cancer comes from prospective cohort studies such as the Alpha-Tocopherol, Beta-Carotene (ATBC) Cancer Prevention Study in Finland. Comparing subjects who developed noncardia gastric cancer with cancer-free control subjects, the researchers found that *H. pylori*-infected individuals had a nearly eightfold increased risk for noncardia gastric cancer.

What Is the Evidence That H. pylori *Infection May Reduce the Risk of Some Cancers?*

Several studies have detected an inverse relationship between *H. pylori* infection and gastric cardia cancer, although the evidence is not entirely consistent. The possibility of an inverse relationship between the bacterium and gastric cardia cancer is supported by the corresponding decrease in *H. pylori* infection rates in Western countries during the past century—the result of improved hygiene and widespread antibiotic use—and the increase in rates of gastric cardia cancer in these same regions.

Similar epidemiologic evidence suggests that *H. pylori* infection may be associated with a lower risk of esophageal adenocarcinoma. For example, a large case–control study in Sweden showed that the risk of esophageal adenocarcinoma in *H. pylori*-infected individuals was one-third that of uninfected individuals. A meta-analysis of 13 studies, including the Swedish study, found a 45 percent reduction in risk of esophageal adenocarcinoma with *H. pylori* infection. Moreover, as with gastric cardia cancer, dramatic increases in esophageal adenocarcinoma rates in several Western countries parallel the declines in *H. pylori* infection rates.

How Might H. pylori *Infection Decrease the Risk of Some Cancers but Increase the Risk of Other Cancers?*

Although it is not known for certain how *H. pylori* infection increases the risk of noncardia gastric cancer, some researchers speculate that the long-term presence of an inflammatory response predisposes cells in the stomach lining to become cancerous. This idea is supported by the finding that increased expression of a single cytokine (interleukin-1-beta) in the stomach of transgenic mice causes sporadic gastric inflammation and cancer. The increased cell turnover resulting from ongoing cellular damage could increase the likelihood that cells will develop harmful mutations.

One hypothesis that may explain reduced risks of gastric cardia cancer and esophageal adenocarcinoma in *H. pylori*-infected individuals relates to the decline in stomach acidity that is often seen after decades of *H. pylori* colonization. This decline would reduce acid reflux into the esophagus, a major risk factor for adenocarcinomas affecting the upper stomach and esophagus.

What Is CagA-Positive H. pylori *and How Does It Affect the Risk of Gastric and Esophageal Cancers?*

Some *H. pylori* bacteria use a needle-like appendage to inject a toxin produced by a gene called cytotoxin-associated gene A (*cagA*) into the junctions where cells of the stomach lining meet. This toxin (known as CagA) alters the structure of stomach cells and allows the bacteria to attach to them more easily. Long-term exposure to the toxin causes chronic inflammation. However, not all strains of *H. pylori* carry the *cagA* gene; those that do are classified as *cagA*-positive.

Epidemiologic evidence suggests that infection with *cagA*-positive strains is especially associated with an increased risk of noncardia gastric cancer and with reduced risks of gastric cardia cancer and esophageal adenocarcinoma. For example, a meta-analysis of 16 case–control studies conducted around the world showed that individuals infected with *cagA*-positive *H. pylori* had twice the risk of noncardia gastric cancer than individuals infected with *cagA*-negative *H. pylori*. Conversely, a case–control study conducted in Sweden found that people infected with *cagA*-positive *H. pylori* had a statistically significantly reduced risk of esophageal adenocarcinoma. Similarly, another case–control study conducted in the United States found that infection with *cagA*-positive *H. pylori* was associated with a reduced risk of esophageal adenocarcinoma and gastric cardia cancer combined, but that infection with *cagA*-negative strains was not associated with risk.

Research has suggested a potential mechanism by which CagA could contribute to gastric carcinogenesis. In three studies, infection with CagA-positive *H. pylori* was associated with inactivation of tumor suppressor proteins, including p53.

What Is Gastric Mucosa-Associated Lymphoid Tissue (MALT) Lymphoma, and What Is the Evidence That It Can Be Caused by H. pylori *Infection?*

Gastric MALT lymphoma is a rare type of non-Hodgkin lymphoma that is characterized by the slow multiplication of B lymphocytes, a type of immune cell, in the stomach lining. This cancer represents approximately 12 percent of the extranodal (outside of lymph nodes) non-Hodgkin lymphoma that occurs among men and approximately 18 percent of extranodal non-Hodgkin lymphoma among women. During the period 1999–2003, the annual incidence of gastric MALT lymphoma in the United States was about one case for every 100,000 persons in the population.

Normally, the lining of the stomach lacks lymphoid (immune system) tissue, but development of this tissue is often stimulated in response to colonization of the lining by *H. pylori*. Only in rare cases does this tissue give rise to MALT lymphoma. However, nearly all patients with gastric MALT lymphoma show signs of *H. pylori* infection, and the risk of developing this tumor is more than six times higher in infected people than in uninfected people.

Is H. pylori *Infection Associated with Any Other Cancer?*

Whether *H. pylori* infection is associated with risk of other cancers remains unclear. Some studies have found a possible association between *H. pylori* infection and pancreatic cancer, but the evidence is conflicting. Studies investigating the possibility that *H. pylori* as a risk factor for colorectal adenocarcinoma and lung cancer have found no evidence that it is associated with the risk of either type of cancer.

Can Treatment to Eradicate H. pylori *Infection Reduce Gastric Cancer Rates?*

Long-term follow-up of data from a randomized clinical trial carried out in Shandong, China—an area where rates of gastric cancer are very high—found that short-term treatment with antibiotics to eradicate *H. pylori* reduced the incidence of gastric cancer. During a nearly 15-year period after treatment, gastric cancer incidence was reduced by almost 40 percent. When the results of this trial were pooled with those of several smaller trials examining the effects on gastric cancer incidence of antimicrobial treatment to eradicate *H. pylori*, a similar reduction was seen.

Who Should Seek Diagnosis and Treatment of an H. pylori *Infection?*

According to the CDC, people who have active gastric or duodenal ulcers or a documented history of ulcers should be tested for *H. pylori*, and, if they are infected, should be treated. Testing for and treating *H. pylori* infection is also recommended after resection of early gastric cancer and for low-grade gastric MALT lymphoma. However, most experts agree that the available evidence does not support widespread testing for and eradication of *H. pylori* infection.

Chapter 7

Hormonal Therapies and Cancer Risk

Chapter Contents

Section 7.1

Oral Contraceptives and Cancer Risk

This section includes text excerpted from "Oral Contraceptives and Cancer Risk," National Cancer Institute (NCI), February 22, 2018.

What Are Oral Contraceptives?

Oral contraceptives (birth control pills) are hormone-containing medications that are taken by mouth to prevent pregnancy. They prevent pregnancy by inhibiting ovulation and also by preventing sperm from penetrating through the cervix.

By far the most commonly prescribed type of oral contraceptive in the United States contains synthetic versions of the natural female hormones estrogen and progesterone. This type of birth control pill is often called a combined oral contraceptive. Another type of oral contraceptive, sometimes called the mini pill, contains only progestin, which is a man-made version of progesterone.

What Is Known about the Relationship between Oral Contraceptive Use and Cancer?

Nearly all the research on the link between oral contraceptives and cancer risk comes from observational studies, both large prospective cohort studies and population-based case–control studies. Data from observational studies cannot definitively establish that an exposure—in this case, oral contraceptives—causes (or prevents) cancer. That is because women who take oral contraceptives may differ from those who don't take them in ways other than their oral contraceptive use, and it is possible that these other differences—rather than oral contraceptive use—are what explains their different cancer risk.

Overall, however, these studies have provided consistent evidence that the risks of breast and cervical cancers are increased in women who use oral contraceptives, whereas the risks of endometrial, ovarian, and colorectal cancers are reduced.

- **Breast cancer:** An analysis of data from more than 150,000 women who participated in 54 epidemiologic studies showed that, overall, women who had ever used oral contraceptives had a slight (7%) increase in the relative risk of breast cancer compared with women who had never used oral contraceptives. Women who were currently using oral contraceptives had a 24 percent increase in risk that did not increase with the duration of use. Risk declined after use of oral contraceptives stopped, and no risk increase was evident by 10 years after use had stopped.

An analysis of data from the Nurses' Health Study (NHS), which has been following more than 116,000 female nurses who were 24–43 years old when they enrolled in the study in 1989, also found that participants who used oral contraceptives had a slight increase in breast cancer risk. However, nearly all of the increased risk was seen among women who took a specific type of oral contraceptive, a "triphasic" pill, in which the dose of hormones is changed in three stages over the course of a woman's monthly cycle. An elevated risk associated with specific triphasic formulations was also reported in a nested case–control study that used electronic medical records to verify oral contraceptive use.

In 2017, a large prospective Danish study reported breast cancer risks associated with more recent formulations of oral contraceptives. Overall, women who were using or had recently stopped using oral combined hormone contraceptives had a modest (about 20%) increase in the relative risk of breast cancer compared with women who had never used oral contraceptives. The risk increase varied from 0–60 percent, depending on the specific type of oral combined hormone contraceptive. The risk of breast cancer also increased the longer oral contraceptives were used.

- **Cervical cancer:** Women who have used oral contraceptives for 5 or more years have a higher risk of cervical cancer than women who have never used oral contraceptives. The longer a woman uses oral contraceptives, the greater the increase in her risk of cervical cancer. One study found a 10 percent increased risk for less than 5 years of use, a 60 percent increased risk with 5–9 years of use, and a doubling of the risk with 10 or more years of use. However, the risk of cervical cancer has been found to decline over time after women stop using oral contraceptives.
- **Endometrial cancer:** Women who have ever used oral contraceptives have a lower risk of endometrial cancer than women who have never used oral contraceptives. Risk is reduced by at least 30 percent, with a greater risk reduction the longer oral

contraceptives were used. The protective effect persists for many years after a woman stops using oral contraceptives. An analysis of women participating in the prospective National Institutes of Health (NIH)-American Association of Retired Persons (AARP) Diet and Health Study found that the risk reduction was especially pronounced in those long-time users of oral contraceptives who were smokers, obese, or exercised rarely.

- **Ovarian cancer:** Women who have ever used oral contraceptives have a 30–50 percent lower risk of ovarian cancer than women who have never used oral contraceptives. This protection has been found to increase with the length of time oral contraceptives are used and to continue for up to 30 years after a woman stops using oral contraceptives. A reduction in ovarian cancer risk with use of oral contraceptives is also seen among women who carry a harmful mutation in the *BRCA1* or *BRCA2* gene.
- **Colorectal cancer:** Oral contraceptive use is associated with 15–20 percent lower risks of colorectal cancer.

How Could Oral Contraceptives Influence Cancer Risk?

Naturally occurring estrogen and progesterone stimulate the development and growth of some cancers (e.g., cancers that express receptors for these hormones, such as breast cancer). Because birth control pills contain synthetic versions of these female hormones, they could potentially also increase cancer risk.

In addition, oral contraceptives might increase the risk of cervical cancer by changing the susceptibility of cervical cells to persistent infection with high-risk HPV types (the cause of virtually all cervical cancers).

Researchers have proposed multiple ways that oral contraceptives may lower the risks of some cancers, including:

- suppressing endometrial cell proliferation (endometrial cancer)
- reducing the number of ovulations a woman experiences in her lifetime, thereby reducing exposure to naturally occurring female hormones (ovarian cancer)
- lowering the levels of bile acids in the blood for women taking oral conjugated estrogens (colorectal cancer)

Section 7.2

Menopausal Hormone Replacement Therapy and Cancer

This section includes text excerpted from "Menopausal Hormone Therapy and Cancer," National Cancer Institute (NCI), December 5, 2011. Reviewed March 2018.

What Is Menopausal Hormone Therapy?

Menopausal hormone therapy (MHT) is a treatment that doctors may recommend to relieve common symptoms of menopause and to address long-term biological changes, such as bone loss, that result from declining levels of the natural hormones estrogen and progesterone in a woman's body during and after the completion of menopause.

MHT usually involves treatment with estrogen alone, estrogen plus progesterone, or estrogen plus progestin, which is a synthetic hormone with effects similar to those of progesterone. Women who have had a hysterectomy are generally prescribed estrogen alone. Women who have not had this surgery are prescribed estrogen plus progestin, because estrogen alone is associated with an increased risk of endometrial cancer, whereas research has suggested that estrogen plus progestin may not be.

How Do the Hormones Used in MHT Differ from the Hormones Produced by a Woman's Body?

The hormones used in MHT come from a variety of plants and animals, or they can be made in a laboratory. The chemical structure of these hormones is similar, although usually not identical, to those of hormones produced by women's bodies.

The U.S. Food and Drug Administration (FDA) has approved many hormone products for use in MHT. FDA-approved products have undergone extensive testing and are produced under standardized conditions to ensure that every dose—whether in a pill, a skin patch, or a cream—contains the proper amount of the appropriate hormones. These FDA-approved products are available only with a doctor's prescription.

Non FDA-approved hormone products, sometimes referred to as "bio-identical hormones," are widely promoted and sold without a prescription on the Internet. Claims that these products are "safer" or more "natural" than FDA-approved hormonal products are not supported by credible scientific evidence.

Where Does Evidence about Risks and Benefits of MHT Come From?

The most comprehensive evidence about risks and benefits of MHT comes from two randomized clinical trials that were sponsored by the National Institutes of Health (NIH) as part of the Women's Health Initiative (WHI):

- The **WHI Estrogen-plus-Progestin study,** in which women with a uterus were randomly assigned to receive either a hormone medication containing both estrogen and progestin (Prempro™) or a placebo.
- The **WHI Estrogen-alone study**, in which women without a uterus were randomly assigned to receive either a hormone medication containing estrogen alone (Premarin™) or a placebo.

More than 27,000 healthy women who were 50–79 years of age at the time of enrollment took part in the two trials. Although both trials were stopped early (in 2002 and 2004, respectively) when it was determined that both types of therapy were associated with specific health risks, longer-term follow-up of the participants continues to provide new information about the health effects of MHT.

What Are the Benefits of Menopausal Hormone Therapy?

Research from the WHI Estrogen-plus-Progestin study has shown that women taking combined hormone therapy had the following benefits:

- One-third fewer hip and vertebral fractures than women taking the placebo. In absolute terms, this meant 10 fractures per 10,000 women per year who took hormone therapy compared with 15 fractures per 10,000 women per year who took the placebo.

- One-third lower risk of colorectal cancer than women taking the placebo. In absolute terms, this meant 10 cases of colorectal cancer per 10,000 women per year who took hormone therapy compared with 16 cases of colorectal cancer per 10,000 women per year who took the placebo.

However, a follow-up study found that neither benefit persisted after the study participants stopped taking combined hormone therapy medication.

Women taking estrogen alone experienced the following benefits:

- One-third lower risk for hip and vertebral fractures than women taking the placebo. In absolute terms, this meant 11 hip and 11 vertebral fractures per 10,000 women per year who took estrogen compared with 17 hip and 17 vertebral fractures per 10,000 women per year who took the placebo.
- A 23 percent reduced risk of breast cancer than women taking the placebo. In absolute terms, this meant 26 cases of invasive breast cancer per 10,000 women per year who took estrogen compared with 33 cases of invasive breast cancer per 10,000 women per year who took the placebo.

After 10.7 years of follow-up, however, the risk of hip fractures was slightly higher in the estrogen-alone group, but the risk of breast cancer remained lower than that among women who took the placebo.

What Are the Health Risks of MHT?

Before the WHI studies began, it was known that MHT with estrogen alone increased the risk of endometrial cancer in women with an intact uterus. It was for this reason that, in the WHI trials, women randomly assigned to receive hormone therapy took estrogen plus progestin if they had a uterus and estrogen alone if they didn't have one.

Research from the WHI studies has shown that MHT is associated with the following harms:

- **Urinary incontinence.** Use of estrogen plus progestin increased the risk of urinary incontinence.
- **Dementia.** Use of estrogen plus progestin doubled the risk of developing dementia among postmenopausal women age 65 and older.

- **Stroke, blood clots, and heart attack.** Women who took either combined hormone therapy or estrogen alone had an increased risk of stroke, blood clots, and heart attack. Fin both groups, however, this risk returned to normal levels after they stopped taking the medication.
- **Breast cancer.** Women who took estrogen plus progestin were more likely to be diagnosed with breast cancer. The breast cancers in these women were larger and more likely to have spread to the lymph nodes by the time they were diagnosed. The number of breast cancers in this group of women increased with the length of time that they took the hormones and decreased after they stopped taking the hormones.

These studies also showed that both combination and estrogen-alone hormone use made mammography less effective for the early detection of breast cancer. Women taking hormones had more repeat mammograms to check on abnormalities found in a screening mammogram and more breast biopsies to determine whether abnormalities detected in mammograms were cancer.

The rate of death from breast cancer among those taking estrogen plus progestin was 2.6 per 10,000 women per year, compared with 1.3 per 10,000 women per year among those taking the placebo. The rate of death from any cause after a diagnosis of breast cancer was 5.3 per 10,000 women per year among women taking combined hormone therapy, compared with 3.4 per 10,000 women per year among those taking the placebo.

- **Lung cancer.** Women who took combined hormone therapy had the same risk of lung cancer as women who took the placebo. However, among those who were diagnosed with lung cancer, women who took estrogen plus progestin were more likely to die of the disease than those who took the placebo.

  There were no differences in the number of cases or the number of deaths from lung cancer among women who took estrogen alone compared with those among women who took the placebo.
- **Colorectal cancer.** In the initial study report, women taking combined hormone therapy had a lower risk of colorectal cancer than women who took the placebo. However, the colorectal tumors that arose in the combined hormone therapy group were more advanced at detection than those in the placebo group. There was no difference in either the risk of colorectal cancer or

the stage of disease at diagnosis between women who took estrogen alone and those who took the placebo.

However, a subsequent analysis of the WHI trials found no strong evidence that either estrogen alone or estrogen plus progestin had any effect on the risk of colorectal cancer, tumor stage at diagnosis, or death from colorectal cancer.

Does Hysterectomy Affect the Cancer Risks Associated with MHT?

Women who had a hysterectomy and who are prescribed MHT generally take estrogen alone. In 2004, when the WHI Estrogen-Alone Study was stopped early, women taking estrogen alone had a 23 percent reduced risk of breast cancer compared with those who took the placebo. An analysis conducted after study participants had been followed for an average of 10.7 years found that women who had taken estrogen alone still had a lower risk of breast cancer than women who had taken the placebo.

Do the Cancer Risks from MHT Change Over Time?

Women who have had a hysterectomy and who use estrogen-alone MHT have a reduced risk of breast cancer that continues for at least 5 years after they stop taking MHT. Women who take combined hormone therapy have an increased risk of breast cancer that continues after they stop taking the medication. In the WHI study, where women took the combined hormone therapy for an average of 5.6 years, this increased risk persisted after an average follow-up period of 11 years. Breast cancers diagnosed in this group of women were larger and more likely to have spread to the lymph nodes (a sign of more advanced disease). Studies have documented a decline in breast cancer diagnoses in the United States after the sharp reduction in the use of MHT that followed publication of the initial results of the Estrogen-plus-Progestin Study in July 2002. Additional factors, such as a reduction in the use of mammography, may also have contributed to this decline.

Is It Safe for Women Who Have Had a Cancer Diagnosis to Take MHT?

One of the roles of naturally occurring estrogen is to promote the normal growth of cells in the breast and uterus. For this reason, it is generally believed that MHT may promote further tumor growth in women who have already been diagnosed with breast cancer. However, studies of hormone use to treat menopausal symptoms in breast cancer survivors have produced conflicting results, with some showing an increased risk of breast cancer recurrence and others showing no increased risk of recurrence.

What Should Women Do If They Have Symptoms of Menopause but Are Concerned about Taking MHT?

Although MHT provides short-term benefits, such as relief from hot flashes and vaginal dryness, several health concerns are associated with its use. Women should discuss whether to take MHT and what alternatives may be appropriate for them with their healthcare provider. The FDA currently advises women to use MHT for the shortest time and at the lowest dose possible to control menopausal symptoms.

Are There Alternatives for Women Who Choose Not to Take Menopausal Hormone Therapy?

Women who are concerned about the health effects that occur naturally with the decline in hormone production that occurs during menopause can make changes in their lifestyle and diet to reduce certain risks. For example, eating foods that are rich in calcium and vitamin D or taking dietary supplements containing these nutrients may help to prevent osteoporosis. FDA-approved drugs such as alendronate (Fosamax®), raloxifene (Evista®), and risedronate (Actonel®) have been shown in randomized trials to prevent bone loss.

Medications approved by the FDA for treating depression and seizures may help to relieve menopausal symptoms such as hot flashes. Those that have been shown in randomized clinical trials to be effective in treating hot flashes include the following:

- Venlafaxine (Effexor®)
- Desvenlafaxine (Pristiq®)
- Paroxetine (Paxil®)
- Fluoxetine (Prozac®)
- Citalopram (Celexa®)
- Gabapentin (Neurontin®)
- Pregabalin (Lyrica®)

Some women seek relief from the symptoms of menopause with over-the-counter complementary and alternative therapies. Some of these remedies contain estrogen-like compounds derived from sources such as soy products, whole-grain cereals, oilseeds (primarily flaxseed), legumes, or the plant black cohosh. To date, however, randomized clinical trials have not shown that any of these remedies is superior to a placebo in relieving hot flashes. Trials of other herbal remedies, such as evening primrose oil, ginseng, and wild yam, have also not shown that they effectively reduce menopausal symptoms.

Section 7.3

Diethylstilbestrol (DES) and Cancer Risk

This section includes text excerpted from documents published by two public domain sources: Text under the headings marked 1 are excerpted from "Diethylstilbestrol (DES) and Cancer," National Cancer Institute (NCI), October 5, 2011. Reviewed March 2018; Text under the heading marked 2 is excerpted from "Women Exposed to DES in the Womb Face Increased Cancer Risk," National Institutes of Health (NIH), October 5, 2011. Reviewed March 2018.

What Is Diethylstilbestrol (DES)?[1]

Diethylstilbestrol (DES) is a synthetic form of the female hormone estrogen. It was prescribed to pregnant women between 1940–1971 to prevent miscarriage, premature labor, and related complications of pregnancy. The use of DES declined after studies in the 1950s showed that it was not effective in preventing these problems.

Women Exposed to DES in the Womb Face Increased Cancer Risk[2]

National Institutes of Health (NIH) study followed daughters of women given diethylstilbestrol during pregnancy and found increased fertility problems and cancer risks.

A large study of the daughters of women who had been given DES, the first synthetic form of estrogen, during pregnancy has found that exposure to the drug while in the womb (in utero) is associated with many reproductive problems and an increased risk of certain cancers and precancerous conditions. The results of this analysis, conducted by researchers at the National Cancer Institute (NCI), part of the National Institutes of Health, and collaborators across the country, were published October 6, 2011, in the *New England Journal of Medicine*.

Beginning in 1940, diethylstilbestrol, known as DES, was used clinically to prevent certain complications of pregnancy. In the 1950s, clinical studies showed DES was ineffective for this purpose. In the late 1960s, an unusual occurrence of a rare cancer of the vagina among young women, called clear cell adenocarcinoma (CCA), was observed and subsequently linked to their exposure to DES while in the womb.

In 1971, the U.S. Food and Drug Administration (FDA) notified physicians that DES should not be prescribed to pregnant women. However, between 5 million and 10 million pregnant women and babies had been exposed to the drug. It was manufactured under many different product names, and came in various forms, including pills, creams, and vaginal suppositories.

"Our study carefully documents elevated risk for DES-exposed daughters for a host of medical problems—many of them also quite common in the general population," said study author Robert N. Hoover, M.D., director of the Epidemiology and Biostatistics Program in NCI's Division of Cancer Epidemiology and Genetics (DCEG). "Without the sentinel finding of a very rare cancer in young women, and without the sustained follow-up of those who were exposed, we would not know the full extent of harm caused by DES exposure in the womb."

In this study, which included over 6,500 women (4,600 exposed and 1,900 unexposed), the researchers found that the daughters with exposure to DES while in the womb had an increased risk of 12 medical conditions, including a twofold higher risk of infertility and a fivefold increased risk of having a preterm delivery. (See table below for complete list of increased risks.) This study is also the first to estimate the cumulative proportion of all DES-exposed women who developed these conditions because of their exposure. Of all DES-exposed women, 1 in 5 will experience some level of infertility because of their exposure. And of all those exposed women who are successful in having at least one birth, 1 in 3 will have a preterm delivery due to DES.

Although DES-exposed daughters have about 40 times the risk of developing CCA than unexposed women, CCA is still a rare disease, occurring in 1 in 1,000 DES-exposed daughters. While the first women diagnosed with this condition in the late 1960s were adolescents and young adults at the time of their diagnosis, the research now shows that the risk for DES-exposed daughters continues through at least age 40. In addition, these women are more than twice as likely to develop precancerous cells in the cervix or vagina (called cervical intraepithelial neoplasia) and have an 80 percent higher chance of developing breast cancer after age 40. According to the results of this study, by age 55, 1 in 25 DES-exposed daughters will develop abnormal cellular changes in the cervix or vagina, and 1 in 50 will develop breast cancer due to their DES exposure.

This study was the first to assess risk based on the presence of vaginal epithelial changes as a biomarker of timing and dose of DES exposure. Exposed daughters with higher total dose of DES and younger age of the embryo at first exposure had evidence of these changes in the lining of the vagina. Women with these changes were at even greater risk for 9 of the 12 conditions compared to exposed women who did not have the biomarker.

This study did not evaluate sons with DES exposure in the womb, but previous reports have indicated an increased risk for certain

Table 7.1. Risks for DES-Exposed Daughters Compared to Nonexposed

Outcome	Increased Risk
Clear-cell adenocarcinoma	40 times higher
Neonatal death	8 times higher
Preterm delivery	4.7 times higher
Loss of 2nd-trimester pregnancy	3.8 times higher
Ectopic pregnancy	3.7 times higher
Stillbirth	2.4 times higher
Infertility	2.4 times higher
Early menopause	2.4 times higher
Cervical intraepithelial neoplasia	2.3 times higher
Breast cancer	1.8 times higher
First-trimester miscarriage	1.6 times higher
Pre-eclampsia	1.4 times higher

testicular abnormalities, including undescended testicles or the development of cysts in the epididymis, tightly coiled tubes connected to the testicles. As DES-exposed sons grow older, more data will be available to assess their cancer risk. So far, research has shown no decreased fertility for these men, even with testicular abnormalities.

The women in this study were followed as part of the NCI's DES follow-up study, which began in 1992. NCI researchers will continue to study DES-exposed daughters as they move into menopausal years. The cancer risks for exposed daughters, as well as sons, are continually being studied to determine if they differ from an unexposed population. In addition, researchers are studying possible health effects on the grandchildren of mothers who took DES during pregnancy, because some of the genetic changes caused by DES exposure in the womb may be inherited.

The other research centers involved in this work are Boston University Slone Epidemiology Center, Boston; Cedars-Sinai Medical Center DES Project, Los Angeles; University of Chicago Department of Obstetrics and Gynecology; Dartmouth-Hitchcock Medical Center, Lebanon, N.H.; The Mayo Clinic DES Project, Rochester, Minn; The Methodist Hospital-Research Institute Department of Obstetrics and Gynecology, Houston; and Tufts Medical Center, Boston.

What Health Problems Might Women Who Took DES during Pregnancy Have?[1]

Women who used DES may have a slight increase in the risk of developing and dying from breast cancer compared with women who did not use DES. No evidence exists to suggest that women who took DES are at higher risk for any other type of cancer.

What Health Problems Might DES-Exposed Grandchildren Have?[1]

Researchers are also studying possible health effects among women and men who are the children of DES daughters. These groups are called DES granddaughters and DES grandsons, or the third generation. Researchers are studying these groups because studies in animal models suggest that DES may cause deoxyribonucleic acid (DNA) changes (i.e., altered patterns of methylation) in mice exposed to the chemical during early development. These changes can be heritable and have the potential to affect subsequent generations.

A comparison of the results of DES granddaughters' pelvic exams with those of their mothers' first pelvic exams found none of the changes that had been associated with prenatal DES exposure in their mothers. However, another analysis showed that DES granddaughters began their menstrual periods later and were more likely to have menstrual irregularities than other women of the same age. The data also suggested that infertility was greater among DES granddaughters, and that they tended to have fewer live births. However, this association is based on small numbers of events and was not statistically significant. Researchers will continue to follow these women to study the risk of infertility.

Studies have found that DES granddaughters and DES grandsons may have a slightly higher risk of cancer and birth defects, including hypospadias in DES grandsons. However, because each of these associations is based on small numbers of events, researchers will continue to study these groups to clarify the findings.

How Can People Find out If They Took DES during Pregnancy or Were Exposed to DES in Utero?[1]

It is estimated that 5 to 10 million Americans—pregnant women and the children born to them—were exposed to DES between 1940–1971. DES was given widely to pregnant women between 1940–1971 to prevent complications during pregnancy. DES was provided under many different product names and also in various forms, such as pills, creams, and vaginal suppositories. The table below includes examples of products that contained DES.

Table 7.2. DES Product Names

Nonsteroidal Estrogens		
Benzestrol	Gynben	Stil-Rol
Chlorotrianisene	Gyneben	Stilbal
Comestrol	Hexestrol	Stilbestrol
Cyren A.	Hexoestrol	Stilbestronate
Cyren B.	Hi-Bestrol	Stilbetin
Delvinal	Menocrin	Stilbinol
DES	Meprane	Stilboestroform
Desplex	Mestilbol	Silboestrol
Dibestil	Microest	Stilboestrol DP
Diestryl	Methallenestril	Stilestrate
Dienestrol	Mikarol	Stilpalmitate
Dienoestrol	Mikarol forti	Stilphostrol

Table 7.2. Continued

Nonsteroidal Estrogens		
Diethylsteilbestrol dipalmitate Diethylstilbestrol diphosphate Diethylstilbestrol dipropionate Diethylstilbenediol Digestil Dienestrol Domestrol Estilben Estrobene Estrobene DP Estrosyn Fonatol	Milestrol Monomestrol Neo-Oestranol I Neo-Oestranol II Nulabort Oestrogenine Oestromenin Oestromon Orestol Pabestrol D Palestrol Restrol	Stilronate Stilrone Stils Synestrin Synestrol Synthosestrin Tace Vallestril Willestrol

Table 7.3. Nonsteroidal Estrogen-Androgen Combinations

Nonsteroidal Estrogen-Androgen Combinations	
Amperone Di-Erone Estan Metystil	Teserene Tylandril Tylostereone

Table 7.4. Nonsteroidal Estrogen-Progesterone Combinations

Nonsteroidal Estrogen-Progesterone Combinations
Progravidium

Table 7.5. Vaginal Cream Suppositories with Nonsteroidal Estrogens

Vaginal Cream Suppositories with Nonsteroidal Estrogens
AVC Cream with Dienestrol Dienestrol Cream

Women who think they used DES during pregnancy, or people who think that their mother used DES during pregnancy, can try contacting the physician or institution where they received their care to request a review of their medical records. If any pills were taken during pregnancy, obstetrical records could be checked to determine the name of the drug.

However, finding medical records after a long period of time can be difficult. If the doctor has retired or died, another doctor may have taken over the practice as well as the records. The county medical society or health department may know where the records have been stored. Some pharmacies keep records for a long time and can be contacted regarding prescription dispensing information. Military medical records are kept for 25 years. In most cases, however, it may be impossible to determine whether DES was used.

What Should DES-Exposed Daughters Do?[1]

Women who know or believe they were exposed to DES before birth should be aware of the health effects of DES and inform their doctor about their possible exposure. It has been recommended that exposed women have an annual medical examination to check for the adverse health effects of DES. A thorough examination may include the following:

- Pelvic examination
- **Pap test and colposcopy**—A routine cervical Pap test is not adequate for DES daughters. The Pap test must gather cells from the cervix and the vagina. It is also good for a clinician to see the cervix and vaginal walls. They may use a colposcope to follow up if there are any abnormal findings.
- Biopsy
- **Breast examinations**—It is recommended that DES daughters continue to rigorously follow the routine breast cancer screening recommendations for their age group.

What Should DES-Exposed Mothers Do?[1]

A woman who took DES while pregnant or who suspects she may have taken it should inform her doctor. She should try to learn the dosage, when the medication was started, and how it was used. She also should inform her children who were exposed before birth so that this information can be included in their medical records.

It is recommended that DES-exposed mothers have regular breast cancer screenings and yearly medical checkups that include a pelvic examination and a Pap test.

What Should DES-Exposed Sons Do?[1]

Men whose mothers took DES while pregnant should inform their physician of their exposure and be examined periodically. Although the risk of developing testicular cancer among DES-exposed sons is unclear, males with undescended or unusually small testicles have an increased risk of testicular cancer whether or not they were exposed to DES.

Chapter 8

Radiation and Cancer Risk

Chapter Contents

Section 8.1

How Radiation Affects Cancer Risk

This section includes text excerpted from "Radiation Protection—Radiation Health Effects," U.S. Environmental Protection Agency (EPA), February 1, 2018.

Ionizing radiation has sufficient energy to cause chemical changes in cells and damage them. Some cells may die or become abnormal, either temporarily or permanently. By damaging the genetic material deoxyribonucleic acid (DNA) contained in the body's cells, radiation can cause cancer. Fortunately, our bodies are extremely efficient at repairing cell damage. The extent of the damage to the cells depends upon the amount and duration of the exposure, as well as the organs exposed. A very large amount of radiation exposure (acute exposure), can cause sickness or even death within hours or days. Such acute exposures are extremely rare.

Chronic Exposure

In general, the amount and duration of radiation exposure affects the severity or type of health effect. There are two broad categories of health effects: chronic (long term) and acute (short term). Chronic exposure is continuous or intermittent exposure to radiation over a long period of time. With chronic exposure, there is a delay between the exposure and the observed health effect. These effects can include cancer and other health outcomes such as benign tumors, cataracts, and potentially harmful genetic changes.

Low Levels of Radiation Exposure

Science suggests there is some cancer risk from any exposure to radiation. However, it is very hard to tell whether a particular cancer was caused by very low doses of radiation or by something else. While experts disagree over the exact definition and effects of "low dose," U.S. radiation protection standards are based on the premise that any radiation dose carries some risk, and that risk increases directly with dose. This method of estimating risk is called the "linear no-threshold model (LNT)." The risk of cancer from radiation also depends on age, sex, and factors such as tobacco use.

Acute Effects

Acute health effects occur when large parts of the body are exposed to a large amount of radiation. The large exposure can occur all at once or from multiple exposures in a short period of time. Instances of acute effects from environmental sources are very rare. Examples include accidentally handling a strong industrial radiation source or extreme events like nuclear explosions.

It takes a large radiation exposure—more than 75 rad—in a short amount of time to cause acute health effects like radiation sickness. This level of radiation would be equivalent to an X-ray dose of 75,000 millirem. For comparison, the average dose from an adult chest X-ray is about 4 millirem. Exposures between 5–10 rad usually result in no acute health effects. However, exposures in this range slightly increase the risk of getting cancer in the future.

Exposure Pathways

Understanding the type of radiation received (alpha, beta, gamma, X-ray), the way a person is exposed (external versus internal), and for how long a person is exposed are all important in estimating health effects.

The risk from exposure to a particular radioactive element depends on:

- The energy of the radiation it emits.
- Its activity (how often it emits radiation).
- The rate at which the body metabolizes and eliminates the radionuclide following ingestion or inhalation.
- Where the radionuclide concentrates in the body and how long it stays there.

The risk that exposure to a radioactive element will cause a particular health effect also depends on whether exposure is internal or external.

- Internal exposure is when radioactive material gets inside the body by eating, drinking, breathing, or injection (from certain medical procedures). Alpha and beta particles pose a serious health threat if significant quantities are inhaled or ingested. Outside the body, alpha particles are too large to pass through the skin or a thin layer of clothes.

- External exposure (also known as direct exposure) is when the radioactive source is outside of your body. X-rays and gamma rays can pass through your body, depositing energy as they go.

Sensitive Populations

Pregnant women and children are especially sensitive to radiation exposure. The cells in children and fetuses divide rapidly, providing more opportunity for radiation to disrupt the process and cause cell damage. U.S. Environmental Protection Agency (EPA) accounts for these differences in sensitivity due to age and sex when revising radiation protection standards.

Section 8.2

Radon and Cancer Risk

This section includes text excerpted from "Radiation and Your Health—Radon in the Home," Centers for Disease Control and Prevention (CDC), December 7, 2015.

What Is Radon?

Radon is a gas that you cannot smell, taste, or see. Radon forms naturally when uranium, thorium, or radium (radioactive metals) breaks down in rocks, soil, and groundwater. People can be exposed to radon primarily from breathing radon in air that comes through cracks and gaps in buildings and homes. Because radon comes naturally from the earth, people are always exposed to it.

- Having your home tested is the only effective way to determine whether you or your family is at risk of high radon exposure.

- For more information on testing your home, check with your state radon office or call the National Radon Hotline at 800-SOS-RADON (800-767-7236).

How Does Radon Enter Your Home?

The U.S. Environmental Protection Agency (EPA) lists the following ways that radon can get into buildings:

- Cracks in solid floors and walls
- Construction joints
- Gaps in suspended floors
- Gaps around service pipes
- Cavities inside walls
- The water supply

Radon and Your Health

When you breathe in radon, radioactive particles from radon gas can get trapped in your lungs. Over time, these radioactive particles increase the risk of lung cancer. It may take years before health problems appear. Radon is the second leading cause of lung cancer after cigarette smoking. EPA and the Surgeon General's office estimate radon is responsible for more than 20,000 lung cancer deaths each year in the United States.

Smoking and Radon

People who smoke and are exposed to radon are at a greater risk of developing lung cancer. EPA recommends taking action to reduce radon in homes that have a radon level at or above 4 picocuries per liter (pCi/L) of air (a "picocurie" is a common unit for measuring the amount of radioactivity). The chances of getting lung cancer are higher if your home has elevated radon levels and you smoke or burn fuels that increase indoor particles.

Your chances of getting lung cancer from radon depend mostly on:

- How much radon is in your home—the location where you spend most of your time (e.g., the main living and sleeping areas).
- The amount of time you spend in your home

- Whether you are a smoker or have ever smoked
- Whether you burn wood, coal, or other substances that add particles to the indoor air

Protect Yourself and Your Family from Radon

Having your home tested is the only effective way to determine whether you and your family are exposed to high levels of radon. The Surgeon General recommends ALL homes be tested for radon gas.

Steps you can take to measure and reduce radon levels include:

- Purchasing a radon test kit
- Testing your home or office
  - Testing is inexpensive and easy—it should only take a few minutes of your time. It requires opening a package and placing a small measuring device in a room and leaving it there for the desired period. Short-term testing can take from a few days to 90 days. Long-term testing takes more than 90 days. The longer the test, the more relevant the results are to your home and lifestyle.
- Sending the kit to appropriate sources to determine radon level
  - Follow the directions on the test kit packaging to find out where to send the device to get the results.
- Fixing your home if radon levels are high

Additional Ways to Take Action

The U.S. Department of Housing and Urban Development (HUD) recommends additional actions you can take to reduce high radon levels in your home and protect yourself from an increased risk of lung cancer.

- **Stop smoking and discourage smoking in your home.**
  - Smoking significantly increases the risk of lung cancer from radon.
- **Increase airflow in your house by opening windows and using fans and vents to circulate air.**
  - Natural ventilation in any type of house is only a temporary strategy to reduce radon.

- **Seal cracks in floors and walls with plaster, caulk, or other materials designed for this purpose.**
    - Contact your state radon office for a list of qualified contractors in your area and for information on how to fix radon problems yourself. Always test again after finishing to make sure you've fixed your radon problem.
- **Ask about radon-resistant construction techniques if you are building a new home.**
    - It is almost always cheaper and easier to build these features into new homes than to add them later.

Section 8.3

Medical X-Rays and Cancer Risk

This section includes text excerpted from "Medical X-Ray Imaging," U.S. Food and Drug Administration (FDA), March 7, 2018.

Medical imaging has led to improvements in the diagnosis and treatment of numerous medical conditions in children and adults.

There are many types—or modalities—of medical imaging procedures, each of which uses different technologies and techniques. Computed tomography (CT), fluoroscopy, and radiography ("conventional X-ray" including mammography) all use ionizing radiation to generate images of the body. Ionizing radiation is a form of radiation that has enough energy to potentially cause damage to deoxyribonucleic acid (DNA) and may elevate a person's lifetime risk of developing cancer.

CT, radiography, and fluoroscopy all work on the same basic principle: an X-ray beam is passed through the body where a portion of the X-rays are either absorbed or scattered by the internal structures, and the remaining X-ray pattern is transmitted to a detector (e.g., film or a computer screen) for recording or further processing by a computer. These exams differ in their purpose:

- **Radiography**—a single image is recorded for later evaluation. Mammography is a special type of radiography to image the internal structures of breasts.
- **Fluoroscopy**—a continuous X-ray image is displayed on a monitor, allowing for real-time monitoring of a procedure or passage of a contrast agent ("dye") through the body. Fluoroscopy can result in relatively high radiation doses, especially for complex interventional procedures (such as placing stents or other devices inside the body) which require fluoroscopy be administered for a long period of time.
- **CT**—many X-ray images are recorded as the detector moves around the patient's body. A computer reconstructs all the individual images into cross-sectional images or "slices" of internal organs and tissues. A CT exam involves a higher radiation dose than conventional radiography because the CT image is reconstructed from many individual X-ray projections.

Benefits and Risks

Benefits

The discovery of X-rays and the invention of CT represented major advances in medicine. X-ray imaging exams are recognized as a valuable medical tool for a wide variety of examinations and procedures. They are used to:

- noninvasively and painlessly help to diagnose disease and monitor therapy;
- support medical and surgical treatment planning; and
- guide medical personnel as they insert catheters, stents, or other devices inside the body, treat tumors, or remove blood clots or other blockages.

Risks

As in many aspects of medicine, there are risks associated with the use of X-ray imaging, which uses ionizing radiation to generate images of the body. Ionizing radiation is a form of radiation that has enough energy to potentially cause damage to DNA. Risks from exposure to ionizing radiation include:

- A small increase in the possibility that a person exposed to X-rays will develop cancer later in life.
- Tissue effects such as cataracts, skin reddening, and hair loss, which occur at relatively high levels of radiation exposure and are rare for many types of imaging exams. For example, the typical use of a CT scanner or conventional radiography equipment should not result in tissue effects, but the dose to the skin from some long, complex interventional fluoroscopy procedures might, in some circumstances, be high enough to result in such effects.

Another risk of X-ray imaging is possible reactions associated with an intravenously injected contrast agent, or "dye," that is sometimes used to improve visualization.

The risk of developing cancer from medical imaging radiation exposure is generally very small, and it depends on:

- **Radiation dose**—The lifetime risk of cancer increases the larger the dose and the more X-ray exams a patient undergoes.
- **Patient's age**—The lifetime risk of cancer is larger for a patient who receives X-rays at a younger age than for one who receives them at an older age.
- **Patient's sex**—Women are at a somewhat higher lifetime risk than men for developing radiation-associated cancer after receiving the same exposures at the same ages.
- **Body region**—Some organs are more radiosensitive than others.

The above statements are generalizations based on scientific analyses of large population data sets, such as survivors exposed to radiation from the atomic bomb. One of the reports of such analyses is Health Risks from Exposure to Low Levels of Ionizing Radiation: BEIR VII Phase 2 (Committee to Assess Health Risks from Exposure to Low Levels of Ionizing Radiation, National Research Council). While specific individuals or cases may not fit into such generalizations, they are still useful in developing an overall approach to medical imaging radiation safety by identifying at-risk populations or higher-risk procedures.

Because radiation risks are dependent on exposure to radiation, an awareness of the typical radiation exposures involved in different imaging exams is useful for communication between the physician and patient.

The medical community has emphasized radiation dose reduction in CT because of the relatively high radiation dose for CT exams (as compared to radiography) and their increased use, as reported in the National Council on Radiation Protection and Measurements (NCRP) Report No. 160. Because tissue effects are extremely rare for typical use of many X-ray imaging devices (including CT), the primary radiation risk concern for most imaging studies is cancer; however, the long exposure times needed for complex interventional fluoroscopy exams and resulting high skin doses may result in tissue effects, even when the equipment is used appropriately.

Balancing Benefits and Risks

While the benefit of a clinically appropriate X-ray imaging exam generally far outweighs the risk, efforts should be made to minimize this risk by reducing unnecessary exposure to ionizing radiation. To help reduce risk to the patient, all exams using ionizing radiation should be performed only when necessary to answer a medical question, treat a disease, or guide a procedure. If there is a medical need for a particular imaging procedure and other exams using no or less radiation are less appropriate, then the benefits exceed the risks, and radiation risk considerations should not influence the physician's decision to perform the study or the patient's decision to have the procedure. However, the "As Low as Reasonably Achievable" (ALARA) principle should always be followed when choosing equipment settings to minimize radiation exposure to the patient.

Patient factors are important to consider in this balance of benefits and risks. For example:

- Because younger patients are more sensitive to radiation, special care should be taken in reducing radiation exposure to pediatric patients for all types of X-ray imaging exams.
- Special care should also be taken in imaging pregnant patients due to possible effects of radiation exposure to the developing fetus.
- The benefit of possible disease detection should be carefully balanced against the risks of an imaging screening study on healthy, asymptomatic patients.

Section 8.4

Iodine-131 and Cancer Risk

This section includes text excerpted from "Get the Facts about Exposure to I-131 Radiation," National Cancer Institute (NCI), August 3, 2015.

During the Cold War in the mid-1940s through early 1960s, the U.S. government conducted about 100 nuclear weapons (atomic bomb) tests in the atmosphere at a test site in Nevada, more than 100 in the Pacific, and one—the first ever—in New Mexico. The radioactive substances released by these tests are known as "fallout." They were carried thousands of miles away from the test site by winds. As a result, people living in the United States at the time of the testing were exposed to varying levels of radiation.

Among the numerous radioactive substances released in fallout, there has been a great deal of concern about and study of one radioactive form of iodine—called iodine-131, or I-131. I-131 collects in the thyroid gland. People exposed to I-131, especially during childhood, may have an increased risk of thyroid disease, including thyroid cancer. Thyroid cancer is uncommon and is usually curable. Typically, it is a slow-growing cancer that is highly treatable. About 98 out of 100 people who are diagnosed with thyroid cancer survive the disease for at least five years after diagnosis.

The thyroid controls many body processes, including heart rate, blood pressure, and body temperature, as well as childhood growth and development. It is located in the front of the neck, just above the top of the breastbone and overlying the windpipe. Although the potential of developing thyroid cancer from exposure to I-131 from nuclear weapons testing is small, it is important for Americans who grew up during the atomic bomb testing between 1945–1963 to be aware of risks.

How Americans Were Exposed to I-131

Because of wind and rainfall patterns, the distribution of I-131 fallout varied widely after each test. Therefore, although all areas of the United States received fallout from at least one nuclear weapons test, certain areas of North America received more fallout than others.

Scientists estimate that the larger amounts of I-131 from the Nevada test site fell over some parts of Utah, Colorado, Idaho, Nevada, and Montana. But I-131 traveled to all states, particularly those in the Midwestern, Eastern, and Northeastern United States. Some of the I-131 collected on pastures and on grasses. Depending on the location, grazing cows and goats sometimes consumed contaminated grasses resulting in I-131 collecting in the animals' milk. Much of the health risk associated with I-131 occurred among milk-drinkers—usually children. From what is known about thyroid cancer and radiation, scientists think that people who were children during the period of atomic bomb testing are at higher risk for developing thyroid cancer. In addition to nuclear testing in Nevada, the Pacific, and New Mexico, Americans were potentially exposed to I-131 from a number of events, including:

- Nuclear testing by other nations elsewhere in the world (mainly in the 1950s and 1960s)
- Nuclear power plant accidents (such as the Chernobyl accident in 1986 and the Fukushima accident in 2011 (primarily Americans in Japan)
- Releases from atomic weapons production plants (such as the Hanford facility in Washington state from 1944–1957)

Scientists are working to find out more about ways to measure and address potential I-131 exposure. They are also working to find out more about other radioactive substances released by fallout and their possible effects on human health.

The Search for Answers

Congress directed government health agencies to investigate the I-131 problem many years ago, and to make recommendations to Americans who might have related health risks. Gathering information turned out to be very complicated. Record-keeping was incomplete at the time of the bomb testing. Much of the information needed to calculate an individual's dose of I-131 and associated risk is either unreliable or unavailable. Despite such challenges, government agencies organized expert scientific teams that have devoted many years to learning more about I-131. A number of reports have been published documenting what they have learned. This information was put together to educate the American people about the potential health risks from exposure to I-131 from nuclear weapons testing.

I-131's Rapid Breakdown

The "active" in "radioactive" means that unstable substances produced in nuclear reactions break down and change, so that they eventually become stable and no longer release radiation. The rate of breakdown can occur quickly in some radioactive substances, often within a few days. Half of the I-131 released during each atomic bomb test was gone in about 8 days. Almost all of it was gone (less than 1 percent remained) 80 days after the test.

Like all radioactive substances, I-131 releases radiation as it breaks down. It is this radiation that can injure human tissues. But I-131's steady breakdown means that the amount of I-131 present in the environment after a bomb test steadily decreased. Therefore, farm animals that grazed in fields within a few days after a test would have consumed higher levels of I-131 than animals grazing later.

The Milk Connection

People younger than 15 at the time of above-ground testing (between 1945–1963) who drank milk, and who lived in the Mountain West, Midwestern, Eastern, and Northeastern United States, probably have a higher thyroid cancer risk from exposure to I-131 in fallout than people who lived in other parts of the United States, who were over the age of 15 in the 1940s, or who did not drink milk. Their thyroid glands were still developing during the testing period. And they were more likely to have consumed milk contaminated with I-131. The amount of I-131 people absorbed depends on:

- Their age during the testing period (between 1945–1963)
- The amount and source of milk they drank in those years
- Where they lived during the testing period

Age and residence during those years are usually known. But few people can recall the exact amounts or sources of the milk they drank as children. While the amount of milk consumed is important in determining exposure to I-131, it is also important to know the source of the milk. Fresh milk from backyard or farm cows and goats usually contained more I-131 than store-bought milk. This is because processing and shipping milk allowed more time for the I-131 to break down.

About Thyroid Disease

There are two main types of thyroid diseases:

Noncancerous Thyroid Disease

Some thyroid diseases are caused by changes in the amount of thyroid hormones that enter the body from the thyroid gland. Doctors can screen for these with a simple blood test. Noncancerous thyroid disease also includes lumps, or nodules, in the thyroid gland that are benign and not cancerous.

Thyroid Cancer

Thyroid cancer occurs when a lump, or nodule, in the thyroid gland is cancerous.

Thyroid Cancer and I-131

Thyroid cancer accounts for a little less than 4 percent of all cancers diagnosed in the United States. Incidence has been going up in recent years, in part due to increased detection. Researchers suspect that rising rates of obesity are also influencing rates. However, these two factors do not fully explain the increases. Typically, thyroid cancer is slow-growing, highly treatable, and usually curable. About 98 out of 100 people who are diagnosed with thyroid cancer survive the disease for at least five years, and about 92 out of 100 people survive the disease for at least 20 years after diagnosis.

The cause of most cases of thyroid cancer is not known. Exposure to I-131 can increase the risk of thyroid cancer. It is thought that risk is higher for people who have had multiple exposures and for people exposed at a younger age. But even among people who have documented exposures to I-131, few develop this cancer. It is known that children have a higher-than-average risk of developing thyroid cancer many years later if they were exposed to radiation. This knowledge comes from studies of people exposed to X-ray treatments for childhood cancer or noncancerous head and neck conditions, or as a result of direct radiation from the atomic bombings of Hiroshima and Nagasaki. The thyroid gland in adults, however, appears to be more resistant to the effects of radiation. There appears to be little risk of developing thyroid cancer from exposure to I-131 or other radiation sources as an adult.

People at Risk

How can people reach a sound decision about their risk of thyroid cancer? When is it time to visit a doctor?

A "personal risk profile" includes four key points that may influence a person's decision to visit a doctor or other health professional for evaluation:

- **Age**—People who are now 50 years of age or older, particularly those born between 1936 and 1963 and who were children at the time of testing, are at higher risk.
- **Milk drinking**—Childhood milk drinkers, particularly those who drank large quantities of milk or those who drank unprocessed milk from farm or backyard cows and goats, have increased risk.
- **Childhood residence**—The Mountain West, Midwest, East, and Northeast areas of the United States generally were more affected by I-131 fallout from nuclear testing.
- **Medical signs**—A lump or nodule that an individual can see or feel in the area of the thyroid gland requires attention. If you can see or feel a lump or nodule, it is important that you see a doctor.

Key Facts

Scientists know that:

- I-131 breaks down rapidly in the atmosphere and environment
- Exposure was highest in the first few days after each nuclear test explosion
- Most exposure occurred through drinking fresh milk
- People received little exposure from eating fruits and leafy vegetables as compared to drinking fresh milk because although I-131 was deposited on fruits and leafy vegetables, the I-131 in fallout was deposited only on the surface; people generally wash or peel fruits and leafy vegetables
- Thyroid cancer is uncommon, usually curable, and approximately 2–3 times more common in women

Reliable information about I-131's impact on human health has been difficult to collect, but scientists think that:

- Risk for thyroid cancer increases with exposure, but even among people exposed to I-131, few develop this cancer
- People exposed as children have a higher risk than people exposed as adults

Taking Care of Yourself

Key steps to estimating personal risk of thyroid cancer, and taking charge of personal thyroid health include:

- Using the "personal risk profile"
- Using the thyroid dose and risk calculator to estimate radiation dose and risk of developing thyroid cancer from fallout exposure from nuclear tests
- Taking this material to a healthcare professional to discuss dose estimates and steps—if any—required for further evaluation
- Getting more information by calling National Cancer Institute's (NCI) Cancer Information Service at 800-4-CANCER (800-422-6237)

Section 8.5

Electromagnetic Fields and Cancer Risk

This section includes text excerpted from "Electromagnetic Fields and Cancer," National Cancer Institute (NCI), May 27, 2016.

What Are Electric and Magnetic Fields (EMF)?

Electric and magnetic fields are invisible areas of energy (also called radiation) that are produced by electricity, which is the movement of electrons, or current, through a wire. An electric field is produced by voltage, which is the pressure used to push the electrons through the wire, much like water being pushed through a pipe. As the voltage increases, the electric field increases in strength. Electric fields are measured in volts per meter (V/m).

A magnetic field results from the flow of current through wires or electrical devices and increases in strength as the current increases. The strength of a magnetic field decreases rapidly with increasing distance from its source. Magnetic fields are measured in microteslas (μT, or millionths of a tesla).

Electric fields are produced whether or not a device is turned on, whereas magnetic fields are produced only when current is flowing, which usually requires a device to be turned on. Power lines produce magnetic fields continuously because current is always flowing through them. Electric fields are easily shielded or weakened by walls and other objects, whereas magnetic fields can pass through buildings, living things, and most other materials.

Electric and magnetic fields together are referred to as electromagnetic fields, or EMFs. The electric and magnetic forces in EMFs are caused by electromagnetic radiation. There are two main categories of EMFs:

- Higher-frequency EMFs, which include X-rays and gamma rays. These EMFs are in the ionizing radiation part of the electromagnetic spectrum and can damage deoxyribonucleic acid (DNA) or cells directly.
- Low- to mid-frequency EMFs, which include static fields (electric or magnetic fields that do not vary with time), magnetic fields from electric power lines and appliances, radio waves, microwaves, infrared radiation, and visible light. These EMFs are in the nonionizing radiation part of the electromagnetic spectrum and are not known to damage DNA or cells directly. Low- to mid-frequency EMFs include extremely low frequency EMFs (ELF-EMFs) and radiofrequency EMFs. ELF-EMFs have frequencies of up to 300 cycles per second, or hertz (Hz), and radiofrequency EMFs range from 3 kilohertz (3 kHz, or 3,000 Hz) to 300 gigahertz (300 GHz, or 300 billion Hz). Radiofrequency radiation is measured in watts per meter squared (W/m^2).

What Are Common Sources of Nonionizing EMFs?

There are both natural and human-made sources of nonionizing EMFs. The earth's magnetic field, which causes the needle on a compass to point North, is one example of a naturally occurring EMF.

Human-made EMFs fall into both the ELF and radiofrequency categories of nonionizing part of the electromagnetic spectrum. These EMFs can come from a number of sources.

Extremely low frequency EMFs (ELF-EMFs). Sources of ELF-EMFs include power lines, electrical wiring, and electrical appliances such as shavers, hair dryers, and electric blankets.

Radiofrequency radiation. The most common sources of radiofrequency radiation are wireless telecommunication devices and equipment, including cell phones, smart meters, and portable wireless devices, such as tablets and laptop computers. In the United States, cell phones currently operate in a frequency range of about 1.8–2.2 GHz.

Other common sources of radiofrequency radiation include:

- **Radio and television signals.** Amplitude-modulated (AM)/frequency-modulated (FM) radios and older VHF/UHF televisions operate at lower radio frequencies than cell phones. Radio signals are AM or FM. AM radio is used for broadcasting over very long distances, whereas FM radio covers more localized areas. AM signals are transmitted from large arrays of antennas that are placed at high elevation on sites that are off limits to the general public because exposures close to the source can be high. Maintenance workers could receive substantial radiofrequency exposures from AM radio antennas, but the general public would not. FM radio antennas and TV broadcasting antennas, which are much smaller than AM antennas, are generally mounted at the top of high towers. Radiofrequency exposures near the base of these towers are below guideline limits, so exposure of the general population is very low. Sometimes small local radio and TV antennas are mounted on the top of a building; access to the roof of such buildings is usually controlled.
- **Radar, satellite stations, magnetic resonance imaging (MRI) devices, and industrial equipment.** These operate at somewhat higher radiofrequencies than cell phones.
- **Microwave ovens** used in homes, which also operate at somewhat higher radiofrequencies than cell phones. Microwave ovens are manufactured with effective shielding that has reduced the leakage of radiofrequency radiation from these appliances to barely detectable levels.
- **Cordless telephones,** which can operate on analogue or DECT (Digital Enhanced Cordless Telecommunications) technology

and typically emit radiofrequencies similar to those of cell phones. However, because cordless phones have a limited range and require a nearby base, their signal strengths are generally much lower than those of cell phones.

- **Cell phone base stations.** Antenna towers or base stations, including those for mobile phone networks and for broadcasting for radio and for television, emit various types of radiofrequency energy. Because the majority of individuals in the general population are exposed only intermittently to base stations and broadcast antennas, it is difficult to estimate exposures for a population. The strength of these exposures varies based on the population density of the region, the average distance from the source, and the time of day or the day of the week (lower exposures on the weekends or at night). In general, exposures decrease with increasing distance from the source. Exposures among maintenance workers have been found to vary depending on their tasks, the type of antenna, and the location of the worker in relation to the source. Cumulative exposures of such workers are very difficult to estimate.
- **Televisions and computer screens** produce electric and magnetic fields at various frequencies, as well as static electric fields. The liquid crystal displays found in some laptop and desktop computers do not produce substantial electric or magnetic fields. Modern computers have conductive screens that reduce static fields produced by the screen to normal background levels.
- **Wireless local area networks,** commonly known as Wi-Fi. These are specific types of wireless networking systems and an increasingly common source of radiofrequency radiation. Wireless networks use radio waves to connect Wi-Fi–enabled devices to an access point that is connected to the Internet, either physically or through some form of data connection. Most Wi-Fi devices operate at radio frequencies that are broadly similar to cell phones, typically 2.4–2.5 GHz, although in recent years Wi-Fi devices that operate at somewhat higher frequencies (5, 5.3, or 5.8 GHz) have appeared. Radiofrequency radiation exposure from Wi-Fi devices is considerably lower than that from cell phones. Both sources emit levels of radiofrequency radiation that are far below the guideline of 10 W/m^2 as specified by the International Commission on Nonionizing Radiation Protection (ICNIRP).

- **Digital electric and gas meters, also known as "smart meters."** These devices, which operate at about the same radio frequencies as cell phones, transmit information on consumption of electricity or gas to utility companies. Smart meters produce very low-level fields that sometimes cannot be distinguished from the total background radiofrequency radiation levels inside a home.

For household appliances and other devices used in the home that require electricity, magnetic field levels are highest near the source of the field and decrease rapidly the farther away the user is from the source. Magnetic fields drop precipitously at a distance of about 1 foot from most appliances. For computer screens, at a distance of 12–20 inches from the screen that most persons using computers sit, magnetic fields are similarly dramatically lower.

Why Are Nonionizing EMFs Studied in Relation to Cancer?

Power lines and electrical appliances that emit nonionizing EMFs are present everywhere in homes and workplaces. For example, wireless local networks are nearly always "on" and are increasingly commonplace in homes, schools, and many public places.

No mechanism by which ELF-EMFs or radiofrequency radiation could cause cancer has been identified. Unlike high-energy (ionizing) radiation, EMFs in the nonionizing part of the electromagnetic spectrum cannot damage deoxyribonucleic acid (DNA) or cells directly. Some scientists have speculated that ELF-EMFs could cause cancer through other mechanisms, such as by reducing levels of the hormone melatonin. There is some evidence that melatonin may suppress the development of certain tumors.

Studies of animals have not provided any indications that exposure to ELF-EMFs is associated with cancer. The few high-quality studies in animals have provided no evidence that Wi-Fi is harmful to health. The National Institute of Environmental Health Sciences (NIEHS), which is part of the National Institutes of Health (NIH), is carrying out a large-scale study in rodents of exposure to radiofrequency energy (the type used in cell phones). This investigation is being conducted in highly specialized labs that can specify and control sources of radiation and measure their effects. Although there is no known mechanism by which nonionizing EMFs could damage DNA and cause cancer, even a small increase in risk would be of clinical importance given how widespread exposure to these fields is.

What Have Studies Shown about Possible Associations between Nonionizing EMFs and Cancer in Children?

Numerous epidemiologic studies and comprehensive reviews of the scientific literature have evaluated possible associations between exposure to nonionizing EMFs and risk of cancer in children. (Magnetic fields are the component of nonionizing EMFs that are usually studied in relation to their possible health effects.) Most of the research has focused on leukemia and brain tumors, the two most common cancers in children. Studies have examined associations of these cancers with living near power lines, with magnetic fields in the home, and with exposure of parents to high levels of magnetic fields in the workplace. No consistent evidence for an association between any source of nonionizing EMF and cancer has been found.

Exposure from power lines. Although a study in 1979 pointed to a possible association between living near electric power lines and childhood leukemia, more recent studies have had mixed findings. Most of these studies did not find an association or found one only for those children who lived in homes with very high levels of magnetic fields, which are present in few residences.

Several studies have analyzed the combined data from multiple studies of power line exposure and childhood leukemia:

- A pooled analysis of nine studies reported a twofold increase in risk of childhood leukemia among children with exposures of 0.4 μT or higher. Less than 1 percent of the children in the studies experienced this level of exposure.
- A meta-analysis of 15 studies observed a 1.7-fold increase in childhood leukemia among children with exposures of 0.3 μT or higher. A little more than 3 percent of children in the studies experienced this level of exposure.
- More recently, a pooled analysis of seven studies published after 2000 reported a 1.4-fold increase in childhood leukemia among children with exposures of 0.3 μT or higher. However, less than one half of 1 percent of the children in the studies experienced this level of exposure.

For the two pooled studies and the meta-analysis, the number of highly exposed children was too small to provide stable estimates of the dose–response relationship. This means that the findings could be interpreted to reflect linear increases in risk, a threshold effect at 0.3 or 0.4 μT, or no significant increase. The interpretation of the finding of increased childhood leukemia risk among children with the highest exposures (at least 0.3 μT) is unclear.

Exposure from electrical appliances. Another way that children can be exposed to magnetic fields is from household electrical appliances. Although magnetic fields near many electrical appliances are higher than those near power lines, appliances contribute less to a person's total exposure to magnetic fields because most appliances are used for only short periods of time. And moving even a short distance from most electrical appliances reduces exposure dramatically. Again, studies have not found consistent evidence for an association between the use of household electrical appliances and risk of childhood leukemia.

Exposure to Wi-Fi. In view of the widespread use of Wi-Fi in schools, the UK Health Protection Agency (now part of Public Health England) has conducted the largest and most comprehensive measurement studies to assess exposures of children to radiofrequency electromagnetic fields from wireless computer networks. This agency concluded that radiofrequency exposures were well below recommended maximum levels and that there was "no reason why Wi-Fi should not continue to be used in schools and in other places."

A review of the published literature concluded that the few high-quality studies to date provide no evidence of biological effects from Wi-Fi exposures.

Exposure to cell phone base stations. Few studies have examined cancer risk in children living close to cell phone base stations or radio or television transmitters. None of the studies that estimated exposures on an individual level found an increased risk of pediatric tumors.

Parental exposure and risk in offspring. Several studies have examined possible associations between maternal or paternal exposure to high levels of magnetic fields before conception and/or during pregnancy and the risk of cancer in their future children. The results to date have been inconsistent. This question requires further evaluation.

Exposure and cancer survival. A few studies have investigated whether magnetic field exposure is associated with prognosis or survival of children with leukemia. Several small retrospective studies of this question have yielded inconsistent results. An analysis that combined prospective data for more than 3,000 children with acute lymphoid leukemia from eight countries showed that ELF magnetic field exposure was not associated with their survival or risk of relapse.

What Have Studies Shown about Possible Associations between Nonionizing EMFs and Cancer in Adults?

Many studies have examined the association between nonionizing EMF exposure and cancer in adults, of which few studies have reported evidence of increased risk.

Residential exposures. The majority of epidemiologic studies have shown no relationship between breast cancer in women and exposure to extremely low frequency EMFs (ELF-EMFs) in the home, although a few individual studies have suggested an association; only one reported results that were statistically significant.

Workplace exposures to ELF radiation. Several studies conducted in the 1980s and early 1990s reported that people who worked in some electrical occupations that exposed them to ELF radiation (such as power station operators and telephone line workers) had higher-than-expected rates of some types of cancer, particularly leukemia, brain tumors, and male breast cancer. Most of the results were based on participants' job titles and not on actual measurements of their exposures. More recent studies, including some that considered exposure measurements as well as job titles, have generally not shown an increasing risk of leukemia, brain tumors, or female breast cancer with increasing exposure to magnetic fields at work.

Workplace exposures to radiofrequency radiation. A limited number of studies have evaluated risks of cancer in workers exposed to radiofrequency radiation. A large study of U.S. Navy personnel found no excess of brain tumors among those with a high probability of exposure to radar (including electronics technicians, aviation technicians, and fire control technicians); however, nonlymphocytic leukemia, particularly acute myeloid leukemia, was increased in electronics technicians in aviation squadrons, but not in Navy personnel in the other job categories. A case-control study among U.S. Air Force (USAF) personnel found the suggestion of an increased risk of brain cancer among personnel who maintained or repaired radiofrequency or microwave-emitting equipment. A case-control study found the suggestion of an increased risk of death from brain cancer among men occupationally exposed to microwave and/or radiofrequency radiation, with all of the excess risk among workers in electrical and electronics jobs involving design, manufacture, repair, or installation of electrical or electronics equipment. There was no evidence that electrical utility workers who were exposed to pulsed electromagnetic fields produced by power lines were more likely to develop brain tumors or leukemia than the general population. Employees of a large manufacturer of wireless communication products were not more likely to die from brain tumors or cancers of the hematopoietic or lymphatic system than the general population.

What Do Expert Organizations Conclude about the Cancer Risk from EMFs?

In 2002, the International Agency for Research on Cancer (IARC), a component of the World Health Organization (WHO), appointed an expert Working Group to review all available evidence on static and extremely low frequency electric and magnetic fields. The Working Group classified ELF-EMFs as "possibly carcinogenic to humans," based on limited evidence from human studies in relation to childhood leukemia. Static electric and magnetic fields and extremely low frequency electric fields were determined "not classifiable as to their carcinogenicity to humans."

In 2015, the European Commission Scientific Committee on Emerging and Newly Identified Health Risks (SCENIHR) reviewed electromagnetic fields in general, as well as cell phones in particular. It found that, overall, epidemiologic studies of extremely low frequency fields show an increased risk of childhood leukemia with estimated daily average exposures above 0.3–0.4 μT, although no mechanisms have been identified and there is no support from experimental studies that explains these findings. It also found that the epidemiologic studies on radiofrequency exposure do not show an increased risk of brain tumors or other cancers of the head and neck region, although the possibility of an association with acoustic neuroma remains open.

Section 8.6

Cell Phones and Cancer Risk

This section includes text excerpted from "Cell Phones and Cancer Risk," National Cancer Institute (NCI), February 16, 2018.

Why Is There Concern That Cell Phones May Cause Cancer or Other Health Problems?

There are three main reasons why people are concerned that cell phones (also known as "mobile" or "wireless" telephones) might have the potential to cause certain types of cancer or other health problems:

- Cell phones emit radiofrequency energy (radio waves), a form of nonionizing radiation, from their antennas. Tissues nearest to the antenna can absorb this energy.
- The number of cell phone users has increased rapidly. As of December 2014, there were more than 327.5 million cell phone subscribers in the United States, according to the Cellular Telecommunications and Internet Association (CTIA). This is a nearly threefold increase from the 110 million users in 2000. Globally, the number of subscriptions is estimated by the International Telecommunications Union (ITU) to be 5 billion.
- Over time, the number of cell phone calls per day, the length of each call, and the amount of time people use cell phones have increased. However, improvements in cell phone technology have resulted in devices that have lower power outputs than earlier models.

What Is Radiofrequency Energy and How Does It Affect the Body?

Radiofrequency energy is a form of electromagnetic radiation. Electromagnetic radiation can be categorized into two types: ionizing (e.g., X-rays, radon, and cosmic rays) and nonionizing (e.g., radiofrequency and extremely low frequency, or power frequency). Electromagnetic radiation is defined according to its wavelength and frequency, which is the number of cycles of a wave that pass a reference point per second. Electromagnetic frequencies are described in units called hertz (Hz).

The energy of electromagnetic radiation is determined by its frequency; ionizing radiation is high frequency, and therefore high energy, whereas nonionizing radiation is low frequency, and therefore low energy.

The frequency of radiofrequency electromagnetic radiation ranges from 30 kilohertz (30 kHz, or 30,000 Hz) to 300 gigahertz (300 GHz, or 300 billion Hz). Electromagnetic fields in the radiofrequency range are used for telecommunications applications, including cell phones, televisions, and radio transmissions. The human body absorbs energy from devices that emit radiofrequency electromagnetic radiation. The dose of the absorbed energy is estimated using a measure called the specific absorption rate (SAR), which is expressed in watts per kilogram of body weight.

Exposure to ionizing radiation, such as from X-rays, is known to increase the risk of cancer. However, although many studies have examined the potential health effects of nonionizing radiation from radar, microwave ovens, cell phones, and other sources, there is currently no consistent evidence that nonionizing radiation increases cancer risk.

The only consistently recognized biological effect of radiofrequency energy is heating. The ability of microwave ovens to heat food is one example of this effect of radiofrequency energy. Radiofrequency exposure from cell phone use does cause heating to the area of the body where a cell phone or other device is held (ear, head, etc.). However, it is not sufficient to measurably increase body temperature, and there are no other clearly established effects on the body from radiofrequency energy.

It has been suggested that radiofrequency energy might affect glucose metabolism, but two small studies that examined brain glucose metabolism after use of a cell phone showed inconsistent results. Whereas one study showed increased glucose metabolism in the region of the brain close to the antenna compared with tissues on the opposite side of the brain, the other study found reduced glucose metabolism on the side of the brain where the phone was used.

Another study investigated whether exposure to the radiofrequency energy from cell phones affects the flow of blood in the brain and found no evidence of such an effect. The authors of these studies noted that the results are preliminary and that possible health outcomes from changes in glucose metabolism are still unknown. Such inconsistent findings are not uncommon in experimental studies of the biological effects of radiofrequency electromagnetic radiation. Some contributing factors include assumptions used to estimate doses, failure to consider temperature effects, and lack of blinding of investigators to exposure status.

How Is Radiofrequency Energy Exposure Measured in Epidemiologic Studies?

Epidemiologic studies use information from several sources, including questionnaires and data from cell phone service providers. Direct measurements are not yet possible outside of a laboratory setting. Estimates take into account the following:

- How "regularly" study participants use cell phones (the number of calls per week or month)
- The age and the year when study participants first used a cell phone and the age and the year of last use (allows calculation of the duration of use and time since the start of use)
- The average number of cell phone calls per day, week, or month (frequency)
- The average length of a typical cell phone call
- The total hours of lifetime use, calculated from the length of typical call times, the frequency of use, and the duration of use

What Has Research Shown about the Possible Cancer-Causing Effects of Radiofrequency Energy?

Radiofrequency energy, unlike ionizing radiation, does not cause DNA damage that can lead to cancer. It's only consistently observed biological effect in humans is tissue heating. In animal studies, it has not been found to cause cancer or to enhance the cancer-causing effects of known chemical carcinogens. The National Institute of Environmental Health Sciences (NIEHS), which is part of the National Institutes of Health (NIH), is carrying out a large-scale study in rodents of exposure to radiofrequency energy (the type used in cell phones). This investigation is being conducted in highly specialized labs that can specify and control sources of radiation and measure their effects.

Researchers have carried out several types of epidemiologic studies to investigate the possibility of a relationship between cell phone use and the risk of malignant (cancerous) brain tumors, such as gliomas, as well as benign (noncancerous) tumors, such as acoustic neuromas (tumors in the cells of the nerve responsible for hearing), most meningiomas (tumors in the meninges, membranes that cover and protect the brain and spinal cord), and parotid gland tumors (tumors in the salivary glands).

In one type of study, called a case-control study, cell phone use is compared between people with these types of tumors and people without them. In another type of study, called a cohort study, a large group of people who do not have cancer at study entry is followed over time and the rate of these tumors in people who did and didn't use cell phones is compared. Cancer incidence data can also be analyzed over time to see if the rates of cancer changed in large populations during the time that cell phone use increased dramatically. These studies have not shown clear evidence of a relationship between cell phone use and cancer. However, researchers have reported some statistically significant associations for certain subgroups of people.

Three large epidemiologic studies have examined the possible association between cell phone use and cancer: Interphone, a case-control study; the Danish Study, a cohort study; and the Million Women Study, another cohort study.

Interphone

How the study was done: This is the largest health-related case-control study of cell phone use and the risk of head and neck tumors. It was conducted by a consortium of researchers from 13 countries. The data came from questionnaires that were completed by study participants.

What the study showed: Most published analyses from this study have shown no statistically significant increases in brain or central nervous system cancers related to higher amounts of cell phone use. One analysis showed a statistically significant, although modest, increase in the risk of glioma among the small proportion of study participants who spent the most total time on cell phone calls. However, the researchers considered this finding inconclusive because they felt that the amount of use reported by some respondents was unlikely and because the participants who reported lower levels of use appeared to have a slightly reduced risk of brain cancer compared with people who did not use cell phones regularly. Another recent analysis from this study found no relationship between brain tumor locations and regions of the brain that were exposed to the highest level of radiofrequency energy from cell phones.

Danish Study

How the study was done: This cohort study, conducted in Denmark, linked billing information from more than 358,000 cell phone subscribers with brain tumor incidence data from the Danish Cancer Registry.

What the study showed: No association was observed between cell phone use and the incidence of glioma, meningioma, or acoustic neuroma, even among people who had been cell phone subscribers for 13 or more years.

Million Women Study

How the study was done: This prospective cohort study conducted in the United Kingdom used data obtained from questionnaires that were completed by study participants.

What the study showed: Self-reported cell phone use was not associated with an increased risk of glioma, meningioma, or noncentral nervous system tumors. Although the original published findings reported an association with an increased risk of acoustic neuroma, this association disappeared after additional follow-up of the cohort.

In addition to these three large studies, other, smaller epidemiologic studies have looked for associations between cell phone use and cancer. These include:

- Two National Institute of Cancer (NCI)-sponsored case-control studies, each conducted in multiple U.S. academic medical centers or hospitals between 1994–1998, that used data from questionnaires or computer-assisted personal interviews. Neither study showed a relationship between cell phone use and the risk of glioma, meningioma, or acoustic neuroma.
- The CERENAT study, another case-control study conducted in multiple areas in France from 2004–2006 using data collected in face-to-face interviews using standardized questionnaires. This study found no association for either gliomas or meningiomas when comparing regular cell phone users with nonusers. However, the heaviest users had significantly increased risks of both gliomas and meningiomas.
- A pooled analysis of two case-control studies conducted in Sweden that reported statistically significant trends of increasing brain cancer risk for the total amount of cell phone use and the

years of use among people who began using cell phones before age 20.

- Another case-control study in Sweden, part of the Interphone pooled studies, did not find an increased risk of brain cancer among long-term cell phone users between the ages of 20–69.
- The CEFALO study, an international case-control study of children diagnosed with brain cancer between ages 7–19, which found no relationship between their cell phone use and risk for brain cancer.

Investigators have also conducted analyses of incidence trends to determine whether the incidence of brain or other cancers has changed during the time that cell phone use increased dramatically. These include:

- An analysis of data from NCI's Surveillance, Epidemiology, and End Results (SEER) Program evaluated trends in cancer incidence in the United States. This analysis found no increase in the incidence of brain or other central nervous system (CNS) cancers between 1992–2006, despite the dramatic increase in cell phone use in this country during that time.
- An analysis of incidence data from Denmark, Finland, Norway, and Sweden for the period 1974–2008 similarly revealed no increase in age-adjusted incidence of brain tumors.
- A series of studies testing different scenarios (called simulations by the study authors) were carried out using incidence data from the Nordic countries to determine the likelihood of detecting various levels of risk as reported in studies of cell phone use and brain tumors between 1979–2008. The results were compatible with no increased risks from cell phones, as reported by most epidemiologic studies. The findings did suggest that the increase reported among the subset of heaviest regular users in the Interphone study could not be ruled out but was unlikely. The highly increased risks reported in the Swedish pooled analysis were strongly inconsistent with the observed glioma rates in the Nordic countries.
- A 2012 study by NCI researchers compared observed glioma incidence rates in U.S. SEER data with rates simulated from the small risks reported in the Interphone study and the greatly increased risk of brain cancer among cell phone users reported

in the Swedish pooled analysis. The observed U.S. rates showed no increase, but a small increased risk among the subset of heaviest users in the Interphone study could not be ruled out. The observed incidence trends were inconsistent with the high risks reported in the Swedish pooled study. These findings suggest that the increased risks observed in the Swedish study are not reflected in U.S. incidence trends.

Why Are the Findings from Different Studies of Cell Phone Use and Cancer Risk Inconsistent?

A limited number of studies have shown some evidence of statistical association of cell phone use and brain tumor risks, but most studies have found no association. Reasons for these discrepancies include the following:

- **Recall bias,** which can occur when data about prior habits and exposures are collected from study participants using questionnaires administered after diagnosis of a disease in some of the participants. It is possible that study participants who have brain tumors may remember their cell phone use differently from individuals without brain tumors. Many epidemiologic studies of cell phone use and brain cancer risk lack verifiable data about the total amount of cell phone use over time. In addition, people who develop a brain tumor may have a tendency to recall cell phone use mostly on the same side of the head where their tumor was found, regardless of whether they actually used their phone on that side of the head a lot or only a little.
- **Inaccurate reporting,** which can happen when people say that something has happened more or less often than it actually did. People may not remember how much they used cell phones in a given time period.
- **Morbidity and mortality** among study participants who have brain cancer. Gliomas are particularly difficult to study, for example, because of their high death rate and the short survival of people who develop these tumors. Patients who survive initial treatment are often impaired, which may affect their responses to questions. Furthermore, for people who have died, next-of-kin are often less familiar with the cell phone use patterns of their deceased family member and may not accurately describe their patterns of use to an interviewer.

- **Participation bias,** which can happen when people who are diagnosed with brain tumors are more likely than healthy people (known as controls) to enroll in a research study. Also, controls who did not or rarely used cell phones were less likely to participate in the Interphone study than controls who used cell phones regularly. For example, the Interphone study reported participation rates of 78 percent for meningioma patients (range 56–92 percent for the individual studies), 64 percent for glioma patients (range 36–92 percent), and 53 percent for control subjects (range 42–74 percent).
- **Changing technology and methods of use.** Older studies evaluated radiofrequency energy exposure from analog cell phones. However, most cell phones today use digital technology, which operates at a different frequency and a lower power level than analog phones. Digital cell phones have been in use for more than a decade in the United States, and cellular technology continues to change. Texting, for example, has become a popular way of using a cell phone to communicate that does not require bringing the phone close to the head. Furthermore, the use of hands-free technology, such as wired and wireless headsets, is increasing and may decrease radiofrequency energy exposure to the head and brain.

What Do Expert Organizations Conclude about the Cancer Risk from Cell Phone Use?

In 2011, the International Agency for Research on Cancer (IARC), a component of the World Health Organization (WHO), appointed an expert Working Group to review all available evidence on the use of cell phones. The Working Group classified cell phone use as "possibly carcinogenic to humans," based on limited evidence from human studies, limited evidence from studies of radiofrequency energy and cancer in rodents, and inconsistent evidence from mechanistic studies.

The Working Group indicated that, although the human studies were susceptible to bias, the findings could not be dismissed as reflecting bias alone, and that a causal interpretation could not be excluded. The Working Group noted that any interpretation of the evidence should also consider that the observed associations could reflect chance, bias, or confounding rather than an underlying causal effect. In addition, the Working Group stated that the investigation of risk of cancer of the brain associated with cell phone use poses complex methodologic challenges in the conduct of the research and in the analysis and interpretation of findings.

The American Cancer Society (ACS) states that the IARC classification means that there could be some cancer risk associated with radiofrequency energy, but the evidence is not strong enough to be considered causal and needs to be investigated further. Individuals who are concerned about radiofrequency energy exposure can limit their exposure, including using an earpiece and limiting cell phone use, particularly among children.

The NIEHS states that the weight of the current scientific evidence has not conclusively linked cell phone use with any adverse health problems, but more research is needed.

The U.S. Food and Drug Administration (FDA) notes that studies reporting biological changes associated with radiofrequency energy have failed to be replicated and that the majority of human epidemiologic studies have failed to show a relationship between exposure to radiofrequency energy from cell phones and health problems.

The Centers for Disease Control and Prevention (CDC) states that no scientific evidence definitively answers whether cell phone use causes cancer.

The Federal Communications Commission (FCC) concludes that no scientific evidence establishes a causal link between wireless device use and cancer or other illnesses.

In 2015 the European Commission Scientific Committee on Emerging and Newly Identified Health Risks (SCENIHR) concluded that, overall, the epidemiologic studies on cell phone radiofrequency electromagnetic radiation exposure do not show an increased risk of brain tumors or of other cancers of the head and neck region. The Committee also stated that epidemiologic studies do not indicate increased risk for other malignant diseases, including childhood cancer.

What Studies Are Underway That Will Help Further Our Understanding of the Possible Health Effects of Cell Phone Use?

A large prospective cohort study of cell phone use and its possible long-term health effects was launched in Europe in March 2010. This study, known as Cohort Study of Mobile Phone Use and Health (COSMOS), has enrolled approximately 290,000 cell phone users aged 18 years or older to date and will follow them for 20–30 years.

Participants in COSMOS will complete a questionnaire about their health, lifestyle, and current and past cell phone use. This information will be supplemented with information from health records and cell phone records.

The challenge of this ambitious study is to continue following the participants for a range of health effects over many decades. Researchers will need to determine whether participants who leave the study are somehow different from those who remain throughout the follow-up period.

Although recall bias is minimized in studies such as COSMOS that link participants to their cell phone records, such studies face other problems. For example, it is impossible to know who is using the listed cell phone or whether that individual also places calls using other cell phones. To a lesser extent, it is not clear whether multiple users of a single phone will be represented on a single phone company account.

Do Children Have a Higher Risk of Developing Cancer Due to Cell Phone Use than Adults?

There are theoretical considerations as to why the possible risk should be investigated separately in children. Their nervous systems are still developing and, therefore, more vulnerable to factors that may cause cancer. Their heads are smaller than those of adults and consequently have a greater proportional exposure to the field of radiofrequency radiation that is emitted by cell phones. And, children have the potential of accumulating more years of cell phone exposure than adults do.

Thus far, the data from studies in children with cancer do not support this theory. The first published analysis came from a large case-control study called CEFALO, which was conducted in Denmark, Sweden, Norway, and Switzerland. The study included children who were diagnosed with brain tumors between 2004–2008, when their ages ranged from 7–19. Researchers did not find an association between cell phone use and brain tumor risk either by time since initiation of use, amount of use, or by the location of the tumor.

Several studies that will provide more information are under way. Researchers from the Centre for Research in Environmental Epidemiology (CREAL) in Spain are conducting another international case-control study—Mobi-Kids—that will include 2000 young people (aged 10–24 years) with newly diagnosed brain tumors and 4000 healthy young people. The goal of the study is to learn more about risk factors for childhood brain tumors.

What Can Cell Phone Users Do to Reduce Their Exposure to Radiofrequency Energy?

The U.S. Food and Drug Administration (FDA) has suggested some steps that concerned cell phone users can take to reduce their exposure to radiofrequency energy:

- Reserve the use of cell phones for shorter conversations or for times when a landline phone is not available.
- Use a device with hands-free technology, such as wired headsets, which place more distance between the phone and the head of the user.

Hands-free kits reduce the amount of radiofrequency energy exposure to the head because the antenna, which is the source of energy, is not placed against the head. Exposures decline dramatically when cell phones are used hands-free.

Where Can I Find More Information about Radiofrequency Energy from My Cell Phone?

The FCC provides information about the specific absorption rate (SAR) of cell phones produced and marketed within the last 1–2 years. The SAR corresponds with the relative amount of radiofrequency energy absorbed by the head of a cell phone user. Consumers can access this information using the phone's FCC ID number, which is usually located on the case of the phone, and the FCC's ID search form.

How Common Is Brain Cancer? Has the Incidence of Brain Cancer Changed over Time?

Brain cancer incidence and mortality (death) rates have changed little in the past decade. In the United States, 23,770 new diagnoses and 16,050 deaths from brain and other central nervous system cancers are estimated for 2016. The 5-year relative survival for brain cancers diagnosed from 2005–2011 was 35 percent. This is the percentage of people diagnosed with brain cancer who will still be alive 5 years after diagnosis compared with the survival of a person of the same age and sex who does not have cancer. The risk of developing brain cancer increases with age. From 2008 through 2012, there were fewer than 5 brain cancer cases for every 100,000 people in the United States under age 65, compared with approximately 19 cases for every 100,000 people in the United States who were ages 65 or older.

Chapter 9

Environmental Carcinogens

Few Carcinogens That Cause Cancer

Cancer is caused by changes to certain genes that alter the way our cells function. Some of these genetic changes occur naturally when DNA (deoxyribonucleic acid) is replicated during the process of cell division. But others are the result of environmental exposures that damage DNA. These exposures may include substances, such as the chemicals in tobacco smoke, or radiation, such as ultraviolet rays from the sun.

People can avoid some cancer-causing exposures, such as tobacco smoke and the sun's rays. But others are harder to avoid, especially if they are in the air we breathe, the water we drink, the food we eat, or the materials we use to do our jobs. Scientists are studying which exposures may cause or contribute to the development of cancer. Understanding which exposures are harmful, and where they are found, may help people to avoid them.

The substances listed below are among the most likely carcinogens to affect human health. Simply because a substance has been designated as a carcinogen, however, does not mean that the substance will

---

This chapter contains text excerpted from the following sources: Text under the heading "Few Carcinogens That Cause Cancer" is excerpted from "Cancer-Causing Substances in the Environment," National Cancer Institute (NCI), March 18, 2015; Text under the heading "Occupational Carcinogens" is excerpted from "Workplace Safety and Health Topics—Occupational Cancer," Centers for Disease Control and Prevention (CDC), February 13, 2018.

necessarily cause cancer. Many factors influence whether a person exposed to a carcinogen will develop cancer, including the amount and duration of the exposure and the individual's genetic background.

Aflatoxins

Aflatoxins are a family of toxins produced by certain fungi that are found on agricultural crops such as maize (corn), peanuts, cottonseed, and tree nuts. The main fungi that produce aflatoxins are Aspergillus flavus and Aspergillus parasiticus, which are abundant in warm and humid regions of the world. Aflatoxin-producing fungi can contaminate crops in the field, at harvest, and during storage. Exposure to aflatoxins is associated with an increased risk of liver cancer.

Aristolochic Acids

Aristolochic acids are a group of acids found naturally in many types of plants known as *Aristolochia* (birthworts or pipevines) and some types of plants known as *Asarum* (wild ginger), which grow worldwide. Cancers of the upper urinary tract (renal pelvis and ureter) and bladder have been reported among individuals who had kidney damage caused by the consumption of herbal products containing aristolochic acids.

Arsenic

Arsenic is a naturally occurring substance that can be found in air, water, and soil. It can also be released into the environment by certain agricultural and industrial processes, such as mining and metal smelting. Arsenic comes in two forms (organic and inorganic); the inorganic form is more toxic than the organic form. Prolonged ingestion of arsenic-containing drinking water is associated with an increased risk of bladder cancer. In addition, cancers of the skin, lung, digestive tract, liver, kidney, and lymphatic and hematopoietic systems have been linked to arsenic exposure.

Asbestos

Asbestos is the name given to a group of naturally occurring fibrous minerals that are resistant to heat and corrosion. Because of these properties, asbestos has been used in commercial products such as insulation and fireproofing materials, automotive brakes, and wallboard materials. Exposure to asbestos is associated with an increased risk of lung cancer and mesothelioma, which is a cancer of the thin membranes that line the chest and abdomen. Mesothelioma is the most common form of cancer associated with asbestos exposure, although the disease is relatively rare.

Benzene

Benzene is a colorless or light-yellow liquid chemical at room temperature. It is used primarily as a solvent in the chemical and pharmaceutical industries, as a starting material and an intermediate in the synthesis of numerous chemicals, and in gasoline. Benzene is produced by both natural and man-made processes. It is a natural component of crude oil, which is the main source of benzene produced today. Other natural sources include gas emissions from volcanoes and forest fires. Exposure to benzene may increase the risk of developing leukemia and other blood disorders.

Benzidine

Benzidine is a manufactured chemical that does not occur in nature. In the past, large amounts of benzidine were used to produce dyes for cloth, paper, and leather. It was also used in clinical laboratories for detecting blood, as a rubber-compounding agent, and in the manufacture of plastic films. However, benzidine has not been sold in the United States since the mid-1970s, and it is no longer used in medical laboratories or in the rubber and plastics industries. Occupational exposure to benzidine results in an increased risk of bladder cancer, according to studies of workers in different geographic locations.

Beryllium

Beryllium is a metal that is found in nature, especially in beryl and bertrandite rock. It is extremely lightweight and hard, is a good conductor of electricity and heat, and is nonmagnetic. Because of these properties, beryllium is used in high-technology consumer and commercial products, including aerospace components, transistors, nuclear reactors, and golf clubs. An increased risk of lung cancer has been observed in workers exposed to beryllium or beryllium compounds.

Cadmium

Cadmium is a natural element found in tiny amounts in air, water, soil, and food. All soils and rocks, including coal and mineral fertilizers, contain some cadmium. Most cadmium used in the United States is extracted during the production of other metals such as zinc, lead, and copper. Cadmium does not corrode easily and has been used to manufacture batteries, pigments, metal coatings, and plastics. Occupational exposure to various cadmium compounds is associated with an increased risk of lung cancer.

Coal Tar and Coal-Tar Pitch

Coal tar is derived from coal. It is a byproduct of the production of coke, a solid fuel that contains mostly carbon, and coal gas. Coal tar is used primarily for the production of refined chemicals and coal-tar products, such as creosote and coal-tar pitch. Certain preparations of coal tar have long been used to treat various skin conditions, such as eczema, psoriasis, and dandruff. Occupational exposure to coal tar or coal-tar pitch is associated with an increased risk of skin cancer. Other types of cancer, including lung, bladder, kidney, and digestive tract cancer, have also been linked to occupational exposure to coal tar and coal-tar pitch.

Coke-Oven Emissions

Coke oven emissions come from large ovens that are used to heat coal to produce coke, which is used to manufacture iron and steel. The emissions are complex mixtures of dust, vapors, and gases that typically include carcinogens such as cadmium and arsenic. Chemicals recovered from coke oven emissions are used as raw materials for producing items such as plastics, solvents, dyes, paints, and insulation. Exposure to coke oven emissions is associated with an increased risk of lung cancer.

Crystalline Silica (Respirable Size)

An abundant natural material, crystalline silica is found in stone, soil, and sand. It is also found in concrete, brick, mortar, and other construction materials. Crystalline silica comes in several forms, with quartz being the most common. Quartz dust is respirable crystalline silica, which means it can be taken in by breathing. Exposure of workers to respirable crystalline silica is associated with elevated rates of lung cancer. The strongest link between human lung cancer and exposure to respirable crystalline silica has been seen in studies of quarry and granite workers and workers involved in ceramic, pottery, refractory brick, and certain earth industries.

Erionite

Erionite is a naturally occurring fibrous mineral that belongs to a group of minerals called zeolites. It forms fibrous masses in the hollows of rock formations. Some of the mineral's properties are similar to those of asbestos; for example, the fibers pose a hazard only if they are disturbed and become airborne. Exposure to erionite is associated with increased risks of lung cancer and mesothelioma.

Ethylene Oxide

At room temperature, ethylene oxide is a flammable colorless gas with a sweet odor. It is used primarily to produce other chemicals, including antifreeze. In smaller amounts, ethylene oxide is used as a pesticide and a sterilizing agent. The ability of ethylene oxide to damage DNA makes it an effective sterilizing agent but also accounts for its cancer-causing activity. Lymphoma and leukemia are the cancers most frequently reported to be associated with occupational exposure to ethylene oxide.

Formaldehyde

Formaldehyde is a colorless, strong-smelling, flammable chemical that is produced industrially and used in building materials such as particleboard, plywood, and other pressed-wood products. In addition, it is commonly used as a fungicide, germicide, and disinfectant, and as a preservative in mortuaries and medical laboratories. Formaldehyde also occurs naturally in the environment. It is produced during the decay of plant material in the soil and during normal chemical processes in most living organisms. It is also a combustion product found in tobacco smoke. Studies of workers exposed to high levels of formaldehyde, such as industrial workers and embalmers, have found that formaldehyde causes myeloid leukemia and rare cancers, including cancers of the paranasal sinuses, nasal cavity, and nasopharynx.

Hexavalent Chromium Compounds

Chromium is an odorless and tasteless metallic element that is found in the earth's crust. It is also found in air, water, soil, and food.

Hexavalent chromium compounds are a group of chemicals that have useful properties, such as corrosion resistance, durability, and hardness. These compounds have been used widely as corrosion inhibitors and in the manufacture of pigments, metal finishing and chrome plating, stainless steel production, leather tanning, and wood preservatives. They have also been used in textile-dyeing processes, printing inks, drilling muds, fireworks, water treatment, and chemical synthesis.

Occupational exposure to these compounds is associated with increased risks of lung cancer and cancer of the paranasal sinuses and nasal cavity.

Indoor Emissions from the Household Combustion of Coal

Burning coal inside the home for the purposes of heating or cooking produces particulate and gas emissions that may contain a number of harmful chemicals, such as benzene, carbon monoxide, formaldehyde, and polycyclic aromatic hydrocarbons. Lung cancer is associated with exposure to indoor coal combustion emissions.

Mineral Oils: Untreated and Mildly Treated

The name mineral oil has been used to describe many colorless, odorless liquids. Most often, the term refers to a liquid by-product of the distillation of petroleum to produce gasoline and other petroleum-based products from crude oil. These oils, including lubricant base oils and products derived from them, are used in manufacturing, mining, construction, and other industries.

A complete description of mineral oils should include how the oils are refined. Oils used in cosmetic products are typically highly refined, whereas those used in automotive oils and fluids tend to be unrefined or only mildly treated. Highly refined products are not covered in this section.

Exposure to mineral oils is strongly associated with an increased risk of nonmelanoma skin cancer, particularly of the scrotum.

Nickel Compounds

Nickel is a silvery-white metallic element found in the earth's crust. It can be combined with other elements to form nickel compounds. Because of its unique properties, nickel has many industrial uses. Most nickel is used in metal alloys because it imparts useful properties, such as corrosion resistance, heat resistance, hardness, and strength.

Exposure to various nickel compounds is associated with increased risks of lung cancer and nasal cancer.

1,3-Butadiene

1,3-Butadiene is a colorless gas at room temperature with a gasoline-like odor. It is used to produce synthetic rubber products, such as tires, resins, and plastics, and other chemicals. Studies have consistently shown an association between occupational exposure to 1,3-butadiene and an increased incidence of leukemia.

Radon

Radon is a radioactive gas that is released from the normal decay of the elements uranium, thorium, and radium in rocks and soil. The invisible, odorless gas seeps up through the ground and diffuses into the air. In a few areas, depending on local geology, radon dissolves into groundwater and can be released into the air when the water is used. Radon gas usually exists at very low levels outdoors, but the gas can accumulate in areas without adequate ventilation, such as underground mines.

Radon was identified as a health problem when scientists noted that underground uranium miners who were exposed to it died of lung cancer at high rates. Experimental studies in animals confirmed the results of the miner studies by showing higher rates of lung tumors among rodents exposed to high levels of radon. There has been a suggestion of an increased risk of leukemia associated with radon exposure in adults and children; the evidence, however, is not conclusive.

Secondhand Tobacco Smoke (Environmental Tobacco Smoke)

Secondhand tobacco smoke is the combination of the smoke given off by a burning tobacco product and the smoke exhaled by a smoker. It is also called environmental tobacco smoke, involuntary smoke, and passive smoke.

More than 7,000 chemicals have been identified in secondhand tobacco smoke. At least 69 of these chemicals are carcinogens, including arsenic, benzene, beryllium, chromium, and formaldehyde.

Inhaling secondhand smoke causes lung cancer in nonsmokers. Some research also suggests that secondhand smoke may increase the risk of some other cancers as well, though more research is needed on this subject.

Soot

Soot is a byproduct of the incomplete burning of organic (carbon-containing) materials, such as wood, fuel oil, plastics, and household refuse. The fine black or brown powder that makes up soot may contain a number of carcinogens, including arsenic, cadmium, and chromium. Exposure to soot was first associated with skin cancer of the scrotum among British chimney sweeps in 1775. Since then, many studies have found that chimney sweeps have an increased risk of scrotal and other skin cancers. Studies of chimney sweeps in several European countries have also found associations with other cancers, including lung, esophageal, and bladder cancers.

Strong Inorganic Acid Mists Containing Sulfuric Acid

At room temperature, sulfuric acid is a clear, colorless, oily, corrosive liquid. Strong inorganic acid mists containing sulfuric acid may be generated during various manufacturing processes.

Occupational exposure to strong inorganic acid mists containing sulfuric acid is associated with increased risks of laryngeal and lung cancer.

Thorium

Thorium is a naturally occurring radioactive metal that is found in soil, rock, and water. It is formed by the radioactive decay of uranium. Minerals such as monazite, thorite, and thorianite are rich in thorium and may be mined for the metal.

Thorium has coloring properties that have made it useful in ceramic glazes. Thorium also has been widely used in lantern mantles for the brightness it imparts (though alternatives are replacing it), and in welding rods, which burn better with small amounts of added thorium. Until the 1950s, thorium dioxide was used as a contrast agent (called Thorotrast) in medical radiology.

Studies of patients who received intravascular injections of Thorotrast found an increased risk of liver tumors among these individuals. And there is research evidence that inhaling thorium dust increases the risk of lung and pancreatic cancer. Individuals exposed to thorium also have an increased risk of bone cancer because thorium may be stored in bone.

Vinyl Chloride

Vinyl chloride is a colorless gas that burns easily. It does not occur naturally and must be produced industrially for its commercial uses. Vinyl chloride is used primarily to make polyvinyl chloride (PVC); PVC is used to make a variety of plastic products, including pipes, wire and cable coatings, and packaging materials. Vinyl chloride is also produced as a combustion product in tobacco smoke.

Vinyl chloride exposure is associated with an increased risk of a rare form of liver cancer (hepatic angiosarcoma), as well as brain and lung cancers, lymphoma, and leukemia.

Wood Dust

Wood dust is created when machines or tools are used to cut or shape wood. High amounts of wood dust are produced in sawmills, and in the furniture-making, cabinet-making, and carpentry industries. Strong and consistent associations with cancers of the paranasal sinuses and nasal cavity have been observed both in studies of people whose occupations were associated with wood-dust exposure and in studies that directly estimated wood-dust exposure.

Occupational Carcinogens

The following is a list of substances National Institute for Occupational Safety and Health (NIOSH) considers to be potential occupational carcinogens.

A number of the carcinogen classifications deal with groups of substances: aniline and homologs, chromates, dinitrotoluenes, arsenic and inorganic arsenic compounds, beryllium and beryllium compounds, cadmium compounds, nickel compounds, and crystalline forms of silica. There are also substances of variable or unclear chemical makeup that are considered carcinogens, coal tar pitch volatiles, coke oven emissions, diesel exhaust, and environmental tobacco smoke.

Some of the potential carcinogens listed in may be re-evaluated by NIOSH as new data become available and the NIOSH recommendations on these carcinogens either as to their status as a potential occupational carcinogen or as to the appropriate recommended exposure limit may change.

- Acetaldehyde
- 2-Acetylaminofluorene
- Acrylamide
- Acrylonitrile
- Aldrin
- 4-Aminodiphenyl
- Amitrole
- Aniline and homologs
- *o*-Anisidine
- Arsenic compounds
- Arsine
- Asbestos

- Asphalt fumes
- Benzene
- Benzidine
- Benzidine-based dyes
- Beryllium
- Butadiene
- *tert*-Butyl chromate
- Cadmium dust and fume
- Captafol
- Captan
- Carbon black
- Carbon tetrachloride
- Chlordane
- Chlorinated camphene
- Chlorodiphenyl
- Chloroform
- Chloromethyl methyl ether
- bis (Chloromethyl) ether
- *B*-Chloroprene
- Chromium
- Chromyl chloride
- Chrysene
- Coal tar pitch volatiles
- Coke oven emissions
- DDT (dichlorodiphenyltri-chloroethane)
- Di-2-ethylhexyl phthalate (DEHP)
- 2,4-Diaminoanisoleo
- o-Dianisidine-based dyes
- 1,2-Dibromo-3-chloropropane (DBCP)
- Dichloroacetylene
- *p*-Dichlorobenzene
- 3,3′-Dichlorobenzidine
- Dichloroethyl ether
- 1,3-Dichloropropene
- Dieldrin
- Diesel exhaust
- Diglycidyl ether (DGE)
- 4-Dimethylaminoazobenzene
- Dimethylcarbomoyl chloride
- 1,1-Dimethylhydrazine
- Dimethyl sulfate
- Dinitrotoluene
- Dioxane
- Environmental tobacco smoke
- Epichlorohydrin
- Ethyl acrylate
- Ethylene dibromide
- Ethylene dichloride
- Ethylene oxide
- Ethyleneimine
- Ethylene thiourea
- Formaldehyde
- Gallium arsenide
- Gasoline
- Heptachlor
- Hexachlorobutadiene
- Hexachloroethane

- Hydrazine
- Kepone
- Malonaldehyde
- Methoxychlor
- Methyl bromide
- Methyl chloride
- Methyl iodide
- Methyl hydrazine
- Methylene chloride
- 4,4-Methylenedianiline (MDA)
- α-Naphthylamine
- β-Naphthylamine
- Nickel
- Nickel carbonyl
- Nickel sulfide roasting
- 4-Nitrobiphenyl
- *p*-Nitrochlorobenzene
- 2-Nitronaphthalene
- 2-Nitropropane
- *N*-Nitrosodimethylamine
- Pentachloroethane
- *N*-Phenyl-*b*-naphthylamine
- Phenyl glycidyl ether
- Phenylhydrazine
- Propane Sultone
- *B*-Propiolactone
- Propylene dichloride
- Propyleneimine
- Propylene oxide
- Radon
- Rosin core solder
- Silica, crystalline cristobalite
- Silica, crystalline quartz
- Silica, crystalline tripoli
- Silica, crystalline tridymite
- silica, fused
- Soapstone, total dust silicates
- Tremolite silicates
- 1,1,2,2-Tetrachloroethane
- Tetrachloroethylene
- Titanium dioxide
- *o*-Tolidine-based dyes
- *o*-Tolidine
- Toluene diisocyanate (TDI)
- Toluene diamine (TDA)
- *o*-Toluidine
- *p*-Toluidine
- 1,1,2-Trichloroethane
- Trichloroethylene
- 1,2,3-Trichloropropane
- Uranium compounds
- Vinyl bromide
- Vinyl chloride
- Vinyl cyclohexene dioxide
- Vinylidene chloride
- Welding fumes
- Wood dust
- Zinc chromate

Chapter 10

Common Moles, Dysplastic Nevi, and Risk of Melanoma

What Is a Common Mole?

A common mole is a growth on the skin that develops when pigment cells (melanocytes) grow in clusters. Most adults have between 10–40 common moles. These growths are usually found above the waist on areas exposed to the sun. They are seldom found on the scalp, breast, or buttocks. Although common moles may be present at birth, they usually appear later in childhood. Most people continue to develop new moles until about age 40. In older people, common moles tend to fade away. Another name for a mole is a nevus. The plural is nevi.

What Does a Common Mole Look Like?

A common mole is usually smaller than about 5 millimeters wide (about 1/4 inch, the width of a pencil eraser). It is round or oval, has a smooth surface with a distinct edge, and is often dome-shaped. A common mole usually has an even color of pink, tan, or brown. People who have dark skin or hair tend to have darker moles than people with fair skin or blonde hair.

This chapter includes text excerpted from "Common Moles, Dysplastic Nevi, and Risk of Melanoma," National Cancer Institute (NCI), May 3, 2017.

Can a Common Mole Turn into Melanoma?

Yes, but a common mole rarely turns into melanoma, which is the most serious type of skin cancer. Although common moles are not cancerous, people who have more than 50 common moles have an increased chance of developing melanoma.

People should tell their doctor if they notice any of the following changes in a common mole:

- The color changes.
- The mole gets unevenly smaller or bigger (unlike normal moles in children, which get evenly bigger).
- The mole changes in shape, texture, or height.
- The skin on the surface becomes dry or scaly.
- The mole becomes hard or feels lumpy.
- It starts to itch.
- It bleeds or oozes.

What Is a Dysplastic Nevus?

A dysplastic nevus is a type of mole that looks different from a common mole. (Some doctors use the term "atypical mole" to refer to a dysplastic nevus.) A dysplastic nevus may be bigger than a common mole, and its color, surface, and border may be different. It is usually more than 5 millimeters wide. A dysplastic nevus can have a mixture of several colors, from pink to dark brown. Usually, it is flat with a smooth, slightly scaly, or pebbly surface, and it has an irregular edge that may fade into the surrounding skin.

A dysplastic nevus may occur anywhere on the body, but it is usually seen in areas exposed to the sun, such as on the back. A dysplastic nevus may also appear in areas not exposed to the sun, such as the scalp, breasts, and areas below the waist. Some people have only a couple of dysplastic nevi, but other people have more than 10. People who have dysplastic nevi usually also have an increased number of common moles.

Can a Dysplastic Nevus Turn into Melanoma?

Yes, but most dysplastic nevi do not turn into melanoma. Most remain stable over time. Researchers estimate that the chance of melanoma is about ten times greater for someone with more than five dysplastic nevi than for someone who has none, and the more dysplastic nevi a person has, the greater the chance of developing melanoma.

What Should People Do If They Have a Dysplastic Nevus?

Everyone should protect their skin from the sun and stay away from sunlamps and tanning booths, but for people who have dysplastic nevi, it is even more important to protect the skin and avoid getting a suntan or sunburn.

In addition, many doctors recommend that people with dysplastic nevi check their skin once a month. People should tell their doctor if they see any of the following changes in a dysplastic nevus:

- The color changes.
- It gets smaller or bigger.
- It changes in shape, texture, or height.
- The skin on the surface becomes dry or scaly.
- It becomes hard or feels lumpy.
- It starts to itch.
- It bleeds or oozes.

Another thing that people with dysplastic nevi should do is get their skin examined by a doctor. Sometimes people or their doctors take photographs of dysplastic nevi so changes over time are easier to see. For people with many (more than five) dysplastic nevi, doctors may conduct a skin exam once or twice a year because of the moderately increased chance of melanoma. For people who also have a family history of melanoma, doctors may suggest a more frequent skin exam, such as every 3–6 months.

Should People Have a Doctor Remove a Dysplastic Nevus or a Common Mole to Prevent It from Changing into Melanoma?

No. Normally, people do not need to have a dysplastic nevus or common mole removed. One reason is that very few dysplastic nevi or common moles turn into melanoma. Another reason is that even removing all of the moles on the skin would not prevent the development of melanoma because melanoma can develop as a new colored area on the skin. That is why doctors usually remove only a mole that changes or a new colored area on the skin.

What Is Melanoma?

Melanoma is a type of skin cancer that begins in melanocytes. It is potentially dangerous because it can invade nearby tissues and spread to other parts of the body, such as the lung, liver, bone, or brain. The earlier that melanoma is detected and removed, the more likely that treatment will be successful.

Most melanocytes are in the skin, and melanoma can occur on any skin surface. It can develop from a common mole or dysplastic nevus, and it can also develop in an area of apparently normal skin. In addition, melanoma can also develop in the eye, the digestive tract, and other areas of the body.

When melanoma develops in men, it is often found on the head, neck, or back. When melanoma develops in women, it is often found on the back or on the lower legs.

People with dark skin are much less likely than people with fair skin to develop melanoma. When it does develop in people with dark skin, it is often found under the fingernails, under the toenails, on the palms of the hands, or on the soles of the feet.

What Does Melanoma Look Like?

Often the first sign of melanoma is a change in the shape, color, size, or feel of an existing mole. Melanoma may also appear as a new colored area on the skin.

The "ABCDE" rule describes the features of early melanoma:

- **Asymmetry.** The shape of one half does not match the other half.
- **Border that is irregular.** The edges are often ragged, notched, or blurred in outline. The pigment may spread into the surrounding skin.
- **Color that is uneven.** Shades of black, brown, and tan may be present. Areas of white, gray, red, pink, or blue may also be seen.
- **Diameter.** There is a change in size, usually an increase. Melanomas can be tiny, but most are larger than 6 millimeters wide (about 1/4 inch wide).

- **Evolving.** The mole has changed over the past few weeks or months.

Melanomas can vary greatly in how they look. Many show all of the ABCDE features. However, some may show only one or two of the ABCDE features.

In advanced melanoma, the texture of the mole may change. The skin on the surface may break down and look scraped. It may become hard or lumpy. The surface may ooze or bleed. Sometimes the melanoma is itchy, tender, or painful.

How Is Melanoma Diagnosed?

The only way to diagnose melanoma is to remove tissue and check it for cancer cells. The doctor will remove all or part of the skin that looks abnormal. Usually, this procedure takes only a few minutes and can be done in a doctor's office, clinic, or hospital. The sample will be sent to a lab and a pathologist will look at the tissue under a microscope to check for melanoma.

What Are the Differences between a Common Mole, a Dysplastic Nevus, and a Melanoma?

Common moles, dysplastic nevi, and melanoma vary by size, color, shape, and surface texture. The list below summarizes some differences between moles and cancer. Another important difference is that a common mole or dysplastic nevus will not return after it is removed by a full excisional biopsy from the skin, but melanoma sometimes grows back. Also, melanoma can spread to other parts of the body.

Common Mole (Nevus)

- **Is it cancer?** No. Common moles rarely become cancer.
- **How many people have common moles?** Most American adults—about 300 million people—have common moles.
- **How big are they?** Usually less than 5 millimeters wide, or about 1/4 inch (not as wide as a new pencil eraser).
- **What color are they?** May be pink, tan, brown, black (in people with dark skin), or a color that is very close to a person's normal skin tone. The color is usually even throughout.

- **What shape are they?** Usually round or oval. A common mole has a distinct edge that separates it from the rest of the skin.
- **What is the surface texture?** Begins as a flat, smooth spot on the skin. May become raised and form a smooth bump.

Dysplastic Nevus

- **Is it cancer?** No. A dysplastic nevus is more likely than a common mole to become cancer, but most do not become cancer.
- **How many people have dysplastic nevi?** About 1 in 10 American adults—about 30 million people—have at least one dysplastic nevus.
- **How big are they?** Often wider than 5 millimeters (wider than a new pencil eraser).
- **What color are they?** May be a mixture of tan, brown, and red or pink shades.
- **What shape are they?** Have irregular or notched edges. May fade into the rest of the skin.
- **What is the surface texture?** May have a smooth, slightly scaly, or rough, irregular, and pebbly appearance.

Melanoma

- **Is it cancer?** Yes.
- **How many people have melanoma?** Melanoma is much less common than other kinds of skin cancer. But every year, about 2 in 10,000 Americans—more than 70,000 people—develop melanoma. More than 800,000 Americans alive today have been diagnosed with melanoma.
- **How big are they?** Usually wider than 6 millimeters (wider than a new pencil eraser).
- **What color are they?** Usually uneven in color. May have shades of black, brown, and tan. May also have areas of white, gray, red, pink, or blue.
- **What shape are they?** Often irregular and asymmetrical (the shape of one half does not match the other half). Edges may be ragged, notched, or blurred. May fade into the rest of the skin.
- **What is the surface texture?** May break down and look scraped, become hard or lumpy, or ooze or bleed.

What Should People Do If a Mole Changes, or They Find a New Mole or Some Other Change on Their Skin?

People should tell their doctor if they find a new mole or a change in an existing mole. A family doctor may refer people with an unusual mole or other concerns about their skin to a dermatologist. A dermatologist is a doctor who specializes in diseases of the skin. Also, some plastic surgeons, general surgeons, internists, cancer specialists, and family doctors have special training in moles and melanoma.

What Factors Increase the Chance of Melanoma?

People with the following risk factors have an increased chance of melanoma:

- **Having a dysplastic nevus**
- **Having more than 50 common moles**
- **Sunlight.** Sunlight is a source of ultraviolet (UV) radiation, which causes skin damage that can lead to melanoma and other skin cancers.
  - **Severe, blistering sunburns.** People who have had at least one severe, blistering sunburn have an increased chance of melanoma. Although people who burn easily are more likely to have had sunburns as a child, sunburns during adulthood also increase the chance of melanoma.
  - **Lifetime sun exposure.** The greater the total amount of sun exposure over a lifetime, the greater the chance of melanoma.
  - **Tanning.** Although having skin that tans well lowers the risk of sunburn, even people who tan well without sunburning increase their chance of melanoma by spending time in the sun without protection.

Sunlight can be reflected by sand, water, snow, ice, and pavement. The sun's rays can get through clouds, windshields, windows, and light clothing.

In the United States, skin cancer is more common where the sun is strong. For example, a larger proportion of people in Texas than Minnesota get skin cancer. Also, the sun is strong at higher elevations, such as in the mountains.

- **Sunlamps and tanning booths.** UV radiation from artificial sources, such as sunlamps and tanning booths, can cause skin damage and melanoma. Healthcare providers strongly encourage people, especially young people, to avoid using sunlamps and tanning booths. The risk of skin cancer is greatly increased by using sunlamps and tanning booths before age 30.
- **Personal history.** People who have had melanoma have an increased risk of developing other melanomas.
- **Family history.** Melanoma sometimes runs in families. People who have two or more close relatives (mother, father, sister, brother, or child) with melanoma have an increased chance of melanoma. In rare cases, members of a family will have an inherited disorder, such as xeroderma pigmentosum, that makes the skin extremely sensitive to the sun and greatly increases the chance of melanoma.
- **Skin that burns easily.** People who have fair (pale) skin that burns easily in the sun, blue or gray eyes, red or blond hair, or many freckles have an increased chance of melanoma.
- **Certain medical conditions or medicines.** Medical conditions or medicines (such as some antibiotics, hormones, or antidepressants) that make skin more sensitive to the sun or that suppress the immune system increase the chance of melanoma.

How Can People Protect Their Skin from the Sun?

The best way to prevent melanoma is to limit exposure to sunlight. Having a suntan or sunburn means that the skin has been damaged by the sun, and continued tanning or burning increases the chance of developing melanoma.

Chapter 11

Cancer Vaccines

What Is the Immune System?

The immune system is a complex network of cells, tissues, organs, and the substances they make that helps the body fight infections and other diseases. The immune system's role in defending against disease-causing microbes has long been recognized. Scientists have also discovered that the immune system can protect the body against threats posed by certain damaged, diseased, or abnormal cells, including cancer cells.

White blood cells, or leukocytes, play the main role in immune responses. These cells carry out the many tasks required to protect the body against disease-causing microbes and abnormal cells.

Some types of leukocytes patrol the circulatory system, seeking foreign invaders and diseased, damaged, or dead cells. These white blood cells provide a general—or nonspecific—level of immune protection.

Other types of leukocytes, known as lymphocytes, provide targeted protection against specific threats, whether from a specific microbe or a diseased or abnormal cell. The most important groups of lymphocytes responsible for carrying out immune responses against such threats are B cells (B lymphocytes) and T cells (T lymphocyte).

B cells make antibodies, which are large secreted proteins that bind to, inactivate, and help destroy foreign invaders or abnormal cells. Cytotoxic T cells, which are also known as killer T cells, kill infected

---

This chapter includes text excerpted from "Cancer Vaccines," National Cancer Institute (NCI), December 18, 2015.

or abnormal cells by releasing toxic chemicals or by prompting the cells to self-destruct (in a process known as apoptosis).

Other types of lymphocytes and leukocytes play supporting roles to ensure that B cells and killer T cells do their jobs effectively. These supporting cells include helper T cells and dendritic cells, which help activate both B cells and killer T cells and enable them to respond to specific threats.

Antigens are substances that have the potential to cause the body to mount an immune response against them. They help the immune system determine whether something is foreign, or "nonself." Normal cells in the body have antigens that identify them as "self." Self-antigens tell the immune system that normal cells are not a threat and should be ignored. In contrast, microbes are recognized by the immune system as a potential threat that should be destroyed because they carry foreign, or nonself, antigens.

Are Cancer Cells Recognized by the Immune System?

Cancer cells can carry both self-antigens as well as what are referred to as cancer-associated antigens. Cancer-associated antigens mark cancer cells as abnormal or foreign and can cause killer T cells to mount an attack against them. Cancer-associated antigens may be:

- Self-antigens that are made in much larger amounts by cancer cells than normal cells and, thus, are viewed as foreign by the immune system
- Self-antigens that are not normally made by the tissue in which the cancer developed (for example, antigens that are normally made only by embryonic tissue but are expressed in an adult cancer) and, thus, are viewed as foreign by the immune system
- Newly formed antigens, or neoantigens, that result from gene mutations in cancer cells and have not been seen previously by the immune system

However, several factors may make it difficult for the immune system to target growing cancers for destruction:

- Many cancer-associated antigens are only slightly altered versions of self-antigens and therefore may be hard for the immune system to recognize.
- Cancer cells may undergo genetic changes that may lead to the loss of cancer-associated antigens.

- Cancer cells can evade anticancer immune responses by killer T cells. As a result, even when the immune system recognizes a growing cancer as a threat, the cancer may still escape a strong attack by the immune system.

What Are Vaccines?

Vaccines are medicines that boost the immune system's natural ability to protect the body against "foreign invaders," mainly infectious agents, that may cause disease.

When an infectious microbe invades the body, the immune system recognizes it as foreign, destroys it, and "remembers" it to prevent another infection should the microbe invade the body again in the future. Vaccines take advantage of this defensive memory response.

Most vaccines are made with harmless versions of microbes—killed or weakened microbes, or parts of microbes—that do not cause disease but are able to stimulate an immune response against the microbes. When the immune system encounters these substances through vaccination, it responds to them, eliminates them from the body, and develops a memory of them. This vaccine-induced memory enables the immune system to act quickly to protect the body if it becomes infected by the same microbes in the future.

What Are Cancer Vaccines?

Cancer vaccines belong to a class of substances known as biological response modifiers. Biological response modifiers work by stimulating or restoring the immune system's ability to fight infections and disease. There are two broad types of cancer vaccines:

- **Preventive (or prophylactic) vaccines,** which are intended to prevent cancer from developing in healthy people
- **Treatment (or therapeutic) vaccines,** which are intended to treat an existing cancer by strengthening the body's natural immune response against the cancer. Treatment vaccines are a form of immunotherapy.

Two types of cancer preventive vaccines (human papillomavirus (HPV) vaccines and hepatitis B virus (HBV) vaccines) are available in the United States, and one treatment vaccine (for metastatic prostate cancer) is available.

How Do Cancer Preventive Vaccines Work?

Cancer preventive vaccines target infectious agents that cause or contribute to the development of cancer. They are similar to traditional vaccines, which help prevent infectious diseases, such as measles or polio, by protecting the body against infection. Both cancer preventive vaccines and traditional vaccines are based on antigens that are carried by infectious agents and that are relatively easy for the immune system to recognize as foreign. Most preventive vaccines, including those aimed at cancer-causing viruses (HBV and HPV), stimulate the production of antibodies that bind to specific targeted microbes and block their ability to cause infection.

What Cancer Preventive Vaccines Are Approved in the United States?

- **Human papillomavirus (HPV) vaccines.** Persistent infections with high-risk HPV types can cause cervical cancer, anal cancer, oropharyngeal cancer, and vaginal, vulvar, and penile cancers. Three vaccines are approved by the U.S. Food and Drug Administration (FDA) to prevent HPV infection: Gardasil®, Gardasil 9®, and Cervarix®. Gardasil and Gardasil 9 are approved for use in females ages 9 through 26 for the prevention of HPV-caused cervical, vulvar, vaginal, and anal cancers; precancerous cervical, vulvar, vaginal, and anal lesions; and genital warts. Gardasil and Gardasil 9 are also approved for use in males for the prevention of HPV-caused anal cancer, precancerous anal lesions, and genital warts. Gardasil is approved for use in males ages 9 through 26, and Gardasil 9 is approved for use in males ages 9 through 15. Cervarix is approved for use in females ages 9 through 25 for the prevention of cervical cancer caused by HPV.
- **Hepatitis B virus (HBV) vaccines.** Chronic HBV infection can lead to liver cancer. The FDA has approved multiple vaccines that protect against HBV infection. Two vaccines, Engerix-B and Recombivax HB, protect against HBV infection only. Both vaccines are approved for use in individuals of all ages. Several other vaccines protect against infection with HBV as well as other viruses. Twinrix protects against HBV and hepatitis A virus, and Pediarix against HBV, poliovirus, and the bacteria that cause diphtheria, tetanus, and pertussis. Twinrix is approved for use in persons 18 years of age or older. Pediarix is

approved for use in infants whose mothers are negative for the HBV surface antigen (HBsAg) and is given as early as 6 weeks of age through 6 years of age. The original HBV vaccine was approved by the FDA in 1981, making it the first cancer preventive vaccine to be successfully developed and marketed. Today, most children in the United States are vaccinated against HBV shortly after birth.

How Are Cancer Treatment Vaccines Designed to Work?

Cancer treatment vaccines are used to treat cancers that have already developed. They are intended to delay or stop cancer cell growth; to cause tumor shrinkage; to prevent cancer from coming back; or to eliminate cancer cells that have not been killed by other forms of treatment.

Cancer treatment vaccines are designed to work by activating cytotoxic T cells and directing them to recognize and act against specific types of cancer or by inducing the production of antibodies that bind to molecules on the surface of cancer cells. To do so, treatment vaccines introduce one or more antigens into the body, usually by injection, where they cause an immune response that results in T cell activation or antibody production. Antibodies recognize and bind to antigens on the surface of cancer cells, whereas T cells can also detect cancer antigens inside cancer cells.

Producing effective treatment vaccines has proven more difficult and challenging than developing cancer preventive vaccines. To be effective, cancer treatment vaccines must achieve two goals. First, like preventive vaccines, cancer treatment vaccines must stimulate specific immune responses against the correct target. Second, the immune responses must be powerful enough to overcome the barriers that cancer cells use to protect themselves from attack by killer T cells.

Has the FDA Approved Any Cancer Treatment Vaccines?

In April 2010, the FDA approved the first cancer treatment vaccine. This vaccine, sipuleucel-T (Provenge®), is approved for use in some men with metastatic prostate cancer. It is designed to stimulate an immune response to prostatic acid phosphatase (PAP), an antigen that is found on most prostate cancer cells. In clinical trials, sipuleucel-T increased the survival of men with a certain type of metastatic prostate cancer by about four months.

Unlike some other cancer treatment vaccines, sipuleucel-T is customized to each patient. The vaccine is created by isolating immune system cells called dendritic cells, which are a type of antigen-presenting cell (APC), from a patient's blood through a procedure called leukapheresis. These cells are sent to the vaccine manufacturer, where they are cultured together with a protein called PAP-GM-CSF. This protein consists of PAP linked to a protein called granulocyte-macrophage colony-stimulating factor (GM-CSF). The GM-CSF stimulates the immune system and enhances antigen presentation.

APC cells cultured with PAP-GM-CSF constitute the active component of sipuleucel-T. The cells are returned to the patient's treating physician and infused into the patient. Patients receive three treatments, usually 2 weeks apart, with each round of treatment requiring the same manufacturing process. Although the precise mechanism of action of sipuleucel-T is not known, it appears that the APCs that have taken up PAP-GM-CSF stimulate T cells of the immune system to kill tumor cells that express PAP.

The FDA approved the first oncolytic virus therapy, talimogene laherparepvec (T-VEC, or Imlygic®) for the treatment of some patients with metastatic melanoma that cannot be surgically removed. In addition to infecting and lysing cancer cells when injected directly into melanoma tumors, T-VEC induces responses in noninjected lesions, suggesting that it triggers an antitumor immune response similar to those of other anticancer vaccines.

How Are Cancer Vaccines Made?

All cancer preventive vaccines approved by the FDA to date have been made using antigens from microbes that cause or contribute to the development of cancer. These include antigens from HBV and specific types of HPV. These antigens are proteins that help make up the outer surface of the viruses. Because only part of these microbes is used, the resulting vaccines are not infectious and, therefore, cannot cause disease.

Researchers are also creating synthetic versions of antigens in the laboratory for use in cancer preventive vaccines. In doing this, they often modify the chemical structure of the antigens to stimulate immune responses that are stronger than those caused by the original antigens.

Similarly, cancer treatment vaccines are made using cancer-associated antigens or modified versions of them. Antigens that have been used thus far include proteins, carbohydrates (sugars), glycoproteins or glycopeptides (carbohydrate–protein combinations), and gangliosides (carbohydrate–lipid combinations).

Cancer treatment vaccines are also being developed using weakened or killed cancer cells that carry a specific cancer-associated antigen(s) or immune cells that are modified to present such an antigen(s) on their surface. These cells can come from a patient himself or herself (called an autologous vaccine, such as with sipuleucel-T) or from another patient (called an allogeneic vaccine).

Some cancer vaccines in late-stage development use viruses, yeast, or bacteria as vehicles (or vectors) to deliver one or more antigens into the body. The vectors themselves are naturally immunogenic (that is, they can stimulate an immune response) but are modified so that they cannot cause disease.

Other types of cancer treatment vaccines that are under development include those made using molecules of deoxyribonucleic acid (DNA) or ribonucleic acid (RNA) that contain the genetic instructions for cancer-associated antigens. The DNA or RNA can be injected alone into a patient as a "naked nucleic acid" vaccine, or packaged into a harmless virus. After the naked nucleic acid or virus is injected into the body, the DNA or RNA is taken up by cells, which begin to manufacture the tumor-associated antigens. Researchers hope that the cells will make enough of the tumor-associated antigens to stimulate a strong immune response.

A number of different cancer-associated antigens are now being used to make experimental cancer treatment vaccines. Some of these antigens are found on or in many or most types of cancer cells. Others are unique to specific cancer types.

Are Adjuvants Used with Cancer Vaccines?

Substances known as adjuvants are often added to vaccines to boost their ability to induce potent anticancer immune responses.

Adjuvants used for cancer vaccines come from many different sources. Some microbes, such as the bacterium Bacillus Calmette-Guérin (BCG), can serve as adjuvants. Substances produced by bacteria, such as Detox B (an oil droplet emulsion of monophosphoryl lipid A and mycobacterial cell wall skeleton), are also frequently used as adjuvants. Biological products derived from nonmicrobial organisms can also be used as adjuvants. One example is keyhole limpet hemocyanin (KLH), which is a large protein produced by a marine mollusk. Attaching antigens to KLH has been shown to increase their ability to stimulate immune responses. Even some nonbiological substances, such as an emulsified oil known as montanide ISA–51, can be used as adjuvants.

Natural or synthetic cytokines can also be used as adjuvants. Cytokines are substances that are naturally produced by white blood cells to regulate and fine-tune immune responses. Some cytokines increase the activity of B cells and killer T cells, whereas other cytokines suppress the activities of these cells. Cytokines frequently used in cancer treatment vaccines or given together with them include interleukin 2 (IL2, also known as aldesleukin), interferon alpha, and granulocyte-macrophage colony-stimulating factor (GM–CSF, also known as sargramostim).

Do Cancer Vaccines Have Side Effects?

Before any vaccine is licensed, the FDA must conclude that it is both safe and effective. Vaccines intended to prevent or treat cancer appear to have safety profiles comparable to those of other vaccines. However, the side effects of cancer vaccines can vary among vaccine formulations and from one person to another.

The most commonly reported side effect of cancer vaccines is inflammation at the site of injection, including redness, pain, swelling, warming of the skin, itchiness, and occasionally a rash.

People sometimes experience flu-like symptoms after receiving a cancer vaccine, including fever, chills, weakness, dizziness, nausea or vomiting, muscle ache, fatigue, headache, and occasional breathing difficulties. Blood pressure may also be affected. These side effects, which usually last for only a short time, indicate that the body is responding to the vaccine and making an immune response, as it does when exposed to a virus.

Other, more serious health problems have been reported in smaller numbers of people after receiving a cancer vaccine. These problems may or may not have been caused by the vaccine. The reported problems have included asthma, appendicitis, pelvic inflammatory disease, and certain autoimmune diseases, including arthritis and systemic lupus erythematosus.

Vaccines that use cells or microbes might have additional side effects. For example, serious side effects of sipuleucel-T include infection near the site of injection and blood in the urine.

Vaccines, like any other medication affecting the immune system, can cause adverse effects that may prove life threatening. For example, severe hypersensitivity (allergic) reactions to specific vaccine ingredients have occurred following vaccination. However, such severe reactions are rare.

Can Cancer Treatment Vaccines Be Combined with Other Types of Cancer Therapy?

Yes. In many of the clinical trials of cancer treatment vaccines that are now underway, vaccines are being given with other forms of cancer therapy. Therapies that have been combined with cancer treatment vaccines include surgery, chemotherapy, radiation therapy, and some forms of targeted therapy, including therapies that are intended to boost immune system responses against cancer.

Several studies have suggested that cancer treatment vaccines may be most effective when given in combination with other forms of cancer therapy. For example, preclinical studies and early-phase clinical trials have demonstrated that radiation therapy can enhance the efficacy of cancer treatment vaccines. In addition, in some clinical trials, cancer treatment vaccines have appeared to increase the effectiveness of other cancer therapies.

Additional evidence suggests that surgical removal of large tumors may enhance the effectiveness of cancer treatment vaccines. In patients with extensive disease, the immune system may be overwhelmed by the cancer. Surgical removal of the tumor may make it easier for the body to develop an effective immune response.

Researchers are also designing clinical trials to answer questions such as whether cancer treatment vaccines work best when they are administered before, after, or at the same time as other therapies. Answers to such questions may not only provide information about how best to use a specific cancer treatment vaccine but also reveal additional basic principles to guide the future development of combination therapies involving vaccines.

What Additional Research Is Underway to Improve Cancer Treatment Vaccines?

Advances in understanding how cancer cells escape recognition and attack by the immune system are now giving researchers the knowledge required to design cancer treatment vaccines that can accomplish both goals.

Although researchers have identified many cancer-associated antigens, these molecules vary widely in their ability to stimulate a strong anticancer immune response. Two major areas of research are aimed at addressing this issue. One involves the identification of novel cancer-associated antigens, or neoantigens, that may prove more effective in stimulating immune responses than the already known antigens.

For example, a neoantigen-based personalized vaccine approach that is in early-phase clinical testing involves the identification and targeting of patient-specific mutated antigens to create treatment vaccines for patients with glioblastoma and melanoma. The other major research area involves the development of methods to enhance the ability of cancer-associated antigens to stimulate the immune system. Research is also under way to determine how to combine multiple antigens within a single cancer treatment vaccine to produce optimal anticancer immune responses.

Improving our understanding of the basic biology underlying how immune system cells and cancer cells interact will be very important for developing cancer vaccines. New technologies are being created as part of this effort. For example, a new type of imaging technology allows researchers to observe killer T cells and cancer cells interacting inside the body.

Researchers are also trying to identify the mechanisms by which cancer cells evade or suppress anticancer immune responses. A better understanding of how cancer cells manipulate the immune system could lead to the development of drugs that block those processes, thereby improving the effectiveness of cancer treatment vaccines.

For example, some cancer cells produce chemical signals that attract white blood cells known as regulatory T cells, or T regs, to a tumor site. T regs often release cytokines that suppress the activity of nearby killer T cells. The combination of a cancer treatment vaccine with a drug that prevents the inactivation of killer T cells might improve the vaccine's effectiveness in generating potent killer T cell antitumor responses.

Immune checkpoint modulators may also improve the effectiveness of cancer vaccines. These modulators target another immune regulatory mechanism used by cancer cells to evade destruction, one that involves immune checkpoint proteins such as PD-1, which is expressed on the surface of T cells. The binding of PD1 to specific partner proteins (or ligands), called PD-L1 and PD-L2, on the surface of some normal cells or cancer cells creates an "off" signal that tells the T cell not to mount an immune response against those cells. (This binding keeps the immune system from overreacting against normal cells and prevents autoimmunity.) Some tumor cells express high levels of PD-L1, which causes T cells to shut down and helps the cancer cells evade immune destruction. Antibodies that block the binding of an immune checkpoint protein to its ligand on a cancer cell remove this "off" signal and allows an immune response to proceed against the cancer cells.

Several such antibodies have been approved by the FDA for treatment of some cancers and are showing promising effects in other cancers. Because these agents allow T cells against cancer to be more effective, it is expected that they will also improve the effectiveness of cancer vaccines. Indeed, they have been found to do so in animal models, and clinical trials that combine a vaccine with PD1 or PD-L1 inhibition are ongoing.

A number of vaccines designed to treat specific cancers are currently under development. These include dendritic cell vaccines for metastatic renal cell carcinoma, glioblastoma, and metastatic hormone-refractory prostate cancer; autologous tumor cell vaccines for colorectal cancer and follicular lymphoma; anti-idiotype vaccines for lymphomas and some solid tumors; vaccines designed to stimulate an immune response against hormones required for the growth and survival of gastrointestinal malignancies; allogeneic vaccines for lung cancer; and a DNA-based vaccine for metastatic breast cancer.

Chapter 12

Common Cancer Myths and Misconceptions

Certain popular ideas about how cancer starts and spreads—though scientifically wrong—can seem to make sense, especially when those ideas are rooted in old theories. But wrong ideas about cancer can lead to needless worry and even hinder good prevention and treatment decisions.

Is Cancer a Death Sentence?

In the United States, the likelihood of dying from cancer has dropped steadily since the 1990s. The 5-year survival rates for some cancers, such as breast, prostate, and thyroid cancers, now exceed 90 percent. The 5-year survival rate for all cancers combined is currently about 66 percent.

It is important to note, however, that these rates are based on data from large numbers of people. How long an individual cancer patient will live and whether he or she will die from the disease depend on many factors, including whether the cancer is slow or fast growing, how much the cancer has spread in the body, whether effective treatments are available, the person's overall health, and more.

This chapter includes text excerpted from "Common Cancer Myths and Misconceptions," National Cancer Institute (NCI), February 3, 2014. Reviewed March 2018.

Will Eating Sugar Make My Cancer Worse?

No. Although research has shown that cancer cells consume more sugar (glucose) than normal cells, no studies have shown that eating sugar will make your cancer worse or that, if you stop eating sugar, your cancer will shrink or disappear. However, a high-sugar diet may contribute to excess weight gain, and obesity is associated with an increased risk of developing several types of cancer.

Do Artificial Sweeteners Cause Cancer?

No. Researchers have conducted studies on the safety of the artificial sweeteners (sugar substitutes) saccharin (Sweet 'N Low®, Sweet Twin®, NectaSweet®); cyclamate; aspartame (Equal®, NutraSweet®); acesulfame potassium (Sunett®, Sweet One®); sucralose (Splenda®); and neotame and found no evidence that they cause cancer in humans. All of these artificial sweeteners except for cyclamate have been approved by the U.S. Food and Drug Administration (FDA) for sale in the United States.

Is Cancer Contagious?

In general, no. Cancer is not a contagious disease that easily spreads from person to person. The only situation in which cancer can spread from one person to another is in the case of organ or tissue transplantation. A person who receives an organ or tissue from a donor who had cancer in the past may be at increased risk of developing a transplant-related cancer in the future. However, that risk is extremely low—about two cases of cancer per 10,000 organ transplants. Doctors avoid the use of organs or tissue from donors who have a history of cancer.

In some people, cancers may be caused by certain viruses (some types of human papillomavirus, or HPV, for example) and bacteria (such as *Helicobacter pylori*). While a virus or bacterium can spread from person to person, the cancers they sometimes cause cannot spread from person to person.

Does My Attitude—Positive or Negative—Determine My Risk of, or Likely Recovery from, Cancer?

To date, there is no convincing scientific evidence that links a person's "attitude" to his or her risk of developing or dying from cancer.

If you have cancer, it's normal to feel sad, angry, or discouraged sometimes and positive or upbeat at other times. People with a positive attitude may be more likely to maintain social connections and stay active, and physical activity and emotional support may help you cope with your cancer.

Can Cancer Surgery or a Tumor Biopsy Cause Cancer to Spread in the Body?

The chance that surgery will cause cancer to spread to other parts of the body is extremely low. Following standard procedures, surgeons use special methods and take many steps to prevent cancer cells from spreading during biopsies or surgery to remove tumors. For example, if they must remove tissue from more than one area of the body, they use different surgical tools for each area.

Will Cancer Get Worse If Exposed to Air?

No. Exposure to air will not make tumors grow faster or cause cancer to spread to other parts of the body.

Do Cell Phones Cause Cancer?

No, not according to the best studies completed so far. Cancer is caused by genetic mutations, and cell phones emit a type of low-frequency energy that does not damage genes.

Do Power Lines Cause Cancer?

No, not according to the best studies completed so far. Power lines emit both electric and magnetic energy. The electric energy emitted by power lines is easily shielded or weakened by walls and other objects. The magnetic energy emitted by power lines is a low-frequency form of radiation that does not damage genes.

Are There Herbal Products That Can Cure Cancer?

No. Although some studies suggest that alternative or complementary therapies, including some herbs, may help patients cope with the side effects of cancer treatment, no herbal products have been shown to be effective for treating cancer. In fact, some herbal products may be harmful when taken during chemotherapy or radiation therapy because they may interfere with how these treatments work. Cancer patients should talk with their doctor about any complementary and alternative medicine products—including vitamins and herbal supplements—they may be using.

If Someone in My Family Has Cancer, Am I Likely to Get Cancer, Too?

Not necessarily. Cancer is caused by harmful changes (mutations) in genes. Only about 5–10 percent of cancers are caused by harmful mutations that are inherited from a person's parents. In families with an inherited cancer-causing mutation, multiple family members will often develop the same type of cancer. These cancers are called "familial" or "hereditary" cancers.

The remaining 90–95 percent of cancers are caused by mutations that happen during a person's lifetime as a natural result of aging and exposure to environmental factors, such as tobacco smoke and radiation. These cancers are called "nonhereditary" or "spontaneous" cancers.

If No One in My Family Has Had Cancer, Does That Mean I'm Risk-Free?

No. Based on the most recent data, about 40 percent of men and women will be diagnosed with cancer at some point during their lives. Most cancers are caused by genetic changes that occur throughout a person's lifetime as a natural result of aging and exposure to environmental factors, such as tobacco smoke and radiation. Other factors, such as what kind of food you eat, how much you eat, and whether you exercise, may also influence your risk of developing cancer.

Do Antiperspirants or Deodorants Cause Breast Cancer?

No. The best studies so far have found no evidence linking the chemicals typically found in antiperspirants and deodorants with changes in breast tissue.

Does Hair Dye Use Increase the Risk of Cancer?

There is no convincing scientific evidence that personal hair dye use increases the risk of cancer. Some studies suggest, however, that hairdressers and barbers who are regularly exposed to large quantities of hair dye and other chemical products may have an increased risk of bladder cancer.

Part Two

Common Types of Cancer

Chapter 13

Brain and Spinal Cord Tumors

General Information about Adult Central Nervous System Tumors

Brain and Its Functions

The brain controls many important body functions.
The brain has three major parts:

- The **cerebrum** is the largest part of the brain. It is at the top of the head. The cerebrum controls thinking, learning, problem solving, emotions, speech, reading, writing, and voluntary movement.
- The **cerebellum** is in the lower back of the brain (near the middle of the back of the head). It controls movement, balance, and posture.
- The **brainstem** connects the brain to the spinal cord. It is in the lowest part of the brain (just above the back of the neck). The brainstem controls breathing, heart rate, and the nerves and muscles used to see, hear, walk, talk, and eat.

This chapter includes text excerpted from "Adult Central Nervous System Tumors Treatment (PDQ®)—Patient Version," National Cancer Institute (NCI), January 12, 2018.

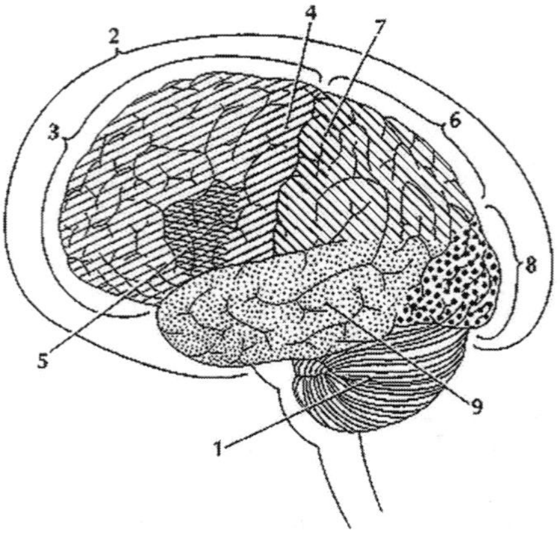

Figure 13.1. *Anatomy of Brain* (Source: "Brain Basics: Know Your Brain," National Institute of Neurological Disorders and Stroke (NINDS).)

Role of Spinal Cord

The spinal cord is a column of nerve tissue that runs from the brainstem down the center of the back. It is covered by three thin layers of tissue called membranes. These membranes are surrounded by the vertebrae (back bones). Spinal cord nerves carry messages between the brain and the rest of the body, such as a message from the brain to cause muscles to move or a message from the skin to the brain to feel touch.

What Is an Adult Central Nervous System Tumor?

An adult central nervous system tumor is a disease in which abnormal cells form in the tissues of the brain and/or spinal cord. There are many types of brain and spinal cord tumors. The tumors are formed by the abnormal growth of cells and may begin in different parts of the brain or spinal cord. Together, the brain and spinal cord make up the central nervous system (CNS).

The tumors may be either benign (not cancer) or malignant (cancer):

- **Benign brain and spinal cord tumors** grow and press on nearby areas of the brain. They rarely spread into other tissues and may recur (come back).
- **Malignant brain and spinal cord tumors** are likely to grow quickly and spread into other brain tissue.

When a tumor grows into or presses on an area of the brain, it may stop that part of the brain from working the way it should. Both benign and malignant brain tumors cause signs and symptoms and need treatment. Brain and spinal cord tumors can occur in both adults and children. However, treatment for children may be different than treatment for adults.

What Is a Metastatic Brain Tumor?

Tumors that start in the brain are called primary brain tumors. Primary brain tumors may spread to other parts of the brain or to the spine. They rarely spread to other parts of the body.

Often, tumors found in the brain have started somewhere else in the body and spread to one or more parts of the brain. These are called metastatic brain tumors (or brain metastases). Metastatic brain tumors are more common than primary brain tumors.

Up to half of metastatic brain tumors are from lung cancer. Other types of cancer that commonly spread to the brain include:

- Melanoma
- Breast cancer
- Colon cancer
- Kidney cancer
- Nasopharyngeal cancer
- Cancer of unknown primary site

Cancer may spread to the leptomeninges (the two innermost membranes covering the brain and spinal cord). This is called leptomeningeal carcinomatosis. The most common cancers that spread to the leptomeninges include:

- Breast cancer
- Lung cancer
- Leukemia
- Lymphoma

What Are the Types of Brain and Spinal Cord Tumors?

There are different types of brain and spinal cord tumors. Brain and spinal cord tumors are named based on the type of cell they formed in and where the tumor first formed in the CNS. The grade of a tumor may be used to tell the difference between slow-growing and fast-growing types of the tumor. The World Health Organization (WHO) tumor grades are based on how abnormal the cancer cells look under a microscope and how quickly the tumor is likely to grow and spread.

WHO Tumor Grading System

- **Grade I (low-grade).** The tumor cells look more like normal cells under a microscope and grow and spread more slowly than grade II, III, and IV tumor cells. They rarely spread into nearby tissues. Grade I brain tumors may be cured if they are completely removed by surgery.
- **Grade II.** The tumor cells grow and spread more slowly than grade III and IV tumor cells. They may spread into nearby tissue and may recur (come back). Some tumors may become a higher-grade tumor.
- **Grade III.** The tumor cells look very different from normal cells under a microscope and grow more quickly than grade I and II tumor cells. They are likely to spread into nearby tissue.
- **Grade IV (high-grade).** The tumor cells do not look like normal cells under a microscope and grow and spread very quickly. There may be areas of dead cells in the tumor. Grade IV tumors usually cannot be cured.

Primary Brain and Spinal Cord Tumors

The following types of primary tumors can form in the brain or spinal cord:

Astrocytic Tumors

An astrocytic tumor begins in star-shaped brain cells called astrocytes, which help keep nerve cells healthy. An astrocyte is a type of glial cell. Glial cells sometimes form tumors called gliomas. Astrocytic tumors include the following:

- **Brainstem glioma (usually high grade).** A brainstem glioma forms in the brainstem, which is the part of the brain connected to the spinal cord. It is often a high-grade tumor, which spreads widely through the brainstem and is hard to cure. Brainstem gliomas are rare in adults.
- **Pineal astrocytic tumor (any grade).** A pineal astrocytic tumor forms in tissue around the pineal gland and may be any grade. The pineal gland is a tiny organ in the brain that makes

melatonin, a hormone that helps control the sleeping and waking cycle.

- **Pilocytic astrocytoma (grade I).** A pilocytic astrocytoma grows slowly in the brain or spinal cord. It may be in the form of a cyst and rarely spreads into nearby tissues. Pilocytic astrocytomas can often be cured.
- **Diffuse astrocytoma (grade II).** A diffuse astrocytoma grows slowly, but often spreads into nearby tissues. The tumor cells look something like normal cells. In some cases, a diffuse astrocytoma can be cured. It is also called a low-grade diffuse astrocytoma.
- **Anaplastic astrocytoma (grade III).** An anaplastic astrocytoma grows quickly and spreads into nearby tissues. The tumor cells look different from normal cells. This type of tumor usually cannot be cured. An anaplastic astrocytoma is also called a malignant astrocytoma or high-grade astrocytoma.
- **Glioblastoma (grade IV).** A glioblastoma grows and spreads very quickly. The tumor cells look very different from normal cells. This type of tumor usually cannot be cured. It is also called glioblastoma multiforme.

Oligodendroglial Tumors

An oligodendroglial tumor begins in brain cells called oligodendrocytes, which help keep nerve cells healthy. An oligodendrocyte is a type of glial cell. Oligodendrocytes sometimes form tumors called oligodendrogliomas. Grades of oligodendroglial tumors include the following:

- **Oligodendroglioma (grade II):** An oligodendroglioma grows slowly, but often spreads into nearby tissues. The tumor cells look something like normal cells. In some cases, an oligodendroglioma can be cured.
- **Anaplastic oligodendroglioma (grade III):** An anaplastic oligodendroglioma grows quickly and spreads into nearby tissues. The tumor cells look different from normal cells. This type of tumor usually cannot be cured.

Mixed Gliomas

A mixed glioma is a brain tumor that has two types of tumor cells in it—oligodendrocytes and astrocytes. This type of mixed tumor is called an oligoastrocytoma.

- **Oligoastrocytoma (grade II).** An oligoastrocytoma is a slow-growing tumor. The tumor cells look something like normal cells. In some cases, an oligoastrocytoma can be cured.
- **Anaplastic oligoastrocytoma (grade III).** An anaplastic oligoastrocytoma grows quickly and spreads into nearby tissues. The tumor cells look different from normal cells. This type of tumor has a worse prognosis than oligoastrocytoma (grade II).

Ependymal Tumors

An ependymal tumor usually begins in cells that line the fluid-filled spaces in the brain and around the spinal cord. An ependymal tumor may also be called an ependymoma. Grades of ependymomas include the following:

- **Ependymoma (grade I or II).** A grade I or II ependymoma grows slowly and has cells that look something like normal cells. There are two types of grade I ependymoma—myxopapillary ependymoma and subependymoma. A grade II ependymoma grows in a ventricle (fluid-filled space in the brain) and its connecting paths or in the spinal cord. In some cases, a grade I or II ependymoma can be cured.
- **Anaplastic ependymoma (grade III).** An anaplastic ependymoma grows quickly and spreads into nearby tissues. The tumor cells look different from normal cells. This type of tumor usually has a worse prognosis than a grade I or II ependymoma.

Medulloblastomas

A medulloblastoma is a type of embryonal tumor. Medulloblastomas are most common in children or young adults.

Pineal Parenchymal Tumors

A pineal parenchymal tumor forms in parenchymal cells or pineocytes, which are the cells that make up most of the pineal gland. These tumors are different from pineal astrocytic tumors. Grades of pineal parenchymal tumors include the following:

- **Pineocytoma (grade II).** A pineocytoma is a slow-growing pineal tumor.
- **Pineoblastoma (grade IV).** A pineoblastoma is a rare tumor that is very likely to spread.

Meningeal Tumors

A meningeal tumor, also called a meningioma, forms in the meninges (thin layers of tissue that cover the brain and spinal cord). It can form from different types of brain or spinal cord cells. Meningiomas are most common in adults. Types of meningeal tumors include the following:

- **Meningioma (grade I).** A grade I meningioma is the most common type of meningeal tumor. A grade I meningioma is a slow-growing tumor. It forms most often in the dura mater. A grade I meningioma can be cured if it is completely removed by surgery.
- **Meningioma (grade II and III).** This is a rare meningeal tumor. It grows quickly and is likely to spread within the brain and spinal cord. The prognosis is worse than a grade I meningioma because the tumor usually cannot be completely removed by surgery.

A hemangiopericytoma is not a meningeal tumor but is treated like a grade II or III meningioma. A hemangiopericytoma usually forms in the dura mater. The prognosis is worse than a grade I meningioma because the tumor usually cannot be completely removed by surgery.

Germ Cell Tumors

A germ cell tumor forms in germ cells, which are the cells that develop into sperm in men or ova (eggs) in women. There are different types of germ cell tumors. These include germinomas, teratomas, embryonal yolk sac carcinomas, and choriocarcinomas. Germ cell tumors can be either benign or malignant.

Craniopharyngioma (Grade I)

A craniopharyngioma is a rare tumor that usually forms in the center of the brain just above the pituitary gland (a pea-sized organ at the bottom of the brain that controls other glands). Craniopharyngiomas can form from different types of brain or spinal cord cells.

What Are the Risk Factors for Central Nervous System Tumor?

Anything that increases your chance of getting a disease is called a risk factor. Having a risk factor does not mean that you will get cancer;

not having risk factors doesn't mean that you will not get cancer. Talk with your doctor if you think you may be at risk. There are few known risk factors for brain tumors. The following conditions may increase the risk of certain types of brain tumors:

- Being exposed to vinyl chloride may increase the risk of glioma
- Infection with the Epstein-Barr virus, having AIDS (acquired immunodeficiency syndrome), or receiving an organ transplant may increase the risk of primary CNS lymphoma
- Having certain genetic syndromes may increase the risk brain tumors:
  - Neurofibromatosis type 1 (NF1) or 2 (NF2)
  - von Hippel-Lindau disease
  - Tuberous sclerosis
  - Li-Fraumeni syndrome
  - Turcot syndrome type 1 or 2
  - Nevoid basal cell carcinoma syndrome

What Causes Adult Brain and Spinal Cord Tumors?

The cause of most adult brain and spinal cord tumors is not known.

What Are the Signs and Symptoms of Adult Brain and Spinal Cord Tumors?

The signs and symptoms of adult brain and spinal cord tumors are not the same in every person.

Signs and symptoms depend on the following:

- Where the tumor forms in the brain or spinal cord
- What the affected part of the brain controls
- The size of the tumor

Signs and symptoms may be caused by CNS tumors or by other conditions, including cancer that has spread to the brain. Check with your doctor if you have any of the following:

Brain Tumor Symptoms

- Morning headache or headache that goes away after vomiting
- Seizures

- Vision, hearing, and speech problems
- Loss of appetite
- Frequent nausea and vomiting
- Changes in personality, mood, ability to focus, or behavior
- Loss of balance and trouble walking
- Weakness
- Unusual sleepiness or change in activity level

Spinal Cord Tumor Symptoms

- Back pain or pain that spreads from the back towards the arms or legs
- A change in bowel habits or trouble urinating
- Weakness or numbness in the arms or legs
- Trouble walking

How Is Adult Brain and Spinal Cord Tumors Diagnosed?

The following tests and procedures may be used:

- **Physical exam and history.** An exam of the body to check general signs of health, including checking for signs of disease, such as lumps or anything else that seems unusual. A history of the patient's health habits and past illnesses and treatments will also be taken.
- **Neurological exam.** A series of questions and tests to check the brain, spinal cord, and nerve function. The exam checks a person's mental status, coordination, and ability to walk normally, and how well the muscles, senses, and reflexes work. This may also be called a neuro exam or a neurologic exam.
- **Visual field exam.** An exam to check a person's field of vision (the total area in which objects can be seen). This test measures both central vision (how much a person can see when looking straight ahead) and peripheral vision (how much a person can see in all other directions while staring straight ahead). Any loss of vision may be a sign of a tumor that has damaged or pressed on the parts of the brain that affect eyesight.

- **Tumor marker test.** A procedure in which a sample of blood, urine, or tissue is checked to measure the amounts of certain substances made by organs, tissues, or tumor cells in the body. Certain substances are linked to specific types of cancer when found in increased levels in the body. These are called tumor markers. This test may be done to diagnose a germ cell tumor.
- **Gene testing.** A laboratory test in which a sample of blood or tissue is tested for changes in a chromosome that has been linked with a certain type of brain tumor. This test may be done to diagnose an inherited syndrome.
- **Computed tomography (CT)/computerized axial tomography (CAT) scan.** A procedure that makes a series of detailed pictures of areas inside the body, taken from different angles. The pictures are made by a computer linked to an X-ray machine. A dye may be injected into a vein or swallowed to help the organs or tissues show up more clearly. This procedure is also called computed tomography, computerized tomography, or computerized axial tomography.
- **Magnetic resonance imaging (MRI) with gadolinium.** A procedure that uses a magnet, radio waves, and a computer to make a series of detailed pictures of the brain and spinal cord. A substance called gadolinium is injected into a vein. The gadolinium collects around the cancer cells so they show up brighter in the picture. This procedure is also called nuclear magnetic resonance imaging (NMRI). MRI is often used to diagnose tumors in the spinal cord. Sometimes a procedure called magnetic resonance spectroscopy (MRS) is done during the MRI scan. An MRS is used to diagnose tumors, based on their chemical makeup.
- **Single photon emission computed tomography (SPECT) scan.** A procedure that uses a special camera linked to a computer to make a 3-dimensional (3D) picture of the brain. A very small amount of a radioactive substance is injected into a vein or inhaled through the nose. As the substance travels through the blood, the camera rotates around the head and takes pictures of the brain. Blood flow and metabolism are higher than normal in areas where cancer cells are growing. These areas will show up brighter in the picture. This procedure may be done just before or after a CT scan. SPECT is used to tell the difference between a primary tumor and a tumor that has spread to the brain from somewhere else in the body.

- **Positron emission tomography (PET) scan.** A procedure to find malignant tumor cells in the body. A small amount of radioactive glucose (sugar) is injected into a vein. The PET scanner rotates around the body and makes a picture of where glucose is being used in the brain. Malignant tumor cells show up brighter in the picture because they are more active and take up more glucose than normal cells do. PET is used to tell the difference between a primary tumor and a tumor that has spread to the brain from somewhere else in the body.

Biopsy

If imaging tests show there may be a brain tumor, a biopsy is usually done. One of the following types of biopsies may be used:

- **Stereotactic biopsy.** When imaging tests show there may be a tumor deep in the brain in a hard to reach place, a stereotactic brain biopsy may be done. This kind of biopsy uses a computer and a 3-dimensional (3D) scanning device to find the tumor and guide the needle used to remove the tissue. A small incision is made in the scalp and a small hole is drilled through the skull. A biopsy needle is inserted through the hole to remove cells or tissues so they can be viewed under a microscope by a pathologist to check for signs of cancer.
- **Open biopsy.** When imaging tests show that there may be a tumor that can be removed by surgery, an open biopsy may be done. A part of the skull is removed in an operation called a craniotomy. A sample of brain tissue is removed and viewed under a microscope by a pathologist. If cancer cells are found, some or all of the tumor may be removed during the same surgery. Tests are done before surgery to find the areas around the tumor that are important for normal brain function. There are also ways to test brain function during surgery. The doctor will use the results of these tests to remove as much of the tumor as possible with the least damage to normal tissue in the brain.

The pathologist checks the biopsy sample to find out the type and grade of brain tumor. The grade of the tumor is based on how the tumor cells look under a microscope and how quickly the tumor is likely to grow and spread.

The following tests may be done on the tumor tissue that is removed:

- **Immunohistochemistry.** A test that uses antibodies to check for certain antigens in a sample of tissue. The antibody is usually linked to a radioactive substance or a dye that causes the tissue to light up under a microscope. This type of test may be used to tell the difference between different types of cancer.
- **Light and electron microscopy.** A laboratory test in which cells in a sample of tissue are viewed under regular and high-powered microscopes to look for certain changes in the cells.
- **Cytogenetic analysis.** A laboratory test in which cells in a sample of tissue are viewed under a microscope to look for certain changes in the chromosomes.

When Biopsy or Surgery Is Not Done

Sometimes a biopsy or surgery cannot be done. For some tumors, a biopsy or surgery cannot be done safely because of where the tumor formed in the brain or spinal cord. These tumors are diagnosed and treated based on the results of imaging tests and other procedures.

Sometimes the results of imaging tests and other procedures show that the tumor is very likely to be benign and a biopsy is not done.

What Is the Prognosis for Adult Brain and Spinal Cord Tumors?

The prognosis (chance of recovery) and treatment options for primary brain and spinal cord tumors depend on the following:

- The type and grade of the tumor
- Where the tumor is in the brain or spinal cord
- Whether the tumor can be removed by surgery
- Whether cancer cells remain after surgery
- Whether there are certain changes in the chromosomes.
- Whether the cancer has just been diagnosed or has recurred (come back)
- The patient's general health

The prognosis and treatment options for metastatic brain and spinal cord tumors depend on the following:

- Whether there are more than two tumors in the brain or spinal cord
- Where the tumor is in the brain or spinal cord
- How well the tumor responds to treatment
- Whether the primary tumor continues to grow or spread

Stages of Adult Central Nervous System Tumors

The extent or spread of cancer is usually described as stages. Brain tumors that begin in the brain may spread to other parts of the brain and spinal cord, but they rarely spread to other parts of the body.

Is There Any Standard Staging System for Adult Brain and Spinal Cord Tumors?

There is no standard staging system for brain and spinal cord tumors.

Treatment Option Overview

Treatment of primary brain and spinal cord tumors is based on the following:

- The type of cell in which the tumor began
- Where the tumor formed in the brain or spinal cord
- The amount of cancer left after surgery
- The grade of the tumor

Treatment of tumors that have spread to the brain from other parts of the body is based on the number of tumors in the brain.

Imaging tests may be repeated after surgery to help plan more treatment. Some of the tests and procedures used to diagnose a brain or spinal cord tumor may be repeated after treatment to find out how much tumor is left.

What Are the Treatment Options for Adult Brain and Spinal Cord Tumors?

Different types of treatment are available for patients with adult brain and spinal cord tumors. Some treatments are standard (the currently used treatment), and some are being tested in clinical trials. A treatment clinical trial is a research study meant to help improve current treatments or obtain information on new treatments for patients with cancer. When clinical trials show that a new treatment is better than the standard treatment, the new treatment may become the standard treatment. Patients may want to think about taking part in a clinical trial. Some clinical trials are open only to patients who have not started treatment.

What Are the Standard Treatment for Adult Brain and Spinal Cord Tumors?

Five types of standard treatment are used:

Active Surveillance

Active surveillance is closely watching a patient's condition but not giving any treatment unless there are changes in test results that show the condition is getting worse. Active surveillance may be used to avoid or delay the need for treatments such as radiation therapy or surgery, which can cause side effects or other problems. During active surveillance, certain exams and tests are done on a regular schedule. Active surveillance may be used for very slow-growing tumors that do not cause symptoms.

Surgery

Surgery may be used to diagnose and treat adult brain and spinal cord tumors. Removing tumor tissue helps decrease pressure of the tumor on nearby parts of the brain.

Even if the doctor removes all the cancer that can be seen at the time of the surgery, some patients may be given chemotherapy or radiation therapy after surgery to kill any cancer cells that are left. Treatment given after the surgery, to lower the risk that the cancer will come back, is called adjuvant therapy.

Radiation Therapy

Radiation therapy is a cancer treatment that uses high-energy X-rays or other types of radiation to kill cancer cells or keep them from growing. There are two types of radiation therapy:

- External radiation therapy uses a machine outside the body to send radiation toward the cancer. Certain ways of giving radiation therapy can help keep radiation from damaging nearby healthy tissue. These types of radiation therapy include the following:

- **Conformal radiation therapy.** Conformal radiation therapy is a type of external radiation therapy that uses a computer to make a 3-dimensional (3D) picture of the tumor and shapes the radiation beams to fit the tumor.
- **Intensity-modulated radiation therapy (IMRT).** IMRT is a type of 3-dimensional (3D) external radiation therapy that uses a computer to make pictures of the size and shape of the tumor. Thin beams of radiation of different intensities (strengths) are aimed at the tumor from many angles.
- **Stereotactic radiosurgery (SRS).** Stereotactic radiosurgery is a type of external radiation therapy. A rigid head frame is attached to the skull to keep the head still during the radiation treatment. A machine aims a single large dose of radiation directly at the tumor. This procedure does not involve surgery. It is also called stereotaxic radiosurgery, radiosurgery, and radiation surgery.

- Internal radiation therapy uses a radioactive substance sealed in needles, seeds, wires, or catheters that are placed directly into or near the cancer.

The way the radiation therapy is given depends on the type and grade of tumor and where it is in the brain or spinal cord. External radiation therapy is used to treat adult central nervous system tumors.

Chemotherapy

Chemotherapy is a cancer treatment that uses drugs to stop the growth of cancer cells, either by killing the cells or by stopping them from dividing. When chemotherapy is taken by mouth or injected into a vein or muscle, the drugs enter the bloodstream and can reach cancer cells throughout the body (systemic chemotherapy). When chemotherapy is placed directly into the cerebrospinal fluid, an organ, or a body cavity such as the abdomen, the drugs mainly affect cancer cells in those areas (regional chemotherapy). Combination chemotherapy is treatment using more than one anticancer drug. To treat brain tumors, a wafer that dissolves may be used to deliver an anticancer drug directly to the brain tumor site after the tumor has been removed by surgery. The way the chemotherapy is given depends on the type and grade of tumor and where it is in the brain.

Anticancer drugs given by mouth or vein to treat brain and spinal cord tumors cannot cross the blood-brain barrier and enter the fluid that surrounds the brain and spinal cord. Instead, an anticancer drug is injected into the fluid-filled space to kill cancer cells there. This is called intrathecal chemotherapy.

Targeted Therapy

Targeted therapy is a type of treatment that uses drugs or other substances to identify and attack specific cancer cells without harming normal cells.

Monoclonal antibody therapy is a type of targeted therapy that uses antibodies made in the laboratory from a single type of immune system cell. These antibodies can identify substances on cancer cells or normal substances that may help cancer cells grow. The antibodies attach to the substances and kill the cancer cells, block their growth, or keep them from spreading. Monoclonal antibodies are given by infusion. They may be used alone or to carry drugs, toxins, or radioactive material directly to cancer cells.

Bevacizumab is a monoclonal antibody that binds to a protein called vascular endothelial growth factor (VEGF) and may prevent the growth of new blood vessels that tumors need to grow. Bevacizumab is used in the treatment of recurrent glioblastoma.

Other types of targeted therapies are being studied for adult brain tumors, including tyrosine kinase inhibitors and new VEGF inhibitors.

What Can Be Done to Lessen the Problems Caused by the Disease or Its Treatment?

Supportive care is given to lessen the problems caused by the disease or its treatment. This therapy controls problems or side effects caused by the disease or its treatment and improves quality of life. For brain tumors, supportive care includes drugs to control seizures and fluid buildup or swelling in the brain.

What Types of Treatment Are Being Tested in Clinical Trials?

New types of treatment are being tested in clinical trials.

Proton Beam Radiation Therapy

Proton beam radiation therapy is a type of high-energy, external radiation therapy that uses streams of protons (small, positively-charged pieces of matter) to make radiation. This type of radiation kills tumor cells with little damage to nearby tissues. It is used to treat cancers of the head, neck, and spine and organs such as the brain, eye, lung, and prostate. Proton beam radiation is different from X-ray radiation.

Biologic Therapy

Biologic therapy is a treatment that uses the patient's immune system to fight cancer. Substances made by the body or made in a laboratory are used to boost, direct, or restore the body's natural defenses against cancer. This type of cancer treatment is also called biotherapy or immunotherapy.

Biologic therapy is being studied for the treatment of some types of brain tumors. Treatments may include the following:

- Dendritic cell vaccine therapy
- Gene therapy

Is There a Need for Follow-Up Tests?

Follow-up tests may be needed. Some of the tests that were done to diagnose the cancer or to find out the stage of the cancer may be repeated. Some tests will be repeated in order to see how well the treatment is working. Decisions about whether to continue, change, or stop treatment may be based on the results of these tests.

Some of the tests will continue to be done from time to time after treatment has ended. The results of these tests can show if your condition has changed or if the cancer has recurred (come back). These tests are sometimes called follow-up tests or check-ups.

The following tests and procedures may be used to check whether a brain tumor has come back after treatment:

- **SPECT scan (single photon emission computed tomography scan).** A procedure that uses a special camera linked to a computer to make a 3D picture of the brain. A very small amount of a radioactive substance is injected into a vein or inhaled through the nose. As the substance travels through the blood, the camera rotates around the head and takes pictures of the brain. Blood flow and metabolism are higher than normal in areas where cancer cells are growing. These areas will show up brighter in the picture. This procedure may be done just before or after a CT scan.

- **PET scan (positron emission tomography scan).** A procedure to find malignant tumor cells in the body. A small amount of radioactive glucose (sugar) is injected into a vein. The PET scanner rotates around the body and makes a picture of where glucose is being used in the brain. Malignant tumor cells show up brighter in the picture because they are more active and take up more glucose than normal cells do.

Chapter 14

Childhood Brain and Spinal Cord Tumors

General Information about Childhood Brain and Spinal Cord Tumors

A childhood brain or spinal cord tumor is a disease in which abnormal cells form in the tissues of the brain or spinal cord. There are many types of childhood brain and spinal cord tumors. The tumors are formed by the abnormal growth of cells and may begin in different areas of the brain or spinal cord. The tumors may be benign (not cancer) or malignant (cancer). Benign brain tumors (BBT) grow and press on nearby areas of the brain. They rarely spread into other tissues. Malignant brain tumors (MBT) are likely to grow quickly and spread into other brain tissue. When a tumor grows into or presses on an area of the brain, it may stop that part of the brain from working the way it should. Both benign and malignant brain tumors can cause signs or symptoms and need treatment.

Together, the brain and spinal cord make up the central nervous system (CNS).

This chapter includes text excerpted from "Childhood Brain and Spinal Cord Tumors Treatment Overview (PDQ®)—Patient Version," National Cancer Institute (NCI), February 5, 2018.

Brain and Its Functions

The brain controls many important body functions
The brain has three major parts:

- The **cerebrum** is the largest part of the brain. It is at the top of the head. The cerebrum controls thinking, learning, problem-solving, emotions, speech, reading, writing, and voluntary movement.
- The **cerebellum** is in the lower back of the brain (near the middle of the back of the head). It controls movement, balance, and posture.
- The **brainstem** connects the brain to the spinal cord. It is in the lowest part of the brain (just above the back of the neck). The brainstem controls breathing, heart rate, and the nerves, and muscles used in seeing, hearing, walking, talking, and eating.

The Spinal Cord and Its Role

The spinal cord connects the brain with nerves in most parts of the body. It is a column of nerve tissue that runs from the brainstem down the center of the back. It is covered by three thin layers of tissue called membranes. These membranes are surrounded by the vertebrae (back bones). Spinal cord nerves carry messages between the brain and the rest of the body, such as a message from the brain to cause muscles to move or a message from the skin to the brain to feel touch.

Brain and Spinal Cord Tumors

Although cancer is rare in children, brain and spinal cord tumors are a common type of childhood cancer. Although cancer is rare in children, brain and spinal cord tumors are the third most common type of childhood cancer, after leukemia and lymphoma. Brain tumors can occur in both children and adults. Treatment for children is usually different than treatment for adults. Metastatic tumors are formed by cancer cells that begin in other parts of the body and spread to the brain or spinal cord. The cause of most childhood brain and spinal cord tumors is unknown.

Signs and Symptoms of Childhood Brain and Spinal Cord Tumors

The signs and symptoms of childhood brain and spinal cord tumors are not the same in every child.

Signs and symptoms depend on the following:

- Where the tumor forms in the brain or spinal cord
- The size of the tumor
- How fast the tumor grows
- The child's age and development

Signs and symptoms may be caused by childhood brain and spinal cord tumors or by other conditions, including cancer that has spread to the brain. Check with your child's doctor if your child has any of the following signs and symptoms of brain tumor:

- Morning headache or headache that goes away after vomiting
- Frequent nausea and vomiting
- Vision, hearing, and speech problems
- Loss of balance and trouble walking
- Unusual sleepiness or change in activity level
- Unusual changes in personality or behavior
- Seizures
- Increase in the head size (in infants)

The signs and symptoms of spinal cord tumor include:

- Back pain or pain that spreads from the back towards the arms or legs
- A change in bowel habits or trouble urinating
- Weakness in the legs
- Trouble walking

In addition to these signs and symptoms of brain and spinal cord tumors, some children are unable to reach certain growth and development milestones such as sitting up, walking, and talking in sentences.

Diagnosis of Childhood Brain and Spinal Cord Tumors

The following tests and procedures may be used:

- **Physical exam and history.** An exam of the body to check general signs of health, including checking for signs of disease,

such as lumps or anything else that seems unusual. A history of the patient's health habits and past illnesses and treatments will also be taken.

- **Neurological exam.** A series of questions and tests to check the brain, spinal cord, and nerve function. The exam checks a person's mental status, coordination, and ability to walk normally, and how well the muscles, senses, and reflexes work. This may also be called a neuro exam or a neurologic exam.
- **Magnetic resonance imaging (MRI) with gadolinium.** A procedure that uses a magnet, radio waves, and a computer to make a series of detailed pictures of the brain and spinal cord. A substance called gadolinium is injected into a vein. The gadolinium collects around the cancer cells so they show up brighter in the picture. This procedure is also called nuclear magnetic resonance imaging (NMRI).
- **Serum tumor marker test.** A procedure in which a sample of blood is examined to measure the amounts of certain substances released into the blood by organs, tissues, or tumor cells in the body. Certain substances are linked to specific types of cancer when found in increased levels in the blood. These are called tumor markers.

Most Childhood Brain Tumors Are Diagnosed and Removed in Surgery

If doctors think there might be a brain tumor, a biopsy may be done to remove a sample of tissue. For tumors in the brain, the biopsy is done by removing part of the skull and using a needle to remove a sample of tissue. A pathologist views the tissue under a microscope to look for cancer cells. If cancer cells are found, the doctor may remove as much tumor as safely possible during the same surgery. The pathologist checks the cancer cells to find out the type and grade of brain tumor. The grade of the tumor is based on how abnormal the cancer cells look under a microscope and how quickly the tumor is likely to grow and spread.

The following test may be done on the sample of tissue that is removed:

- **Immunohistochemistry.** A test that uses antibodies to check for certain antigens in a sample of tissue. The antibody is usually linked to a radioactive substance or a dye that causes the tissue to light up under a microscope. This type of test may be used to tell the difference between different types of cancer.

Some Childhood Brain and Spinal Cord Tumors Are Diagnosed by Imaging Tests

Sometimes a biopsy or surgery cannot be done safely because of where the tumor formed in the brain or spinal cord. These tumors are diagnosed based on the results of imaging tests and other procedures.

Certain Factors Affect Prognosis (Chance of Recovery)

The prognosis (chance of recovery) depends on the following:

- Whether there are any cancer cells left after surgery
- The type of tumor
- Where the tumor is in the body
- The child's age
- Whether the tumor has just been diagnosed or has recurred (come back)

Treatment Option Overview

Different types of treatment are available for children with brain and spinal cord tumors. Some treatments are standard (the currently used treatment), and some are being tested in clinical trials. Because cancer in children is rare, taking part in a clinical trial should be considered.

Three types of standard treatment are used:

- **Surgery.** Surgery may be used to diagnose and treat childhood brain and spinal cord tumors.
- **Radiation Therapy.** Radiation therapy is a cancer treatment that uses high-energy X-rays or other types of radiation to kill cancer cells or keep them from growing. There are two types of radiation therapy:
    - External radiation therapy uses a machine outside the body to send radiation toward the cancer.
    - Internal radiation therapy uses a radioactive substance sealed in needles, seeds, wires, or catheters that are placed directly into or near the cancer.

The way the radiation therapy is given depends on the type of cancer being treated. External radiation therapy is used to treat childhood brain and spinal cord tumors.

- **Chemotherapy.** Chemotherapy is a cancer treatment that uses drugs to stop the growth of cancer cells, either by killing the cells or by stopping them from dividing. When chemotherapy is taken by mouth or injected into a vein or muscle, the drugs enter the bloodstream and can reach cancer cells throughout the body (systemic chemotherapy). When chemotherapy is placed directly in the cerebrospinal fluid, an organ, or a body cavity such as the abdomen, the drugs mainly affect cancer cells in those areas (regional chemotherapy). The way the chemotherapy is given depends on the type and stage of the cancer being treated. Anticancer drugs given by mouth or vein to treat brain and spinal cord tumors cannot cross the blood-brain barrier and enter the fluid that surrounds the brain and spinal cord. Instead, an anticancer drug is injected into the fluid-filled space to kill cancer cells there. This is called intrathecal chemotherapy.

High Dose Chemotherapy with Stem Cell Transplant

High dose chemotherapy with stem cell transplant is a way of giving high doses of chemotherapy and replacing blood-forming cells destroyed by the cancer treatment. Stem cells (immature blood cells) are removed from the blood or bone marrow of the patient or a donor and are frozen and stored. After the chemotherapy is completed, the stored stem cells are thawed and given back to the patient through an infusion. These reinfused stem cells grow into (and restore) the body's blood cells.

Side Effects of Treatment

Some cancer treatments cause side effects months or years after treatment has ended. These are called late effects. Late effects of cancer treatment may include the following:

- Physical problems
- Changes in mood, feelings, thinking, learning, or memory
- Second cancers (new types of cancer)

Some late effects may be treated or controlled. It is important to talk with your child's doctors about the effects cancer treatment can have on your child.

Chapter 15

Neuroblastoma

What Is Neuroblastoma?

Neuroblastoma is a disease in which malignant (cancer) cells form in neuroblasts (immature nerve tissue) in the adrenal gland, neck, chest, or spinal cord. Neuroblastoma often begins in the nerve tissue of the adrenal glands. There are two adrenal glands, one on top of each kidney in the back of the upper abdomen. The adrenal glands make important hormones that help control heart rate, blood pressure, blood sugar, and the way the body reacts to stress.

Neuroblastoma may also begin in nerve tissue in the neck, chest, abdomen or pelvis. Neuroblastoma most often begins in infancy and may be diagnosed in the first month of life. It is found when the tumor begins to grow and cause signs or symptoms. Sometimes it forms before birth and is found during a fetal ultrasound. By the time neuroblastoma is diagnosed, the cancer has usually metastasized (spread). Neuroblastoma spreads most often to the lymph nodes, bones, bone marrow, and liver. In infants, it also spreads to the skin.

What Is the Cause of Neuroblastoma?

Gene mutations that increase the risk of neuroblastoma are sometimes inherited (passed from the parent to the child). In children with

---

This chapter includes text excerpted from "Neuroblastoma Treatment (PDQ®)—Patient Version," National Cancer Institute (NCI), October 6, 2017.

a gene mutation, neuroblastoma usually occurs at a younger age and more than one tumor may form in the adrenal glands.

What Are the Signs and Symptoms of Neuroblastoma?

The most common signs and symptoms of neuroblastoma are caused by the tumor pressing on nearby tissues as it grows or by cancer spreading to the bone. These and other signs and symptoms may be caused by neuroblastoma or by other conditions.

Check with your child's doctor if your child has any of the following:

- Lump in the abdomen, neck, or chest
- Bulging eyes
- Dark circles around the eyes ("black eyes")
- Bone pain
- Swollen stomach and trouble breathing (in infants)
- Painless, bluish lumps under the skin (in infants)
- Weakness or paralysis (loss of ability to move a body part)

Less common signs and symptoms of neuroblastoma include the following:

- Fever
- Shortness of breath
- Feeling tired
- Easy bruising or bleeding
- Petechiae (flat, pinpoint spots under the skin caused by bleeding)
- High blood pressure
- Severe watery diarrhea
- Horner syndrome (droopy eyelid, smaller pupil, and less sweating on one side of the face)
- Jerky muscle movements
- Uncontrolled eye movements

How Is Neuroblastoma Diagnosed?

The following tests and procedures may be used:

- **Physical exam and history.** An exam of the body to check general signs of health, including checking for signs of disease, such as lumps or anything else that seems unusual. A history of the patient's health habits and past illnesses and treatments will also be taken.
- **Neurological exam.** A series of questions and tests to check the brain, spinal cord, and nerve function. The exam checks a person's mental status, coordination, and ability to walk normally, and how well the muscles, senses, and reflexes work. This may also be called a neuro exam or a neurologic exam.
- **Urine catecholamine studies.** A procedure in which a urine sample is checked to measure the amount of certain substances, vanillylmandelic acid (VMA) and homovanillic acid (HVA), that are made when catecholamines break down and are released into the urine. A higher than normal amount of VMA or HVA can be a sign of neuroblastoma.
- **Blood chemistry studies.** A procedure in which a blood sample is checked to measure the amounts of certain substances released into the blood by organs and tissues in the body. An unusual (higher or lower than normal) amount of a substance can be a sign of disease.
- **X-ray.** An X-ray is a type of energy beam that can go through the body and onto film, making a picture of areas inside the body.
- **Computed tomography (CT) scan (Computerized axial tomography (CAT) scan).** A procedure that makes a series of detailed pictures of areas inside the body, take from different angles. The pictures are made by a computer linked to an X-ray machine. A dye may be injected into a vein or swallowed to help the organs or tissues show up more clearly. This procedure is also called computed tomography (CT), or computerized axial tomography (CAT).
- **Magnetic resonance imaging (MRI) with gadolinium.** A procedure that uses a magnet, radio waves, and a computer to make a series of detailed pictures of areas inside the body. A

substance called gadolinium is injected into a vein. The gadolinium collects around the cancer cells so they show up brighter in the picture. This procedure is also called nuclear magnetic resonance imaging (NMRI).

- **Metaiodobenzylguanidine (MIBG) scan.** A procedure used to find neuroendocrine tumors, such as neuroblastoma. A very small amount of a substance called radioactive MIBG is injected into a vein and travels through the bloodstream. Neuroendocrine tumor cells take up the radioactive MIBG and are detected by a scanner. Scans may be taken over 1–3 days. An iodine solution may be given before or during the test to keep the thyroid gland from absorbing too much of the MIBG. This test is also used to find out how well the tumor is responding to treatment. MIBG is used in high doses to treat neuroblastoma.
- **Bone marrow aspiration and biopsy.** The removal of bone marrow, blood, and a small piece of bone by inserting a hollow needle into the hipbone or breastbone. A pathologist views the bone marrow, blood, and bone under a microscope to look for signs of cancer.
- **Ultrasound exam.** A procedure in which high energy sound waves (ultrasound) are bounced off internal tissues or organs and make echoes. The echoes form a picture of body tissues called a sonogram. The picture can be printed to be looked at later. An ultrasound exam is not done if a CT/MRI has been done.

Biopsy

Cells and tissues are removed during a biopsy so they can be viewed under a microscope by a pathologist to check for signs of cancer. The way the biopsy is done depends on where the tumor is in the body. Sometimes the whole tumor is removed at the same time the biopsy is done.

The following tests may be done on the tissue that is removed:

- **Cytogenetic analysis.** A laboratory test in which cells in a sample of tissue are viewed under a microscope to look for certain changes in the chromosomes.
- **Light microscopy.** A laboratory test in which cells in a sample of tissue are viewed under regular and high powered microscopes to look for certain changes in the cells.

- **Immunohistochemistry.** A test that uses antibodies to check for certain antigens in a sample of tissue. The antibody is usually linked to a radioactive substance or a dye that causes the tissue to light up under a microscope. This type of test may be used to tell the difference between different types of cancer.
- **MYCN amplification study.** A laboratory study in which tumor or bone marrow cells are checked for the level of *MYCN*. *MYCN* is important for cell growth. A higher level of *MYCN* (more than 10 copies of the gene) is called *MYCN* amplification. Neuroblastoma with *MYCN* amplification is more likely to spread in the body and less likely to respond to treatment.

Children up to 6 months old may not need a biopsy or surgery to remove the tumor because the tumor may disappear without treatment.

What Treatment Options Are Available for Neuroblastoma?

Different types of treatment are available for patients with neuroblastoma. Some treatments are standard (the currently used treatment), and some are being tested in clinical trials. A treatment clinical trial is a research study meant to help improve current treatments or obtain information on new treatments for patients with cancer. When clinical trials show that a new treatment is better than the standard treatment, the new treatment may become the standard treatment. Because cancer in children is rare, taking part in a clinical trial should be considered. Some clinical trials are open only to patients who have not started treatment.

Seven types of standard treatment are used:

Observation

Observation is closely monitoring a patient's condition without giving any treatment until signs or symptoms appear or change.

Surgery

Surgery is used to treat neuroblastoma unless it has spread to other parts of the body. Depending on where the tumor is, as much of the tumor as is safely possible will be removed. If the tumor cannot be removed, a biopsy may be done instead.

Radiation Therapy

Radiation therapy is a cancer treatment that uses high energy X-rays or other types of radiation to kill cancer cells or keep them from growing. There are two types of radiation therapy:

- External radiation therapy uses a machine outside the body to send radiation toward the cancer.
- Internal radiation therapy uses a radioactive substance sealed in needles, seeds, wires, or catheters that are placed directly into or near the cancer.

The way the radiation therapy is given depends on the type of cancer being treated and the child's risk group. External radiation therapy is used to treat neuroblastoma.

Iodine 131-MIBG Therapy

Iodine 131-MIBG therapy is a treatment with radioactive iodine. The radioactive iodine is given through an intravenous (IV) line and enters the bloodstream which carries radiation directly to tumor cells. Radioactive iodine collects in neuroblastoma cells and kills them with the radiation that is given off. Iodine 131-MIBG therapy is sometimes used to treat high-risk neuroblastoma that comes back after initial treatment.

Chemotherapy

Chemotherapy is a cancer treatment that uses drugs to stop the growth of cancer cells, either by killing the cells or by stopping them from dividing. When chemotherapy is taken by mouth or injected into a vein or muscle, the drugs enter the bloodstream and can reach cancer cells throughout the body (systemic chemotherapy). When chemotherapy is placed directly into the cerebrospinal fluid, an organ, or a body cavity such as the abdomen, the drugs mainly affect cancer cells in those areas (regional chemotherapy). The way the chemotherapy is given depends on the type of cancer being treated and the child's risk group.

The use of two or more anticancer drugs is called combination chemotherapy.

High Dose Chemotherapy (HDC) and Radiation Therapy with Stem Cell Rescue

High dose chemotherapy (HDC) and radiation therapy with stem cell rescue is a way of giving high doses of chemotherapy and radiation therapy and replacing blood-forming cells destroyed by cancer treatment for high-risk neuroblastoma. Stem cells (immature blood cells) are removed from the blood or bone marrow of the patient and are frozen and stored. After chemotherapy and radiation therapy are completed, the stored stem cells are thawed and given back to the patient through an infusion. These reinfused stem cells grow into (and restore) the body's blood cells.

Maintenance therapy is given after high dose chemotherapy and radiation therapy with stem cell rescue to kill any cancer cells that may regrow and cause the disease to come back. Maintenance therapy is given for 6 months and includes the following treatments:

- **Isotretinoin.** A vitamin like drug that slows the cancer's ability to make more cancer cells and changes how these cells look and act. This drug is taken by mouth.
- **Dinutuximab.** A type of monoclonal antibody therapy that uses an antibody made in the laboratory from a single type of immune system cell. Dinutuximab identifies and attaches to a substance, called GD2, on the surface of neuroblastoma cells. Once dinutuximab attaches to the GD2, a signal is sent to the immune system that a foreign substance has been found and needs to be killed. Then the body's immune system kills the neuroblastoma cell. Dinutuximab is given by infusion. It is a type of targeted therapy.
- **Granulocyte macrophage colony stimulating factor (GM-CSF).** A cytokine that helps make more immune system cells, especially granulocytes and macrophages (white blood cells), which can attack and kill cancer cells.
- **Interleukin 2 (IL-2).** A type of immunotherapy that boosts the growth and activity of many immune cells, especially lymphocytes (a type of white blood cell). Lymphocytes can attack and kill cancer cells.

Targeted Therapy

Targeted therapy is a type of treatment that uses drugs or other substances to identify and attack cancer cells with less harm to normal cells.

Tyrosine kinase inhibitors (TKI) are small molecule drugs that go through the cell membrane and work inside cancer cells to block signals that cancer cells need to grow and divide. Crizotinib is used to treat neuroblastoma that has come back after treatment.

Side Effects of Treatment

Children who are treated for neuroblastoma may have late effects, including an increased risk of second cancers. Some cancer treatments cause side effects that continue or appear years after cancer treatment has ended. These are called late effects. Late effects of cancer treatment may include:

- Physical problems
- Changes in mood, feelings, thinking, learning, or memory
- Second cancers (new types of cancer)

Some late effects may be treated or controlled. It is important that parents of children who are treated for neuroblastoma talk with their doctors about the possible late effects caused by some treatments.

What Is the Prognosis for Neuroblastoma?

The prognosis (chance of recovery) and treatment options depend on the following:

- Age of the child at the time of diagnosis
- The child's risk group
- Whether there are certain changes in the genes
- Where in the body the tumor started
- Tumor histology (the shape, function, and structure of the tumor cells)
- Whether there is cancer in the lymph nodes on the same side of the body as the primary cancer or whether there is cancer in the lymph nodes on the opposite side of the body
- How the tumor responds to treatment
- How much time passed between diagnosis and when the cancer recurred (for recurrent cancer)

Prognosis and treatment options for neuroblastoma are also affected by tumor biology, which includes:

- The patterns of the tumor cells
- How different the tumor cells are from normal cells
- How fast the tumor cells are growing

- Whether the tumor shows *MYCN* amplification
- Whether the tumor has changes in the anaplastic lymphoma kinase (*ALK*) gene

The tumor biology is said to be favorable or unfavorable, depending on these factors. A favorable tumor biology means there is a better chance of recovery. In some children up to 6 months old, neuroblastoma may disappear without treatment. This is called spontaneous regression. The child is closely watched for signs or symptoms of neuroblastoma. If signs or symptoms occur, treatment may be needed.

Chapter 16

Primary Central Nervous System Lymphoma

The lymph system is part of the immune system and is made up of the lymph, lymph vessels, lymph nodes, spleen, thymus, tonsils, and bone marrow.

What Is Primary CNS Lymphoma?

Primary CNS lymphoma is a disease in which malignant (cancer) cells form in the lymph tissue of the brain and/or spinal cord. Lymphoma is a disease in which malignant (cancer) cells form in the lymph system. Lymphocytes (carried in the lymph) travel in and out of the CNS. It is thought that some of these lymphocytes become malignant and cause lymphoma to form in the CNS. Primary CNS lymphoma can start in the brain, spinal cord, or meninges (the layers that form the outer covering of the brain). Because the eye is so close to the brain, primary CNS lymphoma can also start in the eye (called ocular lymphoma).

What Are the Risk Factors for Primary CNS Lymphoma?

Anything that increases your chance of getting a disease is called a risk factor. Having a risk factor does not mean that you will get cancer;

This chapter includes text excerpted from "Primary CNS Lymphoma Treatment (PDQ®)—Patient Version," National Cancer Institute (NCI), December 21, 2016.

not having risk factors doesn't mean that you will not get cancer. Talk with your doctor if you think you may be at risk. Having a weakened immune system may increase the risk of developing primary CNS lymphoma. Primary CNS lymphoma may occur in patients who have acquired immunodeficiency syndrome (AIDS) or other disorders of the immune system or who have had a kidney transplant.

How Is Primary CNS Lymphoma Diagnosed?

The following tests and procedures may be used:

- **Physical exam and history.** An exam of the body to check general signs of health, including checking for signs of disease, such as lumps or anything else that seems unusual. A history of the patient's health habits and past illnesses and treatments will also be taken.
- **Neurological exam.** A series of questions and tests to check the brain, spinal cord, and nerve function. The exam checks a person's mental status, coordination, ability to walk normally, and how well the muscles, senses, and reflexes work. This may also be called a neuro exam or a neurologic exam.
- **Slit-lamp eye exam.** An exam that uses a special microscope with a bright, narrow slit of light to check the outside and inside of the eye.
- **Magnetic resonance imaging (MRI).** A procedure that uses a magnet, radio waves, and a computer to make a series of detailed pictures of areas inside the brain and spinal cord. A substance called gadolinium is injected into the patient through a vein. The gadolinium collects around the cancer cells so they show up brighter in the picture. This procedure is also called nuclear magnetic resonance imaging (NMRI).
- **Positron emission tomography (PET).** A procedure to find malignant tumor cells in the body. A small amount of radioactive glucose (sugar) is injected into a vein. The PET scanner rotates around the body and makes a picture of where glucose is being used in the body. Malignant tumor cells show up brighter in the picture because they are more active and take up more glucose than normal cells do.
- **Lumbar puncture (LP).** A procedure used to collect cerebrospinal fluid (CSF) from the spinal column. This is done by

placing a needle between two bones in the spine and into the CSF around the spinal cord and removing a sample of the fluid. The sample of CSF is checked under a microscope for signs of tumor cells. The sample may also be checked for the amounts of protein and glucose. A higher than normal amount of protein or lower than normal amount of glucose may be a sign of a tumor. This procedure is also called an LP or spinal tap.

- **Stereotactic biopsy.** A biopsy procedure that uses a computer and a 3-dimensional (3D) scanning device to find a tumor site and guide the removal of tissue so it can be viewed under a microscope to check for signs of cancer.

The following tests may be done on the samples of tissue that are removed:

Flow cytometry. A laboratory test that measures the number of cells in a sample, the percentage of live cells in a sample, and certain characteristics of cells, such as size, shape, and the presence of tumor markers on the cell surface. The cells are stained with a light-sensitive dye, placed in a fluid, and passed in a stream before a laser or other type of light. The measurements are based on how the light-sensitive dye reacts to the light.

Immunohistochemistry. A test that uses antibodies to check for certain antigens in a sample of tissue. The antibody is usually linked to a radioactive substance or a dye that causes the tissue to light up under a microscope. This type of test may be used to tell the difference between different types of cancer.

Cytogenetic analysis. A laboratory test in which cells in a sample of tissue are viewed under a microscope to look for certain changes in the chromosomes. Other tests, such as fluorescence in situ hybridization (FISH), may also be done to look for certain changes in the chromosomes.

Complete blood count (CBC) with differential: A procedure in which a sample of blood is drawn and checked for the following:

- The number of red blood cells and platelets
- The number and type of white blood cells
- The amount of hemoglobin (the protein that carries oxygen) in the red blood cells
- The portion of the blood sample made up of red blood cells

Blood chemistry studies. A procedure in which a blood sample is checked to measure the amounts of certain substances released into the blood by organs and tissues in the body. An unusual (higher or lower than normal) amount of a substance can be a sign of disease.

Staging Primary CNS Lymphoma

After primary CNS lymphoma has been diagnosed, tests are done to find out if cancer cells have spread within the brain and spinal cord or to other parts of the body. When primary CNS lymphoma continues to grow, it usually does not spread beyond the central nervous system or the eye. The process used to find out if cancer has spread is called staging. It is important to know if cancer has spread to other parts of the body in order to plan treatment. The following tests and procedures may be used in the staging process:

- **Computerized tomography (CT)/computerized axial tomography (CAT) scan.** A procedure that makes a series of detailed pictures of areas inside the body, taken from different angles. The pictures are made by a computer linked to an X-ray machine. A dye may be injected into a vein or swallowed to help the organs or tissues show up more clearly. For primary CNS lymphoma, a CT scan is done of the chest, abdomen, and pelvis (the part of the body between the hips).
- **Positron emission tomography scan (PET).** A procedure to find malignant tumor cells in the body. A small amount of radioactive glucose (sugar) is injected into a vein. The PET scanner rotates around the body and makes a picture of where glucose is being used in the body. Malignant tumor cells show up brighter in the picture because they are more active and take up more glucose than normal cells do. A PET scan and CT scan may be done at the same time. This is called a PET-CT.
- **Magnetic resonance imaging (MRI).** A procedure that uses a magnet, radio waves, and a computer to make a series of detailed pictures of areas inside the body. This procedure is also called nuclear magnetic resonance imaging (NMRI).
- **Bone marrow aspiration and biopsy.** The removal of bone marrow, blood, and a small piece of bone by inserting a hollow needle into the hipbone or breastbone. A pathologist views the bone marrow, blood, and bone under a microscope to look for signs of cancer.

Treatment Option Overview

There are different types of treatment for patients with primary CNS lymphoma. Different types of treatment are available for patients with primary CNS lymphoma. Some treatments are standard (the currently used treatment), and some are being tested in clinical trials. A treatment clinical trial is a research study meant to help improve current treatments or obtain information on new treatments for patients with cancer. When clinical trials show that a new treatment is better than the standard treatment, the new treatment may become the standard treatment. Patients may want to think about taking part in a clinical trial. Some clinical trials are open only to patients who have not started treatment. Surgery is not used to treat primary CNS lymphoma.

Standard Treatment Options Available for People with Primary CNS Lymphoma

Three standard treatments are used:

Radiation Therapy

Radiation therapy is a cancer treatment that uses high-energy X-rays or other types of radiation to kill cancer cells or keep them from growing. There are two types of radiation therapy:

- External radiation therapy uses a machine outside the body to send radiation toward the cancer. Because primary CNS lymphoma spreads throughout the brain, external radiation therapy is given to the whole brain. This is called whole brain radiation therapy.
- Internal radiation therapy uses a radioactive substance sealed in needles, seeds, wires, or catheters that are placed directly into or near the cancer.

The way the radiation therapy is given depends on whether the patient has primary CNS lymphoma and AIDS. External radiation therapy is used to treat primary CNS lymphoma.

High-dose radiation therapy to the brain can damage healthy tissue and cause disorders that can affect thinking, learning, problem solving, speech, reading, writing, and memory. Clinical trials have tested the use of chemotherapy alone or before radiation therapy to reduce the damage to healthy brain tissue that occurs with the use of radiation therapy.

Chemotherapy

Chemotherapy is a cancer treatment that uses drugs to stop the growth of cancer cells, either by killing the cells or by stopping them from dividing. When chemotherapy is taken by mouth or injected into a vein or muscle, the drugs enter the bloodstream and can reach cancer cells throughout the body (systemic chemotherapy). When chemotherapy is placed directly into the cerebrospinal fluid (intrathecal chemotherapy), an organ, or a body cavity such as the abdomen, the drugs mainly affect cancer cells in those areas (regional chemotherapy).

The way the chemotherapy is given depends on where the tumor is in the CNS or eye. Primary CNS lymphoma may be treated with systemic chemotherapy, intrathecal chemotherapy and/or intraventricular chemotherapy, in which anticancer drugs are placed into the ventricles (fluid-filled cavities) of the brain. If primary CNS lymphoma is found in the eye, anticancer drugs are injected directly into the vitreous humor (jelly-like substance) inside the eye.

A network of blood vessels and tissue, called the blood-brain barrier, protects the brain from harmful substances. This barrier can also keep anticancer drugs from reaching the brain. In order to treat CNS lymphoma, certain drugs may be used to make openings between cells in the blood-brain barrier. This is called blood-brain barrier disruption. Anticancer drugs infused into the bloodstream may then reach the brain.

Steroid Therapy

Steroids are hormones made naturally in the body. They can also be made in a laboratory and used as drugs. Glucocorticoids are steroid drugs that have an anticancer effect in lymphomas.

What New Types of Treatment Are Being Tested?

New types of treatment are being tested in clinical trials.

High-Dose Chemotherapy with Stem Cell Transplant

High-dose chemotherapy with stem cell transplant is a method of giving high doses of chemotherapy and replacing blood-forming cells destroyed by the cancer treatment. Stem cells (immature blood cells) are removed from the blood or bone marrow of the patient or a donor and are frozen and stored. After the chemotherapy is completed, the stored stem cells are thawed and given back to the patient through an infusion. These reinfused stem cells grow into (and restore) the body's blood cells.

Targeted Therapy

Targeted therapy is a type of treatment that uses drugs or other substances to attack cancer cells. Targeted therapies usually cause less harm to normal cells than chemotherapy or radiation therapy do. Monoclonal antibody therapy is one type of targeted therapy being studied in the treatment of primary CNS lymphoma.

Monoclonal antibody therapy is a cancer treatment that uses antibodies made in the laboratory from a single type of immune system cell. These antibodies can identify substances on cancer cells or normal substances that may help cancer cells grow. The antibodies attach to the substances and kill the cancer cells, block their growth, or keep them from spreading. Monoclonal antibodies are given by infusion. They may be used alone or to carry drugs, toxins, or radioactive material directly to cancer cells. Rituximab is a type of monoclonal antibody used to treat newly diagnosed primary CNS lymphoma in patients who do not have AIDS.

What Is the Prognosis for Primary CNS Lymphoma?

The prognosis (chance of recovery) depends on the following:

- The patient's age and general health
- The level of certain substances in the blood and CSF
- Where the tumor is in the central nervous system, eye, or both.
- Whether the patient has AIDS

Treatment options depend on the following:

- The stage of the cancer
- Where the tumor is in the central nervous system
- The patient's age and general health
- Whether the cancer has just been diagnosed or has recurred (come back)

Treatment of primary CNS lymphoma works best when the tumor has not spread outside the cerebrum (the largest part of the brain) and the patient is younger than 60 years, able to carry out most daily activities, and does not have acquired immunodeficiency syndrome (AIDS) or other diseases that weaken the immune system.

Chapter 17

Pituitary Tumors

The pituitary gland, a pea-sized organ in the center of the brain, just above the back of the nose. It is sometimes called the "master endocrine gland" because it makes hormones that affect the way many parts of the body work. The pituitary gland hormones control many other glands in the body.

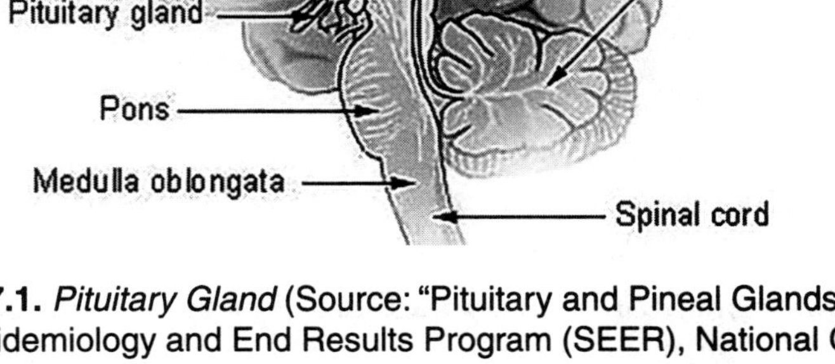

Figure 17.1. *Pituitary Gland* (Source: "Pituitary and Pineal Glands," Surveillance, Epidemiology and End Results Program (SEER), National Cancer Institute (NCI).)

This chapter includes text excerpted from "Pituitary Tumors Treatment (PDQ®)—Patient Version," National Cancer Institute (NCI), August 18, 2017.

Hormones made by the pituitary gland include:

- **Prolactin (PRL).** A hormone that causes a woman's breasts to make milk during and after pregnancy.
- **Adrenocorticotropic hormone (ACTH).** A hormone that causes the adrenal glands to make a hormone called cortisol. Cortisol helps control the use of sugar, protein, and fats in the body and helps the body deal with stress.
- **Growth hormone.** A hormone that helps control body growth and the use of sugar and fat in the body. Growth hormone (GH) is also called somatotropin.
- **Thyroid-stimulating hormone (TSH).** A hormone that causes the thyroid gland to make other hormones that control growth, body temperature, and heart rate. Thyroid-stimulating hormone is also called thyrotropin.
- **Luteinizing hormone (LH) and follicle-stimulating hormone (FSH).** Hormones that control the menstrual cycle in women and the making of sperm in men.

What Are Pituitary Tumors?

A pituitary tumor is a growth of abnormal cells in the tissues of the pituitary gland. Pituitary tumors form in the pituitary gland, a pea-sized organ in the center of the brain, just above the back of the nose. The pituitary gland is sometimes called the "master endocrine gland" because it makes hormones that affect the way many parts of the body work. It also controls hormones made by many other glands in the body.

Pituitary tumors are divided into three groups:

- **Benign pituitary adenomas.** Tumors that are not cancer. These tumors grow very slowly and do not spread from the pituitary gland to other parts of the body.
- **Invasive pituitary adenomas.** Benign tumors that may spread to bones of the skull or the sinus cavity below the pituitary gland.
- **Pituitary carcinomas.** Tumors that are malignant (cancer). These pituitary tumors spread into other areas of the central nervous system (brain and spinal cord) or outside of the central nervous system. Very few pituitary tumors are malignant.

Pituitary tumors may be either nonfunctioning or functioning.

- **Nonfunctioning pituitary tumors** do not make extra amounts of hormones.
- **Functioning pituitary tumors** make more than the normal amount of one or more hormones. Most pituitary tumors are functioning tumors. The extra hormones made by pituitary tumors may cause certain signs or symptoms of disease.

What Are the Risk Factors for Pituitary Tumors?

Having certain genetic conditions increases the risk of developing a pituitary tumor. Anything that increases your risk of getting a disease is called a risk factor. Having a risk factor does not mean that you will get cancer; not having risk factors doesn't mean that you will not get cancer. Talk with your doctor if you think you may be at risk. Risk factors for pituitary tumors include having the following hereditary diseases:

- Multiple endocrine neoplasia type 1 (MEN1) syndrome
- Carney complex
- Isolated familial acromegaly

What Are the Signs and Symptoms of Pituitary Tumors?

Signs of a pituitary tumor include problems with vision and certain physical changes. Signs and symptoms can be caused by the growth of the tumor and/or by hormones the tumor makes or by other conditions. Some tumors may not cause signs or symptoms. Check with your doctor if you have any of these problems.

Signs and Symptoms of a Nonfunctioning Pituitary Tumor

Sometimes, a pituitary tumor may press on or damage parts of the pituitary gland, causing it to stop making one or more hormones. Too little of a certain hormone will affect the work of the gland or organ that the hormone controls. The following signs and symptoms may occur:

- Headache
- Some loss of vision
- Loss of body hair

- In women, less frequent or no menstrual periods or no milk from the breasts
- In men, loss of facial hair, growth of breast tissue, and impotence
- In women and men, lower sex drive
- In children, slowed growth and sexual development

Most of the tumors that make LH and FSH do not make enough extra hormone to cause signs and symptoms. These tumors are considered to be nonfunctioning tumors.

Signs and Symptoms of a Functioning Pituitary Tumor

When a functioning pituitary tumor makes extra hormones, the signs and symptoms will depend on the type of hormone being made.

Too much prolactin (PRL) may cause:

- Headache
- Some loss of vision
- Less frequent or no menstrual periods or menstrual periods with a very light flow
- Trouble becoming pregnant or an inability to become pregnant.
- Impotence in men
- Lower sex drive
- Flow of breast milk in a woman who is not pregnant or breastfeeding

Too much adrenocorticotropic hormone (ACTH) may cause:

- Headache
- Some loss of vision
- Weight gain in the face, neck, and trunk of the body, and thin arms and legs
- A lump of fat on the back of the neck
- Thin skin that may have purple or pink stretch marks on the chest or abdomen
- Easy bruising

- Growth of fine hair on the face, upper back, or arms
- Bones that break easily
- Anxiety, irritability, and depression

Too much growth hormone (GH) may cause:

- Headache
- Some loss of vision
- In adults, acromegaly (growth of the bones in the face, hands, and feet). In children, the whole body may grow much taller and larger than normal.
- Tingling or numbness in the hands and fingers
- Snoring or pauses in breathing during sleep
- Joint pain
- Sweating more than usual
- Dysmorphophobia (extreme dislike of or concern about one or more parts of the body)

Too much thyroid-stimulating hormone (TSH) may cause:

- Irregular heartbeat
- Shakiness
- Weight loss
- Trouble sleeping
- Frequent bowel movements
- Sweating

Other general signs and symptoms of pituitary tumors:

- Nausea and vomiting
- Confusion
- Dizziness
- Seizures
- Runny or "drippy" nose (cerebrospinal fluid that surrounds the brain and spinal cord leaks into the nose)

How Is Pituitary Tumor Diagnosed?

Imaging studies and tests that examine the blood and urine are used to detect (find) and diagnose a pituitary tumor.

The following tests and procedures may be used:

- **Physical exam and history.** An exam of the body to check general signs of health, including checking for signs of disease, such as lumps or anything else that seems unusual. A history of the patient's health habits and past illnesses and treatments will also be taken.
- **Eye exam.** An exam to check vision and the general health of the eyes.
- **Visual field exam.** An exam to check a person's field of vision (the total area in which objects can be seen). This test measures both central vision (how much a person can see when looking straight ahead) and peripheral vision (how much a person can see in all other directions while staring straight ahead). The eyes are tested one at a time. The eye not being tested is covered.
- **Neurological exam.** A series of questions and tests to check the brain, spinal cord, and nerve function. The exam checks a person's mental status, coordination, and ability to walk normally, and how well the muscles, senses, and reflexes work. This may also be called a neuro exam or a neurologic exam.
- **Magnetic resonance imaging (MRI) with gadolinium.** A procedure that uses a magnet, radio waves, and a computer to make a series of detailed pictures of areas inside the brain and spinal cord. A substance called gadolinium is injected into a vein. The gadolinium collects around the cancer cells so they show up brighter in the picture. This procedure is also called nuclear magnetic resonance imaging (NMRI).
- **Blood chemistry study.** A procedure in which a blood sample is checked to measure the amounts of certain substances, such as glucose (sugar), released into the blood by organs and tissues in the body. An unusual (higher or lower than normal) amount of a substance can be a sign of disease.
- **Blood tests.** Tests to measure the levels of testosterone or estrogen in the blood. A higher or lower than normal amount of these hormones may be a sign of pituitary tumor.

- **24-hour urine test.** A test in which urine is collected for 24 hours to measure the amounts of certain substances. An unusual (higher or lower than normal) amount of a substance can be a sign of disease in the organ or tissue that makes it. A higher than normal amount of the hormone cortisol may be a sign of a pituitary tumor and Cushing syndrome.
- **High-dose dexamethasone suppression test.** A test in which one or more high doses of dexamethasone are given. The level of cortisol is checked from a sample of blood or from urine that is collected for three days. This test is done to check if the adrenal gland is making too much cortisol or if the pituitary gland is telling the adrenal glands to make too much cortisol.
- **Low-dose dexamethasone suppression test.** A test in which one or more small doses of dexamethasone are given. The level of cortisol is checked from a sample of blood or from urine that is collected for three days. This test is done to check if the adrenal gland is making too much cortisol.
- **Venous sampling for pituitary tumors.** A procedure in which a sample of blood is taken from veins coming from the pituitary gland. The sample is checked to measure the amount of ACTH released into the blood by the gland. Venous sampling may be done if blood tests show there is a tumor making ACTH, but the pituitary gland looks normal in the imaging tests.
- **Biopsy.** The removal of cells or tissues so they can be viewed under a microscope by a pathologist to check for signs of cancer.

  The following tests may be done on the sample of tissue that is removed:

  - **Immunohistochemistry.** A test that uses antibodies to check for certain antigens in a sample of tissue. The antibody is usually linked to a radioactive substance or a dye that causes the tissue to light up under a microscope. This type of test may be used to tell the difference between different types of cancer.
  - **Immunocytochemistry.** A test that uses antibodies to check for certain antigens in a sample of cells. The antibody is usually linked to a radioactive substance or a dye that causes the cells to light up under a microscope. This type of test may be used to tell the difference between different types of cancer.

- **Light and electron microscopy.** A laboratory test in which cells in a sample of tissue are viewed under regular and high-powered microscopes to look for certain changes in the cells.

Stages of Pituitary Tumors

Once a pituitary tumor has been diagnosed, tests are done to find out if it has spread within the central nervous system (brain and spinal cord) or to other parts of the body. The extent or spread of cancer is usually described as stages. There is no standard staging system for pituitary tumors. Once a pituitary tumor is found, tests are done to find out if the tumor has spread into the brain or to other parts of the body. The following test may be used:

- **Magnetic resonance imaging (MRI).** A procedure that uses a magnet, radio waves, and a computer to make a series of detailed pictures of areas inside the body. This procedure is also called nuclear magnetic resonance imaging (NMRI).

Pituitary tumors are described in several ways. Pituitary tumors are described by their size and grade, whether or not they make extra hormones, and whether the tumor has spread to other parts of the body.

The following sizes are used:

- **Microadenoma:** The tumor is smaller than 1 centimeter.
- **Macroadenoma:** The tumor is 1 centimeter or larger.

Most pituitary adenomas are microadenomas. The grade of a pituitary tumor is based on how far it has grown into the surrounding area of the brain, including the sella (the bone at the base of the skull, where the pituitary gland sits).

Treatment Option Overview

Different types of treatments are available for patients with pituitary tumors. Some treatments are standard (the currently used treatment), and some are being tested in clinical trials. A treatment clinical trial is a research study meant to help improve current treatments or obtain information on new treatments for patients with cancer. When clinical trials show that a new treatment is better than the standard treatment, the new treatment may become the standard treatment.

Patients may want to think about taking part in a clinical trial. Some clinical trials are open only to patients who have not started treatment.

Standard Treatment Available for Patients with Pituitary Tumors

Four types of standard treatment are used:

Surgery

Many pituitary tumors can be removed by surgery using one of the following operations:

- **Transsphenoidal surgery.** A type of surgery in which the instruments are inserted into part of the brain by going through an incision (cut) made under the upper lip or at the bottom of the nose between the nostrils and then through the sphenoid bone (a butterfly-shaped bone at the base of the skull) to reach the pituitary gland. The pituitary gland lies just above the sphenoid bone.
- **Endoscopic transsphenoidal surgery.** A type of surgery in which an endoscope is inserted through an incision (cut) made at the back of the inside of the nose and then through the sphenoid bone to reach the pituitary gland. An endoscope is a thin, tube-like instrument with a light, a lens for viewing, and a tool for removing tumor tissue.
- **Craniotomy.** Surgery to remove the tumor through an opening made in the skull.

Even if the doctor removes all the cancer that can be seen at the time of the surgery, some patients may be given chemotherapy or radiation therapy after surgery to kill any cancer cells that are left. Treatment given after the surgery, to lower the risk that the cancer will come back, is called adjuvant therapy.

Radiation Therapy

Radiation therapy is a cancer treatment that uses high-energy X-rays or other types of radiation to kill cancer cells or keep them from growing. There are two types of radiation therapy:

- External radiation therapy uses a machine outside the body to send radiation toward the cancer. Certain ways of giving radiation therapy can help keep radiation from damaging nearby healthy tissue. This type of radiation therapy may include the following:

- **Stereotactic radiosurgery (SRS).** A rigid head frame is attached to the skull to keep the head still during the radiation treatment. A machine aims a single large dose of radiation directly at the tumor. This procedure does not involve surgery. It is also called stereotaxic radiosurgery, radiosurgery, and radiation surgery.

- Internal radiation therapy uses a radioactive substance sealed in needles, seeds, wires, or catheters that are placed directly into or near the cancer.

The way the radiation therapy is given depends on the type of the cancer being treated. External radiation therapy is used to treat pituitary tumors.

Drug Therapy

Drugs may be given to stop a functioning pituitary tumor from making too many hormones.

Chemotherapy

Chemotherapy may be used as palliative treatment for pituitary carcinomas, to relieve symptoms and improve the patient's quality of life. Chemotherapy uses drugs to stop the growth of cancer cells, either by killing the cells or by stopping them from dividing. When chemotherapy is taken by mouth or injected into a vein or muscle, the drugs enter the bloodstream and can reach cancer cells throughout the body (systemic chemotherapy). When chemotherapy is placed directly into the cerebrospinal fluid, an organ, or a body cavity such as the abdomen, the drugs mainly affect cancer cells in those areas (regional chemotherapy). The way the chemotherapy is given depends on the type of the cancer being treated.

Follow-Up Tests

Some of the tests that were done to diagnose the cancer or to find out the stage of the cancer may be repeated. Some tests will be repeated in order to see how well the treatment is working. Decisions about whether to continue, change, or stop treatment may be based on the results of these tests. Some of the tests will continue to be done from time to time after treatment has ended. The results of these tests can show if your condition has changed or if the cancer has recurred (come back). These tests are sometimes called follow-up tests or check-ups.

What Is the Prognosis for Pituitary Tumors?

The prognosis (chance of recovery) depends on the type of tumor and whether the tumor has spread into other areas of the central nervous system (brain and spinal cord) or outside of the central nervous system to other parts of the body.

Treatment options depend on the following:

- The type and size of the tumor
- Whether the tumor is making hormones
- Whether the tumor is causing problems with vision or other signs or symptoms
- Whether the tumor has spread into the brain around the pituitary gland or to other parts of the body
- Whether the tumor has just been diagnosed or has recurred (come back)

Chapter 18

Thyroid Cancer

Thyroid is a small butterfly-shaped gland found at the base of your neck, just below your Adam's apple. This gland makes thyroid hormone that travels in your blood to all parts of your body. The thyroid hormone controls your body's metabolism in many ways, including how fast you burn calories and how fast your heart beats.

General Information about Thyroid Cancer

Thyroid cancer is a disease in which malignant (cancer) cells form in the tissues of the thyroid gland. The thyroid is a gland at the base of the throat near the trachea (windpipe). It is shaped like a butterfly, with a right lobe and a left lobe. The isthmus, a thin piece of tissue, connects the two lobes. A healthy thyroid is a little larger than a quarter. It usually cannot be felt through the skin.

The thyroid uses iodine, a mineral found in some foods and in iodized salt, to help make several hormones. Thyroid hormones do the following:

- Control heart rate, body temperature, and how quickly food is changed into energy (metabolism)
- Control the amount of calcium in the blood

This chapter contains text excerpted from the following sources: Text in this chapter begins with excerpts from "Thyroid Disease," Office on Women's Health (OWH), U.S. Department of Health and Human Services (HHS), February 6, 2017; Text beginning with the heading "General Information about Thyroid Cancer" is excerpted from "Thyroid Cancer Treatment (Adult) (PDQ®)—Patient Version," National Cancer Institute (NCI), January 12, 2018.

Thyroid nodules are common but usually are not cancer.

Your doctor may find a lump (nodule) in your thyroid during a routine medical exam. A thyroid nodule is an abnormal growth of thyroid cells in the thyroid. Nodules may be solid or fluid-filled. When a thyroid nodule is found, an ultrasound of the thyroid and a fine-needle aspiration biopsy are often done to check for signs of cancer. Blood tests to check thyroid hormone levels and for antithyroid antibodies in the blood may also be done to check for other types of thyroid disease. Thyroid nodules usually don't cause symptoms or need treatment. Sometimes the thyroid nodules become large enough that it is hard to swallow or breathe and more tests and treatment are needed. Only a small number of thyroid nodules are diagnosed as cancer.

Types of Thyroid Cancer

There are different types of thyroid cancer. There are four main types of thyroid cancer:

- Papillary thyroid cancer: The most common type of thyroid cancer
- Follicular thyroid cancer
- Medullary thyroid cancer
- Anaplastic thyroid cancer

Papillary and follicular thyroid cancer are sometimes called differentiated thyroid cancer. Medullary and anaplastic thyroid cancer are sometimes called poorly differentiated or undifferentiated thyroid cancer. Age, gender, and being exposed to radiation can affect the risk of thyroid cancer. Anything that increases your risk of getting a disease is called a risk factor. Having a risk factor does not mean that you will get cancer; not having risk factors doesn't mean that you will not get cancer. Talk with your doctor if you think you may be at risk.

Risk Factors for Thyroid Cancer

Risk factors for thyroid cancer include the following:

- Being between 25 and 65 years old
- Being female
- Being exposed to radiation to the head and neck as an infant or child or being exposed to radiation from an atomic bomb. The cancer may occur as soon as 5 years after exposure.

- Having a history of goiter (enlarged thyroid)
- Having a family history of thyroid disease or thyroid cancer
- Having certain genetic conditions such as familial medullary thyroid cancer (FMTC), multiple endocrine neoplasia type 2A syndrome (MEN2A), and multiple endocrine neoplasia type 2B syndrome (MEN2B)
- Being Asian

Medullary thyroid cancer is sometimes caused by a change in a gene that is passed from parent to child.

The genes in cells carry hereditary information from parent to child. A certain change in the *RET* gene that is passed from parent to child (inherited) may cause medullary thyroid cancer. There is a genetic test that is used to check for the changed gene. The patient is tested first to see if he or she has the changed gene. If the patient has it, other family members may also be tested to find out if they are at increased risk for medullary thyroid cancer. Family members, including young children, who have the changed gene may have a thyroidectomy (surgery to remove the thyroid). This can decrease the chance of developing medullary thyroid cancer.

Signs of Thyroid Cancer

Signs of thyroid cancer include a swelling or lump in the neck. Thyroid cancer may not cause early signs or symptoms. It is sometimes found during a routine physical exam. Signs or symptoms may occur as the tumor gets bigger. Other conditions may cause the same signs or symptoms. Check with your doctor if you have any of the following:

- A lump (nodule) in the neck
- Trouble breathing
- Trouble swallowing
- Pain when swallowing
- Hoarseness

Diagnosis of Thyroid Cancer

Tests that examine the thyroid, neck, and blood are used to detect (find) and diagnose thyroid cancer.

The following tests and procedures may be used:

- **Physical exam and history:** An exam of the body to check general signs of health, including checking for signs of disease, such as lumps (nodules) or swelling in the neck, voice box, and lymph nodes, and anything else that seems unusual. A history of the patient's health habits and past illnesses and treatments will also be taken.
- **Laryngoscopy:** A procedure in which the doctor checks the larynx (voice box) with a mirror or with a laryngoscope. A laryngoscope is a thin, tube-like instrument with a light and a lens for viewing. A thyroid tumor may press on vocal cords. The laryngoscopy is done to see if the vocal cords are moving normally.
- **Blood hormone studies:** A procedure in which a blood sample is checked to measure the amounts of certain hormones released into the blood by organs and tissues in the body. An unusual (higher or lower than normal) amount of a substance can be a sign of disease in the organ or tissue that makes it. The blood may be checked for abnormal levels of thyroid-stimulating hormone (TSH). TSH is made by the pituitary gland in the brain. It stimulates the release of thyroid hormone and controls how fast follicular thyroid cells grow. The blood may also be checked for high levels of the hormone calcitonin and antithyroid antibodies.
- **Blood chemistry studies:** A procedure in which a blood sample is checked to measure the amounts of certain substances, such as calcium, released into the blood by organs and tissues in the body. An unusual (higher or lower than normal) amount of a substance can be a sign of disease.
- **Ultrasound exam:** A procedure in which high-energy sound waves (ultrasound) are bounced off internal tissues or organs in the neck and make echoes. The echoes form a picture of body tissues called a sonogram. The picture can be printed to be looked at later. This procedure can show the size of a thyroid nodule and whether it is solid or a fluid-filled cyst. Ultrasound may be used to guide a fine-needle aspiration biopsy.
- **Computed Tomography (CT) scan:** A procedure that makes a series of detailed pictures of areas inside the body, such as the neck, taken from different angles. The pictures are made by a computer linked to an X-ray machine. A dye may be injected into a vein or swallowed to help the organs or tissues show up more

clearly. This procedure is also called computed tomography, computerized tomography, or computerized axial tomography.

- **Fine-needle aspiration biopsy of the thyroid:** The removal of thyroid tissue using a thin needle. The needle is inserted through the skin into the thyroid. Several tissue samples are removed from different parts of the thyroid. A pathologist views the tissue samples under a microscope to look for cancer cells. Because the type of thyroid cancer can be hard to diagnose, patients should ask to have biopsy samples checked by a pathologist who has experience diagnosing thyroid cancer.
- **Surgical biopsy:** The removal of the thyroid nodule or one lobe of the thyroid during surgery so the cells and tissues can be viewed under a microscope by a pathologist to check for signs of cancer. Because the type of thyroid cancer can be hard to diagnose, patients should ask to have biopsy samples checked by a pathologist who has experience diagnosing thyroid cancer.

Staging of Thyroid Cancer

After thyroid cancer has been diagnosed, tests are done to find out if cancer cells have spread within the thyroid or to other parts of the body. The process used to find out if cancer has spread within the thyroid or to other parts of the body is called staging. The information gathered from the staging process determines the stage of the disease. It is important to know the patient's age and the stage of the cancer in order to plan treatment.

The following tests and procedures may be used in the staging process:

- **CT scan (CAT scan):** A procedure that makes a series of detailed pictures of areas inside the body, such as the chest, abdomen, and brain, taken from different angles. The pictures are made by a computer linked to an X-ray machine. A dye may be injected into a vein or swallowed to help the organs or tissues show up more clearly. This procedure is also called computed tomography, computerized tomography, or computerized axial tomography.
- **Ultrasound exam:** A procedure in which high-energy sound waves (ultrasound) are bounced off internal tissues or organs and make echoes. The echoes form a picture of body tissues called a sonogram. The picture can be printed to be looked at later.

- **Chest X-ray:** An X-ray of the organs and bones inside the chest. An X-ray is a type of energy beam that can go through the body and onto film, making a picture of areas inside the body.
- **Bone scan:** A procedure to check if there are rapidly dividing cells, such as cancer cells, in the bone. A very small amount of radioactive material is injected into a vein and travels through the bloodstream. The radioactive material collects in the bones with cancer and is detected by a scanner.
- **Sentinel lymph node biopsy:** The removal of the sentinel lymph node during surgery. The sentinel lymph node is the first lymph node to receive lymphatic drainage from a tumor. It is the first lymph node the cancer is likely to spread to from the tumor. A radioactive substance and/or blue dye is injected near the tumor. The substance or dye flows through the lymph ducts to the lymph nodes. The first lymph node to receive the substance or dye is removed. A pathologist views the tissue under a microscope to look for cancer cells. If cancer cells are not found, it may not be necessary to remove more lymph nodes.

Ways That Cancer Spreads in the Body

There are three ways that cancer spreads in the body. Cancer can spread through tissue, the lymph system, and the blood:

- **Tissue.** The cancer spreads from where it began by growing into nearby areas.
- **Lymph system.** The cancer spreads from where it began by getting into the lymph system. The cancer travels through the lymph vessels to other parts of the body.
- **Blood.** The cancer spreads from where it began by getting into the blood. The cancer travels through the blood vessels to other parts of the body.

Cancer may spread from where it began to other parts of the body.

When cancer spreads to another part of the body, it is called metastasis. Cancer cells break away from where they began (the primary tumor) and travel through the lymph system or blood.

- **Lymph system.** The cancer gets into the lymph system, travels through the lymph vessels, and forms a tumor (metastatic tumor) in another part of the body.

- **Blood.** The cancer gets into the blood, travels through the blood vessels, and forms a tumor (metastatic tumor) in another part of the body.

The metastatic tumor is the same type of cancer as the primary tumor. For example, if thyroid cancer spreads to the lung, the cancer cells in the lung are actually thyroid cancer cells. The disease is metastatic thyroid cancer, not lung cancer.

Stages of Thyroid Cancer

Stages are used to describe thyroid cancer based on the type of thyroid cancer and the age of the patient:

Papillary and Follicular Thyroid Cancer in Patients Younger than 45 Years

- **Stage I:** In stage I papillary and follicular thyroid cancer, the tumor is any size and may have spread to nearby tissues and lymph nodes. Cancer has not spread to other parts of the body.
- **Stage II:** In stage II papillary and follicular thyroid cancer, the tumor is any size and cancer has spread from the thyroid to other parts of the body, such as the lungs or bone, and may have spread to lymph nodes.

Papillary and Follicular Thyroid Cancer in Patients 45 Years and Older

- **Stage I:** In stage I papillary and follicular thyroid cancer, cancer is found only in the thyroid and the tumor is 2 centimeters or smaller.
- **Stage II:** In stage II papillary and follicular thyroid cancer, cancer is only in the thyroid and the tumor is larger than 2 centimeters but not larger than 4 centimeters.
- **Stage III:** In stage III papillary and follicular thyroid cancer, either of the following is found:
    - the tumor is larger than 4 centimeters and only in the thyroid or the tumor is any size and cancer has spread to tissues just outside the thyroid, but not to lymph nodes; or

    - the tumor is any size and cancer may have spread to tissues just outside the thyroid and has spread to lymph nodes near the trachea or the larynx (voice box).

- **Stage IV:** Stage IV papillary and follicular thyroid cancer is divided into stages IVA, IVB, and IVC.
    - In stage IVA, either of the following is found:
        - the tumor is any size and cancer has spread outside the thyroid to tissues under the skin, the trachea, the esophagus, the larynx (voice box), and/or the recurrent laryngeal nerve (a nerve that goes to the larynx); cancer may have spread to lymph nodes near the trachea or the larynx; or
        - the tumor is any size and cancer may have spread to tissues just outside the thyroid. Cancer has spread to lymph nodes on one or both sides of the neck or between the lungs.
        - In stage IVB, cancer has spread to tissue in front of the spinal column or has surrounded the carotid artery or the blood vessels in the area between the lungs. Cancer may have spread to lymph nodes.
        - In stage IVC, the tumor is any size and cancer has spread to other parts of the body, such as the lungs and bones, and may have spread to lymph nodes.

Medullary Thyroid Cancer for All Ages

- **Stage 0:** Stage 0 medullary thyroid cancer is found only with a special screening test. No tumor can be found in the thyroid.
- **Stage I:** Stage I medullary thyroid cancer is found only in the thyroid and is 2 centimeters or smaller.
- **Stage II:** In stage II medullary thyroid cancer, either of the following is found:
    - the tumor is larger than 2 centimeters and only in the thyroid; or
    - the tumor is any size and has spread to tissues just outside the thyroid, but not to lymph nodes.
- **Stage III:** In stage III medullary thyroid cancer, the tumor is any size, has spread to lymph nodes near the trachea and the larynx (voice box), and may have spread to tissues just outside the thyroid.

- **Stage IV:** Stage IV medullary thyroid cancer is divided into stages IVA, IVB, and IVC.
  - In stage IVA, either of the following is found:
    - the tumor is any size and cancer has spread outside the thyroid to tissues under the skin, the trachea, the esophagus, the larynx (voice box), and/or the recurrent laryngeal nerve (a nerve that goes to the larynx); cancer may have spread to lymph nodes near the trachea or the larynx; or
    - the tumor is any size and cancer may have spread to tissues just outside the thyroid. Cancer has spread to lymph nodes on one or both sides of the neck or between the lungs.
    - In stage IVB, cancer has spread to tissue in front of the spinal column or has surrounded the carotid artery or the blood vessels in the area between the lungs. Cancer may have spread to lymph nodes.
    - In stage IVC, the tumor is any size and cancer has spread to other parts of the body, such as the lungs and bones, and may have spread to lymph nodes.

Anaplastic Thyroid Cancer

Anaplastic thyroid cancer is considered stage IV thyroid cancer. It grows quickly and has usually spread within the neck when it is found. Stage IV anaplastic thyroid cancer is divided into stages IVA, IVB, and IVC.

- In stage IVA, cancer is found in the thyroid and may have spread to lymph nodes
- In stage IVB, cancer has spread to tissue just outside the thyroid and may have spread to lymph nodes
- In stage IVC, cancer has spread to other parts of the body, such as the lungs and bones, and may have spread to lymph nodes

Treatment Option Overview

There are different types of treatment for patients with thyroid cancer. Different types of treatment are available for patients with thyroid cancer. Some treatments are standard (the currently used treatment), and some are being tested in clinical trials. A treatment clinical trial is a research study meant to help improve current treatments or obtain information on new treatments for patients with cancer. When clinical trials show that a new treatment is better than the standard treatment, the new treatment may become the standard treatment. Patients may want to think about taking part in a clinical trial. Some clinical trials are open only to patients who have not started treatment.

Types of Standard Treatments

Six types of standard treatment are used:

Surgery

Surgery is the most common treatment for thyroid cancer. One of the following procedures may be used:

- **Lobectomy:** Removal of the lobe in which thyroid cancer is found. Lymph nodes near the cancer may also be removed and checked under a microscope for signs of cancer.
- **Near-total thyroidectomy:** Removal of all but a very small part of the thyroid. Lymph nodes near the cancer may also be removed and checked under a microscope for signs of cancer.
- **Total thyroidectomy:** Removal of the whole thyroid. Lymph nodes near the cancer may also be removed and checked under a microscope for signs of cancer.
- **Tracheostomy:** Surgery to create an opening (stoma) into the windpipe to help you breathe. The opening itself may also be called a tracheostomy.

Radiation Therapy, Including Radioactive Iodine Therapy

Radiation therapy is a cancer treatment that uses high-energy X-rays or other types of radiation to kill cancer cells or keep them from growing. There are two types of radiation therapy:

- External radiation therapy uses a machine outside the body to send radiation toward the cancer. Sometimes the radiation is aimed directly at the tumor during surgery. This is called intra-operative radiation therapy.
- Internal radiation therapy uses a radioactive substance sealed in needles, seeds, wires, or catheters that are placed directly into or near the cancer.

Radiation therapy may be given after surgery to kill any thyroid cancer cells that were not removed. Follicular and papillary thyroid cancers are sometimes treated with radioactive iodine (RAI) therapy. RAI is taken by mouth and collects in any remaining thyroid tissue, including thyroid cancer cells that have spread to other places in the body. Since only thyroid tissue takes up iodine, the RAI destroys thyroid tissue and thyroid cancer cells without harming other tissue. Before a full treatment dose of RAI is given, a small test-dose is given to see if the tumor takes up the iodine.

The way the radiation therapy is given depends on the type and stage of the cancer being treated. External radiation therapy and RAI therapy are used to treat thyroid cancer.

Chemotherapy

Chemotherapy is a cancer treatment that uses drugs to stop the growth of cancer cells, either by killing the cells or by stopping them from dividing. When chemotherapy is taken by mouth or injected into a vein or muscle, the drugs enter the bloodstream and can reach cancer cells throughout the body (systemic chemotherapy). When chemotherapy is placed directly into the cerebrospinal fluid, an organ, or a body cavity such as the abdomen, the drugs mainly affect cancer cells in those areas (regional chemotherapy). The way the chemotherapy is given depends on the type and stage of the cancer being treated.

Thyroid Hormone Therapy

Hormone therapy is a cancer treatment that removes hormones or blocks their action and stops cancer cells from growing. Hormones are substances made by glands in the body and circulated in the bloodstream. In the treatment of thyroid cancer, drugs may be given to prevent the body from making thyroid-stimulating hormone (TSH), a hormone that can increase the chance that thyroid cancer will grow or recur. Also, because thyroid cancer treatment kills thyroid cells, the thyroid is not able to make enough thyroid hormone. Patients are given thyroid hormone replacement pills.

Targeted Therapy

Targeted therapy is a type of treatment that uses drugs or other substances to identify and attack specific cancer cells without harming normal cells. Tyrosine kinase inhibitor therapy is a type of targeted therapy that blocks signals needed for tumors to grow. Vandetanib and sorafenib are tyrosine kinase inhibitors that are used to treat certain types of thyroid cancer. New types of tyrosine kinase inhibitors are being studied to treat advanced thyroid cancer.

Watchful Waiting

Watchful waiting is closely monitoring a patient's condition without giving any treatment until signs or symptoms appear or change.

Prognosis

Certain factors affect prognosis (chance of recovery) and treatment options. The prognosis (chance of recovery) and treatment options depend on the following:

- The age of the patient at the time of diagnosis
- The type of thyroid cancer
- The stage of the cancer
- Whether the cancer was completely removed by surgery
- Whether the patient has multiple endocrine neoplasia type 2B (MEN 2B)
- The patient's general health
- Whether the cancer has just been diagnosed or has recurred (come back)

Chapter 19

Parathyroid Cancer

The parathyroid glands are four pea-sized organs found in the neck near the thyroid gland. The parathyroid glands make parathyroid hormone (PTH or parathormone). PTH helps the body use and store calcium to keep the calcium in the blood at normal levels.

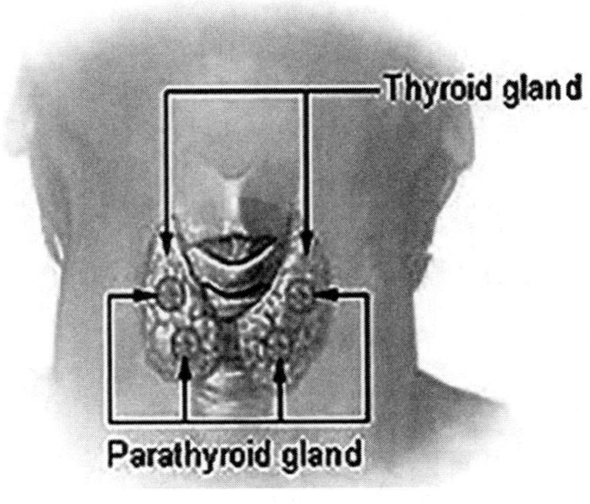

Figure 19.1. *Parathyroid Glands* (Source: "Thyroid and Parathyroid Glands," Surveillance, Epidemiology and End Results Program (SEER), National Cancer Institute (NCI).)

This chapter includes text excerpted from "Parathyroid Cancer Treatment (PDQ®)—Patient Version," National Cancer Institute (NCI), August 18, 2017.

What Is Parathyroid Cancer?

Parathyroid cancer is a rare disease in which malignant (cancer) cells form in the tissues of a parathyroid gland.

What Is Hyperparathyroidism?

A parathyroid gland may become overactive and make too much PTH, a condition called hyperparathyroidism. Hyperparathyroidism can occur when a benign tumor (noncancer), called an adenoma, forms on one of the parathyroid glands, and causes it to grow and become overactive. Sometimes hyperparathyroidism can be caused by parathyroid cancer, but this is very rare.

What Is Hypercalcemia?

The extra PTH causes:

- The calcium stored in the bones to move into the blood
- The intestines to absorb more calcium from the food we eat

This condition is called hypercalcemia (too much calcium in the blood). The hypercalcemia caused by hyperparathyroidism is more serious and life-threatening than parathyroid cancer itself and treating hypercalcemia is as important as treating the cancer.

What Are the Risk Factors for Parathyroid Glands?

Anything that increases the chance of getting a disease is called a risk factor. Risk factors for parathyroid cancer include the following rare disorders that are inherited (passed down from parent to child):

- Familial isolated hyperparathyroidism (FIHP)
- Multiple endocrine neoplasia type 1 (MEN1) syndrome

Having certain inherited disorders can increase the risk of developing parathyroid cancer. Treatment with radiation therapy may increase the risk of developing a parathyroid adenoma.

What Are the Signs and Symptoms of Parathyroid Cancer?

Most parathyroid cancer signs and symptoms are caused by the hypercalcemia that develops. Signs and symptoms of hypercalcemia include the following:

- Weakness
- Feeling very tired
- Nausea and vomiting
- Loss of appetite
- Weight loss for no known reason
- Being much more thirsty than usual
- Urinating much more than usual
- Constipation
- Trouble thinking clearly

Other signs and symptoms of parathyroid cancer include the following:

- Pain in the abdomen, side, or back that doesn't go away
- Pain in the bones
- A broken bone
- A lump in the neck
- Change in voice such as hoarseness
- Trouble swallowing

Other conditions may cause the same signs and symptoms as parathyroid cancer. Check with your doctor if you have any of these problems.

How Is Parathyroid Cancer Diagnosed?

Tests that examine the neck and blood are used to detect (find) and diagnose parathyroid cancer. Once blood tests are done and hyperparathyroidism is diagnosed, imaging tests may be done to help find which of the parathyroid glands is overactive. Sometimes the parathyroid glands are hard to find and imaging tests are done to find exactly where they are. Parathyroid cancer may be hard to diagnose because the cells of a benign parathyroid adenoma and a malignant parathyroid cancer look alike. The patient's symptoms, blood levels of calcium and parathyroid hormone, and characteristics of the tumor are also used to make a diagnosis.

The following tests and procedures may be used:

- **Physical exam and history.** An exam of the body to check general signs of health, including checking for signs of disease, such as lumps or anything else that seems unusual. A history of the patient's health habits and past illnesses and treatments will also be taken.
- **Blood chemistry studies.** A procedure in which a blood sample is checked to measure the amounts of certain substances released into the blood by organs and tissues in the body. An unusual (higher or lower than normal) amount of a substance can be a sign of disease. To diagnose parathyroid cancer, the sample of blood is checked for its calcium level.
- **Parathyroid hormone test.** A procedure in which a blood sample is checked to measure the amount of parathyroid hormone released into the blood by the parathyroid glands. A higher than normal amount of parathyroid hormone can be a sign of disease.
- **Sestamibi scan.** A type of radionuclide scan used to find an overactive parathyroid gland. A very small amount of a radioactive substance called technetium 99 is injected into a vein and travels through the bloodstream to the parathyroid gland. The radioactive substance will collect in the overactive gland and show up brightly on a special camera that detects radioactivity.
- **CT/CAT scan.** A procedure that makes a series of detailed pictures of areas inside the body, taken from different angles. The pictures are made by a computer linked to an X-ray machine. A dye may be injected into a vein or swallowed to help the organs or tissues show up more clearly. This procedure is also called computed tomography, computerized tomography, or computerized axial tomography.
- **Single photon emission computed tomography (SPECT) scan.** A procedure that uses a special camera linked to a computer to make a 3-dimensional (3D) picture. A very small amount of a radioactive substance is injected into a vein. As the substance travels through the blood, the camera rotates around the neck and takes pictures. Blood flow and metabolism are higher than normal in areas where cancer cells are growing. These areas will show up brighter in the picture. This procedure may be done just before or after a computerized tomography (CT) scan.

- **Ultrasound exam.** A procedure in which high-energy sound waves (ultrasound) are bounced off internal tissues or organs and make echoes. The echoes form a picture of body tissues called a sonogram.
- **Angiogram.** A procedure to look at blood vessels and the flow of blood. A contrast dye is injected into the blood vessel. As the contrast dye moves through the blood vessel, X-rays are taken to see if there are any blockages.
- **Venous sampling.** A procedure in which a sample of blood is taken from specific veins and checked to measure the amounts of certain substances released into the blood by nearby organs and tissues. If imaging tests do not show which parathyroid gland is overactive, blood samples may be taken from veins near each parathyroid gland to find which one is making too much PTH.

What Is the Prognosis for Parathyroid Cancer?

The prognosis (chance of recovery) and treatment options depend on the following:

- Whether the calcium level in the blood can be controlled
- The stage of the cancer
- Whether the tumor and the capsule around the tumor can be completely removed by surgery
- The patient's general health

Stages of Parathyroid Cancer

After parathyroid cancer has been diagnosed, tests are done to find out if cancer cells have spread to other parts of the body.

The process used to find out if cancer has spread to other parts of the body is called staging. The following imaging tests may be used to determine if cancer has spread to other parts of the body such as the lungs, liver, bone, heart, pancreas, or lymph nodes:

- **Computed Tomography (CT) scan.** A procedure that makes a series of detailed pictures of areas inside the body, taken from different angles. The pictures are made by a computer linked to an X-ray machine. A dye may be injected into a vein or swallowed to help the organs or tissues show up more clearly. This procedure is also called computed tomography, computerized tomography, or computerized axial tomography.

- **Magnetic resonance imaging (MRI).** A procedure that uses a magnet, radio waves, and a computer to make a series of detailed pictures of areas inside the body. This procedure is also called nuclear magnetic resonance imaging (NMRI).

Are There Any Standard Staging Process for Parathyroid Cancer?

There is no standard staging process for parathyroid cancer. Parathyroid cancer is described as either localized or metastatic:

- **Localized parathyroid cancer** is found in a parathyroid gland and may have spread to nearby tissues.
- **Metastatic parathyroid cancer** has spread to other parts of the body, such as the lungs, liver, bone, sac around the heart, pancreas, or lymph nodes.

Treatment Option Overview

Different types of treatment are available for patients with parathyroid cancer. Some treatments are standard (the currently used treatment), and some are being tested in clinical trials. A treatment clinical trial is a research study meant to help improve current treatments or obtain information on new treatments for patients with cancer. When clinical trials show that a new treatment is better than the standard treatment, the new treatment may become the standard treatment. Patients may want to think about taking part in a clinical trial. Some clinical trials are open only to patients who have not started treatment.

Treatment includes control of hypercalcemia (too much calcium in the blood) in patients who have an overactive parathyroid gland.

In order to reduce the amount of parathyroid hormone that is being made and control the level of calcium in the blood, as much of the tumor as possible is removed in surgery. For patients who cannot have surgery, medication may be used.

Standard Treatment Available for Patients with Parathyroid Cancer

Four types of standard treatment are used:

Surgery

Surgery (removing the cancer in an operation) is the most common treatment for parathyroid cancer that is in the parathyroid glands or has spread to other parts of the body. Because parathyroid cancer grows very slowly, cancer that has spread to other parts of the body may be removed by surgery in order to cure the patient or control the effects of the disease for a long time. Before surgery, treatment is given to control hypercalcemia.

The following surgical procedures may be used:

- **En bloc resection.** Surgery to remove the entire parathyroid gland and the capsule around it. Sometimes lymph nodes, half of the thyroid gland on the same side of the body as the cancer, and muscles, tissues, and a nerve in the neck are also removed.
- **Tumor debulking.** A surgical procedure in which as much of the tumor as possible is removed. Some tumors cannot be completely removed.
- **Metastasectomy.** Surgery to remove any cancer that has spread to distant organs such as the lung.

Surgery for parathyroid cancer sometimes damages nerves of the vocal cords. There are treatments to help with speech problems caused by this nerve damage.

Radiation Therapy

Radiation therapy is a cancer treatment that uses high-energy X-rays or other types of radiation to kill cancer cells or keep them from growing. There are two types of radiation therapy:

- External radiation therapy uses a machine outside the body to send radiation toward the cancer.
- Internal radiation therapy uses a radioactive substance sealed in needles, seeds, wires, or catheters that are placed directly into or near the cancer.

The way the radiation therapy is given depends on the type and stage of the cancer being treated. External radiation therapy is used to treat parathyroid cancer.

Chemotherapy

Chemotherapy is a cancer treatment that uses drugs to stop the growth of cancer cells, either by killing the cells or by stopping them

from dividing. When chemotherapy is taken by mouth or injected into a vein or muscle, the drugs enter the bloodstream and can reach cancer cells throughout the body (systemic chemotherapy). When chemotherapy is placed directly into the cerebrospinal fluid, an organ, or a body cavity such as the abdomen, the drugs mainly affect cancer cells in those areas (regional chemotherapy). The way the chemotherapy is given depends on the type and stage of the cancer being treated.

Supportive Care

Supportive care is given to lessen the problems caused by the disease or its treatment. Supportive care for hypercalcemia caused by parathyroid cancer may include the following:

- Intravenous (IV) fluids
- Drugs that increase how much urine the body makes
- Drugs that stop the body from absorbing calcium from the food we eat
- Drugs that stop the parathyroid gland from making parathyroid hormone

Follow-Up Tests

Some of the tests that were done to diagnose the cancer or to find out the stage of the cancer may be repeated. Some tests will be repeated in order to see how well the treatment is working. Decisions about whether to continue, change, or stop treatment may be based on the results of these tests.

Some of the tests will continue to be done from time to time after treatment has ended. The results of these tests can show if your condition has changed or if the cancer has recurred (come back). These tests are sometimes called follow-up tests or check-ups. Parathyroid cancer often recurs. Patients should have regular check-ups for the rest of their lives, to find and treat recurrences early.

Chapter 20

Adrenocortical Carcinoma

There are two adrenal glands. The adrenal glands are small and shaped like a triangle. One adrenal gland sits on top of each kidney. Each adrenal gland has two parts. The outer layer of the adrenal gland is the adrenal cortex. The center of the adrenal gland is the adrenal medulla.

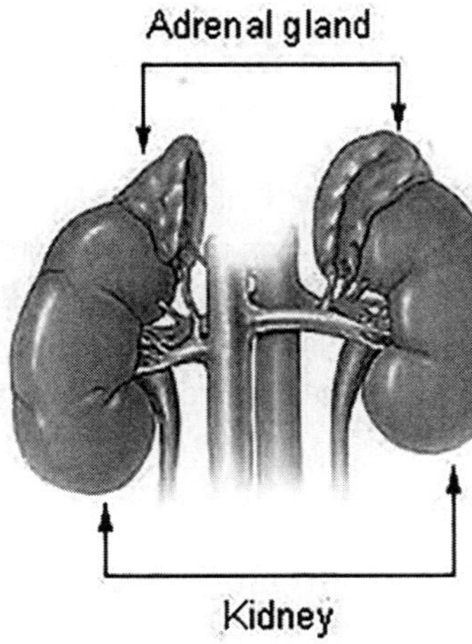

Figure 20.1. *Adrenal Gland* (Source: "Adrenal Gland," Surveillance, Epidemiology and End Results Program (SEER), National Cancer Institute (NCI).)

This chapter includes text excerpted from "Adrenocortical Carcinoma Treatment (PDQ®)—Patient Version," National Cancer Institute (NCI), January 5, 2018.

The adrenal cortex makes important hormones that:

- Balance the water and salt in the body
- Help keep blood pressure normal
- Help control the body's use of protein, fat, and carbohydrates
- Cause the body to have masculine or feminine characteristics

What Is Adrenocortical Carcinoma?

Adrenocortical carcinoma is a rare disease in which malignant (cancer) cells form in the outer layer of the adrenal gland. Adrenocortical carcinoma is also called cancer of the adrenal cortex. A tumor of the adrenal cortex may be functioning (makes more hormones than normal) or nonfunctioning (does not make more hormones than normal). Most adrenocortical tumors are functioning. The hormones made by functioning tumors may cause certain signs or symptoms of disease. The adrenal medulla makes hormones that help the body react to stress. Cancer that forms in the adrenal medulla is called pheochromocytoma. Adrenocortical carcinoma and pheochromocytoma can occur in both adults and children. Treatment for children, however, is different than treatment for adults.

What Are the Risk Factors for Adrenocortical Carcinoma?

Anything that increases your risk of getting a disease is called a risk factor. Having a risk factor does not mean that you will get cancer; not having risk factors doesn't mean that you will not get cancer. Talk with your doctor if you think you may be at risk.

Risk factors for adrenocortical carcinoma include having the following hereditary diseases:

- Li-Fraumeni syndrome
- Beckwith-Wiedemann syndrome
- Carney complex

What Are the Symptoms of Adrenocortical Carcinoma?

Symptoms of adrenocortical carcinoma include pain in the abdomen. These and other signs and symptoms may be caused by adrenocortical carcinoma:

- A lump in the abdomen
- Pain the abdomen or back
- A feeling of fullness in the abdomen

A nonfunctioning adrenocortical tumor may not cause signs or symptoms in the early stages.

A functioning adrenocortical tumor makes too much of one of the following hormones:

- Cortisol
- Aldosterone
- Testosterone
- Estrogen

Too much cortisol may cause:

- Weight gain in the face, neck, and trunk of the body and thin arms and legs
- Growth of fine hair on the face, upper back, or arms
- A round, red, full face
- A lump of fat on the back of the neck
- A deepening of the voice and swelling of the sex organs or breasts in both males and females
- Muscle weakness
- High blood sugar
- High blood pressure

Too much aldosterone may cause:

- High blood pressure
- Muscle weakness or cramps
- Frequent urination
- Feeling thirsty

Too much testosterone (in women) may cause:

- Growth of fine hair on the face, upper back, or arms
- Acne

- Balding
- A deepening of the voice
- No menstrual periods

Men who make too much testosterone do not usually have signs or symptoms.

Too much estrogen (in women) may cause:

- Irregular menstrual periods in women who have not gone through menopause
- Vaginal bleeding in women who have gone through menopause
- Weight gain

Too much estrogen (in men) may cause:

- Growth of breast tissue
- Lower sex drive
- Impotence

These and other signs and symptoms may be caused by adrenocortical carcinoma or by other conditions. Check with your doctor if you have any of these problems.

How Is Adrenocortical Carcinoma Diagnosed?

Imaging studies and tests that examine the blood and urine are used to detect (find) and diagnose adrenocortical carcinoma. The tests and procedures used to diagnose adrenocortical carcinoma depend on the patient's signs and symptoms. The following tests and procedures may be used:

- **Physical exam and history.** An exam of the body to check general signs of health, including checking for signs of disease, such as lumps or anything else that seems unusual. A history of the patient's health habits and past illnesses and treatments will also be taken.
- **24-hour urine test.** A test in which urine is collected for 24 hours to measure the amounts of cortisol or 17-ketosteroids. A higher than normal amount of these in the urine may be a sign of disease in the adrenal cortex.

- **Low-dose dexamethasone suppression test.** A test in which one or more small doses of dexamethasone are given. The level of cortisol is checked from a sample of blood or from urine that is collected for three days. This test is done to check if the adrenal gland is making too much cortisol.
- **High-dose dexamethasone suppression test.** A test in which one or more high doses of dexamethasone are given. The level of cortisol is checked from a sample of blood or from urine that is collected for three days. This test is done to check if the adrenal gland is making too much cortisol or if the pituitary gland is telling the adrenal glands to make too much cortisol.
- **Blood chemistry study.** A procedure in which a blood sample is checked to measure the amounts of certain substances, such as potassium or sodium, released into the blood by organs and tissues in the body. An unusual (higher or lower than normal) amount of a substance can be a sign of disease.
- **Computed tomography (CT)/computerized axial tomography (CAT) scan.** A procedure that makes a series of detailed pictures of areas inside the body, taken from different angles. The pictures are made by a computer linked to an X-ray machine. A dye may be injected into a vein or swallowed to help the organs or tissues show up more clearly.
- **Magnetic resonance imaging (MRI).** A procedure that uses a magnet, radio waves, and a computer to make a series of detailed pictures of areas inside the body. This procedure is also called nuclear magnetic resonance imaging (NMRI). An MRI of the abdomen is done to diagnose adrenocortical carcinoma.
- **Adrenal angiography.** A procedure to look at the arteries and the flow of blood near the adrenal glands. A contrast dye is injected into the adrenal arteries. As the dye moves through the arteries, a series of X-rays are taken to see if any arteries are blocked.
- **Adrenal venography.** A procedure to look at the adrenal veins and the flow of blood near the adrenal glands. A contrast dye is injected into an adrenal vein. As the contrast dye moves through the veins, a series of X-rays are taken to see if any veins are blocked. A catheter (very thin tube) may be inserted into the vein to take a blood sample, which is checked for abnormal hormone levels.

- **Positron emission tomography (PET) scan.** A procedure to find malignant tumor cells in the body. A small amount of radioactive glucose (sugar) is injected into a vein. The PET scanner rotates around the body and makes a picture of where glucose is being used in the body. Malignant tumor cells show up brighter in the picture because they are more active and take up more glucose than normal cells do.
- **Metaiodobenzylguanidine (MIBG) scan.** A very small amount of radioactive material called MIBG is injected into a vein and travels through the bloodstream. Adrenal gland cells take up the radioactive material and are detected by a device that measures radiation. This scan is done to tell the difference between adrenocortical carcinoma and pheochromocytoma.
- **Biopsy.** The removal of cells or tissues so they can be viewed under a microscope by a pathologist to check for signs of cancer. The sample may be taken using a thin needle, called a fine-needle aspiration (FNA) biopsy or a wider needle, called a core biopsy.

What Is the Prognosis for Adrenocortical Carcinoma?

The prognosis (chance of recovery) and treatment options depend on the following:

- The stage of the cancer (the size of the tumor and whether it is in the adrenal gland only or has spread to other places in the body)
- Whether the tumor can be completely removed in surgery
- Whether the cancer has been treated in the past
- The patient's general health
- The grade of tumor cells (how different they look from normal cells under a microscope)

Adrenocortical carcinoma may be cured if treated at an early stage.

Stages of Adrenocortical Carcinoma

After adrenocortical carcinoma has been diagnosed, tests are done to find out if cancer cells have spread within the adrenal gland or to other parts of the body.

The process used to find out if cancer has spread within the adrenal gland or to other parts of the body is called staging. The information gathered from the staging process determines the stage of the disease. It is important to know the stage in order to plan treatment. The following tests and procedures may be used in the staging process:

- **Computed tomography (CT) scan.** A procedure that makes a series of detailed pictures of areas inside the body, such as the abdomen or chest, taken from different angles. The pictures are made by a computer linked to an X-ray machine. A dye may be injected into a vein or swallowed to help the organs or tissues show up more clearly. This procedure is also called computed tomography, computerized tomography, or computerized axial tomography.
- **Magnetic resonance imaging (MRI) with gadolinium.** A procedure that uses a magnet, radio waves, and a computer to make a series of detailed pictures of areas inside the body, such as the abdomen. A substance called gadolinium may be injected into a vein. The gadolinium collects around the cancer cells so they show up brighter in the picture. This procedure is also called nuclear magnetic resonance imaging (NMRI).
- **Positron emission tomography (PET) scan.** A procedure to find malignant tumor cells in the body. A small amount of radioactive glucose (sugar) is injected into a vein. The PET scanner rotates around the body and makes a picture of where glucose is being used in the body. Malignant tumor cells show up brighter in the picture because they are more active and take up more glucose than normal cells do.
- **Ultrasound exam.** A procedure in which high-energy sound waves (ultrasound) are bounced off internal tissues or organs, such as the vena cava, and make echoes. The echoes form a picture of body tissues called a sonogram.
- **Adrenalectomy.** A procedure to remove the affected adrenal gland. A tissue sample is viewed under a microscope by a pathologist to check for signs of cancer.

What Are the Stages of Adrenocortical Carcinoma?

The following stages are used for adrenocortical carcinoma:

- **Stage I.** In stage I, the tumor is 5 centimeters or smaller and is found in the adrenal gland only.

- **Stage II.** In stage II, the tumor is larger than 5 centimeters and is found in the adrenal gland only.
- **Stage III.** In stage III, the tumor is any size and has spread:
  - to nearby lymph nodes; or
  - to nearby tissues or organs (kidney, diaphragm, pancreas, spleen, or liver) or to large blood vessels (renal vein or vena cava) and may have spread to nearby lymph nodes.
- **Stage IV.** In stage IV, the tumor is any size, may have spread to nearby lymph nodes, and has spread to other parts of the body, such as the lung, bone, or peritoneum.

Treatment Option Overview

Different types of treatments are available for patients with adrenocortical carcinoma. Some treatments are standard (the currently used treatment), and some are being tested in clinical trials. A treatment clinical trial is a research study meant to help improve current treatments or obtain information on new treatments for patients with cancer. When clinical trials show that a new treatment is better than the standard treatment, the new treatment may become the standard treatment. Patients may want to think about taking part in a clinical trial. Some clinical trials are open only to patients who have not started treatment.

Standard Treatment for Adrenocortical Carcinoma

Three types of standard treatment are used:

Surgery

Surgery to remove the adrenal gland (adrenalectomy) is often used to treat adrenocortical carcinoma. Sometimes surgery is done to remove the nearby lymph nodes and other tissue where the cancer has spread.

Radiation Therapy

Radiation therapy is a cancer treatment that uses high-energy X-rays or other types of radiation to kill cancer cells or keep them from growing. There are two types of radiation therapy:

- External radiation therapy uses a machine outside the body to send radiation toward the cancer.

- Internal radiation therapy uses a radioactive substance sealed in needles, seeds, wires, or catheters that are placed directly into or near the cancer.

The way the radiation therapy is given depends on the type and stage of the cancer being treated. External radiation therapy is used to treat adrenocortical carcinoma.

Chemotherapy

Chemotherapy is a cancer treatment that uses drugs to stop the growth of cancer cells, either by killing the cells or by stopping them from dividing. When chemotherapy is taken by mouth or injected into a vein or muscle, the drugs enter the bloodstream and can reach cancer cells throughout the body (systemic chemotherapy). When chemotherapy is placed directly into the cerebrospinal fluid, an organ, or a body cavity such as the abdomen, the drugs mainly affect cancer cells in those areas (regional chemotherapy). Combination chemotherapy is treatment using more than one anticancer drug. The way the chemotherapy is given depends on the type and stage of the cancer being treated.

Types of Treatment Being Tested in Clinical Trials

New types of treatment are being tested in clinical trials.

Biologic Therapy

Biologic therapy is a treatment that uses the patient's immune system to fight cancer. Substances made by the body or made in a laboratory are used to boost, direct, or restore the body's natural defenses against cancer. This type of cancer treatment is also called biotherapy or immunotherapy.

Targeted Therapy

Targeted therapy is a type of treatment that uses drugs or other substances to identify and attack specific cancer cells without harming normal cells.

Follow-Up Tests

Some of the tests that were done to diagnose the cancer or to find out the stage of the cancer may be repeated. Some tests will be repeated

in order to see how well the treatment is working. Decisions about whether to continue, change, or stop treatment may be based on the results of these tests. Some of the tests will continue to be done from time to time after treatment has ended. The results of these tests can show if your condition has changed or if the cancer has recurred (come back). These tests are sometimes called follow-up tests or check-ups.

Chapter 21

Islet Cell Tumors

The pancreas is a gland about 6 inches long that is shaped like a thin pear lying on its side. The wider end of the pancreas is called the head, the middle section is called the body, and the narrow end is called the tail. The pancreas lies behind the stomach and in front of the spine.

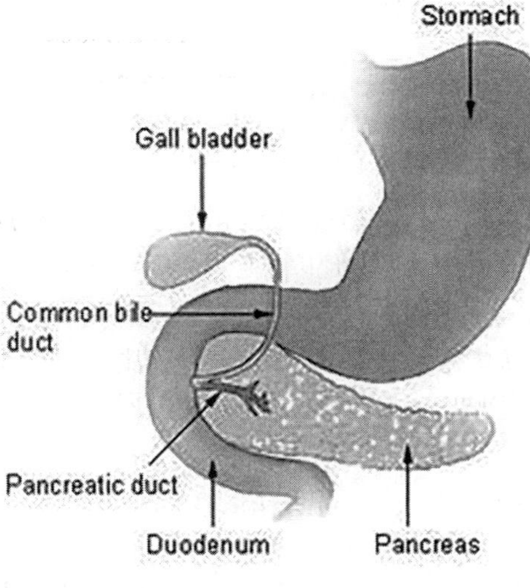

Figure 21.1. *Pancreas* (Source: "Pancreas," Surveillance, Epidemiology and End Results Program (SEER), National Cancer Institute (NCI).)

This chapter includes text excerpted from "Pancreatic Neuroendocrine Tumors (Islet Cell Tumors) Treatment (PDQ®)—Patient Version," National Cancer Institute (NCI), January 29, 2018.

There are two kinds of cells in the pancreas:

- **Endocrine pancreas cells** make several kinds of hormones (chemicals that control the actions of certain cells or organs in the body), such as insulin to control blood sugar. They cluster together in many small groups (islets) throughout the pancreas. Endocrine pancreas cells are also called islet cells or islets of Langerhans. Tumors that form in islet cells are called islet cell tumors, pancreatic endocrine tumors, or pancreatic neuroendocrine tumors (pancreatic NETs).
- **Exocrine pancreas cells** make enzymes that are released into the small intestine to help the body digest food. Most of the pancreas is made of ducts with small sacs at the end of the ducts, which are lined with exocrine cells.

What Are Pancreatic Neuroendocrine Tumors (NETs)?

Pancreatic neuroendocrine tumors (NETs) form in hormone-making cells (islet cells) of the pancreas. Pancreatic NETs may be benign (not cancer) or malignant (cancer). When pancreatic NETs are malignant, they are called pancreatic endocrine cancer or islet cell carcinoma. Pancreatic NETs are much less common than pancreatic exocrine tumors and have a better prognosis.

What Are the Types of Pancreatic NETs?

Pancreatic NETs may be functional or nonfunctional:

- **Functional tumors** make extra amounts of hormones, such as gastrin, insulin, and glucagon, that cause signs and symptoms.
- **Nonfunctional tumors** do not make extra amounts of hormones. Signs and symptoms are caused by the tumor as it spreads and grows. Most nonfunctional tumors are malignant (cancer).

Most pancreatic NETs are functional tumors.

There are different kinds of functional pancreatic NETs.

Pancreatic NETs make different kinds of hormones such as gastrin, insulin, and glucagon. Functional pancreatic NETs include the following:

- **Gastrinoma.** A tumor that forms in cells that make gastrin. Gastrin is a hormone that causes the stomach to release an acid that helps digest food. Both gastrin and stomach acid are increased by gastrinomas. When increased stomach acid, stomach ulcers, and diarrhea are caused by a tumor that makes gastrin, it is called Zollinger-Ellison syndrome. A gastrinoma usually forms in the head of the pancreas and sometimes forms in the small intestine. Most gastrinomas are malignant (cancer).

- **Insulinoma.** A tumor that forms in cells that make insulin. Insulin is a hormone that controls the amount of glucose (sugar) in the blood. It moves glucose into the cells, where it can be used by the body for energy. Insulinomas are usually slow-growing tumors that rarely spread. An insulinoma forms in the head, body, or tail of the pancreas. Insulinomas are usually benign (not cancer).
- **Glucagonoma.** A tumor that forms in cells that make glucagon. Glucagon is a hormone that increases the amount of glucose in the blood. It causes the liver to break down glycogen. Too much glucagon causes hyperglycemia (high blood sugar). A glucagonoma usually forms in the tail of the pancreas. Most glucagonomas are malignant (cancer).
- **Other types of tumors.** There are other rare types of functional pancreatic NETs that make hormones, including hormones that control the balance of sugar, salt, and water in the body. These tumors include:
  - VIPomas, which make vasoactive intestinal peptide. VIPoma may also be called Verner-Morrison syndrome
  - Somatostatinomas, which make somatostatin

These other types of tumors are grouped together because they are treated in much the same way.

What Are the Risk Factors for Pancreatic NETs?

Anything that increases your risk of getting a disease is called a risk factor. Having a risk factor does not mean that you will get cancer; not having risk factors doesn't mean that you will not get cancer. Talk with your doctor if you think you may be at risk. Multiple endocrine neoplasia type 1 (MEN1) syndrome is a risk factor for pancreatic NETs.

What Are the Signs and Symptoms of Pancreatic NETs?

Signs or symptoms can be caused by the growth of the tumor and/or by hormones the tumor makes or by other conditions. Some tumors may not cause signs or symptoms. Check with your doctor if you have any of these problems. Different types of pancreatic NETs have different signs and symptoms.

Signs and Symptoms of a Nonfunctional Pancreatic NET

A nonfunctional pancreatic NET may grow for a long time without causing signs or symptoms. It may grow large or spread to other parts of the body before it causes signs or symptoms, such as:

- Diarrhea
- Indigestion
- A lump in the abdomen
- Pain in the abdomen or back
- Yellowing of the skin and whites of the eyes

Signs and Symptoms of a Functional Pancreatic NET

The signs and symptoms of a functional pancreatic NET depend on the type of hormone being made.

Too much gastrin may cause:

- Stomach ulcers that keep coming back
- Pain in the abdomen, which may spread to the back. The pain may come and go and it may go away after taking an antacid
- The flow of stomach contents back into the esophagus (gastroesophageal reflux)
- Diarrhea

Too much insulin may cause:

- Low blood sugar. This can cause blurred vision, headache, and feeling lightheaded, tired, weak, shaky, nervous, irritable, sweaty, confused, or hungry
- Fast heartbeat

Too much glucagon may cause:

- Skin rash on the face, stomach, or legs
- High blood sugar. This can cause headaches, frequent urination, dry skin and mouth, or feeling hungry, thirsty, tired, or weak
- Blood clots. Blood clots in the lung can cause shortness of breath, cough, or pain in the chest. Blood clots in the arm or leg can cause pain, swelling, warmth, or redness of the arm or leg.
- Diarrhea
- Weight loss for no known reason
- Sore tongue or sores at the corners of the mouth

Too much vasoactive intestinal peptide (VIP) may cause:

- Very large amounts of watery diarrhea
- Dehydration. This can cause feeling thirsty, making less urine, dry skin and mouth, headaches, dizziness, or feeling tired.
- Low potassium level in the blood. This can cause muscle weakness, aching, or cramps, numbness and tingling, frequent urination, fast heartbeat, and feeling confused or thirsty.
- Cramps or pain in the abdomen
- Weight loss for no known reason

Too much somatostatin may cause:

- High blood sugar. This can cause headaches, frequent urination, dry skin and mouth, or feeling hungry, thirsty, tired, or weak.
- Diarrhea
- Steatorrhea (very foul-smelling stool that floats)
- Gallstones
- Yellowing of the skin and whites of the eyes
- Weight loss for no known reason

How is Pancreatic NETs Diagnosed?

Lab tests and imaging tests are used to detect (find) and diagnose pancreatic NETs.

The following tests and procedures may be used:

- **Physical exam and history.** An exam of the body to check general signs of health, including checking for signs of disease, such as lumps or anything else that seems unusual. A history of the patient's health habits and past illnesses and treatments will also be taken.
- **Blood chemistry studies.** A procedure in which a blood sample is checked to measure the amounts of certain substances, such as glucose (sugar), released into the blood by organs and tissues in the body. An unusual (higher or lower than normal) amount of a substance can be a sign of disease.
- **Chromogranin A test.** A test in which a blood sample is checked to measure the amount of chromogranin A in the blood. A higher than normal amount of chromogranin A and normal amounts of hormones such as gastrin, insulin, and glucagon can be a sign of a nonfunctional pancreatic NET.
- **Abdominal CT scan (CAT scan).** A procedure that makes a series of detailed pictures of the abdomen, taken from different angles. The pictures are made by a computer linked to an X-ray machine. A dye may be injected into a vein or swallowed to help the organs or tissues show up more clearly. This procedure is also called computed tomography, computerized tomography, or computerized axial tomography.
- **MRI (magnetic resonance imaging)**. A procedure that uses a magnet, radio waves, and a computer to make a series of detailed pictures of areas inside the body. This procedure is also called nuclear magnetic resonance imaging (NMRI).
- **Somatostatin receptor scintigraphy (SRS).** A type of radionuclide scan that may be used to find small pancreatic NETs. A small amount of radioactive octreotide (a hormone that attaches to tumors) is injected into a vein and travels through the blood. The radioactive octreotide attaches to the tumor and a special camera that detects radioactivity is used to show where the tumors are in the body. This procedure is also called octreotide scan and SRS.
- **Endoscopic ultrasound (EUS).** A procedure in which an endoscope is inserted into the body, usually through the mouth or rectum. An endoscope is a thin, tube-like instrument with a

light and a lens for viewing. A probe at the end of the endoscope is used to bounce high-energy sound waves (ultrasound) off internal tissues or organs and make echoes. The echoes form a picture of body tissues called a sonogram. This procedure is also called endosonography.

- **Endoscopic retrograde cholangiopancreatography (ERCP).** A procedure used to X-ray the ducts (tubes) that carry bile from the liver to the gallbladder and from the gallbladder to the small intestine. Sometimes pancreatic cancer causes these ducts to narrow and block or slow the flow of bile, causing jaundice. An endoscope is passed through the mouth, esophagus, and stomach into the first part of the small intestine. An endoscope is a thin, tube-like instrument with a light and a lens for viewing. A catheter (a smaller tube) is then inserted through the endoscope into the pancreatic ducts. A dye is injected through the catheter into the ducts and an X-ray is taken. If the ducts are blocked by a tumor, a fine tube may be inserted into the duct to unblock it. This tube (or stent) may be left in place to keep the duct open. Tissue samples may also be taken and checked under a microscope for signs of cancer.
- **Angiogram.** A procedure to look at blood vessels and the flow of blood. A contrast dye is injected into the blood vessel. As the contrast dye moves through the blood vessel, X-rays are taken to see if there are any blockages.
- **Laparotomy.** A surgical procedure in which an incision (cut) is made in the wall of the abdomen to check the inside of the abdomen for signs of disease. The size of the incision depends on the reason the laparotomy is being done. Sometimes organs are removed or tissue samples are taken and checked under a microscope for signs of disease.
- **Intraoperative ultrasound.** A procedure that uses high-energy sound waves (ultrasound) to create images of internal organs or tissues during surgery. A transducer placed directly on the organ or tissue is used to make the sound waves, which create echoes. The transducer receives the echoes and sends them to a computer, which uses the echoes to make pictures called sonograms.
- **Biopsy.** The removal of cells or tissues so they can be viewed under a microscope by a pathologist to check for signs of cancer.

There are several ways to do a biopsy for pancreatic NETs. Cells may be removed using a fine or wide needle inserted into the pancreas during an X-ray or ultrasound. Tissue may also be removed during a laparoscopy (a surgical incision made in the wall of the abdomen).

- **Bone scan.** A procedure to check if there are rapidly dividing cells, such as cancer cells, in the bone. A very small amount of radioactive material is injected into a vein and travels through the bloodstream. The radioactive material collects in bones with cancer and is detected by a scanner.

Other kinds of lab tests are used to check for the specific type of pancreatic NETs.

The following tests and procedures may be used:

Gastrinoma

- **Fasting serum gastrin test.** A test in which a blood sample is checked to measure the amount of gastrin in the blood. This test is done after the patient has had nothing to eat or drink for at least 8 hours. Conditions other than gastrinoma can cause an increase in the amount of gastrin in the blood.
- **Basal acid output test.** A test to measure the amount of acid made by the stomach. The test is done after the patient has had nothing to eat or drink for at least 8 hours. A tube is inserted through the nose or throat, into the stomach. The stomach contents are removed and four samples of gastric acid are removed through the tube. These samples are used to find out the amount of gastric acid made during the test and the pH level of the gastric secretions.
- **Secretin stimulation test.** If the basal acid output test result is not normal, a secretin stimulation test may be done. The tube is moved into the small intestine and samples are taken from the small intestine after a drug called secretin is injected. Secretin causes the small intestine to make acid. When there is a gastrinoma, the secretin causes an increase in how much gastric acid is made and the level of gastrin in the blood.
- **Somatostatin receptor scintigraphy.** A type of radionuclide scan that may be used to find small pancreatic NETs. A small amount of radioactive octreotide (a hormone that attaches to tumors) is injected into a vein and travels through the blood.

The radioactive octreotide attaches to the tumor and a special camera that detects radioactivity is used to show where the tumors are in the body. This procedure is also called octreotide scan and SRS.

Insulinoma

- **Fasting serum glucose and insulin test.** A test in which a blood sample is checked to measure the amounts of glucose (sugar) and insulin in the blood. The test is done after the patient has had nothing to eat or drink for at least 24 hours.

Glucagonoma

- **Fasting serum glucagon test.** A test in which a blood sample is checked to measure the amount of glucagon in the blood. The test is done after the patient has had nothing to eat or drink for at least 8 hours.

Other Tumor Types

- **VIPoma**
    - **Serum VIP (vasoactive intestinal peptide) test.** A test in which a blood sample is checked to measure the amount of VIP.
    - **Blood chemistry studies.** A procedure in which a blood sample is checked to measure the amounts of certain substances released into the blood by organs and tissues in the body. An unusual (higher or lower than normal) amount of a substance can be a sign of disease. In VIPoma, there is a lower than normal amount of potassium.
    - **Stool analysis.** A stool sample is checked for a higher than normal sodium (salt) and potassium levels.
- **Somatostatinoma**
    - **Fasting serum somatostatin test.** A test in which a blood sample is checked to measure the amount of somatostatin in the blood. The test is done after the patient has had nothing to eat or drink for at least 8 hours.
    - **Somatostatin receptor scintigraphy.** A type of radionuclide scan that may be used to find small pancreatic NETs. A small amount of radioactive octreotide (a hormone

that attaches to tumors) is injected into a vein and travels through the blood. The radioactive octreotide attaches to the tumor and a special camera that detects radioactivity is used to show where the tumors are in the body. This procedure is also called octreotide scan and SRS.

What Is the Prognosis for Pancreatic NETs?

Pancreatic NETs can often be cured. The prognosis (chance of recovery) and treatment options depend on the following:

- The type of cancer cell
- Where the tumor is found in the pancreas
- Whether the tumor has spread to more than one place in the pancreas or to other parts of the body
- Whether the patient has MEN1 syndrome
- The patient's age and general health
- Whether the cancer has just been diagnosed or has recurred (come back)

Stages of Pancreatic Neuroendocrine Tumors

The process used to find out if cancer has spread within the pancreas or to other parts of the body is called staging. The results of the tests and procedures used to diagnose pancreatic neuroendocrine tumors (NETs) are also used to find out whether the cancer has spread.

Although there is a standard staging system for pancreatic NETs, it is not used to plan treatment. Treatment of pancreatic NETs is based on the following:

- Whether the cancer is found in one place in the pancreas
- Whether the cancer is found in several places in the pancreas
- Whether the cancer has spread to lymph nodes near the pancreas or to other parts of the body such as the liver, lung, peritoneum, or bone

Treatment Option Overview

Different types of treatments are available for patients with pancreatic NETs. Some treatments are standard (the currently used treatment), and some are being tested in clinical trials. A treatment clinical trial is a research study meant to help improve current treatments or obtain information on new treatments for patients with cancer. When clinical trials show that a new treatment is better than the standard treatment, the new treatment may become the standard treatment. Patients may want to think about taking part in a clinical trial. Some clinical trials are open only to patients who have not started treatment.

Standard Treatment for Pancreatic NETs

Six types of standard treatment are used:

Surgery

An operation may be done to remove the tumor. One of the following types of surgery may be used:

- **Enucleation.** Surgery to remove the tumor only. This may be done when cancer occurs in one place in the pancreas.
- **Pancreatoduodenectomy.** A surgical procedure in which the head of the pancreas, the gallbladder, nearby lymph nodes and part of the stomach, small intestine, and bile duct are removed. Enough of the pancreas is left to make digestive juices and insulin. The organs removed during this procedure depend on the patient's condition. This is also called the Whipple procedure.
- **Distal pancreatectomy.** Surgery to remove the body and tail of the pancreas. The spleen may also be removed.
- **Total gastrectomy.** Surgery to remove the whole stomach.
- **Parietal cell vagotomy.** Surgery to cut the nerve that causes stomach cells to make acid.
- **Liver resection.** Surgery to remove part or all of the liver.
- **Radiofrequency ablation.** The use of a special probe with tiny electrodes that kill cancer cells. Sometimes the probe is inserted directly through the skin and only local anesthesia is needed. In other cases, the probe is inserted through an incision in the abdomen. This is done in the hospital with general anesthesia.
- **Cryosurgical ablation.** A procedure in which tissue is frozen to destroy abnormal cells. This is usually done with a special instrument that contains liquid nitrogen or liquid carbon

dioxide. The instrument may be used during surgery or laparoscopy or inserted through the skin. This procedure is also called cryoablation.

Chemotherapy

Chemotherapy is a cancer treatment that uses drugs to stop the growth of cancer cells, either by killing the cells or by stopping them from dividing. When chemotherapy is taken by mouth or injected into a vein or muscle, the drugs enter the bloodstream and can reach cancer cells throughout the body (systemic chemotherapy). When chemotherapy is placed directly into the cerebrospinal fluid, an organ, or a body cavity such as the abdomen, the drugs mainly affect cancer cells in those areas (regional chemotherapy). Combination chemotherapy is the use of more than one anticancer drug. The way the chemotherapy is given depends on the type of the cancer being treated.

Hormone Therapy

Hormone therapy is a cancer treatment that removes hormones or blocks their action and stops cancer cells from growing. Hormones are substances made by glands in the body and circulated in the bloodstream. Some hormones can cause certain cancers to grow. If tests show that the cancer cells have places where hormones can attach (receptors), drugs, surgery, or radiation therapy is used to reduce the production of hormones or block them from working.

Hepatic Arterial Occlusion or Chemoembolization

Hepatic arterial occlusion uses drugs, small particles, or other agents to block or reduce the flow of blood to the liver through the hepatic artery (the major blood vessel that carries blood to the liver). This is done to kill cancer cells growing in the liver. The tumor is prevented from getting the oxygen and nutrients it needs to grow. The liver continues to receive blood from the hepatic portal vein, which carries blood from the stomach and intestine.

Chemotherapy delivered during hepatic arterial occlusion is called chemoembolization. The anticancer drug is injected into the hepatic artery through a catheter (thin tube). The drug is mixed with the substance that blocks the artery and cuts off blood flow to the tumor. Most of the anticancer drug is trapped near the tumor and only a small amount of the drug reaches other parts of the body.

The blockage may be temporary or permanent, depending on the substance used to block the artery.

Targeted Therapy

Targeted therapy is a type of treatment that uses drugs or other substances to identify and attack specific cancer cells without harming normal cells. Certain types of targeted therapies are being studied in the treatment of pancreatic NETs.

Supportive Care

Supportive care is given to lessen the problems caused by the disease or its treatment. Supportive care for pancreatic NETs may include treatment for the following:

- Stomach ulcers may be treated with drug therapy such as:
    - Proton pump inhibitor drugs such as omeprazole, lansoprazole, or pantoprazole
    - Histamine blocking drugs such as cimetidine, ranitidine, or famotidine
    - Somatostatin-type drugs such as octreotide
- Diarrhea may be treated with:
    - Intravenous (IV) fluids with electrolytes such as potassium or chloride
    - Somatostatin-type drugs such as octreotide
- Low blood sugar may be treated by having small, frequent meals or with drug therapy to maintain a normal blood sugar level
- High blood sugar may be treated with drugs taken by mouth or insulin by injection

Follow-Up Tests

Some of the tests that were done to diagnose the cancer or to find out the stage of the cancer may be repeated. Some tests will be repeated in order to see how well the treatment is working. Decisions about whether to continue, change, or stop treatment may be based on the results of these tests.

Some of the tests will continue to be done from time to time after treatment has ended. The results of these tests can show if your condition has changed or if the cancer has recurred (come back). These tests are sometimes called follow-up tests or check-ups.

Chapter 22

Retinoblastoma

The retina is the nerve tissue that lines the inside of the back of the eye. The retina senses light and sends images to the brain by way of the optic nerve.

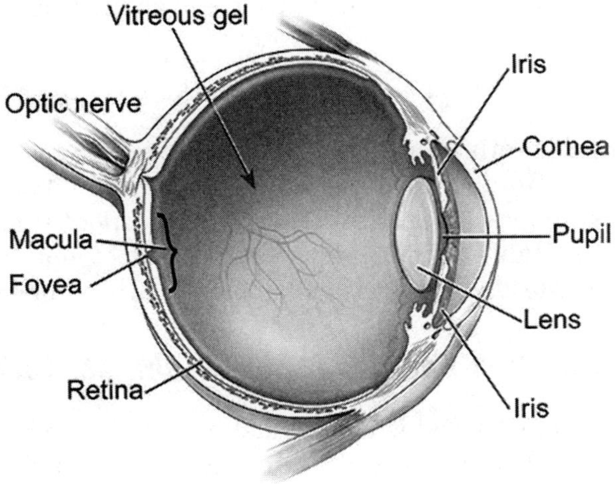

Figure 22.1. *Retina and Other Parts of Eye* (Source: "Diagram of the Eye," National Eye Institute (NEI).)

This chapter includes text excerpted from "Retinoblastoma Treatment (PDQ®)—Patient Version," National Cancer Institute (NCI), January 29, 2018.

What Is Retinoblastoma?

Retinoblastoma Is a Disease in Which Malignant (Cancer) Cells Form in the tissues of the retina. Although retinoblastoma may occur at any age, it occurs most often in children younger than 2 years. The cancer may be in one eye (unilateral) or in both eyes (bilateral). Retinoblastoma rarely spreads from the eye to nearby tissue or other parts of the body. Cavitary retinoblastoma is a rare type of retinoblastoma in which cavities (hollow spaces) form within the tumor.

What Are the Types of Retinoblastoma?

Retinoblastoma occurs in heritable and nonheritable forms. A child is thought to have the heritable form of retinoblastoma when one of the following is true:

- There is a family history of retinoblastoma.
- There is a certain mutation (change) in the *RB1* gene. The mutation in the *RB1* gene may be passed from the parent to the child or it may occur in the egg or sperm before conception or soon after conception.
- There is more than one tumor in the eye or there is a tumor in both eyes.
- There is a tumor in one eye and the child is younger than 1 year.

After heritable retinoblastoma has been diagnosed and treated, new tumors may continue to form for a few years. Regular eye exams to check for new tumors are usually done every 2–4 months for at least 28 months. Nonheritable retinoblastoma is retinoblastoma that is not the heritable form. Most cases of retinoblastoma are the nonheritable form.

What Are the Risk Factors for Retinoblastoma?

A child who has heritable retinoblastoma has an increased risk of trilateral retinoblastoma and other cancers. A child with heritable retinoblastoma has an increased risk of a pineal tumor in the brain. When retinoblastoma and a brain tumor occur at the same time, it is called trilateral retinoblastoma. The brain tumor is usually diagnosed between 20–36 months of age. Regular screening using magnetic resonance imaging (MRI) may be done for a child thought to have heritable retinoblastoma or for a child with retinoblastoma in one eye and a family history of the disease. Computerized tomography (CT) scans are usually not used for routine screening in order to avoid exposing the child to ionizing radiation. Heritable retinoblastoma also increases the child's risk of other types of cancer such as lung cancer, bladder cancer, or melanoma in later years. Regular follow-up exams are important.

What Are the Signs and Symptoms of Retinoblastoma?

Signs and symptoms of retinoblastoma include "white pupil" and eye pain or redness. These and other signs and symptoms may be caused by retinoblastoma or by other conditions. Check with a doctor if your child has any of the following:

- Pupil of the eye appears white instead of red when light shines into it. This may be seen in flash photographs of the child.
- Eyes appear to be looking in different directions (lazy eye)
- Pain or redness in the eye
- Infection around the eye
- Eyeball is larger than normal
- Colored part of the eye and pupil look cloudy

How Is Retinoblastoma Diagnosed?

The following tests and procedures may be used:

- **Physical exam and history.** An exam of the body to check general signs of health, including checking for signs of disease, such as lumps or anything else that seems unusual. A history of the patient's health habits and past illnesses and treatments will also be taken. The doctor will ask if there is a family history of retinoblastoma.
- **Eye exam with dilated pupil.** An exam of the eye in which the pupil is dilated (opened wider) with medicated eye drops to allow the doctor to look through the lens and pupil to the retina. The inside of the eye, including the retina and the optic nerve, is examined with a light. Depending on the age of the child, this exam may be done under anesthesia.

  There are several types of eye exams that are done with the pupil dilated:

  - **Ophthalmoscopy.** An exam of the inside of the back of the eye to check the retina and optic nerve using a small magnifying lens and a light.

    - **Slit-lamp biomicroscopy.** An exam of the inside of the eye to check the retina, optic nerve, and other parts of the eye using a strong beam of light and a microscope.
    - **Fluorescein angiography.** A procedure to look at blood vessels and the flow of blood inside the eye. An orange fluorescent dye called fluorescein is injected into a blood vessel in the arm and goes into the bloodstream. As the dye travels through blood vessels of the eye, a special camera takes pictures of the retina and choroid to find any blood vessels that are blocked or leaking.
- ***RB1* gene test.** A laboratory test in which a sample of blood or tissue is tested for a change in the *RB1* gene.
- **Ultrasound exam of the eye.** A procedure in which high energy sound waves (ultrasound) are bounced off the internal tissues of the eye to make echoes. Eye drops are used to numb the eye and a small probe that sends and receives sound waves is placed gently on the surface of the eye. The echoes make a picture of the inside of the eye and the distance from the cornea to the retina is measured. The picture, called a sonogram, shows on the screen of the ultrasound monitor. The picture can be printed to be looked at later.
- **MRI.** A procedure that uses a magnet, radio waves, and a computer to make a series of detailed pictures of areas inside the body, such as the eye. This procedure is also called nuclear magnetic resonance imaging (NMRI).
- **CT/CAT scan.** A procedure that makes a series of detailed pictures of areas inside the body, such as the eye, taken from different angles. The pictures are made by a computer linked to an X-ray machine. A dye may be injected into a vein or swallowed to help the organs or tissues show up more clearly. This procedure is also called computed tomography, computerized tomography, or computerized axial tomography (CAT).

Retinoblastoma can usually be diagnosed without a biopsy. When retinoblastoma is in one eye, it sometimes forms in the other eye. Exams of the unaffected eye are done until it is known if the retinoblastoma is the heritable form.

What Is the Prognosis for Retinoblastoma?

The prognosis (chance of recovery) and treatment options depend on the following:

- Whether the cancer is in one or both eyes
- The size and number of tumors
- Whether the tumor has spread to the area around the eye, to the brain, or to other parts of the body
- Whether there are symptoms at the time of diagnosis, for trilateral retinoblastoma
- The age of the child
- How likely it is that vision can be saved in one or both eyes
- Whether a second type of cancer has formed

Stages of Retinoblastoma

The process used to find out if cancer has spread within the eye or to other parts of the body is called staging. The information gathered from the staging process determines whether retinoblastoma is only in the eye (intraocular) or has spread outside the eye (extraocular). It is important to know the stage in order to plan treatment. The results of the tests used to diagnose cancer are often also used to stage the disease.

The following tests and procedures may be used in the staging process:

- **Bone scan.** A procedure to check if there are rapidly dividing cells, such as cancer cells, in the bone. A very small amount of radioactive material is injected into a vein and travels through the bloodstream. The radioactive material collects in the bones with cancer and is detected by a scanner that also takes a picture of the body. Areas of bone with cancer show up brighter in the picture because they take up more radioactive material than normal bone cells do.

- **Bone marrow aspiration and biopsy.** The removal of bone marrow and a small piece of bone by inserting a hollow needle into the hipbone or breastbone. A pathologist views the bone marrow under a microscope to look for signs of cancer. A bone marrow aspiration and biopsy is done if the doctor thinks the cancer has spread outside of the eye.

- **Lumbar puncture (LP).** A procedure used to collect cerebrospinal fluid (CSF) from the spinal column. This is done by placing a needle between two bones in the spine and into the CSF around the spinal cord and removing a sample of the fluid. The sample of CSF is checked under a microscope for signs that the cancer has spread to the brain and spinal cord. This procedure is also called an LP or spinal tap.

International Retinoblastoma Staging System (IRSS)

There are several staging systems for retinoblastoma. The International Retinoblastoma Staging System (IRSS) stages are based on how much cancer remains after surgery to remove the tumor and whether the cancer has spread.

- **Stage 0.** The tumor is in the eye only. The eye has not been removed and the tumor was treated without surgery.
- **Stage I.** The tumor is in the eye only. The eye has been removed and no cancer cells remain.
- **Stage II.** The tumor is in the eye only. The eye has been removed and there are cancer cells left that can be seen only with a microscope.
- **Stage III.** Stage III is divided into stages IIIA and IIIB:
  - In stage IIIA, cancer has spread from the eye to tissues around the eye socket.
  - In stage IIIB, cancer has spread from the eye to lymph nodes near the ear or in the neck.
- **Stage IV.** Stage IV is divided into stages IVA and IVB:
  - In stage IVa, cancer has spread to the blood but not to the brain or spinal cord. One or more tumors may have spread to other parts of the body such as the bone or liver.
  - In stage IVb, cancer has spread to the brain or spinal cord. It also may have spread to other parts of the body.

Treatment Option Overview

Different types of treatment are available for patients with retinoblastoma. Some treatments are standard (the currently used treatment), and some are being tested in clinical trials. A treatment clinical trial is a research study meant to help improve current treatments or obtain information on new treatments for patients with cancer. When clinical trials show that a new treatment is better than the standard treatment, the new treatment may become the standard treatment.

Because cancer in children is rare, taking part in a clinical trial should be considered. Some clinical trials are open only to patients who have not started treatment.

Factors on Which Treatment for Retinoblastoma Depends On

Treatment for Retinoblastoma Depends on Whether It Is Intraocular (within the Eye) or Extraocular (outside the Eye).

Intraocular Retinoblastoma

In intraocular retinoblastoma, cancer is found in one or both eyes and may be in the retina only or may also be in other parts of the eye such as the choroid, ciliary body, or part of the optic nerve. Cancer has not spread to tissues around the outside of the eye or to other parts of the body.

Extraocular Retinoblastoma (Metastatic)

In extraocular retinoblastoma, cancer has spread beyond the eye. It may be found in tissues around the eye (orbital retinoblastoma) or it may have spread to the central nervous system (CNS) (brain and spinal cord) or to other parts of the body such as the liver, bones, bone marrow, or lymph nodes.

Treatment for Both Forms of Retinoblastoma Should Include Genetic Counseling

Parents should receive genetic counseling (a discussion with a trained professional about the risk of genetic diseases) to discuss genetic testing to check for a mutation (change) in the *RB1* gene. Genetic counseling also includes a discussion of the risk of retinoblastoma for the child and the child's brothers or sisters.

Children with a Family History of Retinoblastoma Should Have Eye Exams to Check for Retinoblastoma

A child with a family history of retinoblastoma should have regular eye exams beginning early in life to check for retinoblastoma, unless it is known that the child does not have the *RB1* gene change. Early diagnosis of retinoblastoma may mean the child will need less intense treatment. Brothers or sisters of a child with retinoblastoma should have regular eye exams by an ophthalmologist until age 3–5 years, unless it is known that the brother or sister does not have the *RB1* gene change.

Healthcare Team for Treating Children with Retinoblastoma

Children with retinoblastoma should have their treatment planned by a team of healthcare providers who are experts in treating cancer in children. The goals of treatment are to save the child's life, to save vision and the eye, and to prevent serious side effects. Treatment will be overseen by a pediatric oncologist, a doctor who specializes in treating children with cancer. The pediatric oncologist works with other healthcare providers who are experts in treating children with eye cancer and who specialize in certain areas of medicine. These may include a pediatric ophthalmologist (children's eye doctor) who has a lot of experience in treating retinoblastoma and the following specialists:

- Pediatric surgeon
- Radiation oncologist
- Pediatrician
- Pediatric nurse specialist
- Rehabilitation specialist
- Social worker
- Geneticist or genetic counselor

What Are the Side Effects of Treatment for Retinoblastoma?

Treatment for retinoblastoma may cause side effects. Side effects from cancer treatment that begin after treatment and continue for months or years are called late effects. Late effects of treatment for retinoblastoma may include the following:

- Physical problems such as seeing or hearing problems or, if the eye is removed, a change in the shape and size of the bone around the eye
- Changes in mood, feelings, thinking, learning, or memory
- Second cancers (new types of cancer), such as lung and bladder cancers, osteosarcoma, soft tissue sarcoma, or melanoma

The following risk factors may increase the risk of having another cancer:

- Having the heritable form of retinoblastoma
- Past treatment with radiation therapy, especially before age 1 year
- Having already had a previous second cancer

What Are the Standard Treatment for Retinoblastoma?

Six types of standard treatment are used:

Cryotherapy

Cryotherapy is a treatment that uses an instrument to freeze and destroy abnormal tissue. This type of treatment is also called cryosurgery.

Thermotherapy

Thermotherapy is the use of heat to destroy cancer cells. Thermotherapy may be given using a laser beam aimed through the dilated pupil or onto the outside of the eyeball. Thermotherapy may be used alone for small tumors or combined with chemotherapy for larger tumors. This treatment is a type of laser therapy.

Chemotherapy

Chemotherapy is a cancer treatment that uses drugs to stop the growth of cancer cells, either by killing the cells or by stopping them from dividing. The way the chemotherapy is given depends on the stage of the cancer and where the cancer is in the body.

There are different types of chemotherapy:

- **Systemic chemotherapy.** When chemotherapy is taken by mouth or injected into a vein or muscle, the drugs enter the bloodstream and can reach cancer cells throughout the body. Systemic chemotherapy is given to shrink the tumor (chemoreduction) and avoid surgery to remove the eye. After chemoreduction, other treatments may include radiation therapy, cryotherapy, laser therapy, or regional chemotherapy. Systemic chemotherapy may also be given to kill any cancer cells that are left after the initial treatment or to patients with retinoblastoma that occurs outside the eye. Treatment given after the initial treatment, to lower the risk that the cancer will come back, is called adjuvant therapy.

- **Regional chemotherapy.** When chemotherapy is placed directly into the cerebrospinal fluid (intrathecal chemotherapy), an organ (such as the eye), or a body cavity, the drugs mainly affect cancer cells in those areas. Several types of regional chemotherapy are used to treat retinoblastoma.
  - **Ophthalmic artery infusion chemotherapy.** Ophthalmic artery infusion chemotherapy carries anticancer drugs directly to the eye. A catheter is put into an artery that leads to the eye and the anticancer drug is given through the catheter. After the drug is given, a small balloon may be inserted into the artery to block it and keep most of the anticancer drug trapped near the tumor. This type of chemotherapy may be given as the initial treatment when the tumor is in the eye only or when the tumor has not responded to other types of treatment. Ophthalmic artery infusion chemotherapy is given at special retinoblastoma treatment centers.
  - **Intravitreal chemotherapy.** Intravitreal chemotherapy is the injection of anticancer drugs directly into the vitreous humor (jelly-like substance) inside of the eye. It is used to treat cancer that has spread to the vitreous humor and has not responded to treatment or has come back after treatment.

Radiation Therapy

Radiation therapy is a cancer treatment that uses high energy X-rays or other types of radiation to kill cancer cells or keep them from growing. There are two types of radiation therapy:

- External beam radiation therapy uses a machine outside the body to send radiation toward the cancer. Certain ways of giving radiation therapy can help keep radiation from damaging nearby healthy tissue. These types of radiation therapy include the following:
  - **Intensity modulated radiation therapy (IMRT).** IMRT is a type of 3-dimensional (3D) external radiation therapy that uses a computer to make pictures of the size and shape of the tumor. Thin beams of radiation of different intensities (strengths) are aimed at the tumor from many angles.

- **Proton beam radiation therapy.** Proton beam therapy is a type of high energy, external radiation therapy. A radiation therapy machine aims streams of protons (tiny, invisible, positively charged particles) at the cancer cells to kill them.

- Internal radiation therapy uses a radioactive substance sealed in needles, seeds, wires, or catheters that are placed directly into or near the cancer. Certain ways of giving radiation therapy can help keep radiation from damaging nearby healthy tissue. This type of internal radiation therapy may include the following:
  - **Plaque radiotherapy.** Radioactive seeds are attached to one side of a disk, called a plaque, and placed directly on the outside wall of the eye near the tumor. The side of the plaque with the seeds on it faces the eyeball, aiming radiation at the tumor. The plaque helps protect other nearby tissue from the radiation.

The way the radiation therapy is given depends on the type and stage of the cancer being treated and how the cancer responded to other treatments. External and internal radiation therapy are used to treat retinoblastoma.

High Dose Chemotherapy with Stem Cell Rescue

High dose chemotherapy with stem cell rescue is a way of giving high doses of chemotherapy and replacing blood-forming cells destroyed by the cancer treatment. Stem cells (immature blood cells) are removed from the blood or bone marrow of the patient and are frozen and stored. After the chemotherapy is completed, the stored stem cells are thawed and given back to the patient through an infusion. These reinfused stem cells grow into (and restore) the body's blood cells.

Surgery (Enucleation)

Enucleation is surgery to remove the eye and part of the optic nerve. A sample of the eye tissue that is removed will be checked under a microscope to see if there are any signs that the cancer is likely to spread to other parts of the body. This should be done by an experienced pathologist, who is familiar with retinoblastoma and other diseases of the eye. Enucleation is done if there is little or no chance that vision can be saved and when the tumor is large, did not respond to treatment, or comes back after treatment. The patient will be fitted for an artificial eye. Close follow-up is needed for 2 years or more to check for signs of recurrence in the area around the affected eye and to check the other eye.

New Types of Treatment Being Tested in Clinical Trials

New types of treatment are being tested in clinical trials.

Targeted Therapy

Targeted therapy is a type of treatment that uses drugs or other substances to attack cancer cells. Targeted therapies usually cause less harm to normal cells than chemotherapy or radiation therapy do.

Targeted therapy is being studied for the treatment of retinoblastoma that has recurred (come back).

Follow-Up Tests

Some of the tests that were done to diagnose the cancer or to find out the stage of the cancer may be repeated. Some tests will be repeated in order to see how well the treatment is working. Decisions about whether to continue, change, or stop treatment may be based on the results of these tests.

Chapter 23

Lip and Oral Cavity Cancer

The oral cavity includes the following:

- The front two-thirds of the tongue
- The gingiva (gums)
- The buccal mucosa (the lining of the inside of the cheeks)
- The floor (bottom) of the mouth under the tongue
- The hard palate (the roof of the mouth)
- The retromolar trigone (the small area behind the wisdom teeth)

Most lip and oral cavity cancers start in squamous cells, the thin, flat cells that line the lips and oral cavity. These are called squamous cell carcinomas. Cancer cells may spread into deeper tissue as the cancer grows. Squamous cell carcinoma usually develops in areas of leukoplakia (white patches of cells that do not rub off).

- Lip and oral cavity cancer is a type of head and neck cancer.

This chapter includes text excerpted from "Lip and Oral Cavity Cancer Treatment (Adult) (PDQ®)—Patient Version," National Cancer Institute (NCI), February 27, 2018.

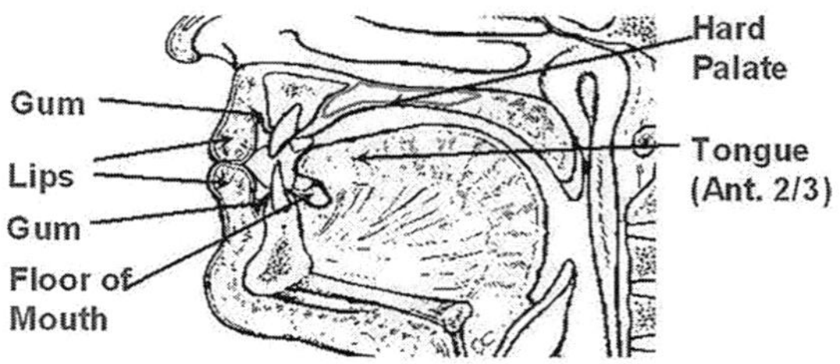

Figure 23.1. *Lip and Oral Cavity* (Source: "Lip and Oral Cavity," Surveillance, Epidemiology and End Results Program (SEER), National Cancer Institute (NCI).)

What Is Lip and Oral Cavity Cancer?

Lip and oral cavity cancer is a disease in which malignant (cancer) cells form in the lips or mouth.

What Are the Risk Factors for Lip and Oral Cavity Cancer?

Anything that increases your risk of getting a disease is called a risk factor. Having a risk factor does not mean that you will get cancer; not having risk factors doesn't mean that you will not get cancer. Talk with your doctor if you think you may be at risk. Risk factors for lip and oral cavity cancer include the following:

- Using tobacco products
- Heavy alcohol use
- Being exposed to natural sunlight or artificial sunlight (such as from tanning beds) over long periods of time
- Being male

What Are the Signs and Symptoms of Lip and Oral Cavity Cancer?

Signs of lip and oral cavity cancer include a sore or lump on the lips or in the mouth. These and other signs and symptoms may be caused by lip and oral cavity cancer or by other conditions. Check with your doctor if you have any of the following:

- A sore on the lip or in the mouth that does not heal

- A lump or thickening on the lips or gums or in the mouth
- A white or red patch on the gums, tongue, or lining of the mouth
- Bleeding, pain, or numbness in the lip or mouth
- Change in voice
- Loose teeth or dentures that no longer fit well
- Trouble chewing or swallowing or moving the tongue or jaw
- Swelling of jaw
- Sore throat or feeling that something is caught in the throat
- Lip and oral cavity cancer may not have any symptoms and is sometimes found during a regular dental exam

How Is Lip and Oral Cavity Cancer Diagnosed?

The following tests and procedures may be used:

- **Physical exam of the lips and oral cavity.** An exam to check the lips and oral cavity for abnormal areas. The medical doctor or dentist will feel the entire inside of the mouth with a gloved finger and examine the oral cavity with a small long-handled mirror and lights. This will include checking the insides of the cheeks and lips; the gums; the roof and floor of the mouth; and the top, bottom, and sides of the tongue. The neck will be felt for swollen lymph nodes. A history of the patient's health habits and past illnesses and medical and dental treatments will also be taken.
- **Endoscopy.** A procedure to look at organs and tissues inside the body to check for abnormal areas. An endoscope is inserted through an incision (cut) in the skin or opening in the body, such as the mouth. An endoscope is a thin, tube-like instrument with a light and a lens for viewing. It may also have a tool to remove tissue or lymph node samples, which are checked under a microscope for signs of disease.
- **Biopsy.** The removal of cells or tissues so they can be viewed under a microscope by a pathologist. If leukoplakia is found, cells taken from the patches are also checked under the microscope for signs of cancer.
- **Exfoliative cytology.** A procedure to collect cells from the lip or oral cavity. A piece of cotton, a brush, or a small wooden stick

is used to gently scrape cells from the lips, tongue, mouth, or throat. The cells are viewed under a microscope to find out if they are abnormal.

- **Magnetic resonance imaging (MRI).** A procedure that uses a magnet, radio waves, and a computer to make a series of detailed pictures of areas inside the body. This procedure is also called nuclear magnetic resonance imaging (NMRI).
- **Computed tomography (CT)/computerized axial tomography (CAT) scan.** A procedure that makes a series of detailed pictures of areas inside the body, taken from different angles. The pictures are made by a computer linked to an X-ray machine. A dye may be injected into a vein or swallowed to help the organs or tissues show up more clearly. This procedure is also called computed tomography, computerized tomography, or computerized axial tomography.
- **Barium swallow.** A series of X-rays of the esophagus and stomach. The patient drinks a liquid that contains barium (a silver-white metallic compound). The liquid coats the esophagus and X-rays are taken. This procedure is also called an upper GI series.
- **Positron emission tomography (PET) scan.** A procedure to find malignant tumor cells in the body. A small amount of radioactive glucose (sugar) is injected into a vein. The PET scanner rotates around the body and makes a picture of where glucose is being used in the body. Malignant tumor cells show up brighter in the picture because they are more active and take up more glucose than normal cells do.
- **Bone scan.** A procedure to check if there are rapidly dividing cells, such as cancer cells, in the bone. A very small amount of radioactive material is injected into a vein and travels through the bloodstream. The radioactive material collects in the bones with cancer and is detected by a scanner.

What Is the Prognosis for Lip and Oral Cavity Cancer?

Prognosis (chance of recovery) depends on the following:

- The stage of the cancer
- Where the tumor is in the lip or oral cavity
- Whether the cancer has spread to blood vessels

- For patients who smoke, the chance of recovery is better if they stop smoking before beginning radiation therapy

Treatment options depend on the following:

- The stage of the cancer
- The size of the tumor and where it is in the lip or oral cavity
- Whether the patient's appearance and ability to talk and eat can stay the same
- The patient's age and general health

Patients who have had lip and oral cavity cancer have an increased risk of developing a second cancer in the head or neck. Frequent and careful follow-up is important.

Stages of Lip and Oral Cavity Cancer

After lip and oral cavity cancer has been diagnosed, tests are done to find out if cancer cells have spread within the lip and oral cavity or to other parts of the body. The process used to find out if cancer has spread within the lip and oral cavity or to other parts of the body is called staging. The information gathered from the staging process determines the stage of the disease. It is important to know the stage in order to plan treatment.

The following stages are used for lip and oral cavity cancer:

Stage 0 (Carcinoma in Situ). In stage 0, abnormal cells are found in the lining of the lips and oral cavity. These abnormal cells may become cancer and spread into nearby normal tissue. Stage 0 is also called carcinoma in situ.

Stage I. In stage I, cancer has formed and the tumor is 2 centimeters or smaller. Cancer has not spread to the lymph nodes.

Stage II. In stage II, the tumor is larger than 2 centimeters but not larger than 4 centimeters, and cancer has not spread to the lymph nodes.

Stage III. In stage III, the tumor:

- may be any size and has spread to one lymph node that is 3 centimeters or smaller, on the same side of the neck as the tumor; or
- is larger than 4 centimeters

Stage IV. Stage IV is divided into stages IVA, IVB, and IVC.

- In stage IVA, the tumor:
    - has spread through tissue in the lip or oral cavity into nearby tissue and/or bone (jaw, tongue, floor of mouth, maxillary sinus, or skin on the chin or nose); cancer may have spread to one lymph node that is 3 centimeters or smaller, on the same side of the neck as the tumor; or
    - is any size or has spread through tissue in the lip or oral cavity into nearby tissue and/or bone (jaw, tongue, floor of mouth, maxillary sinus, or skin on the chin or nose), and cancer has spread:
        - to one lymph node on the same side of the neck as the tumor and the lymph node is larger than 3 centimeters but not larger than 6 centimeters; or
        - to more than one lymph node on the same side of the neck as the tumor and the lymph nodes are not larger than 6 centimeters; or
        - to lymph nodes on the opposite side of the neck as the tumor or on both sides of the neck, and the lymph nodes are not larger than 6 centimeters.
- In stage IVB, the tumor:
    - may be any size and has spread to one or more lymph nodes that are larger than 6 centimeters; or
    - has spread further into the muscles or bones in the oral cavity, or to the base of the skull and/or the carotid artery. Cancer may have spread to one or more lymph nodes anywhere in the neck.
- In stage IVC, the tumor has spread beyond the lip or oral cavity to distant parts of the body, such as the lungs. The tumor may be any size and may have spread to the lymph nodes.

Treatment Option Overview

Different types of treatment are available for patients with lip and oral cavity cancer. Some treatments are standard (the currently used treatment), and some are being tested in clinical trials. A treatment clinical trial is a research study meant to help improve current treatments or obtain information on new treatments for patients with cancer. When clinical trials show that a new treatment is better than the standard treatment, the new treatment may become the standard treatment. Patients may want to think about taking part in a clinical trial. Some clinical trials are open only to patients who have not started treatment.

Healthcare Team for Treating Lip and Oral Cavity Cancer

Treatment will be overseen by a medical oncologist, a doctor who specializes in treating people with cancer. Because the lips and oral cavity are important for breathing, eating, and talking, patients may need special help adjusting to the side effects of the cancer and its treatment. The medical oncologist may refer the patient to other health professionals with special training in the treatment of patients with head and neck cancer. These include the following:

- Head and neck surgeon
- Radiation oncologist
- Dentist
- Speech therapist
- Dietitian
- Psychologist
- Rehabilitation specialist
- Plastic surgeon

Standard Treatment Available for Patients with Lip and Oral Cavity Cancer

Two types of standard treatment are used:

Surgery

Surgery (removing the cancer in an operation) is a common treatment for all stages of lip and oral cavity cancer. Surgery may include the following:

- **Wide local excision.** Removal of the cancer and some of the healthy tissue around it. If cancer has spread into bone, surgery may include removal of the involved bone tissue.

- **Neck dissection.** Removal of lymph nodes and other tissues in the neck. This is done when cancer may have spread from the lip and oral cavity.
- **Plastic surgery.** An operation that restores or improves the appearance of parts of the body. Dental implants, a skin graft, or other plastic surgery may be needed to repair parts of the mouth, throat, or neck after removal of large tumors.

Even if the doctor removes all the cancer that can be seen at the time of the surgery, some patients may be given chemotherapy or radiation therapy after surgery to kill any cancer cells that are left. Treatment given after the surgery, to lower the risk that the cancer will come back, is called adjuvant therapy.

Radiation Therapy

Radiation therapy is a cancer treatment that uses high-energy X-rays or other types of radiation to kill cancer cells or keep them from growing. There are two types of radiation therapy:

- External radiation therapy uses a machine outside the body to send radiation toward the cancer.
- Internal radiation therapy uses a radioactive substance sealed in needles, seeds, wires, or catheters that are placed directly into or near the cancer.

The way the radiation therapy is given depends on the type and stage of the cancer being treated. External and internal radiation therapy are used to treat lip and oral cavity cancer. Radiation therapy may work better in patients who have stopped smoking before beginning treatment. It is also important for patients to have a dental exam before radiation therapy begins, so that existing problems can be treated.

Chapter 24

Laryngeal Cancer

The larynx is a part of the throat, between the base of the tongue and the trachea. The larynx contains the vocal cords, which vibrate and make sound when air is directed against them. The sound echoes through the pharynx, mouth, and nose to make a person's voice.

There are three main parts of the larynx:

- **Supraglottis.** The upper part of the larynx above the vocal cords, including the epiglottis.

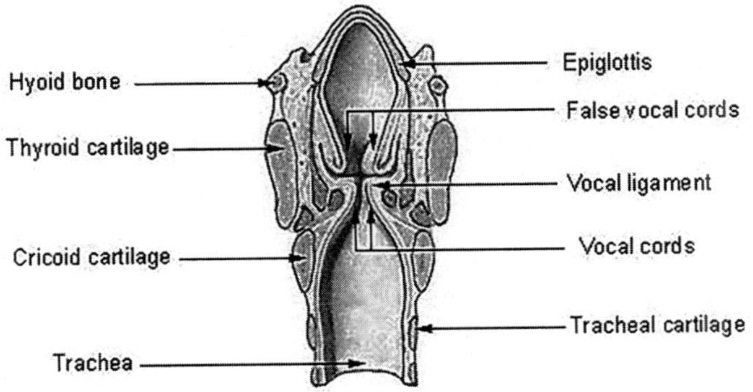

Figure 24.1. *Larynx* (Source: "Larynx and Trachea," Surveillance, Epidemiology and End Results Program (SEER), National Cancer Institute (NCI).)

This chapter includes text excerpted from "Laryngeal Cancer Treatment (Adult) (PDQ®)—Patient Version," National Cancer Institute (NCI), February 27, 2018.

- **Glottis.** The middle part of the larynx where the vocal cords are located.
- **Subglottis.** The lower part of the larynx between the vocal cords and the trachea (windpipe).

What Is Laryngeal Cancer?

Laryngeal cancer is a disease in which malignant (cancer) cells form in the tissues of the larynx. Most laryngeal cancers form in squamous cells, the thin, flat cells lining the inside of the larynx. Laryngeal cancer is a type of head and neck cancer.

What Are the Risk Factors for Laryngeal Cancer?

Anything that increases your risk of getting a disease is called a risk factor. Use of tobacco products and drinking too much alcohol can affect the risk of laryngeal cancer. Having a risk factor does not mean that you will get cancer; not having risk factors doesn't mean that you will not get cancer. Talk with your doctor if you think you may be at risk.

What Are the Signs and Symptoms of Laryngeal Cancer?

Signs and symptoms of laryngeal cancer include a sore throat and ear pain. These and other signs and symptoms may be caused by laryngeal cancer or by other conditions. Check with your doctor if you have any of the following:

- A sore throat or cough that does not go away
- Trouble or pain when swallowing
- Ear pain
- A lump in the neck or throat
- A change or hoarseness in the voice

How Is Laryngeal Cancer Diagnosed?

The following tests and procedures may be used for diagnosis:

- **Physical exam of the throat and neck.** An exam to check the throat and neck for abnormal areas. The doctor will feel the inside of the mouth with a gloved finger and examine the mouth and throat with a small long-handled mirror and light. This will include checking the insides of the cheeks and lips; the gums; the back, roof, and floor of the mouth; the top, bottom, and sides of the tongue; and the throat. The neck will be felt for swollen lymph nodes. A history of the patient's health habits and past illnesses and medical treatments will also be taken.

- **Biopsy.** The removal of cells or tissues so they can be viewed under a microscope by a pathologist to check for signs of cancer. The sample of tissue may be removed during one of the following procedures:
  - **Laryngoscopy.** A procedure to look at the larynx (voice box) for abnormal areas. A mirror or a laryngoscope (a thin, tube-like instrument with a light and a lens for viewing) is inserted through the mouth to see the larynx. A special tool on the laryngoscope may be used to remove samples of tissue.
  - **Endoscopy.** A procedure to look at organs and tissues inside the body, such as the throat, esophagus, and trachea to check for abnormal areas. An endoscope (a thin, lighted tube with a light and a lens for viewing) is inserted through an opening in the body, such as the mouth. A special tool on the endoscope may be used to remove samples of tissue.
- **Computerized tomography (CT)/computerized axial tomography (CAT) scan.** A procedure that makes a series of detailed pictures of areas inside the body, taken from different angles. The pictures are made by a computer linked to an X-ray machine. A dye may be injected into a vein or swallowed to help the organs or tissues show up more clearly.
- **Magnetic resonance imaging (MRI).** A procedure that uses a magnet, radio waves, and a computer to make a series of detailed pictures of areas inside the body. This procedure is also called nuclear magnetic resonance imaging (NMRI).
- **Positron emission tomography (PET) scan.** A procedure to find malignant tumor cells in the body. A small amount of radioactive glucose (sugar) is injected into a vein. The PET scanner rotates around the body and makes a picture of where glucose is being used in the body. Malignant tumor cells show up brighter in the picture because they are more active and take up more glucose than normal cells do.

- **PET-CT scan.** A procedure that combines the pictures from a PET and a CT scan. The PET and CT scans are done at the same time with the same machine. The combined scans give more detailed pictures of areas inside the body than either scan gives by itself. A PET-CT scan may be used to help diagnose disease, such as cancer, plan treatment, or find out how well treatment is working.
- **Bone scan.** A procedure to check if there are rapidly dividing cells, such as cancer cells, in the bone. A very small amount of radioactive material is injected into a vein and travels through the bloodstream. The radioactive material collects in the bones with cancer and is detected by a scanner.
- **Barium swallow.** A series of X-rays of the esophagus and stomach. The patient drinks a liquid that contains barium (a silver-white metallic compound). The liquid coats the esophagus and stomach, and X-rays are taken. This procedure is also called an upper GI series.

What Is the Prognosis for Laryngeal Cancer?

Prognosis (chance of recovery) depends on the following:

- The stage of the disease
- The location and size of the tumor
- The grade of the tumor
- The patient's age, gender, and general health, including whether the patient is anemic

What Are the Factors on Which Treatment Options Depend On?

Treatment options depend on the following:

- The stage of the disease
- The location and size of the tumor
- Keeping the patient's ability to talk, eat, and breathe as normal as possible
- Whether the cancer has come back (recurred)

Smoking tobacco and drinking alcohol decrease the effectiveness of treatment for laryngeal cancer. Patients with laryngeal cancer who continue to smoke and drink are less likely to be cured and more likely to develop a second tumor. After treatment for laryngeal cancer, frequent and careful follow-up is important.

Stages of Laryngeal Cancer

After laryngeal cancer has been diagnosed, tests are done to find out if cancer cells have spread within the larynx or to other parts of the body.

The process used to find out if cancer has spread within the larynx or to other parts of the body is called staging. The information gathered from the staging process determines the stage of the disease. It is important to know the stage of the disease in order to plan treatment. The results of some of the tests used to diagnose laryngeal cancer are often also used to stage the disease.

The following stages are used for laryngeal cancer:

Stage 0 (Carcinoma in Situ). In stage 0, abnormal cells are found in the lining of the larynx. These abnormal cells may become cancer and spread into nearby normal tissue. Stage 0 is also called carcinoma in situ.

Stage I. In stage I, cancer has formed. Stage I laryngeal cancer depends on where cancer began in the larynx:

- Supraglottis: Cancer is in one area of the supraglottis only and the vocal cords can move normally.
- Glottis: Cancer is in one or both vocal cords and the vocal cords can move normally.
- Subglottis: Cancer is in the subglottis only.

Stage II. In stage II, cancer is in the larynx only. Stage II laryngeal cancer depends on where cancer began in the larynx:

- Supraglottis: Cancer is in more than one area of the supraglottis or surrounding tissues.
- Glottis: Cancer has spread to the supraglottis and/or the subglottis and/or the vocal cords cannot move normally.
- Subglottis: Cancer has spread to one or both vocal cords, which may not move normally.

Stage III. Stage III laryngeal cancer depends on whether cancer has spread from the supraglottis, glottis, or subglottis.

In stage III cancer of the supraglottis:

- Cancer is in the larynx only and the vocal cords cannot move, and/or cancer is in tissues next to the larynx. Cancer may have spread to one lymph node on the same side of the neck as the original tumor and the lymph node is 3 centimeters or smaller; or
- Cancer is in one area of the supraglottis and in one lymph node on the same side of the neck as the original tumor; the lymph node is 3 centimeters or smaller and the vocal cords can move normally; or
- Cancer is in more than one area of the supraglottis or surrounding tissues and in one lymph node on the same side of the neck as the original tumor; the lymph node is 3 centimeters or smaller.

In stage III cancer of the glottis:

- Cancer is in the larynx only and the vocal cords cannot move, and/or cancer is in tissues next to the larynx; cancer may have spread to one lymph node on the same side of the neck as the original tumor and the lymph node is 3 centimeters or smaller; or
- Cancer is in one or both vocal cords and in one lymph node on the same side of the neck as the original tumor; the lymph node is 3 centimeters or smaller and the vocal cords can move normally; or
- Cancer has spread to the supraglottis and/or the subglottis and/or the vocal cords cannot move normally. Cancer has also spread to one lymph node on the same side of the neck as the original tumor and the lymph node is 3 centimeters or smaller.

In stage III cancer of the subglottis:

- Cancer is in the larynx and the vocal cords cannot move; cancer may have spread to one lymph node on the same side of the neck as the original tumor and the lymph node is 3 centimeters or smaller; or
- Cancer is in the subglottis and in one lymph node on the same side of the neck as the original tumor; the lymph node is 3 centimeters or smaller; or
- Cancer has spread to one or both vocal cords, which may not move normally. Cancer has also spread to one lymph node on the

same side of the neck as the original tumor and the lymph node is 3 centimeters or smaller.

Stage IV. Stage IV is divided into stage IVA, stage IVB, and stage IVC. Each substage is the same for cancer in the supraglottis, glottis, or subglottis.

- In stage IVA:
  - Cancer has spread through the thyroid cartilage and/or has spread to tissues beyond the larynx such as the neck, trachea, thyroid, or esophagus. Cancer may have spread to one lymph node on the same side of the neck as the original tumor and the lymph node is 3 centimeters or smaller; or
  - Cancer has spread to one lymph node on the same side of the neck as the original tumor and the lymph node is larger than 3 centimeters but not larger than 6 centimeters, or has spread to more than one lymph node anywhere in the neck with none larger than 6 centimeters. Cancer may have spread to tissues beyond the larynx, such as the neck, trachea, thyroid, or esophagus. The vocal cords may not move normally.
- In stage IVB:
  - Cancer has spread to the space in front of the spinal column, surrounds the carotid artery, or has spread to parts of the chest. Cancer may have spread to one or more lymph nodes anywhere in the neck and the lymph nodes may be any size; or
  - Cancer has spread to a lymph node that is larger than 6 centimeters and may have spread as far as the space in front of the spinal column, around the carotid artery, or to parts of the chest. The vocal cords may not move normally.
- In stage IVC, cancer has spread to other parts of the body, such as the lungs, liver, or bone.

Treatment Option Overview

Different types of treatment are available for patients with laryngeal cancer. Some treatments are standard (the currently used treatment), and some are being tested in clinical trials. A treatment clinical trial is a research study meant to help improve current treatments or obtain information on new treatments for patients with cancer. When clinical trials show that a new treatment is better than the standard treatment, the new treatment may become the standard treatment. Patients may want to think about taking part in a clinical trial. Some clinical trials are open only to patients who have not started treatment.

Standard Options for Treating Laryngeal Cancer

Three types of standard treatment are used:

Radiation Therapy

Radiation therapy is a cancer treatment that uses high-energy X-rays or other types of radiation to kill cancer cells or keep them from growing. There are two types of radiation therapy:

- External radiation therapy uses a machine outside the body to send radiation toward the cancer.
- Internal radiation therapy uses a radioactive substance sealed in needles, seeds, wires, or catheters that are placed directly into or near the cancer.

The way the radiation therapy is given depends on the type and stage of the cancer being treated. External radiation therapy is used to treat laryngeal cancer.

Radiation therapy may work better in patients who have stopped smoking before beginning treatment. External radiation therapy to the thyroid or the pituitary gland may change the way the thyroid gland works. A blood test to check the thyroid hormone level in the body may be done before and after therapy to make sure the thyroid gland is working properly.

Hyperfractionated radiation therapy may be used to treat laryngeal cancer. Hyperfractionated radiation therapy is radiation treatment in which a smaller than usual total daily dose of radiation is divided into two doses and the treatments are given twice a day. Hyperfractionated radiation therapy is given over the same period of time (days or weeks) as standard radiation therapy. New types of radiation therapy are being studied in the treatment of laryngeal cancer.

Surgery

Surgery (removing the cancer in an operation) is a common treatment for all stages of laryngeal cancer. The following surgical procedures may be used:

- **Cordectomy:** Surgery to remove the vocal cords only.
- **Supraglottic laryngectomy:** Surgery to remove the supraglottis only.
- **Hemilaryngectomy:** Surgery to remove half of the larynx (voice box). A hemilaryngectomy saves the voice.
- **Partial laryngectomy:** Surgery to remove part of the larynx (voice box). A partial laryngectomy helps keep the patient's ability to talk.
- **Total laryngectomy:** Surgery to remove the whole larynx. During this operation, a hole is made in the front of the neck to allow the patient to breathe. This is called a tracheostomy.
- **Thyroidectomy:** The removal of all or part of the thyroid gland.
- **Laser surgery:** A surgical procedure that uses a laser beam (a narrow beam of intense light) as a knife to make bloodless cuts in tissue or to remove a surface lesion such as a tumor in the larynx.

Even if the doctor removes all the cancer that can be seen at the time of the surgery, some patients may be given chemotherapy or radiation therapy after surgery to kill any cancer cells that are left. Treatment given after the surgery, to lower the risk that the cancer will come back, is called adjuvant therapy.

Chemotherapy

Chemotherapy is a cancer treatment that uses drugs to stop the growth of cancer cells, either by killing the cells or by stopping the cells from dividing. When chemotherapy is taken by mouth or injected into a vein or muscle, the drugs enter the bloodstream and can reach cancer cells throughout the body (systemic chemotherapy). When chemotherapy is placed directly into the cerebrospinal fluid, an organ, or a body cavity such as the abdomen, the drugs mainly affect cancer cells in those areas (regional chemotherapy). The way the chemotherapy is given depends on the type and stage of the cancer being treated.

New Types of Treatment Being Tested in Clinical Trials

Targeted Therapy

Targeted therapy is a type of treatment that uses drugs or other substances to attack specific cancer cells. Targeted therapies usually cause less harm to normal cells than chemotherapy or radiation therapy do.

Monoclonal antibodies are a type of targeted therapy being studied in the treatment of laryngeal cancer. Monoclonal antibody therapy is a cancer treatment that uses antibodies made in the laboratory from a single type of immune system cell. These antibodies can identify substances on cancer cells or normal substances in the blood or tissues that may help cancer cells grow. The antibodies attach to the substances and kill the cancer cells, block their growth, or keep them from spreading. Monoclonal antibodies are given by infusion. They may be used alone or to carry drugs, toxins, or radioactive material directly to cancer cells.

Cetuximab is a type of monoclonal antibody that is being studied in the treatment of laryngeal cancer. It works by binding to a protein on the surface of the cancer cells and stops the cells from growing and dividing.

Radiosensitizers

Radiosensitizers are drugs that make tumor cells more sensitive to radiation therapy. Combining radiation therapy with radiosensitizers may kill more tumor cells.

Follow-Up Tests

Some of the tests that were done to diagnose the cancer or to find out the stage of the cancer may be repeated. Some tests will be repeated in order to see how well the treatment is working. Decisions about whether to continue, change, or stop treatment may be based on the results of these tests. Some of the tests will continue to be done from time to time after treatment has ended. The results of these tests can show if your condition has changed or if the cancer has recurred (come back). These tests are sometimes called follow-up tests or check-ups.

Chapter 25

Lung Cancer: An Overview

Lung cancer is the leading cause of cancer death and the second most common cancer among both men and women in the United States. The most important thing you can do to lower your lung cancer risk is to quit smoking and avoid secondhand smoke. The second leading cause of lung cancer is radon, a naturally occurring gas that comes

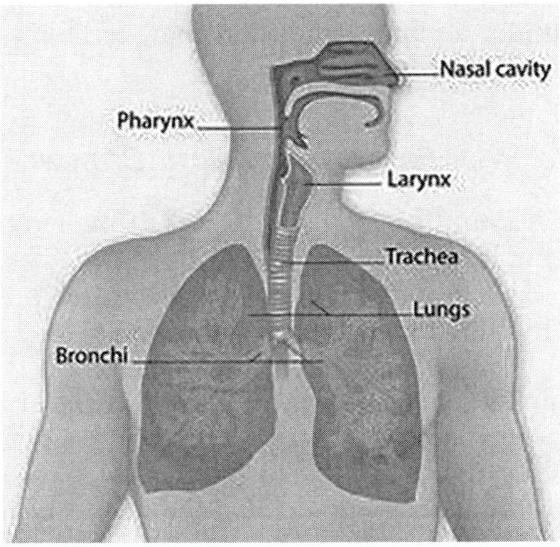

Figure 25.1. *Lungs*

This chapter includes text excerpted from "Lung Cancer," Centers for Disease Control and Prevention (CDC), February 8, 2018.

from rocks and dirt and can get trapped in houses and buildings. Get your home tested for radon. People who have smoked for many years may want to think about screening for lung cancer with low-dose computed tomography (LDCT). Talk to your doctor about lung cancer screening and the possible benefits and harms. Lung cancer screening is not a substitute for quitting smoking.

What Is Lung Cancer?

Cancer is a disease in which cells in the body grow out of control. When cancer starts in the lungs, it is called lung cancer. Lung cancer begins in the lungs and may spread to lymph nodes or other organs in the body, such as the brain. Cancer from other organs also may spread to the lungs. When cancer cells spread from one organ to another, they are called metastases. Lung cancers usually are grouped into two main types called small cell and nonsmall cell. These types of lung cancer grow differently and are treated differently. Nonsmall cell lung cancer is more common than small cell lung cancer.

Types of Lung Cancer

There two main types of lung cancer are small cell lung cancer and nonsmall cell lung cancer. These categories refer to what the cancer cells look like under a microscope. Nonsmall cell lung cancer is more common than small cell lung cancer.

What Are the Risk Factors for Lung Cancer?

Research has found several risk factors that may increase your chances of getting lung cancer.

Smoking

Cigarette smoking is the number one risk factor for lung cancer. In the United States, cigarette smoking is linked to about 80–90 percent of lung cancers. Using other tobacco products such as cigars or pipes also increases the risk for lung cancer. Tobacco smoke is a toxic mix of more than 7,000 chemicals. Many are poisons. At least 70 are known to cause cancer in people or animals.

People who smoke cigarettes are 15–30 times more likely to get lung cancer or die from lung cancer than people who do not smoke. Even smoking a few cigarettes a day or smoking occasionally increases the risk of lung cancer. The more years a person smokes and the more cigarettes smoked each day, the more risk goes up.

People who quit smoking have a lower risk of lung cancer than if they had continued to smoke, but their risk is higher than the risk for people who never smoked. Quitting smoking at any age can lower the risk of lung cancer.

Cigarette smoking can cause cancer almost anywhere in the body. Cigarette smoking causes cancer of the mouth and throat, esophagus, stomach, colon, rectum, liver, pancreas, voice box (larynx), trachea, bronchus, kidney and renal pelvis, urinary bladder, and cervix, and causes acute myeloid leukemia.

Secondhand Smoke

Smoke from other people's cigarettes, pipes, or cigars (secondhand smoke) also causes lung cancer. When a person breathes in secondhand smoke, it is like he or she is smoking. In the United States, two out of five adults who don't smoke and half of the children are exposed to secondhand smoke, and about 7,300 people who never smoked die from lung cancer due to secondhand smoke every year.

Radon

Radon is a naturally occurring gas that comes from rocks and dirt and can get trapped in houses and buildings. It cannot be seen, tasted, or smelled. According to the U.S. Environmental Protection Agency (EPA), radon causes about 20,000 cases of lung cancer each year, making it the second leading cause of lung cancer. Nearly one out of every 15 homes in the United States is thought to have high radon levels. The EPA recommends testing homes for radon and using proven ways to lower high radon levels.

Other Substances

Examples of substances found at some workplaces that increase risk include asbestos, arsenic, diesel exhaust, and some forms of silica and chromium. For many of these substances, the risk of getting lung cancer is even higher for those who smoke.

Personal or Family History of Lung Cancer

If you are a lung cancer survivor, there is a risk that you may develop another lung cancer, especially if you smoke. Your risk of lung cancer may be higher if your parents, brothers or sisters, or children have had lung cancer. This could be true because they also smoke, or they live or work in the same place where they are exposed to radon and other substances that can cause lung cancer.

Radiation Therapy to the Chest

Cancer survivors who had radiation therapy to the chest are at higher risk of lung cancer.

Diet

Scientists are studying many different foods and dietary supplements to see whether they change the risk of getting lung cancer. There is still much needed to know. It's not known that smokers who take beta-carotene supplements have increased risk of lung cancer.

What Are the Symptoms of Lung Cancer?

Different people have different symptoms for lung cancer. Some people have symptoms related to the lungs. Some people whose lung cancer has spread to other parts of the body (metastasized) have symptoms specific to that part of the body. Some people just have general symptoms of not feeling well. Most people with lung cancer don't have symptoms until the cancer is advanced. Lung cancer symptoms may include:

- Coughing that gets worse or doesn't go away
- Chest pain
- Shortness of breath
- Wheezing
- Coughing up blood
- Feeling very tired all the time
- Weight loss with no known cause

Other changes that can sometimes occur with lung cancer may include repeated bouts of pneumonia and swollen or enlarged lymph nodes (glands) inside the chest in the area between the lungs. These symptoms can happen with other illnesses, too. If you have some of these symptoms, talk to your doctor, who can help find the cause.

What Can I Do to Reduce My Risk of Lung Cancer?

You can help lower your risk of lung cancer in the following ways:

- **Don't smoke.** Cigarette smoking causes about 90 percent of lung cancer deaths in the United States. The most important thing you can do to prevent lung cancer is to not start smoking, or to quit if you smoke.
- **Avoid secondhand smoke.** Smoke from other people's cigarettes, cigars, or pipes is called secondhand smoke. Make your home and car smoke-free.
- **Get your home tested for radon.** The U.S. Environmental Protection Agency (EPA) recommends that all homes be tested for radon.
- **Be careful at work.** Health and safety guidelines in the workplace can help workers avoid carcinogens—things that can cause cancer.

What Screening Tests Are There?

Screening means testing for a disease when there are no symptoms or history of that disease. Doctors recommend a screening test to find a disease early, when treatment may work better. The only recommended screening test for lung cancer is low-dose computed tomography (also called a low-dose CT scan, or LDCT). In this test, an X-ray machine scans the body and uses low doses of radiation to make detailed pictures of the lungs.

Who Should Be Screened?

The U.S. Preventive Services Task Force (USPSTF) recommends yearly lung cancer screening with LDCT for people who:

- Have a history of heavy smoking, and
- Smoke now or have quit within the past 15 years, and
- Are between 55–80 years old.

Heavy smoking means a smoking history of 30 pack years or more. A pack year is smoking an average of one pack of cigarettes per day for one year. For example, a person could have a 30 pack-year history by smoking one pack a day for 30 years or two packs a day for 15 years.

Risks of Screening

Lung cancer screening has at least three risks:

- A lung cancer screening test can suggest that a person has lung cancer when no cancer is present. This is called a false-positive result. False-positive results can lead to follow-up tests and surgeries that are not needed and may have more risks.
- A lung cancer screening test can find cases of cancer that may never have caused a problem for the patient. This is called overdiagnosis. Overdiagnosis can lead to treatment that is not needed.
- Radiation from repeated LDCT tests can cause cancer in otherwise healthy people.

That is why lung cancer screening is recommended only for adults who have no symptoms but who are at high risk for developing the disease because of their smoking history and age.

If you are thinking about getting screened, talk to your doctor. If lung cancer screening is right for you, your doctor can refer you to a high-quality treatment facility.

The best way to reduce your risk of lung cancer is to not smoke and to avoid secondhand smoke. Lung cancer screening is not a substitute for quitting smoking.

When Should Screening Stop?

The Task Force recommends that yearly lung cancer screening stop when the person being screened:

- Turns 81 years old, or
- Has not smoked in 15 years, or
- Develops a health problem that makes him or her unwilling or unable to have surgery if lung cancer is found.

Staging

If lung cancer is diagnosed, other tests are done to find out how far it has spread through the lungs, lymph nodes, and the rest of the body. This process is called staging. The type and stage of lung cancer tells doctors what kind of treatment you need.

Treatment Option Overview

Lung cancer is treated in several ways, depending on the type of lung cancer and how far it has spread. People with nonsmall cell lung cancer can be treated with surgery, chemotherapy, radiation therapy, targeted therapy, or a combination of these treatments. People with small cell lung cancer are usually treated with radiation therapy and chemotherapy.

- **Surgery.** An operation where doctors cut out cancer tissue.
- **Chemotherapy.** Using special medicines to shrink or kill the cancer. The drugs can be pills you take or medicines given in your veins, or sometimes both.
- **Radiation therapy.** Using high-energy rays (similar to X-rays) to kill the cancer.
- **Targeted therapy.** Using drugs to block the growth and spread of cancer cells. The drugs can be pills you take or medicines given in your veins.

Doctors from different specialties often work together to treat lung cancer. Pulmonologists are doctors who are experts in diseases of the lungs. Surgeons are doctors who perform operations. Thoracic surgeons specialize in chest, heart, and lung surgery. Medical oncologists are doctors who treat cancer with medicines. Radiation oncologists are doctors who treat cancers with radiation.

Complementary and alternative medicine. Complementary and alternative medicine are medicines and health practices that are not standard cancer treatments. Complementary medicine is used in addition to standard treatments, and alternative medicine is used instead of standard treatments. Meditation, yoga, and supplements like vitamins and herbs are some examples.

Many kinds of complementary and alternative medicine have not been tested scientifically and may not be safe. Talk to your doctor about the risks and benefits before you start any kind of complementary or alternative medicine.

Which Treatment Is Right for Me?

Choosing the treatment that is right for you may be hard. Talk to your cancer doctor about the treatment options available for your type and stage of cancer. Your doctor can explain the risks and benefits of each treatment and their side effects. Side effects are how your body reacts to drugs or other treatments.

Sometimes people get an opinion from more than one cancer doctor. This is called a "second opinion." Getting a second opinion may help you choose the treatment that is right for you.

Chapter 26

Small Cell Lung Cancer

The lungs are a pair of cone-shaped breathing organs that are found in the chest. The lungs bring oxygen into the body when you breathe in and take out carbon dioxide when you breathe out. Each lung has sections called lobes. The left lung has two lobes. The right lung, which is slightly larger, has three. A thin membrane called the pleura surrounds the lungs. Two tubes called bronchi lead from the trachea (windpipe) to the right and left lungs. Small tubes called bronchioles and tiny air sacs called alveoli make up the inside of the lungs. There are two types of lung cancer: small cell lung cancer and nonsmall cell lung cancer.

What Is Small Cell Lung Cancer?

Small cell lung cancer is a disease in which malignant (cancer) cells form in the tissues of the lung. There are two main types of small cell lung cancer. These two types include many different types of cells. The cancer cells of each type grow and spread in different ways. The types of small cell lung cancer are named for the kinds of cells found in the cancer and how the cells look when viewed under a microscope:

- Small cell carcinoma (oat cell cancer)
- Combined small cell carcinoma

This chapter includes text excerpted from "Small Cell Lung Cancer Treatment (PDQ®)—Patient Version," National Cancer Institute (NCI), January 29, 2018.

What Are the Risk Factors for Small Cell Lung Cancer?

Anything that increases your chance of getting a disease is called a risk factor. Having a risk factor does not mean that you will get cancer; not having risk factors doesn't mean that you will not get cancer. Talk to your doctor if you think you may be at risk for lung cancer.

Risk factors for lung cancer include the following:

- Smoking cigarettes, pipes, or cigars, now or in the past. This is the most important risk factor for lung cancer. The earlier in life a person starts smoking, the more often a person smokes, and the more years a person smokes, the greater the risk of lung cancer.
- Being exposed to secondhand smoke
- Being exposed to radiation from any of the following:
    - Radiation therapy to the breast or chest
    - Radon in the home or workplace
    - Imaging tests such as computed tomography (CT) scans
    - Atomic bomb radiation
- Being exposed to asbestos, chromium, nickel, beryllium, arsenic, soot, or tar in the workplace
- Living where there is air pollution
- Having a family history of lung cancer
- Being infected with the human immunodeficiency virus (HIV)
- Taking beta-carotene supplements and being a heavy smoker

Older age is the main risk factor for most cancers. The chance of getting cancer increases as you get older. Smoking is the major risk factor for small cell lung cancer. When smoking is combined with other risk factors, the risk of lung cancer is increased.

What Are the Signs and Symptoms of Small Cell Lung Cancer?

Signs and symptoms of small cell lung cancer include coughing, shortness of breath, and chest pain. These and other signs and symptoms may be caused by small cell lung cancer or by other conditions. Check with your doctor if you have any of the following:

- Chest discomfort or pain
- A cough that doesn't go away or gets worse over time
- Trouble breathing
- Wheezing
- Blood in sputum (mucus coughed up from the lungs)
- Hoarseness
- Trouble swallowing
- Loss of appetite
- Weight loss for no known reason
- Feeling very tired
- Swelling in the face and/or veins in the neck

How Is Small Cell Lung Cancer Diagnosed?

Tests and procedures that examine the lungs are used to detect (find), diagnose, and stage small cell lung cancer. The following tests and procedures may be used:

- **Physical exam and history.** An exam of the body to check general signs of health, including checking for signs of disease, such as lumps or anything else that seems unusual. A history of the patient's health habits, including smoking, and past jobs, illnesses, and treatments will also be taken.
- **Laboratory tests.** Medical procedures that test samples of tissue, blood, urine, or other substances in the body. These tests help to diagnose disease, plan and check treatment, or monitor the disease over time.
- **Chest X-ray.** An X-ray of the organs and bones inside the chest. An X-ray is a type of energy beam that can go through the body and onto film, making a picture of areas inside the body.
- **Computed tomography (CT)/computerized axial tomography (CAT) scan of the brain, chest, and abdomen.** A procedure that makes a series of detailed pictures of areas inside the body, taken from different angles. The pictures are made by a computer linked to an X-ray machine. A dye may be injected into a vein or swallowed to help the organs or tissues show up more clearly.

- **Sputum cytology.** A microscope is used to check for cancer cells in the sputum (mucus coughed up from the lungs).
- **Biopsy.** The removal of cells or tissues so they can be viewed under a microscope by a pathologist to check for signs of cancer. The different ways a biopsy can be done include the following:
    - **Fine needle aspiration (FNA) biopsy of the lung.** The removal of tissue or fluid from the lung, using a thin needle. A CT scan, ultrasound, or other imaging procedure is used to find the abnormal tissue or fluid in the lung. A small incision may be made in the skin where the biopsy needle is inserted into the abnormal tissue or fluid. A sample is removed with the needle and sent to the laboratory. A pathologist then views the sample under a microscope to look for cancer cells. A chest X-ray is done after the procedure to make sure no air is leaking from the lung into the chest.
    - **Bronchoscopy.** A procedure to look inside the trachea and large airways in the lung for abnormal areas. A bronchoscope is inserted through the nose or mouth into the trachea and lungs. A bronchoscope is a thin, tube-like instrument with a light and a lens for viewing. It may also have a tool to remove tissue samples, which are checked under a microscope for signs of cancer.
    - **Thoracoscopy.** A surgical procedure to look at the organs inside the chest to check for abnormal areas. An incision (cut) is made between two ribs, and a thoracoscope is inserted into the chest. A thoracoscope is a thin, tube-like instrument with a light and a lens for viewing. It may also have a tool to remove tissue or lymph node samples, which are checked under a microscope for signs of cancer. In some cases, this procedure is used to remove part of the esophagus or lung. If certain tissues, organs, or lymph nodes can't be reached, a thoracotomy may be done. In this procedure, a larger incision is made between the ribs and the chest is opened.
    - **Thoracentesis.** The removal of fluid from the space between the lining of the chest and the lung, using a needle. A pathologist views the fluid under a microscope to look for cancer cells.
    - **Mediastinoscopy.** A surgical procedure to look at the organs, tissues, and lymph nodes between the lungs for

abnormal areas. An incision (cut) is made at the top of the breastbone and a mediastinoscope is inserted into the chest. A mediastinoscope is a thin, tube-like instrument with a light and a lens for viewing. It may also have a tool to remove tissue or lymph node samples, which are checked under a microscope for signs of cancer.

- **Light and electron microscopy.** A laboratory test in which cells in a sample of tissue are viewed under regular and high powered microscopes to look for certain changes in the cells.
- **Immunohistochemistry.** A test that uses antibodies to check for certain antigens in a sample of tissue. The antibody is usually linked to a radioactive substance or a dye that causes the tissue to light up under a microscope. This type of test may be used to tell the difference between different types of cancer.

What Is the Prognosis for Small Cell Lung Cancer?

The prognosis (chance of recovery) and treatment options depend on the following:

- The stage of the cancer (whether it is in the chest cavity only or has spread to other places in the body)
- The patient's age, gender, and general health

For certain patients, prognosis also depends on whether the patient is treated with both chemotherapy and radiation.

Stages of Small Cell Lung Cancer

After small cell lung cancer has been diagnosed, tests are done to find out if cancer cells have spread within the chest or to other parts of the body. The process used to find out if cancer has spread within the chest or to other parts of the body is called staging. The information gathered from the staging process determines the stage of the disease. It is important to know the stage in order to plan treatment. Some of the tests used to diagnose small cell lung cancer are also used to stage the disease.

Other tests and procedures that may be used in the staging process include the following:

- **Magnetic resonance imaging (MRI) of the brain:** A procedure that uses a magnet, radio waves, and a computer to make a series of detailed pictures of areas inside the body. This procedure is also called nuclear magnetic resonance imaging (NMRI).

- **Computed tomography (CT)/computerized axial tomography (CAT) scan.** A procedure that makes a series of detailed pictures of areas inside the body, such as the brain, chest or upper abdomen, taken from different angles. The pictures are made by a computer linked to an X-ray machine. A dye may be injected into a vein or swallowed to help the organs or tissues show up more clearly. This procedure is also called computed tomography, computerized tomography, or computerized axial tomography.
- **Positron emission tomography (PET) scan.** A procedure to find malignant tumor cells in the body. A small amount of radioactive glucose (sugar) is injected into a vein. The PET scanner rotates around the body and makes a picture of where glucose is being used in the body. Malignant tumor cells show up brighter in the picture because they are more active and take up more glucose than normal cells do. A PET scan and CT scan may be done at the same time. This is called a PET-CT.
- **Bone scan.** A procedure to check if there are rapidly dividing cells, such as cancer cells, in the bone. A very small amount of radioactive material is injected into a vein and travels through the bloodstream. The radioactive material collects in the bones with cancer and is detected by a scanner.

The following stages are used for small cell lung cancer:

- **Limited stage small cell lung cancer:** In limited stage, cancer is in the lung where it started and may have spread to the area between the lungs or to the lymph nodes above the collarbone.
- **Extensive stage small cell lung cancer:** In extensive stage, cancer has spread beyond the lung or the area between the lungs or the lymph nodes above the collarbone to other places in the body.

Treatment Option Overview

Different types of treatment are available for patients with small cell lung cancer. Some treatments are standard (the currently used treatment), and some are being tested in clinical trials. A treatment clinical trial is a research study meant to help improve current treatments or obtain information on new treatments for patients with cancer. When clinical trials show that a new treatment is better than the standard treatment, the new treatment may become the standard treatment. Patients may want to think about taking part in a clinical trial. Some clinical trials are open only to patients who have not started treatment.

Five types of standard treatment are used:

Surgery

Surgery may be used if the cancer is found in one lung and in nearby lymph nodes only. Because this type of lung cancer is usually found in both lungs, surgery alone is not often used. During surgery, the doctor will also remove lymph nodes to find out if they have cancer in them. Sometimes, surgery may be used to remove a sample of lung tissue to find out the exact type of lung cancer. Even if the doctor removes all the cancer that can be seen at the time of the operation, some patients may be given chemotherapy or radiation therapy after surgery to kill any cancer cells that are left. Treatment given after the surgery, to lower the risk that the cancer will come back, is called adjuvant therapy (AD).

Chemotherapy

Chemotherapy is a cancer treatment that uses drugs to stop the growth of cancer cells, either by killing the cells or by stopping them from dividing. When chemotherapy is taken by mouth or injected into a vein or muscle, the drugs enter the bloodstream and can reach cancer cells throughout the body (systemic chemotherapy). When chemotherapy is placed directly into the cerebrospinal fluid, an organ, or a body cavity such as the abdomen, the drugs mainly affect cancer cells in those areas (regional chemotherapy). The way the chemotherapy is given depends on the type and stage of the cancer being treated.

Radiation Therapy

Radiation therapy is a cancer treatment that uses high energy X-rays or other types of radiation to kill cancer cells or keep them from growing. There are two types of radiation therapy:

- External radiation therapy uses a machine outside the body to send radiation toward the cancer.

- Internal radiation therapy uses a radioactive substance sealed in needles, seeds, wires, or catheters that are placed directly into or near the cancer.

The way the radiation therapy is given depends on the type and stage of the cancer being treated. External radiation therapy is used to treat small cell lung cancer, and may also be used as palliative therapy to relieve symptoms and improve quality of life. Radiation therapy to the brain to lessen the risk that cancer will spread to the brain may also be given.

Laser Therapy

Laser therapy is a cancer treatment that uses a laser beam (a narrow beam of intense light) to kill cancer cells.

Endoscopic Stent Placement

An endoscope is a thin, tube-like instrument used to look at tissues inside the body. An endoscope has a light and a lens for viewing and may be used to place a stent in a body structure to keep the structure open. An endoscopic stent can be used to open an airway blocked by abnormal tissue.

Follow-Up Tests

Some of the tests that were done to diagnose the cancer or to find out the stage of the cancer may be repeated. Some tests will be repeated in order to see how well the treatment is working. Decisions about whether to continue, change, or stop treatment may be based on the results of these tests. Some of the tests will continue to be done from time to time after treatment has ended. The results of these tests can show if your condition has changed or if the cancer has recurred (come back). These tests are sometimes called follow-up tests or check-ups.

Chapter 27

Nonsmall Cell Lung Cancer

The lungs are a pair of cone-shaped breathing organs in the chest. The lungs bring oxygen into the body as you breathe in. They release carbon dioxide, a waste product of the body's cells, as you breathe out. Each lung has sections called lobes. The left lung has two lobes. The right lung is slightly larger and has three lobes. Two tubes called bronchi lead from the trachea (windpipe) to the right and left lungs. The bronchi are sometimes also involved in lung cancer. Tiny air sacs called alveoli and small tubes called bronchioles make up the inside of the lungs. A thin membrane called the pleura covers the outside of each lung and lines the inside wall of the chest cavity. This creates a sac called the pleural cavity. The pleural cavity normally contains a small amount of fluid that helps the lungs move smoothly in the chest when you breathe.

What Is Nonsmall Cell Lung Cancer?

Nonsmall cell lung cancer is a disease in which malignant (cancer) cells form in the tissues of the lung.

This chapter includes text excerpted from "Non-Small Cell Lung Cancer Treatment (PDQ®)—Patient Version," National Cancer Institute (NCI), November 9, 2017.

How Many Types of Nonsmall Cell Lung Cancer Are There?

There are two main types of lung cancer: nonsmall cell lung cancer and small cell lung cancer. There are several types of nonsmall cell lung cancer. Each type of nonsmall cell lung cancer has different kinds of cancer cells. The cancer cells of each type grow and spread in different ways. The types of nonsmall cell lung cancer are named for the kinds of cells found in the cancer and how the cells look under a microscope:

- **Squamous cell carcinoma.** Cancer that begins in squamous cells, which are thin, flat cells that look like fish scales. This is also called epidermoid carcinoma.
- **Large cell carcinoma.** Cancer that may begin in several types of large cells.
- **Adenocarcinoma.** Cancer that begins in the cells that line the alveoli and make substances such as mucus.

Other less common types of nonsmall cell lung cancer are: pleomorphic, carcinoid tumor, salivary gland carcinoma, and unclassified carcinoma.

What Are the Risk Factors for Nonsmall Cell Lung Cancer?

Anything that increases your chance of getting a disease is called a risk factor. Having a risk factor does not mean that you will get cancer; not having risk factors doesn't mean that you will not get cancer. Talk to your doctor if you think you may be at risk for lung cancer. Smoking Is the major risk factor for nonsmall cell lung cancer.

Risk factors for lung cancer include the following:

- Smoking cigarettes, pipes, or cigars, now or in the past. This is the most important risk factor for lung cancer. The earlier in life a person starts smoking, the more often a person smokes, and the more years a person smokes, the greater the risk of lung cancer.
- Being exposed to secondhand smoke
- Being exposed to radiation from any of the following:
    - Radiation therapy to the breast or chest

  - Radon in the home or workplace
  - Imaging tests such as computed tomography (CT) scans
  - Atomic bomb radiation
- Being exposed to asbestos, chromium, nickel, beryllium, arsenic, soot, or tar in the workplace
- Living where there is air pollution
- Having a family history of lung cancer
- Being infected with the human immunodeficiency virus (HIV)
- Taking beta-carotene supplements and being a heavy smoker

Older age is the main risk factor for most cancers. The chance of getting cancer increases as you get older. When smoking is combined with other risk factors, the risk of lung cancer is increased.

What Are the Signs and Symptoms of Nonsmall Cell Lung Cancer?

Signs of nonsmall cell lung cancer include a cough that doesn't go away and shortness of breath. Sometimes lung cancer does not cause any signs or symptoms. It may be found during a chest X-ray done for another condition. Signs and symptoms may be caused by lung cancer or by other conditions. Check with your doctor if you have any of the following:

- Chest discomfort or pain
- A cough that doesn't go away or gets worse over time
- Trouble breathing
- Wheezing
- Blood in sputum (mucus coughed up from the lungs)
- Hoarseness
- Loss of appetite
- Weight loss for no known reason
- Feeling very tired
- Trouble swallowing
- Swelling in the face and/or veins in the neck

How Is Nonsmall Cell Lung Cancer Diagnosed?

Tests and procedures to detect, diagnose, and stage nonsmall cell lung cancer are often done at the same time. Some of the following tests and procedures may be used:

- **Physical exam and history.** An exam of the body to check general signs of health, including checking for signs of disease, such as lumps or anything else that seems unusual. A history of the patient's health habits, including smoking, and past jobs, illnesses, and treatments will also be taken.
- **Laboratory tests.** Medical procedures that test samples of tissue, blood, urine, or other substances in the body. These tests help to diagnose disease, plan and check treatment, or monitor the disease over time.
- **Chest X-ray.** An X-ray of the organs and bones inside the chest. An X-ray is a type of energy beam that can go through the body and onto film, making a picture of areas inside the body.
- **Computed tomography (CT)/computerized axial tomography (CAT) scan.** A procedure that makes a series of detailed pictures of areas inside the body, such as the chest, taken from different angles. The pictures are made by a computer linked to an X-ray machine. A dye may be injected into a vein or swallowed to help the organs or tissues show up more clearly. This procedure is also called computed tomography, computerized tomography, or computerized axial tomography.
- **Sputum cytology.** A procedure in which a pathologist views a sample of sputum (mucus coughed up from the lungs) under a microscope, to check for cancer cells.
- **Fine needle aspiration (FNA) biopsy of the lung.** The removal of tissue or fluid from the lung using a thin needle. A CT scan, ultrasound, or other imaging procedure is used to locate the abnormal tissue or fluid in the lung. A small incision may be made in the skin where the biopsy needle is inserted into the abnormal tissue or fluid. A sample is removed with the needle and sent to the laboratory. A pathologist then views the sample under a microscope to look for cancer cells. A chest X-ray is done after the procedure to make sure no air is leaking from the lung into the chest.
- **Bronchoscopy.** A procedure to look inside the trachea and large airways in the lung for abnormal areas. A bronchoscope is

inserted through the nose or mouth into the trachea and lungs. A bronchoscope is a thin, tube-like instrument with a light and a lens for viewing. It may also have a tool to remove tissue samples, which are checked under a microscope for signs of cancer.

- **Thoracoscopy.** A surgical procedure to look at the organs inside the chest to check for abnormal areas. An incision (cut) is made between two ribs, and a thoracoscope is inserted into the chest. A thoracoscope is a thin, tube-like instrument with a light and a lens for viewing. It may also have a tool to remove tissue or lymph node samples, which are checked under a microscope for signs of cancer. In some cases, this procedure is used to remove part of the esophagus or lung. If certain tissues, organs, or lymph nodes can't be reached, a thoracotomy may be done. In this procedure, a larger incision is made between the ribs and the chest is opened.
- **Thoracentesis.** The removal of fluid from the space between the lining of the chest and the lung, using a needle. A pathologist views the fluid under a microscope to look for cancer cells.
- **Light and electron microscopy.** A laboratory test in which cells in a sample of tissue are viewed under regular and high powered microscopes to look for certain changes in the cells.
- **Immunohistochemistry.** A test that uses antibodies to check for certain antigens in a sample of tissue. The antibody is usually linked to a radioactive substance or a dye that causes the tissue to light up under a microscope. This type of test may be used to tell the difference between different types of cancer.

What Is the Prognosis for Nonsmall Cell Lung Cancer Diagnosed?

The prognosis (chance of recovery) and treatment options depend on the following:

- The stage of the cancer (the size of the tumor and whether it is in the lung only or has spread to other places in the body)
- The type of lung cancer
- Whether the cancer has mutations (changes) in certain genes, such as the epidermal growth factor receptor (*EGFR*) gene or the anaplastic lymphoma kinase (*ALK*) gene

- Whether there are signs and symptoms such as coughing or trouble breathing
- The patient's general health

Stages of Nonsmall Cell Lung Cancer

After lung cancer has been diagnosed, tests are done to find out if cancer cells have spread within the lungs or to other parts of the body. The process used to find out if cancer has spread within the lungs or to other parts of the body is called staging. The information gathered from the staging process determines the stage of the disease. It is important to know the stage in order to plan treatment. Some of the tests used to diagnose nonsmall cell lung cancer are also used to stage the disease.

Other tests and procedures that may be used in the staging process include the following:

- **Magnetic resonance imaging (MRI).** A procedure that uses a magnet, radio waves, and a computer to make a series of detailed pictures of areas inside the body, such as the brain. This procedure is also called nuclear magnetic resonance imaging (NMRI).
- **Computed tomography (CT)/computerized axial tomography (CAT) scan.** A procedure that makes a series of detailed pictures of areas inside the body, such as the brain and abdomen, taken from different angles. The pictures are made by a computer linked to an X-ray machine. A dye may be injected into a vein or swallowed to help the organs or tissues show up more clearly.
- **Positron emission tomography (PET) scan.** A procedure to find malignant tumor cells in the body. A small amount of radioactive glucose (sugar) is injected into a vein. The PET scanner rotates around the body and makes a picture of where glucose is being used in the body. Malignant tumor cells show up brighter in the picture because they are more active and take up more glucose than normal cells do.
- **Radionuclide bone scan.** A procedure to check if there are rapidly dividing cells, such as cancer cells, in the bone. A very small amount of radioactive material is injected into a vein and travels through the bloodstream. The radioactive material collects in the bones and is detected by a scanner.

- **Pulmonary function test (PFT).** A test to see how well the lungs are working. It measures how much air the lungs can hold and how quickly air moves into and out of the lungs. It also measures how much oxygen is used and how much carbon dioxide is given off during breathing. This is also called lung function test.
- **Endoscopic ultrasound (EUS).** A procedure in which an endoscope is inserted into the body. An endoscope is a thin, tube-like instrument with a light and a lens for viewing. A probe at the end of the endoscope is used to bounce high energy sound waves (ultrasound) off internal tissues or organs and make echoes. The echoes form a picture of body tissues called a sonogram. This procedure is also called endosonography. EUS may be used to guide fine needle aspiration (FNA) biopsy of the lung, lymph nodes, or other areas.
- **Mediastinoscopy.** A surgical procedure to look at the organs, tissues, and lymph nodes between the lungs for abnormal areas. An incision (cut) is made at the top of the breastbone and a mediastinoscope is inserted into the chest. A mediastinoscope is a thin, tube-like instrument with a light and a lens for viewing. It may also have a tool to remove tissue or lymph node samples, which are checked under a microscope for signs of cancer.
- **Anterior mediastinotomy.** A surgical procedure to look at the organs and tissues between the lungs and between the breastbone and heart for abnormal areas. An incision (cut) is made next to the breastbone and a mediastinoscope is inserted into the chest. A mediastinoscope is a thin, tube-like instrument with a light and a lens for viewing. It may also have a tool to remove tissue or lymph node samples, which are checked under a microscope for signs of cancer. This is also called the Chamberlain procedure.
- **Lymph node biopsy.** The removal of all or part of a lymph node. A pathologist views the tissue under a microscope to look for cancer cells.
- **Bone marrow aspiration and biopsy.** The removal of bone marrow, blood, and a small piece of bone by inserting a hollow needle into the hipbone or breastbone. A pathologist views the bone marrow, blood, and bone under a microscope to look for signs of cancer.

The following stages are used for nonsmall cell lung cancer:

Occult (hidden) stage: In the occult (hidden) stage, cancer cannot be seen by imaging or bronchoscopy. Cancer cells are found in sputum (mucus coughed up from the lungs) or bronchial washing (a sample of cells taken from inside the airways that lead to the lung). Cancer may have spread to other parts of the body.

Stage 0 (carcinoma in situ): In stage 0, abnormal cells are found in the lining of the airways. These abnormal cells may become cancer and spread into nearby normal tissue. Stage 0 is also called carcinoma in situ.

Stage I. In stage I, cancer has formed. Stage I is divided into stages IA and IB:

- **Stage IA.** The tumor is in the lung only and is 3 centimeters or smaller.
- **Stage IB.** Cancer has not spread to the lymph nodes and one or more of the following is true:
    - The tumor is larger than 3 centimeters but not larger than 5 centimeters.
    - Cancer has spread to the main bronchus and is at least 2 centimeters below where the trachea joins the bronchus.
    - Cancer has spread to the innermost layer of the membrane that covers the lung.
    - Part of the lung has collapsed or developed pneumonitis (inflammation of the lung) in the area where the trachea joins the bronchus.

Stage II. Stage II is divided into stages IIA and IIB. Stage IIA, and IIB are each divided into two sections depending on the size of the tumor, where the tumor is found, and whether there is cancer in the lymph nodes.

Stage IIA:

1. Cancer has spread to lymph nodes on the same side of the chest as the tumor. The lymph nodes with cancer are within the lung or near the bronchus. Also, one or more of the following is true:

    - The tumor is not larger than 5 centimeters.

- Cancer has spread to the main bronchus and is at least 2 centimeters below where the trachea joins the bronchus.
- Cancer has spread to the innermost layer of the membrane that covers the lung.
- Part of the lung has collapsed or developed pneumonitis (inflammation of the lung) in the area where the trachea joins the bronchus.

or

2. Cancer has not spread to lymph nodes and one or more of the following is true:
   - The tumor is larger than 5 centimeters but not larger than 7 centimeters.
   - Cancer has spread to the main bronchus and is at least 2 centimeters below where the trachea joins the bronchus.
   - Cancer has spread to the innermost layer of the membrane that covers the lung.
   - Part of the lung has collapsed or developed pneumonitis (inflammation of the lung) in the area where the trachea joins the bronchus.

Stage IIB:

1. Cancer has spread to nearby lymph nodes on the same side of the chest as the tumor. The lymph nodes with cancer are within the lung or near the bronchus. Also, one or more of the following is true:
   - The tumor is larger than 5 centimeters but not larger than 7 centimeters.
   - Cancer has spread to the main bronchus and is at least 2 centimeters below where the trachea joins the bronchus.
   - Cancer has spread to the innermost layer of the membrane that covers the lung.
   - Part of the lung has collapsed or developed pneumonitis (inflammation of the lung) in the area where the trachea joins the bronchus.

   or

2. Cancer has not spread to lymph nodes and one or more of the following is true:
   - The tumor is larger than 7 centimeters.
   - Cancer has spread to the main bronchus (and is less than 2 centimeters below where the trachea joins the bronchus), the chest wall, the diaphragm, or the nerve that controls the diaphragm.
   - Cancer has spread to the membrane around the heart or lining the chest wall.
   - The whole lung has collapsed or developed pneumonitis (inflammation of the lung).
   - There are one or more separate tumors in the same lobe of the lung.

Stage IIIA. Stage IIIA is divided into three sections depending on the size of the tumor, where the tumor is found, and which lymph nodes have cancer (if any).

1. Cancer has spread to lymph nodes on the same side of the chest as the tumor. The lymph nodes with cancer are near the sternum (chest bone) or where the bronchus enters the lung. Also:
   - The tumor may be any size
   - Part of the lung (where the trachea joins the bronchus) or the whole lung may have collapsed or developed pneumonitis (inflammation of the lung)
   - There may be one or more separate tumors in the same lobe of the lung
   - Cancer may have spread to any of the following:
     - Main bronchus, but not the area where the trachea joins the bronchus
     - Chest wall
     - Diaphragm and the nerve that controls it
     - Membrane around the lung or lining the chest wall
     - Membrane around the heart

2. Cancer has spread to lymph nodes on the same side of the chest as the tumor. The lymph nodes with cancer are within the lung or near the bronchus. Also:
   - The tumor may be any size
   - The whole lung may have collapsed or developed pneumonitis (inflammation of the lung)
   - There may be one or more separate tumors in any of the lobes of the lung with cancer
   - Cancer may have spread to any of the following:
     - Main bronchus, but not the area where the trachea joins the bronchus
     - Chest wall
     - Diaphragm and the nerve that controls it
     - Membrane around the lung or lining the chest wall
     - Heart or the membrane around it
     - Major blood vessels that lead to or from the heart
     - Trachea
     - Esophagus
     - Nerve that controls the larynx (voice box)
     - Sternum (chest bone) or backbone
     - Carina (where the trachea joins the bronchi)

   or

3. Cancer has not spread to the lymph nodes and the tumor may be any size. Cancer has spread to any of the following:
   - Heart
   - Major blood vessels that lead to or from the heart
   - Trachea
   - Esophagus
   - Nerve that controls the larynx (voice box)
   - Sternum (chest bone) or backbone
   - Carina (where the trachea joins the bronchi)

Stage IIIB. Stage IIIB is divided into two sections depending on the size of the tumor, where the tumor is found, and which lymph nodes have cancer.

1. Cancer has spread to lymph nodes above the collarbone or to lymph nodes on the opposite side of the chest as the tumor. Also:
   - The tumor may be any size
   - Part of the lung (where the trachea joins the bronchus) or the whole lung may have collapsed or developed pneumonitis (inflammation of the lung)
   - There may be one or more separate tumors in any of the lobes of the lung with cancer
   - Cancer may have spread to any of the following:
     - Main bronchus
     - Chest wall
     - Diaphragm and the nerve that controls it
     - Membrane around the lung or lining the chest wall
     - Heart or the membrane around it
     - Major blood vessels that lead to or from the heart
     - Trachea
     - Esophagus
     - Nerve that controls the larynx (voice box)
     - Sternum (chest bone) or backbone
     - Carina (where the trachea joins the bronchi)

   or

2. Cancer has spread to lymph nodes on the same side of the chest as the tumor. The lymph nodes with cancer are near the sternum (chest bone) or where the bronchus enters the lung. Also:
   - The tumor may be any size
   - There may be separate tumors in different lobes of the same lung

- Cancer has spread to any of the following:
    - Heart
    - Major blood vessels that lead to or from the heart
    - Trachea
    - Esophagus
    - Nerve that controls the larynx (voice box)
    - Sternum (chest bone) or backbone
    - Carina (where the trachea joins the bronchi)

Stage IV. In stage IV, the tumor may be any size and cancer may have spread to lymph nodes. One or more of the following is true:

- There are one or more tumors in both lungs
- Cancer is found in fluid around the lungs or the heart
- Cancer has spread to other parts of the body, such as the brain, liver, adrenal glands, kidneys, or bone

Treatment Option Overview

Different types of treatments are available for patients with nonsmall cell lung cancer. Some treatments are standard (the currently used treatment), and some are being tested in clinical trials. A treatment clinical trial is a research study meant to help improve current treatments or obtain information on new treatments for patients with cancer. When clinical trials show that a new treatment is better than the standard treatment, the new treatment may become the standard treatment. Patients may want to think about taking part in a clinical trial. Some clinical trials are open only to patients who have not started treatment.

Standard Treatments Available for People with Nonsmall Cell Lung Cancer

Nine types of standard treatment are used:

Surgery

Four types of surgery are used to treat lung cancer:

- Wedge resection. Surgery to remove a tumor and some of the normal tissue around it. When a slightly larger amount of tissue is taken, it is called a segmental resection.

- Lobectomy. Surgery to remove a whole lobe (section) of the lung.
- Pneumonectomy. Surgery to remove one whole lung.
- Sleeve resection. Surgery to remove part of the bronchus.

Even if the doctor removes all the cancer that can be seen at the time of the surgery, some patients may be given chemotherapy or radiation therapy after surgery to kill any cancer cells that are left. Treatment given after the surgery, to lower the risk that the cancer will come back, is called adjuvant therapy.

Radiation Therapy

Radiation therapy is a cancer treatment that uses high energy X-rays or other types of radiation to kill cancer cells or keep them from growing. There are two types of radiation therapy:

- External radiation therapy uses a machine outside the body to send radiation toward the cancer.
- Internal radiation therapy uses a radioactive substance sealed in needles, seeds, wires, or catheters that are placed directly into or near the cancer.

Stereotactic body radiation therapy (SRT) is a type of external radiation therapy. Special equipment is used to place the patient in the same position for each radiation treatment. Once a day for several days, a radiation machine aims a larger than usual dose of radiation directly at the tumor. By having the patient in the same position for each treatment, there is less damage to nearby healthy tissue. This procedure is also called stereotactic external beam radiation therapy (EBRT) and SRT.

Stereotactic radiosurgery is a type of external radiation therapy used to treat lung cancer that has spread to the brain. A rigid head frame is attached to the skull to keep the head still during the radiation treatment. A machine aims a single large dose of radiation directly at the tumor in the brain. This procedure does not involve surgery. It is also called stereotaxic radiosurgery, radiosurgery, and radiation surgery.

For tumors in the airways, radiation is given directly to the tumor through an endoscope.

The way the radiation therapy is given depends on the type and stage of the cancer being treated. It also depends on where the cancer is found. External and internal radiation therapy are used to treat nonsmall cell lung cancer.

Chemotherapy

Chemotherapy is a cancer treatment that uses drugs to stop the growth of cancer cells, either by killing the cells or by stopping them from dividing. When chemotherapy is taken by mouth or injected into a vein or muscle, the drugs enter the bloodstream and can reach cancer cells throughout the body (systemic chemotherapy). When chemotherapy is placed directly into the cerebrospinal fluid, an organ, or a body cavity such as the abdomen, the drugs mainly affect cancer cells in those areas (regional chemotherapy).

The way the chemotherapy is given depends on the type and stage of the cancer being treated.

Targeted Therapy

Targeted therapy is a type of treatment that uses drugs or other substances to attack specific cancer cells. Targeted therapies usually cause less harm to normal cells than chemotherapy or radiation therapy do. Monoclonal antibodies and tyrosine kinase inhibitors (TKI) are the two main types of targeted therapy being used to treat advanced, metastatic, or recurrent nonsmall cell lung cancer.

Monoclonal Antibodies

Monoclonal antibody therapy is a cancer treatment that uses antibodies made in the laboratory from a single type of immune system cell. These antibodies can identify substances on cancer cells or normal substances in the blood or tissues that may help cancer cells grow. The antibodies attach to the substances and kill the cancer cells, block their growth, or keep them from spreading. Monoclonal antibodies are given by infusion. They may be used alone or to carry drugs, toxins, or radioactive material directly to cancer cells.

There are different types of monoclonal antibody therapy:

- **Vascular endothelial growth factor (VEGF) inhibitor therapy.** Cancer cells make a substance called VEGF, which causes new blood vessels to form (angiogenesis) and helps the cancer grow. VEGF inhibitors block VEGF and stop new blood vessels from forming. This may kill cancer cells because they need new blood vessels to grow. Bevacizumab and ramucirumab are VEGF inhibitors and angiogenesis inhibitors.
- **Epidermal growth factor receptor (EGFR) inhibitor therapy.** EGFRs are proteins found on the surface of certain cells,

including cancer cells. Epidermal growth factor attaches to the EGFR on the surface of the cell and causes the cells to grow and divide. EGFR inhibitors block the receptor and stop the epidermal growth factor from attaching to the cancer cell. This stops the cancer cell from growing and dividing. Cetuximab and necitumumab are EGFR inhibitors.

- **Immune checkpoint inhibitor therapy.** PD-1 is a protein on the surface of T cells that helps keep the body's immune responses in check. When PD-1 attaches to another protein called PDL-1 on a cancer cell, it stops the T cell from killing the cancer cell. PD-1 inhibitors attach to PDL-1 and allow the T cells to kill cancer cells. Nivolumab, pembrolizumab, and atezolizumab are types of immune checkpoint inhibitors.

Tyrosine Kinase Inhibitors

Tyrosine kinase inhibitors are small molecule drugs that go through the cell membrane and work inside cancer cells to block signals that cancer cells need to grow and divide. Some tyrosine kinase inhibitors also have angiogenesis inhibitor effects.

There are different types of tyrosine kinase inhibitors:

- **EGFR tyrosine kinase inhibitors.** EGFRs are proteins found on the surface and inside certain cells, including cancer cells. Epidermal growth factor attaches to the EGFR inside the cell and sends signals to the tyrosine kinase area of the cell, which tells the cell to grow and divide. EGFR tyrosine kinase inhibitors stop these signals and stop the cancer cell from growing and dividing. Erlotinib, gefitinib, and afatinib are types of EGFR tyrosine kinase inhibitors. Some of these drugs work better when there is also a mutation (change) in the *EGFR* gene.
- **Kinase inhibitors that affect cells with certain gene change.** Certain changes in the *ALK* and *ROS1* genes cause too much protein to be made. Blocking these proteins may stop the cancer from growing and spreading. Crizotinib is used to stop proteins from being made by the *ALK* and *ROS1* gene. Ceritinib is used to stop proteins from being made by the *ALK* gene.

Laser Therapy

Laser therapy is a cancer treatment that uses a laser beam (a narrow beam of intense light) to kill cancer cells.

Photodynamic Therapy (PDT)

Photodynamic therapy (PDT) is a cancer treatment that uses a drug and a certain type of laser light to kill cancer cells. A drug that is not active until it is exposed to light is injected into a vein. The drug collects more in cancer cells than in normal cells. Fiberoptic tubes are then used to carry the laser light to the cancer cells, where the drug becomes active and kills the cells. PDT causes little damage to healthy tissue. It is used mainly to treat tumors on or just under the skin or in the lining of internal organs. When the tumor is in the airways, PDT is given directly to the tumor through an endoscope.

Cryosurgery

Cryosurgery is a treatment that uses an instrument to freeze and destroy abnormal tissue, such as carcinoma in situ. This type of treatment is also called cryotherapy. For tumors in the airways, cryosurgery is done through an endoscope.

Electrocautery

Electrocautery is a treatment that uses a probe or needle heated by an electric current to destroy abnormal tissue. For tumors in the airways, electrocautery is done through an endoscope.

Watchful Waiting

Watchful waiting is closely monitoring a patient's condition without giving any treatment until signs or symptoms appear or change. This may be done in certain rare cases of nonsmall cell lung cancer.

New Types of Treatment Are Being Tested in Clinical Trials

- **Chemoprevention:** Chemoprevention is the use of drugs, vitamins, or other substances to reduce the risk of cancer or to reduce the risk cancer will recur (come back). For lung cancer, chemoprevention is used to lessen the chance that a new tumor will form in the lung.
- **Radiosensitizers:** Radiosensitizers are substances that make tumor cells easier to kill with radiation therapy. The combination of chemotherapy and radiation therapy given with a radiosensitizer is being studied in the treatment of nonsmall cell lung cancer.
- **New Combinations:** New combinations of treatments are being studied in clinical trials.

Chapter 28

Malignant Mesothelioma

What Is Malignant Mesothelioma?

Malignant mesothelioma is a disease in which malignant (cancer) cells are found in the pleura (the thin layer of tissue that lines the chest cavity and covers the lungs) or the peritoneum (the thin layer of tissue that lines the abdomen and covers most of the organs in the abdomen). Malignant mesothelioma may also form in the heart or testicles, but this is rare.

What Are the Risk Factors for Malignant Mesothelioma?

Anything that increases your chance of getting a disease is called a risk factor. Having a risk factor does not mean that you will get cancer; not having risk factors doesn't mean that you will not get cancer. Talk to your doctor if you think you may be at risk. Being exposed to asbestos can affect the risk of malignant mesothelioma. Most people with malignant mesothelioma have worked or lived in places where they inhaled or swallowed asbestos. After being exposed to asbestos, it usually takes a long time for malignant mesothelioma to form. Living with a person who works near asbestos is also a risk factor for malignant mesothelioma.

This chapter includes text excerpted from "Malignant Mesothelioma Treatment (PDQ®)—Patient Version," National Cancer Institute (NCI), November 9, 2017.

What Are the Signs and Symptoms of Malignant Mesothelioma?

Sometimes the cancer causes fluid to collect in the chest or in the abdomen. Signs and symptoms may be caused by the fluid, malignant mesothelioma, or other conditions. It may also include shortness of breath and pain under the rib cage. Check with your doctor if you have any of the following:

- Trouble breathing
- Cough
- Pain under the rib cage
- Pain or swelling in the abdomen
- Lumps in the abdomen
- Constipation
- Problems with blood clots (clots form when they shouldn't)
- Weight loss for no known reason
- Feeling very tired

How Is Malignant Mesothelioma Diagnosed?

Sometimes it is hard to tell the difference between malignant mesothelioma in the chest and lung cancer. The following tests and procedures may be used to diagnose malignant mesothelioma in the chest or peritoneum:

- **Physical exam and history.** An exam of the body to check general signs of health, including checking for signs of disease, such as lumps or anything else that seems unusual. A history of the patient's health habits, exposure to asbestos, and past illnesses and treatments will also be taken.
- **Chest X-ray.** An X-ray of the organs and bones inside the chest. An X-ray is a type of energy beam that can go through the body and onto film, making a picture of areas inside the body.
- **Computed tomography (CT)/computerized axial tomography (CAT) scan.** A procedure that makes a series of detailed pictures of the chest and abdomen, taken from different angles. The pictures are made by a computer linked to an X-ray machine. A dye may be injected into a vein or swallowed to help the organs or tissues show up more clearly.

- **Biopsy.** The removal of cells or tissues from the pleura or peritoneum so they can be viewed under a microscope by a pathologist to check for signs of cancer.

  Procedures used to collect the cells or tissues include the following:

  - **Fine needle (FNA) aspiration biopsy of the lung.** The removal of tissue or fluid using a thin needle. An imaging procedure is used to locate the abnormal tissue or fluid in the lung. A small incision may be made in the skin where the biopsy needle is inserted into the abnormal tissue or fluid, and a sample is removed.
  - **Thoracoscopy.** An incision (cut) is made between two ribs and a thoracoscope (a thin, tube-like instrument with a light and a lens for viewing) is inserted into the chest.
  - **Thoracotomy.** An incision (cut) is made between two ribs to check inside the chest for signs of disease.
  - **Peritoneoscopy.** An incision (cut) is made in the abdominal wall and a peritoneoscope (a thin, tube-like instrument with a light and a lens for viewing) is inserted into the abdomen.
  - **Laparotomy.** An incision (cut) is made in the wall of the abdomen to check the inside of the abdomen for signs of disease.
  - **Open biopsy.** A procedure in which an incision (cut) is made through the skin to expose and remove tissues to check for signs of disease.

The following tests may be done on the cells and tissue samples that are taken:

- **Cytologic exam.** An exam of cells under a microscope to check for anything abnormal. For mesothelioma, fluid is taken from the chest or from the abdomen. A pathologist checks the fluid for signs of cancer.
- **Immunohistochemistry.** A test that uses antibodies to check for certain antigens in a sample of tissue. The antibody is usually linked to a radioactive substance or a dye that causes the tissue to light up under a microscope. This type of test may be used to tell the difference between different types of cancer.
- **Electron microscopy.** A laboratory test in which cells in a sample of tissue are viewed under a high powered microscope

to look for certain changes in the cells. An electron microscope shows tiny details better than other types of microscopes.

What Factors Affect Prognosis and Treatment Options for People with Malignant Mesothelioma?

The prognosis (chance of recovery) and treatment options depend on the following:

- The stage of the cancer
- The size of the tumor
- Whether the tumor can be removed completely by surgery
- The amount of fluid in the chest or abdomen
- The patient's age
- The patient's activity level
- The patient's general health, including lung and heart health
- The type of mesothelioma cells and how they look under a microscope
- The number of white blood cells and how much hemoglobin is in the blood
- Whether the patient is male or female
- Whether the cancer has just been diagnosed or has recurred (come back)

Stages of Malignant Mesothelioma

After malignant mesothelioma has been diagnosed, tests are done to find out if cancer cells have spread to other parts of the body.

The process used to find out if cancer has spread outside the pleura or peritoneum is called staging. The information gathered from the staging process determines the stage of the disease. It is important to know whether the cancer has spread in order to plan treatment.

The following tests and procedures may be used in the staging process:

- **Computed tomography (CT)/computerized axial tomography (CAT) scan.** A procedure that makes a series of detailed pictures of the chest and abdomen, taken from different angles.

The pictures are made by a computer linked to an X-ray machine. A dye may be injected into a vein or swallowed to help the organs or tissues show up more clearly.

- **Positron emission tomography (PET) scan.** A procedure to find malignant tumor cells in the body. A small amount of radioactive glucose (sugar) is injected into a vein. The PET scanner rotates around the body and makes a picture of where glucose is being used in the body. Malignant tumor cells show up brighter in the picture because they are more active and take up more glucose than normal cells do.
- **Endoscopic ultrasound (EUS).** A procedure in which an endoscope is inserted into the body. An endoscope is a thin, tube-like instrument with a light and a lens for viewing. A probe at the end of the endoscope is used to bounce high energy sound waves (ultrasound) off internal tissues or organs and make echoes. The echoes form a picture of body tissues called a sonogram. This procedure is also called endosonography. EUS may be used to guide fine needle aspiration (FNA) biopsy of the lung, lymph nodes, or other areas.
- **Pulmonary function (PFT) test.** A test to see how well the lungs are working. It measures how much air the lungs can hold and how quickly air moves into and out of the lungs. It also measures how much oxygen is used and how much carbon dioxide is given off during breathing. This is also called lung function test.

The following stages are used for malignant mesothelioma:
Stage I (Localized). Stage I is divided into stages IA and IB:

- In stage IA, cancer is found in one side of the chest in the lining of the chest wall and may also be found in the lining of the chest cavity between the lungs and/or the lining that covers the diaphragm. Cancer has not spread to the lining that covers the lung.
- In stage IB, cancer is found in one side of the chest in the lining of the chest wall and the lining that covers the lung. Cancer may also be found in the lining of the chest cavity between the lungs and/or the lining that covers the diaphragm.

Stage II (Advanced). In stage II, cancer is found in one side of the chest in the lining of the chest wall, the lining of the chest cavity between the lungs, the lining that covers the diaphragm, and the lining that covers the lung. Also, cancer has spread into one or both of the following:

- Lung tissue
- Diaphragm

Stage III (Advanced). In stage III, either of the following is true:

Cancer is found in one side of the chest in the lining of the chest wall. Cancer may have spread to:

- the lining of the chest cavity between the lungs
- the lining that covers the diaphragm
- the lining that covers the lung
- the lung tissue
- the diaphragm

Cancer has spread to lymph nodes where the lung joins the bronchus, along the trachea and esophagus, between the lung and diaphragm, or below the trachea.

or

Cancer is found in one side of the chest in the lining of the chest wall, the lining of the chest cavity between the lungs, the lining that covers the diaphragm, and the lining that covers the lung. Cancer has spread into one or more of the following:

- Tissue between the ribs and the lining of the chest wall
- Fat in the area between the lungs
- Soft tissues of the chest wall
- Sac around the heart

Cancer may have spread to lymph nodes where the lung joins the bronchus, along the trachea and esophagus, between the lung and diaphragm, or below the trachea.

Stage IV (Advanced). In stage IV, cancer cannot be removed by surgery and is found in one or both sides of the body. Cancer may have spread to lymph nodes anywhere in the chest or above the collarbone. Cancer has spread in one or more of the following ways:

- Through the diaphragm into the peritoneum (the thin layer of tissue that lines the abdomen and covers most of the organs in the abdomen)

- To the tissue lining the chest on the opposite side of the body as the tumor
- To the chest wall and may be found in the rib
- Into the organs in the center of the chest cavity
- Into the spine
- Into the sac around the heart or into the heart muscle
- To distant parts of the body such as the brain, spine, thyroid, or prostate

Treatment Option Overview

Different types of treatments are available for patients with malignant mesothelioma. Some treatments are standard (the currently used treatment), and some are being tested in clinical trials. A treatment clinical trial is a research study meant to help improve current treatments or obtain information on new treatments for patients with cancer. When clinical trials show that a new treatment is better than the standard treatment, the new treatment may become the standard treatment. Patients may want to think about taking part in a clinical trial. Some clinical trials are open only to patients who have not started treatment.

Standard Treatments for People with Malignant Mesothelioma

Four types of standard treatment are used:

Surgery

The following surgical treatments may be used for malignant mesothelioma in the chest:

- **Wide local excision:** Surgery to remove the cancer and some of the healthy tissue around it.
- **Pleurectomy and decortication:** Surgery to remove part of the covering of the lungs and lining of the chest and part of the outside surface of the lungs.
- **Extrapleural pneumonectomy:** Surgery to remove one whole lung and part of the lining of the chest, the diaphragm, and the lining of the sac around the heart.

- **Pleurodesis:** A surgical procedure that uses chemicals or drugs to make a scar in the space between the layers of the pleura. Fluid is first drained from the space using a catheter or chest tube and the chemical or drug is put into the space. The scarring stops the buildup of fluid in the pleural cavity.

Even if the doctor removes all the cancer that can be seen at the time of the surgery, some patients may be given chemotherapy or radiation therapy after surgery to kill any cancer cells that are left. Treatment given after surgery, to lower the risk that the cancer will come back, is called adjuvant therapy.

Radiation Therapy

Radiation therapy is a cancer treatment that uses high-energy X-rays or other types of radiation to kill cancer cells or keep them from growing. There are two types of radiation therapy:

- External radiation therapy uses a machine outside the body to send radiation toward the cancer.
- Internal radiation therapy uses a radioactive substance sealed in needles, seeds, wires, or catheters that are placed directly into or near the cancer.

The way the radiation therapy is given depends on the type and stage of the cancer being treated. External radiation therapy is used to treat malignant mesothelioma, and may also be used as palliative therapy to relieve symptoms and improve quality of life.

Chemotherapy

Chemotherapy is a cancer treatment that uses drugs to stop the growth of cancer cells, either by killing the cells or by stopping them from dividing. When chemotherapy is taken by mouth or injected into a vein or muscle, the drugs enter the bloodstream and can reach cancer cells throughout the body (systemic chemotherapy). When chemotherapy is placed directly into the cerebrospinal fluid, an organ, or a body cavity such as the chest or peritoneum, the drugs mainly affect cancer cells in those areas (regional chemotherapy). Combination chemotherapy is the use of more than one anticancer drug.

Hyperthermic intraperitoneal chemotherapy is used in the treatment of mesothelioma that has spread to the peritoneum (tissue that lines the abdomen and covers most of the organs in the abdomen).

After the surgeon removes all the cancer that can be seen, a solution containing anticancer drugs is heated and pumped into and out of the abdomen to kill cancer cells that remain. Heating the anticancer drugs may kill more cancer cells.

Targeted Therapy

Targeted therapy is a type of treatment that uses drugs or other substances to attack specific cancer cells. Targeted therapies usually cause less harm to normal cells than chemotherapy or radiation therapy do. Monoclonal antibody therapy is a type of targeted therapy that uses antibodies made in the laboratory, from a single type of immune system cell. These antibodies can identify substances on cancer cells or normal substances that may help cancer cells grow. The antibodies attach to the substances and kill the cancer cells, block their growth, or keep them from spreading. Monoclonal antibodies are given by infusion. They may be used alone or to carry drugs, toxins, or radioactive material directly to cancer cells.

Bevacizumab is a monoclonal antibody used to treat advanced malignant mesothelioma. It binds to a protein called vascular endothelial growth factor (VEGF). This may prevent the growth of new blood vessels that tumors need to grow. Other monoclonal antibodies are being studied in malignant mesothelioma. Kinase inhibitors are a type of targeted therapy being studied in the treatment of malignant mesothelioma. Kinase inhibitors are targeted therapy drugs that block signals needed for tumors to grow.

Chapter 29

Esophageal Cancer

The esophagus is the hollow, muscular tube that moves food and liquid from the throat to the stomach. The wall of the esophagus is made up of several layers of tissue, including mucous membrane, muscle, and connective tissue.

What Is Esophageal Cancer?

Esophageal cancer is a disease in which malignant (cancer) cells form in the tissues of the esophagus. It starts on the inside lining of the esophagus and spreads outward through the other layers as it grows. The two most common forms of esophageal cancer are named for the type of cells that become malignant (cancerous):

- **Squamous cell carcinoma:** Cancer that forms in squamous cells, the thin, flat cells lining the esophagus. This cancer is most often found in the upper and middle part of the esophagus, but can occur anywhere along the esophagus. This is also called epidermoid carcinoma.
- **Adenocarcinoma:** Cancer that begins in glandular (secretory) cells. Glandular cells in the lining of the esophagus produce and release fluids such as mucus. Adenocarcinomas usually form in the lower part of the esophagus, near the stomach.

This chapter includes text excerpted from "Esophageal Cancer Treatment (PDQ®)—Patient Version," National Cancer Institute (NCI), December 7, 2017.

What Are the Risk Factors for Esophageal Cancer?

Anything that increases your risk of getting a disease is called a risk factor. Having a risk factor does not mean that you will get cancer; not having risk factors doesn't mean that you will not get cancer. Talk with your doctor if you think you may be at risk. Smoking, heavy alcohol use, and Barrett esophagus can increase the risk of esophageal cancer. Risk factors include the following:

- Tobacco use
- Heavy alcohol use
- Barrett esophagus: A condition in which the cells lining the lower part of the esophagus have changed or been replaced with abnormal cells that could lead to cancer of the esophagus. Gastric reflux (the backing up of stomach contents into the lower section of the esophagus) may irritate the esophagus and, over time, cause Barrett esophagus
- Older age

What Are the Signs and Symptoms of Esophageal Cancer?

Signs and symptoms of esophageal cancer are weight loss and painful or difficult swallowing. These and other signs and symptoms may be caused by esophageal cancer or by other conditions. Check with your doctor if you have any of the following:

- Painful or difficult swallowing
- Weight loss
- Pain behind the breastbone
- Hoarseness and cough
- Indigestion and heartburn

How Is Esophageal Cancer Diagnosed?

The following tests and procedures may be used:

- **Physical exam and history:** An exam of the body to check general signs of health, including checking for signs of disease, such as lumps or anything else that seems unusual. A history

of the patient's health habits and past illnesses and treatments will also be taken.

- **Chest X-ray:** An X-ray of the organs and bones inside the chest. An X-ray is a type of energy beam that can go through the body and onto film, making a picture of areas inside the body.
- **Barium swallow:** A series of X-rays of the esophagus and stomach. The patient drinks a liquid that contains barium (a silver-white metallic compound). The liquid coats the esophagus and stomach, and X-rays are taken. This procedure is also called an upper GI series.
- **Esophagoscopy:** A procedure to look inside the esophagus to check for abnormal areas. An esophagoscope is inserted through the mouth or nose and down the throat into the esophagus. An esophagoscope is a thin, tube-like instrument with a light and a lens for viewing. It may also have a tool to remove tissue samples, which are checked under a microscope for signs of cancer. When the esophagus and stomach are looked at, it is called an upper endoscopy.
- **Biopsy:** The removal of cells or tissues so they can be viewed under a microscope by a pathologist to check for signs of cancer. The biopsy is usually done during an esophagoscopy. Sometimes a biopsy shows changes in the esophagus that are not cancer but may lead to cancer.

What Is the Prognosis for Esophageal Cancer?

The prognosis (chance of recovery) and treatment options depend on the following:

- The stage of the cancer (whether it affects part of the esophagus, involves the whole esophagus, or has spread to other places in the body).
- Whether the tumor can be completely removed by surgery.
- The patient's general health.

When esophageal cancer is found very early, there is a better chance of recovery. Esophageal cancer is often in an advanced stage when it is diagnosed. At later stages, esophageal cancer can be treated but rarely can be cured. Taking part in one of the clinical trials being done to improve treatment should be considered.

Stages of Esophageal Cancer

After esophageal cancer has been diagnosed, tests are done to find out if cancer cells have spread within the esophagus or to other parts of the body. The process used to find out if cancer cells have spread within the esophagus or to other parts of the body is called staging. The information gathered from the staging process determines the stage of the disease. It is important to know the stage in order to plan treatment.

The following tests and procedures may be used in the staging process:

- **Endoscopic ultrasound (EUS):** A procedure in which an endoscope is inserted into the body, usually through the mouth or rectum. For esophageal cancer, the endoscope is inserted through the mouth. An endoscope is a thin, tube-like instrument with a light and a lens for viewing. A probe at the end of the endoscope is used to bounce high-energy sound waves (ultrasound) off internal tissues or organs and make echoes. The echoes form a picture of body tissues called a sonogram. This procedure is also called endosonography.
- **Computed tomography (CT)/computerized axial tomography (CAT) scan:** A procedure that makes a series of detailed pictures of areas inside the body, such as the chest, abdomen, and pelvis, taken from different angles. The pictures are made by a computer linked to an X-ray machine. A dye may be injected into a vein or swallowed to help the organs or tissues show up more clearly. This procedure is also called computed tomography, computerized tomography, or computerized axial tomography.
- **Positron emission tomography (PET) scan:** A procedure to find malignant tumor cells in the body. A small amount of radioactive glucose (sugar) is injected into a vein. The PET scanner rotates around the body and makes a picture of where glucose is being used in the body. Malignant tumor cells show up brighter in the picture because they are more active and take up more glucose than normal cells do. A PET scan and CT scan may be done at the same time. This is called a PET-CT.
- **Magnetic resonance imaging (MRI):** A procedure that uses a magnet, radio waves, and a computer to make a series of detailed pictures of areas inside the body. This procedure is also called nuclear magnetic resonance imaging (NMRI).

- **Thoracoscopy:** A surgical procedure to look at the organs inside the chest to check for abnormal areas. An incision (cut) is made between two ribs and a thoracoscope is inserted into the chest. A thoracoscope is a thin, tube-like instrument with a light and a lens for viewing. It may also have a tool to remove tissue or lymph node samples, which are checked under a microscope for signs of cancer. In some cases, this procedure may be used to remove part of the esophagus or lung.
- **Laparoscopy:** A surgical procedure to look at the organs inside the abdomen to check for signs of disease. Small incisions (cuts) are made in the wall of the abdomen and a laparoscope (a thin, lighted tube) is inserted into one of the incisions. Other instruments may be inserted through the same or other incisions to perform procedures such as removing organs or taking tissue samples to be checked under a microscope for signs of disease.

Tumor Grade

The grade of the tumor describes how abnormal the cancer cells look under a microscope and how quickly the tumor is likely to grow and spread. Grades 1–3 are used to describe esophageal cancer:

- In grade 1, the cancer cells look more like normal cells under a microscope and grow and spread more slowly than grade 2 and 3 cancer cells.
- In grade 2, the cancer cells look more abnormal under a microscope and grow and spread more quickly than grade 1 cancer cells.
- In grade 3, the cancer cells look more abnormal under a microscope and grow and spread more quickly than grade 1 and 2 cancer cells.

Squamous Cell Carcinoma of the Esophagus

The following stages are used for squamous cell carcinoma of the esophagus:

Stage 0 (High-grade dysplasia). In stage 0, abnormal cells are found in the mucosa or submucosa layer of the esophagus wall. These abnormal cells may become cancer and spread into nearby normal tissue. Stage 0 is also called high-grade dysplasia.

Stage I squamous cell carcinoma of the esophagus. Stage I is divided into Stage IA and Stage IB, depending on where the cancer is found.

- **Stage IA:** Cancer has formed in the mucosa or submucosa layer of the esophagus wall. The cancer cells are grade 1. Grade 1 cancer cells look more like normal cells under a microscope and grow and spread more slowly than grade 2 and 3 cancer cells.
- **Stage IB:** Cancer has formed:
  - in the mucosa or submucosa layer of the esophagus wall. The cancer cells are grade 2 and 3; or
  - in the mucosa or submucosa layer and spread into the muscle layer or the connective tissue layer of the esophagus wall. The cancer cells are grade 1. The tumor is in the lower esophagus or it is not known where the tumor is.

Grade 1 cancer cells look more like normal cells under a microscope and grow and spread more slowly than grade 2 and 3 cancer cells.

Stage II squamous cell carcinoma of the esophagus. Stage II is divided into Stage IIA and Stage IIB, depending on where the cancer has spread.

- **Stage IIA:** Cancer has spread:
  - into the muscle layer or the connective tissue layer of the esophagus wall. The cancer cells are grade 1. The tumor is in either the upper or middle esophagus; or
  - into the muscle layer or the connective tissue layer of the esophagus wall. The cancer cells are grade 2 and 3. The tumor is in the lower esophagus or it is not known where the tumor is.

Grade 1 cancer cells look more like normal cells under a microscope and grow and spread more slowly than grade 2 and 3 cancer cells.

- **Stage IIB:** Cancer:
  - has spread into the muscle layer or the connective tissue layer of the esophagus wall. The cancer cells are grade 2 and 3. Grade 2 and 3 cancer cells look more abnormal under a microscope and grow and spread more quickly than grade 1 cancer cells. The tumor is in either the upper or middle esophagus; or

    - is in the mucosa or submucosa layer and may have spread into the muscle layer of the esophagus wall. Cancer is found in 1 or 2 lymph nodes near the tumor.

Stage III squamous cell carcinoma of the esophagus. Stage III is divided into Stage IIIA, Stage IIIB, and Stage IIIC, depending on where the cancer has spread.

- **Stage IIIA:** Cancer:
    - is in the mucosa or submucosa layer and may have spread into the muscle layer of the esophagus wall. Cancer is found in 3–6 lymph nodes near the tumor; or
    - has spread into the connective tissue layer of the esophagus wall. Cancer is found in 1 or 2 lymph nodes near the tumor; or
    - has spread into the diaphragm, pleura (tissue that covers the lungs and lines the inner wall of the chest cavity), or sac around the heart. The cancer can be removed by surgery.
- **Stage IIIB:** Cancer has spread into the connective tissue layer of the esophagus wall. Cancer is found in 3–6 lymph nodes near the tumor.
- **Stage IIIC:** Cancer has spread:
    - into the diaphragm, pleura (tissue that covers the lungs and lines the inner wall of the chest cavity), or sac around the heart. The cancer can be removed by surgery. Cancer is found in 1–6 lymph nodes near the tumor; or
    - into other nearby organs such as the aorta, trachea, or spine, and the cancer cannot be removed by surgery; or
    - to 7 or more lymph nodes near the tumor.

Stage IV squamous cell carcinoma of the esophagus
In Stage IV, cancer has spread to other parts of the body.

Stages for Adenocarcinoma of the Esophagus

The following stages are used for adenocarcinoma of the esophagus:

Stage 0 (High-grade Dysplasia). In stage 0, abnormal cells are found in the mucosa or submucosa layer of the esophagus wall. These abnormal cells may become cancer and spread into nearby normal tissue. Stage 0 is also called high-grade dysplasia.

Stage I adenocarcinoma of the esophagus. Stage I is divided into Stage IA and Stage IB, depending on where the cancer is found.

- **Stage IA:** Cancer has formed in the mucosa or submucosa layer of the esophagus wall. The cancer cells are grade 1 or 2. Grade 1 and 2 cancer cells look more like normal cells under a microscope and grow and spread more slowly than grade 3 cancer cells.
- **Stage IB:** Cancer has formed:
    - in the mucosa or submucosa layer of the esophagus wall. The cancer cells are grade 3; or
    - in the mucosa or submucosa layer and spread into the muscle layer of the esophagus wall. The cancer cells are grade 1 or 2.

Grade 1 and 2 cancer cells look more like normal cells under a microscope and grow and spread more slowly than grade 3 cancer cells.

Stage II adenocarcinoma of the esophagus. Stage II is divided into Stage IIA and Stage IIB, depending on where the cancer has spread.

- **Stage IIA:** Cancer has spread into the muscle layer of the esophagus wall. The cancer cells are grade 3. Grade 3 cancer cells look more abnormal under a microscope and grow and spread more quickly than grade 1 and 2 cancer cells.
- **Stage IIB:** Cancer:
    - has spread into the connective tissue layer of the esophagus wall; or
    - is in the mucosa or submucosa layer and may have spread into the muscle layer of the esophagus wall. Cancer is found in 1 or 2 lymph nodes near the tumor.

Stage III adenocarcinoma of the esophagus. Stage III is divided into Stage IIIA, Stage IIIB, and Stage IIIC, depending on where the cancer has spread.

- **Stage IIIA:** Cancer:
    - is in the mucosa or submucosa layer and may have spread into the muscle layer of the esophagus wall. Cancer is found in 3–6 lymph nodes near the tumor; or

- has spread into the connective tissue layer of the esophagus wall. Cancer is found in 1 or 2 lymph nodes near the tumor; or
- has spread into the diaphragm, pleura (tissue that covers the lungs and lines the inner wall of the chest cavity), or sac around the heart. The cancer can be removed by surgery.

- **Stage IIIB:** Cancer has spread into the connective tissue layer of the esophagus wall. Cancer is found in 3–6 lymph nodes near the tumor.
- **Stage IIIC:** Cancer has spread:
  - into the diaphragm, pleura (tissue that covers the lungs and lines the inner wall of the chest cavity), or sac around the heart. The cancer can be removed by surgery. Cancer is found in 1–6 lymph nodes near the tumor; or
  - into other nearby organs such as the aorta, trachea, or spine, and the cancer cannot be removed by surgery; or
  - to 7 or more lymph nodes near the tumor.

Stage IV adenocarcinoma of the esophagus. In Stage IV, cancer has spread to other parts of the body.

Treatment Option Overview

Different types of treatment are available for patients with esophageal cancer. Some treatments are standard (the currently used treatment), and some are being tested in clinical trials. A treatment clinical trial is a research study meant to help improve current treatments or obtain information on new treatments for patients with cancer. When clinical trials show that a new treatment is better than the standard treatment, the new treatment may become the standard treatment. Patients may want to think about taking part in a clinical trial. Some clinical trials are open only to patients who have not started treatment.

Patients have special nutritional needs during treatment for esophageal cancer. Many people with esophageal cancer find it hard to eat because they have trouble swallowing. The esophagus may be narrowed by the tumor or as a side effect of treatment. Some patients may receive nutrients directly into a vein. Others may need a feeding tube (a flexible plastic tube that is passed through the nose or mouth into the stomach) until they are able to eat on their own.

Standard Treatments for Esophageal Cancer

Six types of standard treatment are used:

Surgery

Surgery is the most common treatment for cancer of the esophagus. Part of the esophagus may be removed in an operation called an esophagectomy.

The doctor will connect the remaining healthy part of the esophagus to the stomach so the patient can still swallow. A plastic tube or part of the intestine may be used to make the connection. Lymph nodes near the esophagus may also be removed and viewed under a microscope to see if they contain cancer. If the esophagus is partly blocked by the tumor, an expandable metal stent (tube) may be placed inside the esophagus to help keep it open. Small, early-stage cancer and high-grade dysplasia of the esophagus may be removed by endoscopic resection. An endoscope (a thin, tube-like instrument with a light and a lens for viewing) is inserted through a small incision (cut) in the skin or through an opening in the body, such as the mouth. A tool attached to the endoscope is used to remove tissue.

Radiation Therapy

Radiation therapy is a cancer treatment that uses high-energy X-rays or other types of radiation to kill cancer cells or keep them from growing. There are two types of radiation therapy:

- External radiation therapy uses a machine outside the body to send radiation toward the cancer.
- Internal radiation therapy uses a radioactive substance sealed in needles, seeds, wires, or catheters that are placed directly into or near the cancer.

The way the radiation therapy is given depends on the type and stage of the cancer being treated. External and internal radiation therapy are used to treat esophageal cancer. A plastic tube may be inserted into the esophagus to keep it open during radiation therapy. This is called intraluminal intubation and dilation.

Chemotherapy

Chemotherapy is a cancer treatment that uses drugs to stop the growth of cancer cells, either by killing the cells or by stopping them

from dividing. When chemotherapy is taken by mouth or injected into a vein or muscle, the drugs enter the bloodstream and can reach cancer cells throughout the body (systemic chemotherapy). When chemotherapy is placed directly into the cerebrospinal fluid, an organ, or a body cavity such as the abdomen, the drugs mainly affect cancer cells in those areas (regional chemotherapy). The way the chemotherapy is given depends on the type and stage of the cancer being treated.

Chemoradiation Therapy

Chemoradiation therapy combines chemotherapy and radiation therapy to increase the effects of both.

Laser Therapy

Laser therapy is a cancer treatment that uses a laser beam (a narrow beam of intense light) to kill cancer cells.

Electrocoagulation

Electrocoagulation is the use of an electric current to kill cancer cells.

New Treatments That Are Tested

New types of treatment are being tested in clinical trials.

Targeted Therapy

Targeted therapy is a type of treatment that uses drugs or other substances to identify and attack specific cancer cells. Targeted therapies usually cause less harm to normal cells than chemotherapy or radiation therapy do. Monoclonal antibody therapy is a type of targeted therapy used in the treatment of esophageal cancer.

Monoclonal antibody therapy uses antibodies made in the laboratory from a single type of immune system cell. These antibodies can identify substances on cancer cells or normal substances that may help cancer cells grow. The antibodies attach to the substances and kill the cancer cells, block their growth, or keep them from spreading. Monoclonal antibodies are given by infusion. They may be used alone or to carry drugs, toxins, or radioactive material directly to cancer cells. Trastuzumab is a monoclonal antibody being studied in esophageal cancer. It may be given to block the effect of the growth factor protein HER2, which sends growth signals to esophageal cancer cells. Treatment for esophageal cancer may cause side effects.

Follow-Up Tests

Some of the tests that were done to diagnose the cancer or to find out the stage of the cancer may be repeated. Some tests will be repeated in order to see how well the treatment is working. Decisions about whether to continue, change, or stop treatment may be based on the results of these tests. Some of the tests will continue to be done from time to time after treatment has ended. The results of these tests can show if your condition has changed or if the cancer has recurred (come back). These tests are sometimes called follow-up tests or check-ups.

Chapter 30

Stomach (Gastric) Cancer

The stomach is a J-shaped organ in the upper abdomen. It is part of the digestive system, which processes nutrients (vitamins, minerals, carbohydrates, fats, proteins, and water) in foods that are eaten and helps pass waste material out of the body. Food moves from the throat to the stomach through a hollow, muscular tube called the esophagus. After leaving the stomach, partly digested food passes into the small intestine and then into the large intestine. The wall of the stomach is made up of 3 layers of tissue: the mucosal (innermost) layer, the muscularis (middle) layer, and the serosal (outermost) layer.

What Is Gastric Cancer?

Gastric cancer is a disease in which malignant (cancer) cells form in the lining of the stomach. It begins in the cells lining the mucosal layer and spreads through the outer layers as it grows.

What Are the Risk Factors for Gastric Cancer?

Anything that increases your risk of getting a disease is called a risk factor. Having a risk factor does not mean that you will get cancer; not having risk factors doesn't mean that you will not get cancer. Talk with your doctor if you think you may be at risk. Age, diet, and

---

This chapter includes text excerpted from "Gastric Cancer Treatment (PDQ®)—Patient Version," National Cancer Institute (NCI), February 16, 2018.

stomach disease can affect the risk of developing gastric cancer. Risk factors for gastric cancer include the following:

- Having any of the following medical conditions:
    - *Helicobacter pylori (H. pylori)* infection of the stomach
    - Chronic gastritis (inflammation of the stomach)
    - Pernicious anemia
    - Intestinal metaplasia (a condition in which the normal stomach lining is replaced with the cells that line the intestines)
    - Familial adenomatous polyposis (FAP) or gastric polyps
- Eating a diet high in salted, smoked foods and low in fruits and vegetables
- Eating foods that have not been prepared or stored properly
- Being older or male
- Smoking cigarettes
- Having a mother, father, sister, or brother who has had stomach cancer

What Are the Signs and Symptoms of Gastric Cancer?

Symptoms of gastric cancer include indigestion and stomach discomfort or pain. These and other signs and symptoms may be caused by gastric cancer or by other conditions.

In the early stages of gastric cancer, the following symptoms may occur:

- Indigestion and stomach discomfort
- A bloated feeling after eating
- Mild nausea
- Loss of appetite
- Heartburn

In more advanced stages of gastric cancer, the following signs and symptoms may occur:

- Blood in the stool
- Vomiting

- Weight loss for no known reason
- Stomach pain
- Jaundice (yellowing of eyes and skin)
- Ascites (buildup of fluid in the abdomen)
- Trouble swallowing

How Is Gastric Cancer Diagnosed?

- **Physical exam and history:** An exam of the body to check general signs of health, including checking for signs of disease, such as lumps or anything else that seems unusual. A history of the patient's health habits and past illnesses and treatments will also be taken.
- **Blood chemistry studies:** A procedure in which a blood sample is checked to measure the amounts of certain substances released into the blood by organs and tissues in the body. An unusual (higher or lower than normal) amount of a substance can be a sign of disease.
- **Complete blood count (CBC):** A procedure in which a sample of blood is drawn and checked for the following:
  - The number of red blood cells, white blood cells, and platelets
  - The amount of hemoglobin (the protein that carries oxygen) in the red blood cells
  - The portion of the sample made up of red blood cells
- **Upper endoscopy:** A procedure to look inside the esophagus, stomach, and duodenum (first part of the small intestine) to check for abnormal areas. An endoscope (a thin, lighted tube) is passed through the mouth and down the throat into the esophagus.
- **Barium swallow:** A series of X-rays of the esophagus and stomach. The patient drinks a liquid that contains barium (a silver-white metallic compound). The liquid coats the esophagus and stomach, and X-rays are taken. This procedure is also called an upper GI series.
- **Computed tomography (CT)/computerized axial tomography (CAT) scan:** A procedure that makes a series of detailed

pictures of areas inside the body, taken from different angles. The pictures are made by a computer linked to an X-ray machine. A dye may be injected into a vein or swallowed to help the organs or tissues show up more clearly.

- **Biopsy:** The removal of cells or tissues so they can be viewed under a microscope to check for signs of cancer. A biopsy of the stomach is usually done during the endoscopy.

The sample of tissue may be checked to measure how many *HER2* genes there are and how much HER2 protein is being made. If there are more *HER2* genes or higher levels of HER2 protein than normal, the cancer is called HER2 positive. HER2-positive gastric cancer may be treated with a monoclonal antibody that targets the HER2 protein.

What Is the Prognosis for Gastric Cancer?

The prognosis (chance of recovery) and treatment options depend on the following:

- The stage of the cancer (whether it is in the stomach only or has spread to lymph nodes or other places in the body)
- The patient's general health

When gastric cancer is found very early, there is a better chance of recovery. Gastric cancer is often in an advanced stage when it is diagnosed. At later stages, gastric cancer can be treated but rarely can be cured.

Stages of Gastric Cancer

After gastric cancer has been diagnosed, tests are done to find out if cancer cells have spread within the stomach or to other parts of the body. The process used to find out if cancer has spread within the stomach or to other parts of the body is called staging. The information gathered from the staging process determines the stage of the disease. It is important to know the stage in order to plan treatment.

The following tests and procedures may be used in the staging process:

- **CEA (carcinoembryonic antigen) assay:** Tests that measure the level of CEA in the blood. This substance is released into the bloodstream from both cancer cells and normal cells. When found in higher than normal amounts, it can be a sign of gastric cancer or other conditions.

- **Endoscopic ultrasound (EUS):** A procedure in which an endoscope is inserted into the body, usually through the mouth or rectum. An endoscope is a thin, tube-like instrument with a light and a lens for viewing. A probe at the end of the endoscope is used to bounce high energy sound waves (ultrasound) off internal tissues or organs and make echoes. The echoes form a picture of body tissues called a sonogram. This procedure is also called endosonography.
- **CT/CAT scan:** A procedure that makes a series of detailed pictures of areas inside the body, taken from different angles. The pictures are made by a computer linked to an X-ray machine. A dye may be injected into a vein or swallowed to help the organs or tissues show up more clearly. This procedure is also called computed tomography, computerized tomography, or computerized axial tomography.
- **Positron emission tomography (PET) scan:** A procedure to find malignant tumor cells in the body. A small amount of radioactive glucose (sugar) is injected into a vein. The PET scanner rotates around the body and makes a picture of where glucose is being used in the body. Malignant tumor cells show up brighter in the picture because they are more active and take up more glucose than normal cells do. A PET scan and CT scan may be done at the same time. This is called a PET-CT.

The following stages are used for gastric cancer:

Stage 0 (carcinoma in situ). In stage 0, abnormal cells are found in the inside lining of the mucosa (innermost layer) of the stomach wall. These abnormal cells may become cancer and spread into nearby normal tissue. Stage 0 is also called carcinoma in situ.

Stage I. In stage I, cancer has formed in the inside lining of the mucosa (innermost layer) of the stomach wall. Stage I is divided into stage IA and stage IB, depending on where the cancer has spread.

- **Stage IA:** Cancer may have spread into the submucosa (layer of tissue next to the mucosa) of the stomach wall.

- **Stage IB:** Cancer:
    - may have spread into the submucosa (layer of tissue next to the mucosa) of the stomach wall and is found in 1 or 2 lymph nodes near the tumor; or
    - has spread to the muscle layer of the stomach wall.

Stage II. Stage II gastric cancer is divided into stage IIA and stage IIB, depending on where the cancer has spread.

Stage IIA: Cancer:

- has spread to the subserosa (layer of tissue next to the serosa) of the stomach wall; or
- has spread to the muscle layer of the stomach wall and is found in 1 or 2 lymph nodes near the tumor; or
- may have spread to the submucosa (layer of tissue next to the mucosa) of the stomach wall and is found in 3–6 lymph nodes near the tumor.

Stage IIB: Cancer:

- has spread to the serosa (outermost layer) of the stomach wall; or
- has spread to the subserosa (layer of tissue next to the serosa) of the stomach wall and is found in 1 or 2 lymph nodes near the tumor; or
- has spread to the muscle layer of the stomach wall and is found in 3–6 lymph nodes near the tumor; or
- may have spread to the submucosa (layer of tissue next to the mucosa) of the stomach wall and is found in 7 or more lymph nodes near the tumor.

Stage III. Stage III gastric cancer is divided into stage IIIA, stage IIIB, and stage IIIC, depending on where the cancer has spread.

Stage IIIA: Cancer has spread to:

- the serosa (outermost) layer of the stomach wall and is found in 1 or 2 lymph nodes near the tumor; or
- the subserosa (layer of tissue next to the serosa) of the stomach wall and is found in 3–6 lymph nodes near the tumor; or

- the muscle layer of the stomach wall and is found in 7 or more lymph nodes near the tumor.

Stage IIIB: Cancer has spread to:

- nearby organs such as the spleen, transverse colon, liver, diaphragm, pancreas, kidney, adrenal gland, or small intestine, and may be found in 1 or 2 lymph nodes near the tumor; or
- the serosa (outermost layer) of the stomach wall and is found in 3–6 lymph nodes near the tumor; or
- the subserosa (layer of tissue next to the serosa) of the stomach wall and is found in 7 or more lymph nodes near the tumor.

Stage IIIC: Cancer has spread to:

- nearby organs such as the spleen, transverse colon, liver, diaphragm, pancreas, kidney, adrenal gland, or small intestine, and may be found in 3 or more lymph nodes near the tumor; or
- the serosa (outermost layer) of the stomach wall and is found in 7 or more lymph nodes near the tumor.

Stage IV. In stage IV, cancer has spread to distant parts of the body.

Treatment Option Overview

Different types of treatments are available for patients with gastric cancer. Some treatments are standard (the currently used treatment), and some are being tested in clinical trials. A treatment clinical trial is a research study meant to help improve current treatments or obtain information on new treatments for patients with cancer. When clinical trials show that a new treatment is better than the standard treatment, the new treatment may become the standard treatment. Patients may want to think about taking part in a clinical trial. Some clinical trials are open only to patients who have not started treatment.

Standard Treatment Options Available for Patients with Gastric Cancer

Five types of standard treatment are used:

Surgery

Surgery is a common treatment of all stages of gastric cancer. The following types of surgery may be used:

- **Subtotal gastrectomy:** Removal of the part of the stomach that contains cancer, nearby lymph nodes, and parts of other tissues and organs near the tumor. The spleen may be removed. The spleen is an organ in the upper abdomen that filters the blood and removes old blood cells.
- **Total gastrectomy:** Removal of the entire stomach, nearby lymph nodes, and parts of the esophagus, small intestine, and other tissues near the tumor. The spleen may be removed. The esophagus is connected to the small intestine so the patient can continue to eat and swallow.

If the tumor is blocking the stomach but the cancer cannot be completely removed by standard surgery, the following procedures may be used:

- **Endoluminal stent placement:** A procedure to insert a stent (a thin, expandable tube) in order to keep a passage (such as arteries or the esophagus) open. For tumors blocking the passage into or out of the stomach, surgery may be done to place a stent from the esophagus to the stomach or from the stomach to the small intestine to allow the patient to eat normally.
- **Endoluminal laser therapy:** A procedure in which an endoscope (a thin, lighted tube) with a laser attached is inserted into the body. A laser is an intense beam of light that can be used as a knife.
- **Gastrojejunostomy:** Surgery to remove the part of the stomach with cancer that is blocking the opening into the small intestine. The stomach is connected to the jejunum (a part of the small intestine) to allow food and medicine to pass from the stomach into the small intestine.

Chemotherapy

Chemotherapy is a cancer treatment that uses drugs to stop the growth of cancer cells, either by killing the cells or by stopping them from dividing. When chemotherapy is taken by mouth or injected into a vein or muscle, the drugs enter the bloodstream and can reach cancer cells throughout the body (systemic chemotherapy). When chemotherapy is placed directly into the cerebrospinal fluid, an organ, or a body cavity such as the abdomen, the drugs mainly affect cancer cells in those areas (regional chemotherapy). The way the chemotherapy is given depends on the type and stage of the cancer being treated.

Radiation Therapy

Radiation therapy is a cancer treatment that uses high-energy X-rays or other types of radiation to kill cancer cells or keep them from growing. There are two types of radiation therapy:

- External radiation therapy uses a machine outside the body to send radiation toward the cancer.
- Internal radiation therapy uses a radioactive substance sealed in needles, seeds, wires, or catheters that are placed directly into or near the cancer.

The way the radiation therapy is given depends on the type and stage of the cancer being treated. External radiation therapy is used to treat gastric cancer.

Chemoradiation

Chemoradiation therapy combines chemotherapy and radiation therapy to increase the effects of both. Chemoradiation given after surgery, to lower the risk that the cancer will come back, is called adjuvant therapy. Chemoradiation given before surgery, to shrink the tumor (neoadjuvant therapy), is being studied.

Targeted Therapy

Targeted therapy is a type of treatment that uses drugs or other substances to identify and attack specific cancer cells without harming normal cells. Monoclonal antibody therapy is a type of targeted therapy used in the treatment of gastric cancer.

Monoclonal antibody therapy uses antibodies made in the laboratory from a single type of immune system cell. These antibodies can identify substances on cancer cells or normal substances that may help cancer cells grow. The antibodies attach to the substances and kill the cancer cells, block their growth, or keep them from spreading. Monoclonal antibodies are given by infusion. They may be used alone or to carry drugs, toxins, or radioactive material directly to cancer cells. For stage IV gastric cancer and gastric cancer that has recurred, monoclonal antibodies, such as trastuzumab or ramucirumab, may be given. Trastuzumab blocks the effect of the growth factor protein HER2, which sends growth signals to gastric cancer cells. Ramucirumab blocks the effect of the protein VEGF and may prevent the growth of new blood vessels that tumors need to grow. Treatment for gastric cancer may cause side effects.

Chapter 31

Gallbladder Cancer

The gallbladder is a pear-shaped organ that lies just under the liver in the upper abdomen. The gallbladder stores bile, a fluid made by the liver to digest fat. When food is being broken down in the stomach and intestines, bile is released from the gallbladder through a tube called the common bile duct, which connects the gallbladder and liver to the first part of the small intestine.

The wall of the gallbladder has 4 main layers of tissue:

- Mucosal (inner) layer
- Muscle layer
- Connective tissue layer
- Serosal (outer) layer

What Is Gallbladder Cancer?

Gallbladder cancer is a rare disease in which malignant (cancer) cells are found in the tissues of the gallbladder. Primary gallbladder cancer starts in the inner layer and spreads through the outer layers as it grows.

This chapter includes text excerpted from "Gallbladder Cancer Treatment (PDQ®)—Patient Version," National Cancer Institute (NCI), February 16, 2018.

What Are the Risk Factors for Gallbladder Cancer?

Anything that increases your chance of getting a disease is called a risk factor. Having a risk factor does not mean that you will get cancer; not having risk factors doesn't mean that you will not get cancer. Talk with your doctor if you think you may be at risk.

Being female can increase the risk of developing gallbladder cancer. Risk factors for gallbladder cancer include the following:

- Being female
- Being Native American

What Are the Signs and Symptoms of Gallbladder Cancer?

Signs and symptoms of gallbladder cancer include jaundice, fever, and pain. These and other signs and symptoms may be caused by gallbladder cancer or by other conditions. Check with your doctor if you have any of the following:

- Jaundice (yellowing of the skin and whites of the eyes)
- Pain above the stomach
- Fever
- Nausea and vomiting
- Bloating
- Lumps in the abdomen

How Is Gallbladder Cancer Diagnosed?

Gallbladder cancer is difficult to detect (find) and diagnose early. It is difficult to detect and diagnose for the following reasons:

- There are no signs or symptoms in the early stages of gallbladder cancer.
- The symptoms of gallbladder cancer, when present, are like the symptoms of many other illnesses.
- The gallbladder is hidden behind the liver.

Gallbladder cancer is sometimes found when the gallbladder is removed for other reasons. Patients with gallstones rarely develop gallbladder cancer.

Procedures that make pictures of the gallbladder and the area around it help diagnose gallbladder cancer and show how far the cancer has spread. The process used to find out if cancer cells have spread within and around the gallbladder is called staging.

In order to plan treatment, it is important to know if the gallbladder cancer can be removed by surgery. Tests and procedures to detect, diagnose, and stage gallbladder cancer are usually done at the same time. The following tests and procedures may be used:

- **Physical exam and history:** An exam of the body to check general signs of health, including checking for signs of disease, such as lumps or anything else that seems unusual. A history of the patient's health habits and past illnesses and treatments will also be taken.
- **Liver function tests:** A procedure in which a blood sample is checked to measure the amounts of certain substances released into the blood by the liver. A higher than normal amount of a substance can be a sign of liver disease that may be caused by gallbladder cancer.
- **Blood chemistry studies:** A procedure in which a blood sample is checked to measure the amounts of certain substances released into the blood by organs and tissues in the body. An unusual (higher or lower than normal) amount of a substance can be a sign of disease.
- **Computed tomography (CT)/computerized axial tomography (CAT) scan:** A procedure that makes a series of detailed pictures of areas inside the body, such as the chest, abdomen, and pelvis, taken from different angles. The pictures are made by a computer linked to an X-ray machine. A dye may be injected into a vein or swallowed to help the organs or tissues show up more clearly.
- **Ultrasound exam:** A procedure in which high-energy sound waves (ultrasound) are bounced off internal tissues or organs and make echoes. The echoes form a picture of body tissues called a sonogram. An abdominal ultrasound is done to diagnose gallbladder cancer.
- **Percutaneous transhepatic cholangiography (PTC):** A procedure used to X-ray the liver and bile ducts. A thin needle is inserted through the skin below the ribs and into the liver. Dye is injected into the liver or bile ducts and an X-ray is taken. If

a blockage is found, a thin, flexible tube called a stent is sometimes left in the liver to drain bile into the small intestine or a collection bag outside the body.

- **Endoscopic retrograde cholangiopancreatography (ERCP):** A procedure used to X-ray the ducts (tubes) that carry bile from the liver to the gallbladder and from the gallbladder to the small intestine. Sometimes gallbladder cancer causes these ducts to narrow and block or slow the flow of bile, causing jaundice. An endoscope (a thin, lighted tube) is passed through the mouth, esophagus, and stomach into the first part of the small intestine. A catheter (a smaller tube) is then inserted through the endoscope into the bile ducts. A dye is injected through the catheter into the ducts and an X-ray is taken. If the ducts are blocked by a tumor, a fine tube may be inserted into the duct to unblock it. This tube (or stent) may be left in place to keep the duct open. Tissue samples may also be taken.
- **Magnetic resonance imaging (MRI) with gadolinium:** A procedure that uses a magnet, radio waves, and a computer to make a series of detailed pictures of areas inside the body. A substance called gadolinium is injected into a vein. The gadolinium collects around the cancer cells so they show up brighter in the picture. This procedure is also called nuclear magnetic resonance imaging (NMRI).
- **Endoscopic ultrasound (EUS):** A procedure in which an endoscope is inserted into the body, usually through the mouth or rectum. An endoscope is a thin, tube-like instrument with a light and a lens for viewing. A probe at the end of the endoscope is used to bounce high-energy sound waves (ultrasound) off internal tissues or organs and make echoes. The echoes form a picture of body tissues called a sonogram. This procedure is also called endosonography.
- **Laparoscopy:** A surgical procedure to look at the organs inside the abdomen to check for signs of disease. Small incisions (cuts) are made in the wall of the abdomen and a laparoscope (a thin, lighted tube) is inserted into one of the incisions. Other instruments may be inserted through the same or other incisions to perform procedures such as removing organs or taking tissue samples for biopsy. The laparoscopy helps to find out if the cancer is within the gallbladder only or has spread to nearby tissues and if it can be removed by surgery.

- **Biopsy:** The removal of cells or tissues so they can be viewed under a microscope by a pathologist to check for signs of cancer. The biopsy may be done after surgery to remove the tumor. If the tumor clearly cannot be removed by surgery, the biopsy may be done using a fine needle to remove cells from the tumor.

What Is the Prognosis for Gallbladder Cancer?

The prognosis (chance of recovery) and treatment options depend on the following:

- The stage of the cancer (whether the cancer has spread from the gallbladder to other places in the body)
- Whether the cancer can be completely removed by surgery
- The type of gallbladder cancer (how the cancer cell looks under a microscope)
- Whether the cancer has just been diagnosed or has recurred (come back)

Treatment may also depend on the age and general health of the patient and whether the cancer is causing signs or symptoms. Gallbladder cancer can be cured only if it is found before it has spread, when it can be removed by surgery. If the cancer has spread, palliative treatment can improve the patient's quality of life by controlling the symptoms and complications of this disease. Taking part in one of the clinical trials being done to improve treatment should be considered.

Stages of Gallbladder Cancer

The following stages are used for gallbladder cancer:

Stage 0 (carcinoma in situ). In stage 0, abnormal cells are found in the mucosa (innermost layer) of the gallbladder wall. These abnormal cells may become cancer and spread into nearby normal tissue. Stage 0 is also called carcinoma in situ.

Stage I. In stage I, cancer has formed in the mucosa (innermost layer) of the gallbladder wall and may have spread to the muscle layer of the gallbladder wall.

Stage II. Stage II is divided into stages IIA and IIB, depending on where the cancer has spread in the gallbladder.

- In stage IIA, cancer has spread through the muscle layer to the connective tissue layer of the gallbladder wall on the side of the gallbladder that is not near the liver.
- In stage IIB, cancer has spread through the muscle layer to the connective tissue layer of the gallbladder wall on the same side as the liver. Cancer has not spread to the liver.

Stage III. Stage III is divided into stages IIIA and IIIB, depending on where the cancer has spread.

- In stage IIIA, cancer has spread through the connective tissue layer of the gallbladder wall and one or more of the following is true:
    - Cancer has spread to the serosa (layer of tissue that covers the gallbladder)
    - Cancer has spread to the liver
    - Cancer has spread to one nearby organ or structure (such as the stomach, small intestine, colon, pancreas, or the bile ducts outside the liver)
- In stage IIIB, cancer has formed in the mucosa (innermost layer) of the gallbladder wall and may have spread to the muscle, connective tissue, or serosa (layer of tissue that covers the gallbladder) and may have also spread to the liver or to one nearby organ or structure (such as the stomach, small intestine, colon, pancreas, or the bile ducts outside the liver). Cancer has spread to one to three nearby lymph nodes.

Stage IV. Stage IV is divided into stages IVA and IVB.

- In stage IVA, cancer has spread to the portal vein or hepatic artery or to two or more organs or structures other than the liver. Cancer may have spread to 1–3 nearby lymph nodes.
- In stage IVB, cancer may have spread to nearby organs or structures. Cancer has spread:
    - to four or more nearby lymph nodes; or
    - to other parts of the body, such as the peritoneum and liver.

For gallbladder cancer, stages are also grouped according to how the cancer may be treated. There are two treatment groups:

Localized (Stage I): Cancer is found in the wall of the gallbladder and can be completely removed by surgery.

Unresectable, recurrent, or metastatic (stage II, stage III, and stage IV): Unresectable cancer cannot be removed completely by surgery. Most patients with gallbladder cancer have unresectable cancer.

Recurrent cancer is cancer that has recurred (come back) after it has been treated. Gallbladder cancer may come back in the gallbladder or in other parts of the body.

Metastasis is the spread of cancer from the primary site (place where it started) to other places in the body. Metastatic gallbladder cancer may spread to surrounding tissues, organs, throughout the abdominal cavity, or to distant parts of the body.

Treatment Option Overview

Different types of treatments are available for patients with gallbladder cancer. Some treatments are standard (the currently used treatment), and some are being tested in clinical trials. A treatment clinical trial is a research study meant to help improve current treatments or obtain information on new treatments for patients with cancer. When clinical trials show that a new treatment is better than the standard treatment, the new treatment may become the standard treatment. Patients may want to think about taking part in a clinical trial. Some clinical trials are open only to patients who have not started treatment.

Standard Treatment for Gallbladder Cancer

Three types of standard treatment are used:

Surgery

Gallbladder cancer may be treated with a cholecystectomy, surgery to remove the gallbladder and some of the tissues around it. Nearby lymph nodes may be removed. A laparoscope is sometimes used to guide gallbladder surgery. The laparoscope is attached to a video camera and inserted through an incision (port) in the abdomen. Surgical instruments are inserted through other ports to perform the surgery. Because there is a risk that gallbladder cancer cells may spread to these ports, tissue surrounding the port sites may also be removed.

If the cancer has spread and cannot be removed, the following types of palliative surgery may relieve symptoms:

- **Surgical biliary bypass:** If the tumor is blocking the small intestine and bile is building up in the gallbladder, a biliary bypass may be done. During this operation, the gallbladder or bile duct will be cut and sewn to the small intestine to create a new pathway around the blocked area.
- **Endoscopic stent placement:** If the tumor is blocking the bile duct, surgery may be done to put in a stent (a thin, flexible tube) to drain bile that has built up in the area. The stent may be placed through a catheter that drains to the outside of the body or the stent may go around the blocked area and drain the bile into the small intestine.
- **Percutaneous transhepatic biliary drainage:** A procedure done to drain bile when there is a blockage and endoscopic stent placement is not possible. An X-ray of the liver and bile ducts is done to locate the blockage. Images made by ultrasound are used to guide placement of a stent, which is left in the liver to drain bile into the small intestine or a collection bag outside the body. This procedure may be done to relieve jaundice before surgery.

Radiation Therapy

Radiation therapy is a cancer treatment that uses high-energy X-rays or other types of radiation to kill cancer cells or keep them from growing. There are two types of radiation therapy:

- External radiation therapy uses a machine outside the body to send radiation toward the cancer.
- Internal radiation therapy uses a radioactive substance sealed in needles, seeds, wires, or catheters that are placed directly into or near the cancer.

The way the radiation therapy is given depends on the type and stage of the cancer being treated. External radiation therapy is used to treat gallbladder cancer.

Chemotherapy

Chemotherapy is a cancer treatment that uses drugs to stop the growth of cancer cells, either by killing the cells or by stopping the cells from dividing. When chemotherapy is taken by mouth or injected into a vein or muscle, the drugs enter the bloodstream and can reach cancer cells throughout the body (systemic chemotherapy). When chemotherapy is placed directly into the cerebrospinal fluid, an organ, or a body cavity such as the abdomen, the drugs mainly affect cancer cells in those areas (regional chemotherapy). The way the chemotherapy is given depends on the type and stage of the cancer being treated.

New Types of Treatment Tested

Radiation Sensitizers

Clinical trials are studying ways to improve the effect of radiation therapy on tumor cells, including the following:

- **Hyperthermia therapy:** A treatment in which body tissue is exposed to high temperatures to damage and kill cancer cells or to make cancer cells more sensitive to the effects of radiation therapy and certain anticancer drugs.
- **Radiosensitizers:** Drugs that make tumor cells more sensitive to radiation therapy. Giving radiation therapy together with radiosensitizers may kill more tumor cells.

Chapter 32

Pancreatic Cancer

The pancreas is a gland about 6 inches long that is shaped like a thin pear lying on its side. The wider end of the pancreas is called the head, the middle section is called the body, and the narrow end is called the tail. The pancreas lies between the stomach and the spine.

The pancreas has two main jobs in the body:

- To make juices that help digest (break down) food
- To make hormones, such as insulin and glucagon, that help control blood sugar levels. Both of these hormones help the body use and store the energy it gets from food

The digestive juices are made by exocrine pancreas cells and the hormones are made by endocrine pancreas cells. About 95 percent of pancreatic cancers begin in exocrine cells

What Is Pancreatic Cancer?

Pancreatic cancer is a disease in which malignant (cancer) cells form in the tissues of the pancreas.

This chapter includes text excerpted from "Pancreatic Cancer Treatment (PDQ®)—Patient Version," National Cancer Institute (NCI), February 16, 2018.

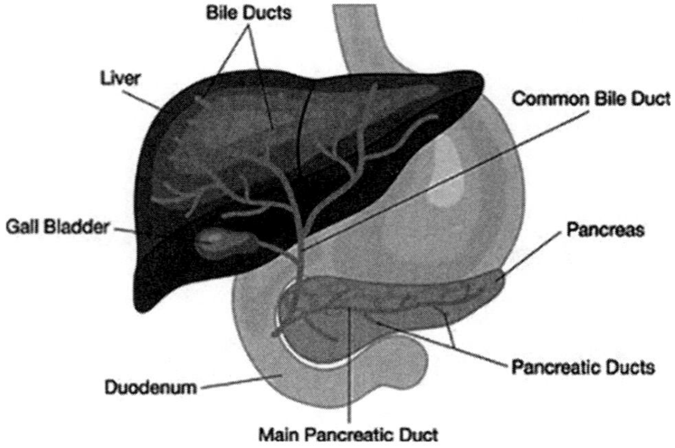

Figure 32.1. *Pancreas and Surrounding Organs* (Source: "Endoscopic Retrograde Cholangiopancreatography (ERCP)," National Institute of Diabetes and Digestive and Kidney Diseases (NIDDK).)

What Are the Risk Factors for Pancreatic Cancer?

Anything that increases your risk of getting a disease is called a risk factor. Having a risk factor does not mean that you will get cancer; not having risk factors doesn't mean that you will not get cancer. Talk with your doctor if you think you may be at risk.

Smoking and health history can affect the risk of pancreatic cancer. Risk factors for pancreatic cancer include the following:

- Smoking
- Being very overweight
- Having a personal history of diabetes or chronic pancreatitis
- Having a family history of pancreatic cancer or pancreatitis
- Having certain hereditary conditions, such as:
    - Multiple endocrine neoplasia type 1 (MEN1) syndrome
    - Hereditary nonpolyposis colon cancer (HNPCC; Lynch syndrome)
    - von Hippel-Lindau syndrome (VHL)
    - Peutz-Jeghers syndrome (PJS)
    - Hereditary breast and ovarian cancer syndrome (HBOC)
    - Familial atypical multiple mole melanoma (FAMMM) syndrome

What Are the Signs and Symptoms of Pancreatic Cancer?

Pancreatic cancer may not cause early signs or symptoms. Signs and symptoms may be caused by pancreatic cancer or by other conditions. Check with your doctor if you have any of the following:

- Jaundice (yellowing of the skin and whites of the eyes)
- Light-colored stools
- Dark urine
- Pain in the upper or middle abdomen and back
- Weight loss for no known reason
- Loss of appetite
- Feeling very tired

How Is Pancreatic Cancer Diagnosed?

Pancreatic cancer is difficult to detect and diagnose for the following reasons:

- There aren't any noticeable signs or symptoms in the early stages of pancreatic cancer
- The signs and symptoms of pancreatic cancer, when present, are like the signs and symptoms of many other illnesses
- The pancreas is hidden behind other organs such as the stomach, small intestine, liver, gallbladder, spleen, and bile ducts

Pancreatic cancer is usually diagnosed with tests and procedures that make pictures of the pancreas and the area around it. The process used to find out if cancer cells have spread within and around the pancreas is called staging. Tests and procedures to detect, diagnose, and stage pancreatic cancer are usually done at the same time. In order to plan treatment, it is important to know the stage of the disease and whether or not the pancreatic cancer can be removed by surgery.

The following tests and procedures may be used:

- **Physical exam and history:** An exam of the body to check general signs of health, including checking for signs of disease, such as lumps or anything else that seems unusual. A history

of the patient's health habits and past illnesses and treatments will also be taken.

- **Blood chemistry studies:** A procedure in which a blood sample is checked to measure the amounts of certain substances, such as bilirubin, released into the blood by organs and tissues in the body. An unusual (higher or lower than normal) amount of a substance can be a sign of disease.
- **Tumor marker test:** A procedure in which a sample of blood, urine, or tissue is checked to measure the amounts of certain substances, such as CA 19-9, and carcinoembryonic antigen (CEA), made by organs, tissues, or tumor cells in the body. Certain substances are linked to specific types of cancer when found in increased levels in the body. These are called tumor markers.
- **Magnetic resonance imaging (MRI):** A procedure that uses a magnet, radio waves, and a computer to make a series of detailed pictures of areas inside the body. This procedure is also called nuclear magnetic resonance imaging (NMRI).
- **Computed tomography (CT)/computerized axial tomography (CAT) scan:** A procedure that makes a series of detailed pictures of areas inside the body, taken from different angles. The pictures are made by a computer linked to an X-ray machine. A dye may be injected into a vein or swallowed to help the organs or tissues show up more clearly. This procedure is also called computed tomography, computerized tomography, or computerized axial tomography. A spiral or helical CT scan makes a series of very detailed pictures of areas inside the body using an X-ray machine that scans the body in a spiral path.
- **Positron emission tomography (PET) scan:** A procedure to find malignant tumor cells in the body. A small amount of radioactive glucose (sugar) is injected into a vein. The PET scanner rotates around the body and makes a picture of where glucose is being used in the body. Malignant tumor cells show up brighter in the picture because they are more active and take up more glucose than normal cells do. A PET scan and CT scan may be done at the same time. This is called a PET-CT.
- **Abdominal ultrasound:** An ultrasound exam used to make pictures of the inside of the abdomen. The ultrasound transducer is pressed against the skin of the abdomen and directs high energy sound waves (ultrasound) into the abdomen. The sound

waves bounce off the internal tissues and organs and make echoes. The transducer receives the echoes and sends them to a computer, which uses the echoes to make pictures called sonograms. The picture can be printed to be looked at later.

- **Endoscopic ultrasound (EUS):** A procedure in which an endoscope is inserted into the body, usually through the mouth or rectum. An endoscope is a thin, tube-like instrument with a light and a lens for viewing. A probe at the end of the endoscope is used to bounce high energy sound waves (ultrasound) off internal tissues or organs and make echoes. The echoes form a picture of body tissues called a sonogram. This procedure is also called endosonography.
- **Endoscopic retrograde cholangiopancreatography (ERCP):** A procedure used to X-ray the ducts (tubes) that carry bile from the liver to the gallbladder and from the gallbladder to the small intestine. Sometimes pancreatic cancer causes these ducts to narrow and block or slow the flow of bile, causing jaundice. An endoscope (a thin, lighted tube) is passed through the mouth, esophagus, and stomach into the first part of the small intestine. A catheter (a smaller tube) is then inserted through the endoscope into the pancreatic ducts. A dye is injected through the catheter into the ducts and an X-ray is taken. If the ducts are blocked by a tumor, a fine tube may be inserted into the duct to unblock it. This tube (or stent) may be left in place to keep the duct open. Tissue samples may also be taken.
- **Percutaneous transhepatic cholangiography (PTC):** A procedure used to X-ray the liver and bile ducts. A thin needle is inserted through the skin below the ribs and into the liver. Dye is injected into the liver or bile ducts and an X-ray is taken. If a blockage is found, a thin, flexible tube called a stent is sometimes left in the liver to drain bile into the small intestine or a collection bag outside the body. This test is done only if ERCP cannot be done.
- **Laparoscopy:** A surgical procedure to look at the organs inside the abdomen to check for signs of disease. Small incisions (cuts) are made in the wall of the abdomen and a laparoscope (a thin, lighted tube) is inserted into one of the incisions. The laparoscope may have an ultrasound probe at the end in order to bounce high-energy sound waves off internal organs, such as the pancreas. This is called laparoscopic ultrasound. Other

instruments may be inserted through the same or other incisions to perform procedures such as taking tissue samples from the pancreas or a sample of fluid from the abdomen to check for cancer.

- **Biopsy:** The removal of cells or tissues so they can be viewed under a microscope by a pathologist to check for signs of cancer. There are several ways to do a biopsy for pancreatic cancer. A fine needle or a core needle may be inserted into the pancreas during an X-ray or ultrasound to remove cells. Tissue may also be removed during a laparoscopy.

What Is the Prognosis for Pancreatic Cancer?

The prognosis (chance of recovery) and treatment options depend on the following:

- Whether or not the tumor can be removed by surgery
- The stage of the cancer (the size of the tumor and whether the cancer has spread outside the pancreas to nearby tissues or lymph nodes or to other places in the body)
- The patient's general health
- Whether the cancer has just been diagnosed or has recurred (come back)

Pancreatic cancer can be controlled only if it is found before it has spread, when it can be completely removed by surgery. If the cancer has spread, palliative treatment can improve the patient's quality of life by controlling the symptoms and complications of this disease.

Stages of Pancreatic Cancer

The process used to find out if cancer has spread within the pancreas or to other parts of the body is called staging. The information gathered from the staging process determines the stage of the disease. It is important to know the stage of the disease in order to plan treatment. The results of some of the tests used to diagnose pancreatic cancer are often also used to stage the disease.

The following stages are used for pancreatic cancer:

Stage 0 (carcinoma in situ). In stage 0, abnormal cells are found in the lining of the pancreas. These abnormal cells may become cancer and spread into nearby normal tissue. Stage 0 is also called carcinoma in situ.

Stage I. In stage I, cancer has formed and is found in the pancreas only. Stage I is divided into stage IA and stage IB, based on the size of the tumor.

- **Stage IA:** The tumor is 2 centimeters or smaller.
- **Stage IB:** The tumor is larger than 2 centimeters.

Stage II. In stage II, cancer may have spread to nearby tissue and organs, and may have spread to lymph nodes near the pancreas. Stage II is divided into stage IIA and stage IIB, based on where the cancer has spread.

- **Stage IIA:** Cancer has spread to nearby tissue and organs but has not spread to nearby lymph nodes.
- **Stage IIB:** Cancer has spread to nearby lymph nodes and may have spread to nearby tissue and organs.

Stage III. In stage III, cancer has spread to the major blood vessels near the pancreas and may have spread to nearby lymph nodes.

Stage IV. In stage IV, cancer may be of any size and has spread to distant organs, such as the liver, lung, and peritoneal cavity. It may have also spread to organs and tissues near the pancreas or to lymph nodes.

Treatment Option Overview

Different types of treatment are available for patients with pancreatic cancer. Some treatments are standard (the currently used treatment), and some are being tested in clinical trials. A treatment clinical trial is a research study meant to help improve current treatments or obtain information on new treatments for patients with cancer. When clinical trials show that a new treatment is better than the standard treatment, the new treatment may become the standard treatment. Patients may want to think about taking part in a clinical trial. Some clinical trials are open only to patients who have not started treatment.

Standard Treatment Available for Patients with Pancreatic Cancer

Five types of standard treatment are used:

Surgery

One of the following types of surgery may be used to take out the tumor:

- **Whipple procedure:** A surgical procedure in which the head of the pancreas, the gallbladder, part of the stomach, part of the small intestine, and the bile duct are removed. Enough of the pancreas is left to produce digestive juices and insulin.
- **Total pancreatectomy:** This operation removes the whole pancreas, part of the stomach, part of the small intestine, the common bile duct, the gallbladder, the spleen, and nearby lymph nodes.
- **Distal pancreatectomy:** The body and the tail of the pancreas and usually the spleen are removed.

If the cancer has spread and cannot be removed, the following types of palliative surgery may be done to relieve symptoms and improve quality of life:

- **Surgical biliary bypass:** If cancer is blocking the small intestine and bile is building up in the gallbladder, a biliary bypass may be done. During this operation, the doctor will cut the gallbladder or bile duct and sew it to the small intestine to create a new pathway around the blocked area.
- **Endoscopic stent placement:** If the tumor is blocking the bile duct, surgery may be done to put in a stent (a thin tube) to drain bile that has built up in the area. The doctor may place the stent through a catheter that drains to the outside of the body or the stent may go around the blocked area and drain the bile into the small intestine.
- **Gastric bypass:** If the tumor is blocking the flow of food from the stomach, the stomach may be sewn directly to the small intestine so the patient can continue to eat normally.

Radiation Therapy

Radiation therapy is a cancer treatment that uses high energy X-rays or other types of radiation to kill cancer cells or keep them from growing. There are two types of radiation therapy:

- External radiation therapy uses a machine outside the body to send radiation toward the cancer.

- Internal radiation therapy uses a radioactive substance sealed in needles, seeds, wires, or catheters that are placed directly into or near the cancer.

The way the radiation therapy is given depends on the type and stage of the cancer being treated. External radiation therapy is used to treat pancreatic cancer.

Chemotherapy

Chemotherapy is a cancer treatment that uses drugs to stop the growth of cancer cells, either by killing the cells or by stopping them from dividing. When chemotherapy is taken by mouth or injected into a vein or muscle, the drugs enter the bloodstream and can reach cancer cells throughout the body (systemic chemotherapy). When chemotherapy is placed directly into the cerebrospinal fluid, an organ, or a body cavity such as the abdomen, the drugs mainly affect cancer cells in those areas (regional chemotherapy). Combination chemotherapy is treatment using more than one anticancer drug. The way the chemotherapy is given depends on the type and stage of the cancer being treated.

Chemotherapy for pancreatic cancer may cause side effects.

Chemoradiation Therapy

Chemoradiation therapy combines chemotherapy and radiation therapy to increase the effects of both.

Targeted Therapy

Targeted therapy is a type of treatment that uses drugs or other substances to identify and attack specific cancer cells without harming normal cells. Tyrosine kinase inhibitors (TKIs) are targeted therapy drugs that block signals needed for tumors to grow. Erlotinib is a type of TKI used to treat pancreatic cancer.

How to Manage the Pain Caused by the Treatment for Pancreatic Cancer

There are treatments for pain caused by pancreatic cancer. Pain can occur when the tumor presses on nerves or other organs near the pancreas. When pain medicine is not enough, there are treatments that act on nerves in the abdomen to relieve the pain. The doctor may inject medicine into the area around affected nerves or may cut the nerves to block the feeling of pain. Radiation therapy with or without chemotherapy can also help relieve pain by shrinking the tumor.

Are There Any Special Nutritional Needs for Patients with Pancreatic Cancer?

Patients with pancreatic cancer have special nutritional needs. Surgery to remove the pancreas may affect its ability to make pancreatic enzymes that help to digest food. As a result, patients may have problems digesting food and absorbing nutrients into the body. To prevent malnutrition, the doctor may prescribe medicines that replace these enzymes.

What Are the New Types of Treatment Are Being Tested in Clinical Trials?

Biologic Therapy

Biologic therapy is a treatment that uses the patient's immune system to fight cancer. Substances made by the body or made in a laboratory are used to boost, direct, or restore the body's natural defenses against cancer. This type of cancer treatment is also called biotherapy or immunotherapy.

Chapter 33

Liver Cancer

The liver is the largest organ in the human body, located on the upper right side of the body, behind the lower ribs. The liver does many jobs, including:

- Storing nutrients
- Removing waste products and worn out cells from the blood
- Filtering and processing chemicals in food, alcohol, and medications
- Producing bile, a solution that helps digest fats and eliminate waste products

What Is Liver Cancer?

Cancer is a disease in which cells in the body grow out of control. When cancer starts in the liver, it is called liver cancer. Each year in the United States, about 22,000 men and 9,000 women get liver cancer, and about 16,000 men and 8,000 women die from the disease. The percentage of Americans who get liver cancer has been rising for several decades. To lower your risk for liver cancer, get vaccinated against Hepatitis B, get tested for Hepatitis C, and don't drink too much alcohol.

This chapter includes text excerpted from "Liver Cancer," Centers for Disease Control and Prevention (CDC), February 8, 2018.

What Causes Liver Cancer?

Many liver cancer cases are related to the hepatitis B virus or hepatitis C virus. More than 4 million people are living with chronic Hepatitis B or chronic Hepatitis C in the United States. Most people don't know they have the virus.

What Are the Risk Factors for Liver Cancer?

Other behaviors and conditions that increase risk for getting liver cancer are:

- Heavy alcohol use
- Cirrhosis (scarring of the liver, which can also be caused by hepatitis and alcohol use)
- Obesity
- Diabetes
- Having hemochromatosis, a condition where the body takes up and stores more iron than it needs
- Eating foods that have aflatoxin (a fungus that can grow on foods, such as grains and nuts that have not been stored properly)

What Are the Symptoms of Liver Cancer?

In its early stages, liver cancer may not have symptoms that can be seen or felt. However, as the cancer grows larger, people may notice one or more of these common symptoms. It's important to remember that these symptoms could also be caused by other health conditions. If you have any of these symptoms, talk to your doctor.

Liver cancer symptoms may include:

- Discomfort in the upper abdomen on the right side
- A swollen abdomen
- A hard lump on the right side just below the rib cage
- Pain near the right shoulder blade or in the back
- Jaundice (yellowing of the skin and whites of the eyes)
- Easy bruising or bleeding
- Unusual tiredness

- Nausea and vomiting
- Loss of appetite
- Weight loss for no known reason

How Can I Reduce My Risk for Liver Cancer?

You can lower your risk of getting liver cancer in the following ways:

- Get vaccinated against Hepatitis B infection. The Hepatitis B vaccine is recommended for all infants at birth and for adults who may be at increased risk.
- Get tested for Hepatitis C, and get treated if you have it.
- Avoid drinking too much alcohol.

Chapter 34

Bile Duct Cancer

A network of tubes, called ducts, connects the liver, gallbladder, and small intestine. This network begins in the liver where many small ducts collect bile (a fluid made by the liver to break down fats during digestion). The small ducts come together to form the right and left hepatic ducts, which lead out of the liver. The two ducts join outside the liver and form the common hepatic duct. The cystic duct connects the gallbladder to the common hepatic duct. Bile from the liver passes through the hepatic ducts, common hepatic duct, and cystic duct and is stored in the gallbladder. When food is being digested, bile stored in the gallbladder is released and passes through the cystic duct to the common bile duct and into the small intestine.

What Is Bile Duct Cancer?

Bile duct cancer is a rare disease in which malignant (cancer) cells form in the bile ducts. Bile duct cancer is also called cholangiocarcinoma.

There are two types of bile duct cancer:

- **Intrahepatic bile duct cancer:** This type of cancer forms in the bile ducts inside the liver. Only a small number of bile duct cancers are intrahepatic. Intrahepatic bile duct cancers are also called intrahepatic cholangiocarcinomas.

This chapter includes text excerpted from "Bile Duct Cancer (Cholangiocarcinoma) Treatment (PDQ®)—Patient Version," National Cancer Institute (NCI), March 2, 2018.

- **Extrahepatic bile duct cancer:** The extrahepatic bile duct is made up of the hilum region and the distal region. Cancer can form in either region:
  - **Perihilar bile duct cancer:** This type of cancer is found in the hilum region, the area where the right and left bile ducts exit the liver and join to form the common hepatic duct. Perihilar bile duct cancer is also called a Klatskin tumor or perihilar cholangiocarcinoma.
  - **Distal extrahepatic bile duct cancer:** This type of cancer is found in the distal region. The distal region is made up of the common bile duct which passes through the pancreas and ends in the small intestine. Distal extrahepatic bile duct cancer is also called extrahepatic cholangiocarcinoma.

What Are the Risk Factors for Bile Duct Cancer?

Anything that increases your risk of getting a disease is called a risk factor. Having a risk factor does not mean that you will get cancer; not having risk factors doesn't mean that you will not get cancer. People who think they may be at risk should discuss this with their doctor. Having colitis or certain liver diseases can increase the risk of bile duct cancer. Risk factors for bile duct cancer include the following conditions:

- Primary sclerosing cholangitis (a progressive disease in which the bile ducts become blocked by inflammation and scarring)
- Chronic ulcerative colitis
- Cysts in the bile ducts (cysts block the flow of bile and can cause swollen bile ducts, inflammation, and infection)
- Infection with a Chinese liver fluke parasite

What Are the Signs and Symptoms of Bile Duct Cancer?

Signs of bile duct cancer include jaundice and pain in the abdomen. These and other signs and symptoms may be caused by bile duct cancer or by other conditions. Check with your doctor if you have any of the following:

- Jaundice (yellowing of the skin or whites of the eyes)

- Dark urine
- Clay-colored stool
- Pain in the abdomen
- Fever
- Itchy skin
- Nausea and vomiting
- Weight loss for an unknown reason

How Is Bile Duct Cancer Diagnosed?

Procedures that make pictures of the bile ducts and the nearby area help diagnose bile duct cancer and show how far the cancer has spread. The process used to find out if cancer cells have spread within and around the bile ducts or to distant parts of the body is called staging. In order to plan treatment, it is important to know if the bile duct cancer can be removed by surgery. Tests and procedures to detect, diagnose, and stage bile duct cancer are usually done at the same time.

The following tests and procedures may be used:

- **Physical exam and history:** An exam of the body to check general signs of health, including checking for signs of disease, such as lumps or anything else that seems unusual. A history of the patient's health habits and past illnesses and treatments will also be taken.
- **Liver function tests:** A procedure in which a blood sample is checked to measure the amounts of bilirubin and alkaline phosphatase released into the blood by the liver. A higher than normal amount of these substances can be a sign of liver disease that may be caused by bile duct cancer.
- **Laboratory tests:** Medical procedures that test samples of tissue, blood, urine, or other substances in the body. These tests help to diagnose disease, plan and check treatment, or monitor the disease over time.
- **Carcinoembryonic antigen (CEA) and CA 19-9 tumor marker test:** A procedure in which a sample of blood, urine, or tissue is checked to measure the amounts of certain substances made by organs, tissues, or tumor cells in the body. Certain substances are linked to specific types of cancer when found in

increased levels in the body. These are called tumor markers. Higher than normal levels of carcinoembryonic antigen (CEA) and CA 19-9 may mean there is bile duct cancer.

- **Ultrasound exam:** A procedure in which high-energy sound waves (ultrasound) are bounced off internal tissues or organs, such as the abdomen, and make echoes. The echoes form a picture of body tissues called a sonogram. The picture can be printed to be looked at later.
- **Computed tomography (CT)/computerized axial tomography (CAT) scan:** A procedure that makes a series of detailed pictures of areas inside the body, such as the abdomen, taken from different angles. The pictures are made by a computer linked to an X-ray machine. A dye may be injected into a vein or swallowed to help the organs or tissues show up more clearly. This procedure is also called computed tomography, computerized tomography, or computerized axial tomography.
- **Magnetic resonance imaging (MRI):** A procedure that uses a magnet, radio waves, and a computer to make a series of detailed pictures of areas inside the body. This procedure is also called nuclear magnetic resonance imaging (NMRI).
- **Magnetic resonance cholangiopancreatography (MRCP):** A procedure that uses a magnet, radio waves, and a computer to make a series of detailed pictures of areas inside the body such as the liver, bile ducts, gallbladder, pancreas, and pancreatic duct.

Procedures Used to Obtain a Sample of Tissue and Diagnose Bile Duct Cancer

Cells and tissues are removed during a biopsy so they can be viewed under a microscope by a pathologist to check for signs of cancer. Different procedures may be used to obtain the sample of cells and tissue. The type of procedure used depends on whether the patient is well enough to have surgery.

Types of biopsy procedures include the following:

- **Laparoscopy:** A surgical procedure to look at the organs inside the abdomen, such as the bile ducts and liver, to check for signs of cancer. Small incisions (cuts) are made in the wall of the abdomen and a laparoscope (a thin, lighted tube) is inserted into one of the incisions. Other instruments may be inserted through the same or other incisions to perform procedures such as taking tissue samples to be checked for signs of cancer.

- **Percutaneous transhepatic cholangiography (PTC):** A procedure used to X-ray the liver and bile ducts. A thin needle is inserted through the skin below the ribs and into the liver. Dye is injected into the liver or bile ducts and an X-ray is taken. A sample of tissue is removed and checked for signs of cancer. If the bile duct is blocked, a thin, flexible tube called a stent may be left in the liver to drain bile into the small intestine or a collection bag outside the body. This procedure may be used when a patient cannot have surgery.
- **Endoscopic retrograde cholangiopancreatography (ERCP):** A procedure used to X-ray the ducts (tubes) that carry bile from the liver to the gallbladder and from the gallbladder to the small intestine. Sometimes bile duct cancer causes these ducts to narrow and block or slow the flow of bile, causing jaundice. An endoscope is passed through the mouth and stomach and into the small intestine. Dye is injected through the endoscope (thin, tube-like instrument with a light and a lens for viewing) into the bile ducts and an X-ray is taken. A sample of tissue is removed and checked for signs of cancer. If the bile duct is blocked, a thin tube may be inserted into the duct to unblock it. This tube (or stent) may be left in place to keep the duct open. This procedure may be used when a patient cannot have surgery.

What Is the Prognosis for Bile Duct Cancer?

The prognosis (chance of recovery) and treatment options depend on the following:

- Whether the cancer is in the upper or lower part of the bile duct system
- The stage of the cancer (whether it affects only the bile ducts or has spread to the liver, lymph nodes, or other places in the body)
- Whether the cancer has spread to nearby nerves or veins
- Whether the cancer can be completely removed by surgery
- Whether the patient has other conditions, such as primary sclerosing cholangitis

- Whether the level of CA 19-9 is higher than normal
- Whether the cancer has just been diagnosed or has recurred (come back)

Treatment options may also depend on the symptoms caused by the cancer. Bile duct cancer is usually found after it has spread and can rarely be completely removed by surgery. Palliative therapy may relieve symptoms and improve the patient's quality of life.

Stages of Bile Duct Cancer

The process used to find out if cancer has spread to other parts of the body is called staging. For bile duct cancer, the information gathered from tests and procedures is used to plan treatment, including whether the tumor can be removed by surgery.

Stages that are used to describe the different types of bile duct cancer are as follows:

Intrahepatic Bile Duct Cancer

- **Stage 0:** Abnormal cells are found in the innermost layer of tissue lining the intrahepatic bile duct. These abnormal cells may become cancer and spread into nearby normal tissue. Stage 0 is also called carcinoma in situ.
- **Stage I:** There is one tumor that has spread into the intrahepatic bile duct and it has not spread into any blood vessels.
- **Stage II:** There is one tumor that has spread through the wall of the bile duct and into a blood vessel, or there are multiple tumors that may have spread into a blood vessel.
- **Stage III:** The tumor has spread through the tissue that lines the abdominal wall or has spread to organs or tissues near the liver such as the duodenum, colon, and stomach.
- **Stage IV:** Stage IV is divided into stage IVA and stage IVB.
    - **Stage IVA:** The cancer has spread along the outside of the intrahepatic bile ducts or the cancer has spread to nearby lymph nodes.
    - **Stage IVB:** The cancer has spread to organs in other parts of the body.

Perihilar Bile Duct Cancer

- **Stage 0:** Abnormal cells are found in the innermost layer of tissue lining the perihilar bile duct. These abnormal cells may become cancer and spread into nearby normal tissue. Stage 0 is also called carcinoma in situ.
- **Stage I:** Cancer has formed in the innermost layer of the wall of the perihilar bile duct and has spread into the muscle layer or fibrous tissue layer of the wall.
- **Stage II:** Cancer has spread through the wall of the perihilar bile duct to nearby fatty tissue or to the liver.
- **Stage III:** Stage III is divided into stage IIIA and stage IIIB.
    - **Stage IIIA:** Cancer has spread to branches on one side of the hepatic artery or of the portal vein.
    - **Stage IIIB:** Cancer has spread to nearby lymph nodes. Cancer may have spread into the wall of the perihilar bile duct or through the wall to nearby fatty tissue, the liver, or to branches on one side of the hepatic artery or of the portal vein.
- **Stage IV:** Stage IV is divided into stage IVA and stage IVB.
    - **Stage IVA:** Cancer has spread to one or more of the following:
        - the main part of the portal vein and/or common hepatic artery;
        - the branches of the portal vein and/or common hepatic artery on both sides;
        - the right hepatic duct and the left branch of the hepatic artery or of the portal vein;
        - the left hepatic duct and the right branch of the hepatic artery or of the portal vein.
        - Cancer may have spread to nearby lymph nodes.
    - **Stage IVB:** Cancer has spread to lymph nodes in more distant parts of the abdomen, or to organs in other parts of the body.

Distal Extrahepatic Bile Duct Cancer

- **Stage 0:** Abnormal cells are found in the innermost layer of tissue lining the distal extrahepatic bile duct. These abnormal cells may become cancer and spread into nearby normal tissue. Stage 0 is also called carcinoma in situ.
- **Stage I:** Stage I is divided into stage IA and stage IB.
    - **Stage IA:** Cancer has formed and is found in the distal extrahepatic bile duct wall only.
    - **Stage IB:** Cancer has formed and has spread through the wall of the distal extrahepatic bile duct but has not spread to nearby organs.
- **Stage II:** Stage II is divided into stage IIA and stage IIB.
    - **Stage IIA:** Cancer has spread from the distal extrahepatic bile duct to the gallbladder, pancreas, duodenum, or other nearby organs.
    - **Stage IIB:** Cancer has spread from the distal extrahepatic bile duct to nearby lymph nodes. Cancer may have spread through the wall of the duct or to nearby organs.
- **Stage III:** Cancer has spread to the large vessels that carry blood to the organs in the abdomen. Cancer may have spread to nearby lymph nodes.
- **Stage IV:** Cancer has spread to organs in distant parts of the body.

The following groups are used to plan treatment:

Resectable (Localized) Bile Duct Cancer

The cancer is in an area, such as the lower part of the common bile duct or perihilar area, where it can be removed completely by surgery.

Unresectable, Metastatic, or Recurrent Bile Duct Cancer

Unresectable cancer cannot be removed completely by surgery. Most patients with bile duct cancer cannot have their cancer completely removed by surgery.

Metastasis is the spread of cancer from the primary site (place where it started) to other places in the body. Metastatic bile duct cancer may have spread to the liver, other parts of the abdominal cavity, or to distant parts of the body. Recurrent bile duct cancer is cancer that has recurred (come back) after it has been treated. The cancer may come back in the bile ducts, liver, or gallbladder. Less often, it may come back in distant parts of the body.

Treatment Option Overview

Different types of treatments are available for patients with bile duct cancer. Some treatments are standard (the currently used treatment), and some are being tested in clinical trials. A treatment clinical trial is a research study meant to help improve current treatments or obtain information on new treatments for patients with cancer. When clinical trials show that a new treatment is better than the standard treatment, the new treatment may become the standard treatment. Patients may want to think about taking part in a clinical trial. Some clinical trials are open only to patients who have not started treatment.

Standard Treatments Available for Patients with Bile Duct Cancer

Three types of standard treatment are used:

Surgery

The following types of surgery are used to treat bile duct cancer:

- **Removal of the bile duct:** A surgical procedure to remove part of the bile duct if the tumor is small and in the bile duct only. Lymph nodes are removed and tissue from the lymph nodes is viewed under a microscope to see if there is cancer.
- **Partial hepatectomy:** A surgical procedure in which the part of the liver where cancer is found is removed. The part removed may be a wedge of tissue, an entire lobe, or a larger part of the liver, along with some normal tissue around it.
- **Whipple procedure:** A surgical procedure in which the head of the pancreas, the gallbladder, part of the stomach, part of the small intestine, and the bile duct are removed. Enough of the pancreas is left to make digestive juices and insulin.

Even if the doctor removes all the cancer that can be seen at the time of the operation, some patients may be given chemotherapy or radiation therapy after surgery to kill any cancer cells that are left.

Treatment given after the surgery, to lower the risk that the cancer will come back, is called adjuvant therapy. It is not yet known whether chemotherapy or radiation therapy given after surgery helps keep the cancer from coming back.

The following types of palliative surgery may be done to relieve symptoms caused by a blocked bile duct and improve quality of life:

- **Biliary bypass:** A surgical procedure in which the part of the bile duct before the blockage is connected with part of the bile duct that is past the blockage or to the small intestine. This allows bile to flow to the gallbladder or small intestine.
- **Stent placement:** A surgical procedure in which a stent (a thin, flexible tube or metal tube) is placed in the bile duct to open it and allow bile to flow into the small intestine or through a catheter that goes to a collection bag outside of the body.
- **Percutaneous transhepatic biliary drainage:** A procedure used to X-ray the liver and bile ducts. A thin needle is inserted through the skin below the ribs and into the liver. Dye is injected into the liver or bile ducts and an X-ray is taken. If the bile duct is blocked, a thin, flexible tube called a stent may be left in the liver to drain bile into the small intestine or a collection bag outside the body.

Radiation Therapy

Radiation therapy is a cancer treatment that uses high-energy X-rays or other types of radiation to kill cancer cells or keep them from growing. There are two types of radiation therapy:

- External radiation therapy uses a machine outside the body to send radiation toward the cancer.
- Internal radiation therapy uses a radioactive substance sealed in needles, seeds, wires, or catheters that are placed directly into or near the cancer.

External and internal radiation therapy are used to treat bile duct cancer.

It is not yet known whether external radiation therapy helps in the treatment of resectable bile duct cancer. In unresectable, metastatic, or recurrent bile duct cancer, new ways to improve the effect of external radiation therapy on cancer cells are being studied:

- **Hyperthermia therapy:** A treatment in which body tissue is exposed to high temperatures to make cancer cells more sensitive to the effects of radiation therapy and certain anticancer drugs.

- **Radiosensitizers:** Drugs that make cancer cells more sensitive to radiation therapy. Combining radiation therapy with radiosensitizers may kill more cancer cells.

Chemotherapy

Chemotherapy is a cancer treatment that uses drugs to stop the growth of cancer cells, either by killing the cells or by stopping them from dividing. When chemotherapy is taken by mouth or injected into a vein or muscle, the drugs enter the bloodstream and can reach cancer cells throughout the body (systemic chemotherapy). When chemotherapy is placed directly into the cerebrospinal fluid, an organ, or a body cavity such as the abdomen, the drugs mainly affect cancer cells in those areas (regional chemotherapy).

Systemic chemotherapy is used to treat unresectable, metastatic, or recurrent bile duct cancer. It is not yet known whether systemic chemotherapy helps in the treatment of resectable bile duct cancer. In unresectable, metastatic, or recurrent bile duct cancer, intra-arterial embolization is being studied. It is a procedure in which the blood supply to a tumor is blocked after anticancer drugs are given in blood vessels near the tumor. Sometimes, the anticancer drugs are attached to small beads that are injected into an artery that feeds the tumor. The beads block blood flow to the tumor as they release the drug. This allows a higher amount of drug to reach the tumor for a longer period of time, which may kill more cancer cells. Treatment for bile duct cancer may cause side effects.

New Types of Treatment Are Being Tested in Clinical Trials

Liver Transplant

In a liver transplant, the entire liver is removed and replaced with a healthy donated liver. A liver transplant may be done in patients with perihilar bile duct cancer. If the patient has to wait for a donated liver, other treatment is given as needed.

Follow-Up Tests

Some of the tests that were done to diagnose the cancer or to find out the stage of the cancer may be repeated. Some tests will be repeated in order to see how well the treatment is working. Decisions about whether to continue, change, or stop treatment may be based on the results of these tests.

Some of the tests will continue to be done from time to time after treatment has ended. The results of these tests can show if your condition has changed or if the cancer has recurred (come back). These tests are sometimes called follow-up tests or check-ups.

Chapter 35

Gastrointestinal Carcinoid Tumors

The gastrointestinal (GI) tract is part of the body's digestive system. It helps to digest food, takes nutrients (vitamins, minerals, carbohydrates, fats, proteins, and water) from food to be used by the body and helps pass waste material out of the body. The GI tract is made up of these and other organs:

- Stomach
- Small intestine (duodenum, jejunum, and ileum)
- Colon
- Rectum

What Is Gastrointestinal (GI) Carcinoid Tumors?

A GI carcinoid tumor is cancer that forms in the lining of the GI tract. GI carcinoid tumors form from a certain type of neuroendocrine cell (a type of cell that is like a nerve cell and a hormone-making cell). These cells are scattered throughout the chest and abdomen but most are found in the GI tract. Neuroendocrine cells make hormones that help

---

This chapter includes text excerpted from "Gastrointestinal Carcinoid Tumors Treatment (PDQ®)—Patient Version," National Cancer Institute (NCI), January 29, 2018.

control digestive juices and the muscles used in moving food through the stomach and intestines. A GI carcinoid tumor may also make hormones and release them into the body. GI carcinoid tumors are rare and most grow very slowly. Most of them occur in the small intestine, rectum, and appendix. Sometimes more than one tumor will form.

What Are the Risk Factors for GI Carcinoid Tumor?

Anything that increases a person's chance of developing a disease is called a risk factor. Having a risk factor does not mean that you will get cancer; not having risk factors doesn't mean that you will not get cancer. Talk to your doctor if you think you may be at risk.

Health history can affect the risk of GI carcinoid tumors. Risk factors for GI carcinoid tumors include the following:

- Having a family history of multiple endocrine neoplasia type 1 (MEN1) syndrome or neurofibromatosis type 1 (NF1) syndrome
- Having certain conditions that affect the stomach's ability to make stomach acid, such as atrophic gastritis, pernicious anemia, or Zollinger-Ellison syndrome

What Are the Signs and Symptoms of GI Carcinoid Tumor?

Some GI carcinoid tumors have no signs or symptoms in the early stages. Signs and symptoms may be caused by the growth of the tumor and/or the hormones the tumor makes. Some tumors, especially tumors of the stomach or appendix, may not cause signs or symptoms. Carcinoid tumors are often found during tests or treatments for other conditions.

Carcinoid tumors in the small intestine (duodenum, jejunum, and ileum), colon, and rectum sometimes cause signs or symptoms as they grow or because of the hormones they make. Other conditions may cause the same signs or symptoms. Check with your doctor if you have any of the following:

Duodenum

Signs and symptoms of GI carcinoid tumors in the duodenum (first part of the small intestine, that connects to the stomach) may include the following:

- Abdominal pain
- Constipation

- Diarrhea
- Change in stool color
- Nausea
- Vomiting
- Jaundice (yellowing of the skin and whites of the eyes)
- Heartburn

Jejunum and Ileum

Signs and symptoms of GI carcinoid tumors in the jejunum (middle part of the small intestine) and ileum (last part of the small intestine, that connects to the colon) may include the following:

- Abdominal pain
- Weight loss for no known reason
- Feeling very tired
- Feeling bloated
- Diarrhea
- Nausea
- Vomiting

Colon

Signs and symptoms of GI carcinoid tumors in the colon may include the following:

- Abdominal pain
- Weight loss for no known reason

Rectum

Signs and symptoms of GI carcinoid tumors in the rectum may include the following:

- Blood in the stool
- Pain in the rectum
- Constipation

What Causes Carcinoid Syndrome?

Carcinoid syndrome may occur if the tumor spreads to the liver or other parts of the body. The hormones made by gastrointestinal carcinoid tumors are usually destroyed by liver enzymes in the blood. If the tumor has spread to the liver and the liver enzymes cannot destroy the extra hormones made by the tumor, high amounts of these hormones may remain in the body and cause carcinoid syndrome. This can also happen if tumor cells enter the blood. Signs and symptoms of carcinoid syndrome include the following:

- Redness or a feeling of warmth in the face and neck
- Abdominal pain
- Feeling bloated
- Diarrhea
- Wheezing or other trouble breathing
- Fast heartbeat

These signs and symptoms may be caused by GI carcinoid tumors or by other conditions. Talk to your doctor if you have any of these signs or symptoms.

How Is GI Carcinoid Tumor Diagnosed?

Imaging studies and tests that examine the blood and urine are used to detect (find) and diagnose GI carcinoid tumors.

The following tests and procedures may be used:

- **Physical exam and history:** An exam of the body to check general signs of health, including checking for signs of disease, such as lumps or anything else that seems unusual. A history of the patient's health habits and past illnesses and treatments will also be taken.
- **Blood chemistry studies:** A procedure in which a blood sample is checked to measure the amounts of certain substances, such as hormones, released into the blood by organs and tissues in the body. An unusual (higher or lower than normal) amount of a substance can be a sign of disease. The blood sample is checked to see if it contains a hormone produced by carcinoid tumors. This test is used to help diagnose carcinoid syndrome.

- **Tumor marker test:** A procedure in which a sample of blood, urine, or tissue is checked to measure the amounts of certain substances, such as chromogranin A, made by organs, tissues, or tumor cells in the body. Chromogranin A is a tumor marker. It has been linked to neuroendocrine tumors when found in increased levels in the body.
- **24-hour urine test:** A test in which urine is collected for 24 hours to measure the amounts of certain substances, such as 5-hydroxyindoleacetic acid (5-HIAA) or serotonin (hormone). An unusual (higher or lower than normal) amount of a substance can be a sign of disease in the organ or tissue that makes it. This test is used to help diagnose carcinoid syndrome.
- **Metaiodobenzylguanidine (MIBG) scan:** A procedure used to find neuroendocrine tumors, such as carcinoid tumors. A very small amount of radioactive material called MIBG is injected into a vein and travels through the bloodstream. Carcinoid tumors take up the radioactive material and are detected by a device that measures radiation.
- **Computerized tomography (CT)/computerized axial tomography (CAT) scan:** A procedure that makes a series of detailed pictures of areas inside the body, taken from different angles. The pictures are made by a computer linked to an X-ray machine. A dye may be injected into a vein or swallowed to help the organs or tissues show up more clearly.
- **Magnetic resonance imaging (MRI):** A procedure that uses a magnet, radio waves, and a computer to make a series of detailed pictures of areas inside the body. This procedure is also called nuclear magnetic resonance imaging
- **Positron emission tomography (PET) scan:** A procedure to find malignant tumor cells in the body. A small amount of radioactive glucose (sugar) is injected into a vein. The PET scanner rotates around the body and makes a picture of where glucose is being used in the body. Malignant tumor cells show up brighter in the picture because they are more active and take up more glucose than normal cells.
- **Endoscopic ultrasound (EUS):** A procedure in which an endoscope is inserted into the body, usually through the mouth or rectum. An endoscope is a thin, tube-like instrument with a

light and a lens for viewing. A probe at the end of the endoscope is used to bounce high-energy sound waves (ultrasound) off internal tissues or organs, such as the stomach, small intestine, colon, or rectum, and make echoes. The echoes form a picture of body tissues called a sonogram. This procedure is also called endosonography.

- **Upper endoscopy:** A procedure to look at organs and tissues inside the body to check for abnormal areas. An endoscope is inserted through the mouth and passed through the esophagus into the stomach. Sometimes the endoscope also is passed from the stomach into the small intestine. An endoscope is a thin, tube-like instrument with a light and a lens for viewing. It may also have a tool to remove tissue or lymph node samples, which are checked under a microscope for signs of disease.
- **Colonoscopy:** A procedure to look inside the rectum and colon for polyps, abnormal areas, or cancer. A colonoscope is inserted through the rectum into the colon. A colonoscope is a thin, tube-like instrument with a light and a lens for viewing. It may also have a tool to remove polyps or tissue samples, which are checked under a microscope for signs of cancer.
- **Capsule endoscopy:** A procedure used to see all of the small intestine. The patient swallows a capsule that contains a tiny camera. As the capsule moves through the gastrointestinal tract, the camera takes pictures and sends them to a receiver worn on the outside of the body.
- **Biopsy:** The removal of cells or tissues so they can be viewed under a microscope to check for signs of cancer. Tissue samples may be taken during endoscopy and colonoscopy.

What Is the Prognosis for GI Carcinoid Tumor?

The prognosis (chance of recovery) and treatment options depend on the following:

- Where the tumor is in the GI intestinal tract
- The size of the tumor
- Whether the cancer has spread from the stomach and intestines to other parts of the body, such as the liver or lymph nodes
- Whether the patient has carcinoid syndrome or has carcinoid heart syndrome

- Whether the cancer can be completely removed by surgery
- Whether the cancer is newly diagnosed or has recurred

Stages of GI Carcinoid Tumors

After a gastrointestinal carcinoid tumor has been diagnosed, tests are done to find out if cancer cells have spread within the stomach and intestines or to other parts of the body. Staging is the process used to find out how far the cancer has spread. The information gathered from the staging process determines the stage of the disease. The results of tests and procedures used to diagnose GI carcinoid tumors may also be used for staging. A bone scan may be done to check if there are rapidly dividing cells, such as cancer cells, in the bone. A very small amount of radioactive material is injected into a vein and travels through the bloodstream.

The radioactive material collects in the bones with cancer and is detected by a scanner.

What Does GI Carcinoid Tumors Depend Upon?

The plan for cancer treatment depends on where the carcinoid tumor is found and whether it can be removed by surgery. For many cancers it is important to know the stage of the cancer in order to plan treatment. However, the treatment of GI carcinoid tumors is not based on the stage of the cancer. Treatment depends mainly on whether the tumor can be removed by surgery and if the tumor has spread.

Treatment is based on whether the tumor:

- Can be completely removed by surgery
- Has spread to other parts of the body
- Has come back after treatment. The tumor may come back in the stomach or intestines or in other parts of the body.
- Has not gotten better with treatment

Treatment Option Overview

Different types of treatment are available for patients with GI carcinoid tumor. Some treatments are standard (the currently used treatment), and some are being tested in clinical trials. A treatment clinical trial is a research study meant to help improve current treatments or obtain information on new treatments for patients with cancer. When clinical trials show that a new treatment is better than the standard treatment, the new treatment may become the standard treatment. Patients may want to think about taking part in a clinical trial. Some clinical trials are open only to patients who have not started treatment.

Standard Treatments Available for Patients with GI Carcinoid Tumors

Four types of standard treatment are used:

Surgery

Treatment of GI carcinoid tumors usually includes surgery. One of the following surgical procedures may be used:

- **Endoscopic resection:** Surgery to remove a small tumor that is on the inside lining of the GI tract. An endoscope is inserted through the mouth and passed through the esophagus to the stomach and sometimes, the duodenum. An endoscope is a thin, tube-like instrument with a light, a lens for viewing, and a tool for removing tumor tissue.
- **Local excision:** Surgery to remove the tumor and a small amount of normal tissue around it.
- **Resection:** Surgery to remove part or all of the organ that contains cancer. Nearby lymph nodes may also be removed.
- **Cryosurgery:** A treatment that uses an instrument to freeze and destroy carcinoid tumor tissue. This type of treatment is also called cryotherapy. The doctor may use ultrasound to guide the instrument.
- **Radiofrequency ablation:** The use of a special probe with tiny electrodes that release high-energy radio waves (similar to microwaves) that kill cancer cells. The probe may be inserted through the skin or through an incision (cut) in the abdomen.
- **Liver transplant:** Surgery to remove the whole liver and replace it with a healthy donated liver.
- **Hepatic artery embolization:** A procedure to embolize (block) the hepatic artery, which is the main blood vessel that brings blood into the liver. Blocking the flow of blood to the liver helps kill cancer cells growing there.

Radiation Therapy

Radiation therapy is a cancer treatment that uses high-energy X-rays or other types of radiation to kill cancer cells or keep them from growing. There are two types of radiation therapy:

- External radiation therapy uses a machine outside the body to send radiation toward the cancer.
- Internal radiation therapy uses a radioactive substance sealed in needles, seeds, wires, or catheters that are placed directly into or near the cancer.

Radiopharmaceutical therapy is a type of internal radiation therapy. Radiation is given to the tumor using a drug that has a radioactive substance, such as iodine I 131, attached to it. The radioactive substance kills the tumor cells.

External and internal radiation therapy are used to treat GI carcinoid tumors that have spread to other parts of the body.

Chemotherapy

Chemotherapy is a cancer treatment that uses drugs to stop the growth of cancer cells, either by killing the cells or by stopping the cells from dividing. When chemotherapy is taken by mouth or injected into a vein or muscle, the drugs enter the bloodstream and can reach cancer cells throughout the body (systemic chemotherapy). When chemotherapy is placed directly into the cerebrospinal fluid, an organ, or a body cavity such as the abdomen, the drugs mainly affect cancer cells in those areas (regional chemotherapy).

Chemoembolization of the hepatic artery is a type of regional chemotherapy that may be used to treat a GI carcinoid tumor that has spread to the liver. The anticancer drug is injected into the hepatic artery through a catheter (thin tube). The drug is mixed with a substance that embolizes (blocks) the artery, and cuts off blood flow to the tumor. Most of the anticancer drug is trapped near the tumor and only a small amount of the drug reaches other parts of the body. The blockage may be temporary or permanent, depending on the substance used to block the artery. The tumor is prevented from getting the oxygen and nutrients it needs to grow. The liver continues to receive blood from the hepatic portal vein, which carries blood from the stomach and intestine.

The way the chemotherapy is given depends on the type and stage of the cancer being treated.

Hormone Therapy

Hormone therapy with a somatostatin analogue is a treatment that stops extra hormones from being made. GI carcinoid tumors are treated with octreotide or lanreotide which are injected under the skin or into the muscle. Octreotide and lanreotide may also have a small effect on stopping tumor growth.

Treatment for Carcinoid Syndrome

Treatment for carcinoid syndrome may also be needed. It may include the following:

- Hormone therapy with a somatostatin analogue stops extra hormones from being made. Carcinoid syndrome is treated with octreotide or lanreotide to lessen flushing and diarrhea. Octreotide and lanreotide may also help slow tumor growth.
- Interferon therapy stimulates the body's immune system to work better and lessens flushing and diarrhea. Interferon may also help slow tumor growth.
- Taking medicine for diarrhea
- Taking medicine for skin rashes
- Taking medicine to breathe easier
- Taking medicine before having anesthesia for a medical procedure

Other ways to help treat carcinoid syndrome include avoiding things that cause flushing or difficulty breathing such as alcohol, nuts, certain cheeses and foods with capsaicin, such as chili peppers. Avoiding stressful situations and certain types of physical activity can also help treat carcinoid syndrome.

For some patients with carcinoid heart syndrome, a heart valve replacement may be done.

New Types of Treatment Being Tested in Clinical Trials

Targeted Therapy

Targeted therapy is a type of treatment that uses drugs or other substances to identify and attack specific cancer cells without harming normal cells. Several types of targeted therapy are being studied in the treatment of GI carcinoid tumors.

Follow-Up Tests

Some of the tests that were done to diagnose the cancer or to find out the stage of the cancer may be repeated. Some tests will be repeated in order to see how well the treatment is working. Decisions about whether to continue, change, or stop treatment may be based on the results of these tests.

Some of the tests will continue to be done from time to time after treatment has ended. The results of these tests can show if your condition has changed or if the cancer has recurred (come back). These tests are sometimes called follow-up tests or check-ups.

Chapter 36

Small Intestine Cancer

The small intestine is part of the body's digestive system, which also includes the esophagus, stomach, and large intestine. The digestive system removes and processes nutrients (vitamins, minerals, carbohydrates, fats, proteins, and water) from foods and helps pass waste material out of the body. The small intestine is a long tube that connects the stomach to the large intestine. It folds many times to fit inside the abdomen.

What Is Small Intestine Cancer?

Small intestine cancer is a rare disease in which malignant (cancer) cells form in the tissues of the small intestine.

How Many Types of Small Intestine Cancer Are There?

There are five types of small intestine cancer. They are adenocarcinoma, sarcoma, carcinoid tumors, gastrointestinal stromal tumor, and lymphoma. This chapter discusses adenocarcinoma and leiomyosarcoma (a type of sarcoma). Adenocarcinoma starts in glandular cells in the lining of the small intestine and is the most common type of small intestine cancer. Most of these tumors occur in the part of the small intestine near the stomach. They may grow and block the intestine.

This chapter includes text excerpted from "Small Intestine Cancer Treatment (PDQ®)—Patient Version," National Cancer Institute (NCI), February 16, 2018.

Leiomyosarcoma starts in the smooth muscle cells of the small intestine. Most of these tumors occur in the part of the small intestine near the large intestine.

What Are the Risk Factors for Small Intestine Cancer?

Anything that increases your risk of getting a disease is called a risk factor. Having a risk factor does not mean that you will get cancer; not having risk factors doesn't mean that you will not get cancer. Talk with your doctor if you think you may be at risk.

Diet and health history can affect the risk of developing small intestine cancer. Risk factors for small intestine cancer include the following:

- Eating a high-fat diet
- Having Crohn disease
- Having celiac disease
- Having familial adenomatous polyposis (FAP)

What Are the Signs and Symptoms of Small Intestine Cancer?

Signs and symptoms of small intestine cancer include unexplained weight loss and abdominal pain. These and other signs and symptoms may be caused by small intestine cancer or by other conditions. Check with your doctor if you have any of the following:

- Pain or cramps in the middle of the abdomen
- Weight loss with no known reason
- A lump in the abdomen
- Blood in the stool

How Is Small Intestine Cancer Diagnosed?

Tests that examine the small intestine are used to detect (find), diagnose, and stage small intestine cancer. Procedures that make pictures of the small intestine and the area around it help diagnose small intestine cancer and show how far the cancer has spread. The process used to find out if cancer cells have spread within and around the small intestine is called staging.

In order to plan treatment, it is important to know the type of small intestine cancer and whether the tumor can be removed by surgery. Tests and procedures to detect, diagnose, and stage small intestine cancer are usually done at the same time. The following tests and procedures may be used:

- **Physical exam and history:** An exam of the body to check general signs of health, including checking for signs of disease, such as lumps or anything else that seems unusual. A history of the patient's health habits and past illnesses and treatments will also be taken.
- **Blood chemistry studies:** A procedure in which a blood sample is checked to measure the amounts of certain substances released into the blood by organs and tissues in the body. An unusual (higher or lower than normal) amount of a substance can be a sign of disease.
- **Liver function tests:** A procedure in which a blood sample is checked to measure the amounts of certain substances released into the blood by the liver. A higher than normal amount of a substance can be a sign of liver disease that may be caused by small intestine cancer.
- **Endoscopy:** A procedure to look at organs and tissues inside the body to check for abnormal areas. There are different types of endoscopy:
    - **Upper endoscopy:** A procedure to look at the inside of the esophagus, stomach, and duodenum (first part of the small intestine, near the stomach). An endoscope is inserted through the mouth and into the esophagus, stomach, and duodenum. An endoscope is a thin, tube-like instrument with a light and a lens for viewing. It may also have a tool to remove tissue samples, which are checked under a microscope for signs of cancer.
    - **Capsule endoscopy:** A procedure to look at the inside of the small intestine. A capsule that is about the size of a large pill and contains a light and a tiny wireless camera is swallowed by the patient. The capsule travels through the digestive tract, including the small intestine, and sends many pictures of the inside of the digestive tract to a recorder that is worn around the waist or over the shoulder. The pictures are sent from the recorder to a computer and viewed by the

doctor who checks for signs of cancer. The capsule passes out of the body during a bowel movement.

- **Double balloon endoscopy:** A procedure to look at the inside of the small intestine. A special instrument made up of two tubes (one inside the other) is inserted through the mouth or rectum and into the small intestine. The inside tube (an endoscope with a light and lens for viewing) is moved through part of the small intestine and a balloon at the end of it is inflated to keep the endoscope in place. Next, the outer tube is moved through the small intestine to reach the end of the endoscope, and a balloon at the end of the outer tube is inflated to keep it in place. Then, the balloon at the end of the endoscope is deflated and the endoscope is moved through the next part of the small intestine. These steps are repeated many times as the tubes move through the small intestine. The doctor is able to see the inside of the small intestine through the endoscope and use a tool to remove samples of abnormal tissue. The tissue samples are checked under a microscope for signs of cancer. This procedure may be done if the results of a capsule endoscopy are abnormal. This procedure is also called double balloon enteroscopy.

- **Laparotomy:** A surgical procedure in which an incision (cut) is made in the wall of the abdomen to check the inside of the abdomen for signs of disease. The size of the incision depends on the reason the laparotomy is being done. Sometimes organs or lymph nodes are removed or tissue samples are taken and checked under a microscope for signs of disease.
- **Biopsy:** The removal of cells or tissues so they can be viewed under a microscope to check for signs of cancer. This may be done during an endoscopy or laparotomy. The sample is checked by a pathologist to see if it contains cancer cells.
- **Upper gastrointestinal (GI) series with small bowel follow-through:** A series of X-rays of the esophagus, stomach, and small bowel. The patient drinks a liquid that contains barium (a silver-white metallic compound). The liquid coats the esophagus, stomach, and small bowel. X-rays are taken at different times as the barium travels through the upper GI tract and small bowel.
- **Computed tomography (CT)/computerized axial tomography(CAT) scan:** A procedure that makes a series of detailed

pictures of areas inside the body, taken from different angles. The pictures are made by a computer linked to an X-ray machine. A dye may be injected into a vein or swallowed to help the organs or tissues show up more clearly. This procedure is also called computed tomography, computerized tomography, or computerized axial tomography.

- **Magnetic resonance imaging (MRI):** A procedure that uses a magnet, radio waves, and a computer to make a series of detailed pictures of areas inside the body. This procedure is also called nuclear magnetic resonance imaging (NMRI).

What Is the Prognosis for Small Intestine Cancer?

The prognosis (chance of recovery) and treatment options depend on the following:

- The type of small intestine cancer
- Whether the cancer is in the inner lining of the small intestine only or has spread into or beyond the wall of the small intestine
- Whether the cancer has spread to other places in the body, such as the lymph nodes, liver, or peritoneum (tissue that lines the wall of the abdomen and covers most of the organs in the abdomen)
- Whether the cancer can be completely removed by surgery
- Whether the cancer is newly diagnosed or has recurred

Stages of Small Intestine Cancer

Tests and procedures to stage small intestine cancer are usually done at the same time as diagnosis. Staging is used to find out how far the cancer has spread, but treatment decisions are not based on stage. Small intestine cancer is grouped according to whether or not the tumor can be completely removed by surgery. Treatment depends on whether the tumor can be removed by surgery and if the cancer is being treated as a primary tumor or is metastatic cancer.

Treatment Option Overview

Different types of treatments are available for patients with small intestine cancer. Some treatments are standard (the currently used treatment), and some are being tested in clinical trials. A treatment clinical trial is a research study meant to help improve current treatments or obtain information on new treatments for patients with cancer. When clinical trials show that a new treatment is better than the standard treatment, the new treatment may become the standard treatment. Patients may want to think about taking part in a clinical trial. Some clinical trials are open only to patients who have not started treatment.

Standard Treatment Options Available for Patients with Small Intestine Cancer

Three types of standard treatment are used:

Surgery

Surgery is the most common treatment of small intestine cancer. One of the following types of surgery may be done:

- **Resection:** Surgery to remove part or all of an organ that contains cancer. The resection may include the small intestine and nearby organs (if the cancer has spread). The doctor may remove the section of the small intestine that contains cancer and perform an anastomosis (joining the cut ends of the intestine together). The doctor will usually remove lymph nodes near the small intestine and examine them under a microscope to see whether they contain cancer.
- **Bypass:** Surgery to allow food in the small intestine to go around (bypass) a tumor that is blocking the intestine but cannot be removed.

Even if the doctor removes all the cancer that can be seen at the time of the surgery, some patients may be given radiation therapy after surgery to kill any cancer cells that are left. Treatment given after the surgery, to lower the risk that the cancer will come back, is called adjuvant therapy.

Radiation Therapy

Radiation therapy is a cancer treatment that uses high-energy X-rays or other types of radiation to kill cancer cells or keep them from growing. There are two types of radiation therapy:

- External radiation therapy uses a machine outside the body to send radiation toward the cancer.

- Internal radiation therapy uses a radioactive substance sealed in needles, seeds, wires, or catheters that are placed directly into or near the cancer.

The way the radiation therapy is given depends on the type of the cancer being treated. External radiation therapy is used to treat small intestine cancer.

Chemotherapy

Chemotherapy is a cancer treatment that uses drugs to stop the growth of cancer cells, either by killing the cells or by stopping them from dividing. When chemotherapy is taken by mouth or injected into a vein or muscle, the drugs enter the bloodstream and can reach cancer cells throughout the body (systemic chemotherapy). When chemotherapy is placed directly into the cerebrospinal fluid, an organ, or a body cavity such as the abdomen, the drugs mainly affect cancer cells in those areas (regional chemotherapy). The way the chemotherapy is given depends on the type and stage of the cancer being treated.

What New Types of Treatment Are Being Tested in Clinical Trials?

Biologic Therapy

Biologic therapy is a treatment that uses the patient's immune system to fight cancer. Substances made by the body or made in a laboratory are used to boost, direct, or restore the body's natural defenses against cancer. This type of cancer treatment is also called biotherapy or immunotherapy.

Radiation Therapy with Radiosensitizers

Radiosensitizers are drugs that make tumor cells more sensitive to radiation therapy. Combining radiation therapy with radiosensitizers may kill more tumor cells.

Follow-Up Tests

Some of the tests that were done to diagnose the cancer or to find out the stage of the cancer may be repeated. Some tests will be repeated in order to see how well the treatment is working. Decisions about whether to continue, change, or stop treatment may be based on the results of these tests.

Some of the tests will continue to be done from time to time after treatment has ended. The results of these tests can show if your condition has changed or if the cancer has recurred (come back). These tests are sometimes called follow-up tests or check-ups.

Chapter 37

Colorectal Cancer

The colon is part of the body's digestive system. The digestive system removes and processes nutrients (vitamins, minerals, carbohydrates, fats, proteins, and water) from foods and helps pass waste material out of the body. The digestive system is made up of the mouth, throat, esophagus, stomach, and the small and large intestines. The colon (large bowel) is the first part of the large intestine and is about 5 feet long. Together, the rectum and anal canal make up the last part of the large intestine and are 6–8 inches long. The anal canal ends at the anus (the opening of the large intestine to the outside of the body).

Cancer that begins in the colon is called colon cancer, and cancer that begins in the rectum is called rectal cancer. Cancer that affects either of these organs may also be called colorectal cancer.

Colorectal cancer is the second leading cause of death from cancer in the United States. The number of new colorectal cancer cases and

---

This chapter contains text excerpted from the following sources: Text in this chapter begins with excerpts from "Colorectal Cancer Prevention (PDQ®)—Patient Version," National Cancer Institute (NCI), March 9, 2018; Text beginning with the heading "What Are the Risk Factors for Colorectal Cancer?" is excerpted from "Colorectal (Colon) Cancer—Basic Information about Colorectal Cancer," Centers for Disease Control and Prevention (CDC), April 25, 2016; Text under the heading "Colon Cancer Treatment" is excerpted from "Colon Cancer Treatment (PDQ®)—Patient Version," National Cancer Institute (NCI), December 7, 2017; Text under the heading "Rectal Cancer Treatment" is excerpted from "Rectal Cancer Treatment (PDQ®)—Patient Version," National Cancer Institute (NCI), February 16, 2018.

the number of deaths from colorectal cancer are both decreasing a little bit each year. However, in adults younger than 50 years, the number of new colorectal cancer cases has slowly increased since 1998. The number of new colorectal cancers and deaths from colorectal cancer are higher in African Americans than in other races.

Finding and treating colorectal cancer early may prevent death from colorectal cancer. Screening tests may be used to help find colorectal cancer.

What Are the Risk Factors for Colorectal Cancer?

Your risk of getting colorectal cancer increases as you get older. Other risk factors include:

having:

- Inflammatory bowel disease such as Crohn's disease or ulcerative colitis
- A personal or family history of colorectal cancer or colorectal polyps
- A genetic syndrome such as familial adenomatous polyposis (FAP) or hereditary nonpolyposis colorectal cancer (Lynch syndrome)

Lifestyle factors that may contribute to an increased risk of colorectal cancer include:

- Lack of regular physical activity
- A diet low in fruit and vegetables
- A low-fiber and high-fat diet
- Overweight and obesity
- Alcohol consumption
- Tobacco use

What Can I Do to Reduce My Risk of Colorectal Cancer?

Almost all colorectal cancers begin as precancerous polyps (abnormal growths) in the colon or rectum. Such polyps can be present in the colon for years before invasive cancer develops. They may not cause any symptoms. Colorectal cancer screening can find precancerous polyps so they can be removed before they turn into cancer. In this way, colorectal cancer is prevented. Screening can also find colorectal cancer early, when there is a greater chance that treatment will be most effective and lead to a cure.

Research is underway to find out if changes to your diet can reduce your colorectal cancer risk. Medical experts don't agree on the role of diet in preventing colorectal cancer, but often recommend a diet low in animal fats and high in fruits, vegetables, and whole grains to reduce the risk of other chronic diseases, such as coronary artery disease and diabetes. This diet also may reduce the risk of colorectal cancer. Also, researchers are examining the role of certain medicines and supplements in preventing colorectal cancer.

The U.S. Preventive Services Task Force (USPSTF) found that taking low-dose aspirin can help prevent cardiovascular disease and colorectal cancer in some adults, depending on age and risk factors.

Some studies suggest that people may reduce their risk of developing colorectal cancer by increasing physical activity, limiting alcohol consumption, and avoiding tobacco.

What Are the Symptoms of Colorectal Cancer?

Colorectal polyps and colorectal cancer don't always cause symptoms, especially at first. Someone could have polyps or colorectal cancer and not know it. That is why getting screened regularly for colorectal cancer is so important.

If you have symptoms, they may include:

- Blood in or on your stool (bowel movement)
- Stomach pain, aches, or cramps that don't go away
- Losing weight and you don't know why

If you have any of these symptoms, talk to your doctor. They may be caused by something other than cancer. The only way to know what is causing them is to see your doctor.

What Is Colorectal Cancer Screening?

A screening test is used to look for a disease when a person doesn't have symptoms. (When a person has symptoms, diagnostic tests are used to find out the cause of the symptoms.) Colorectal cancer almost always develops from precancerous polyps (abnormal growths) in the colon or rectum. Screening tests can find precancerous polyps, so that they can be removed before they turn into cancer. Screening tests can also find colorectal cancer early, when treatment works best.

When Should I Begin to Get Screened?

You should begin screening for colorectal cancer soon after turning 50, then continue getting screened at regular intervals. However, you may need to be tested earlier than 50, or more often than other people, if:

- You or a close relative have had colorectal polyps or colorectal cancer
- You have an inflammatory bowel disease such as Crohn's disease or ulcerative colitis
- You have a genetic syndrome such as familial adenomatous polyposis (FAP) or hereditary nonpolyposis colorectal cancer (Lynch syndrome)

If you think you are at increased risk for colorectal cancer, speak with your doctor about:

- When to begin screening
- Which test is right for you
- How often to get tested

Free or Low-Cost Screening

Six states in Centers for Disease Control and Prevention's (CDC) Colorectal Cancer Control Program (CRCCP) provide colorectal cancer screening to some people. Those eligible are low-income men and women aged 50–64 years who are underinsured or uninsured for screening, when resources are available and there is no other payment option.

Colorectal cancer screening tests may be covered by your health insurance policy without a deductible or copay.

Colon Cancer Treatment

Six types of standard treatment are used:

Surgery

Surgery (removing the cancer in an operation) is the most common treatment for all stages of colon cancer. A doctor may remove the cancer using one of the following types of surgery:

- **Local excision:** If the cancer is found at a very early stage, the doctor may remove it without cutting through the abdominal wall. Instead, the doctor may put a tube with a cutting tool through the rectum into the colon and cut the cancer out. This is called a local excision. If the cancer is found in a polyp (a small bulging area of tissue), the operation is called a polypectomy.
- **Resection of the colon with anastomosis:** If the cancer is larger, the doctor will perform a partial colectomy (removing the cancer and a small amount of healthy tissue around it). The doctor may then perform an anastomosis (sewing the healthy parts of the colon together). The doctor will also usually remove lymph nodes near the colon and examine them under a microscope to see whether they contain cancer.
- **Resection of the colon with colostomy:** If the doctor is not able to sew the 2 ends of the colon back together, a stoma (an opening) is made on the outside of the body for waste to pass through. This procedure is called a colostomy. A bag is placed around the stoma to collect the waste. Sometimes the colostomy is needed only until the lower colon has healed, and then it can be reversed. If the doctor needs to remove the entire lower colon, however, the colostomy may be permanent.

Even if the doctor removes all the cancer that can be seen at the time of the operation, some patients may be given chemotherapy or radiation therapy after surgery to kill any cancer cells that are left. Treatment given after the surgery, to lower the risk that the cancer will come back, is called adjuvant therapy.

Radiofrequency Ablation

Radiofrequency ablation is the use of a special probe with tiny electrodes that kill cancer cells. Sometimes the probe is inserted directly through the skin and only local anesthesia is needed. In other cases, the probe is inserted through an incision in the abdomen. This is done in the hospital with general anesthesia.

Cryosurgery

Cryosurgery is a treatment that uses an instrument to freeze and destroy abnormal tissue. This type of treatment is also called cryotherapy.

Chemotherapy

Chemotherapy is a cancer treatment that uses drugs to stop the growth of cancer cells, either by killing the cells or by stopping them from dividing. When chemotherapy is taken by mouth or injected into a vein or muscle, the drugs enter the bloodstream and can reach cancer cells throughout the body (systemic chemotherapy). When chemotherapy is placed directly into the cerebrospinal fluid, an organ, or a body cavity such as the abdomen, the drugs mainly affect cancer cells in those areas (regional chemotherapy).

Chemoembolization of the hepatic artery may be used to treat cancer that has spread to the liver. This involves blocking the hepatic artery (the main artery that supplies blood to the liver) and injecting anticancer drugs between the blockage and the liver. The liver's arteries then deliver the drugs throughout the liver. Only a small amount of the drug reaches other parts of the body. The blockage may be temporary or permanent, depending on what is used to block the artery. The liver continues to receive some blood from the hepatic portal vein, which carries blood from the stomach and intestine.

The way the chemotherapy is given depends on the type and stage of the cancer being treated.

Radiation Therapy

Radiation therapy is a cancer treatment that uses high-energy X-rays or other types of radiation to kill cancer cells or keep them from growing. There are two types of radiation therapy:

- External radiation therapy uses a machine outside the body to send radiation toward the cancer.
- Internal radiation therapy uses a radioactive substance sealed in needles, seeds, wires, or catheters that are placed directly into or near the cancer.

The way the radiation therapy is given depends on the type and stage of the cancer being treated. External radiation therapy is used as palliative therapy to relieve symptoms and improve quality of life.

Targeted Therapy

Targeted therapy is a type of treatment that uses drugs or other substances to identify and attack specific cancer cells without harming normal cells.

Types of targeted therapies used in the treatment of colon cancer include the following:

- **Monoclonal antibodies:** Monoclonal antibodies are made in the laboratory from a single type of immune system cell. These antibodies can identify substances on cancer cells or normal substances that may help cancer cells grow. The antibodies attach to the substances and kill the cancer cells, block their growth, or keep them from spreading. Monoclonal antibodies are given by infusion. They may be used alone or to carry drugs, toxins, or radioactive material directly to cancer cells.
    - Bevacizumab and ramucirumab are types of monoclonal antibodies that bind to a protein called vascular endothelial growth factor (VEGF). This may prevent the growth of new blood vessels that tumors need to grow.
    - Cetuximab and panitumumab are types of monoclonal antibodies that bind to a protein called epidermal growth factor receptor (EGFR) on the surface of some types of cancer cells. This may stop cancer cells from growing and dividing.
- **Angiogenesis inhibitors:** Angiogenesis inhibitors stop the growth of new blood vessels that tumors need to grow.
    - Ziv-aflibercept is a vascular endothelial growth factor trap that blocks an enzyme needed for the growth of new blood vessels in tumors.
    - Regorafenib is used to treat colorectal cancer that has spread to other parts of the body and has not gotten better with other treatment. It blocks the action of certain proteins, including vascular endothelial growth factor. This may help keep cancer cells from growing and may kill them. It may also prevent the growth of new blood vessels that tumors need to grow.

Rectal Cancer Treatment

Five types of standard treatment are used:

Surgery

Surgery is the most common treatment for all stages of rectal cancer. The cancer is removed using one of the following types of surgery:

- **Polypectomy:** If the cancer is found in a polyp (a small piece of bulging tissue), the polyp is often removed during a colonoscopy.

- **Local excision:** If the cancer is found on the inside surface of the rectum and has not spread into the wall of the rectum, the cancer and a small amount of surrounding healthy tissue is removed.
- **Resection:** If the cancer has spread into the wall of the rectum, the section of the rectum with cancer and nearby healthy tissue is removed. Sometimes the tissue between the rectum and the abdominal wall is also removed. The lymph nodes near the rectum are removed and checked under a microscope for signs of cancer.
- **Radiofrequency ablation:** The use of a special probe with tiny electrodes that kill cancer cells. Sometimes the probe is inserted directly through the skin and only local anesthesia is needed. In other cases, the probe is inserted through an incision in the abdomen. This is done in the hospital with general anesthesia.
- **Cryosurgery:** A treatment that uses an instrument to freeze and destroy abnormal tissue. This type of treatment is also called cryotherapy.
- **Pelvic exenteration:** If the cancer has spread to other organs near the rectum, the lower colon, rectum, and bladder are removed. In women, the cervix, vagina, ovaries, and nearby lymph nodes may be removed. In men, the prostate may be removed. Artificial openings (stoma) are made for urine and stool to flow from the body to a collection bag.

After the cancer is removed, the surgeon will either:

- do an anastomosis (sew the healthy parts of the rectum together, sew the remaining rectum to the colon, or sew the colon to the anus);

or

- make a stoma (an opening) from the rectum to the outside of the body for waste to pass through. This procedure is done if the cancer is too close to the anus and is called a colostomy. A bag is placed around the stoma to collect the waste. Sometimes the colostomy is needed only until the rectum has healed, and then it can be reversed. If the entire rectum is removed, however, the colostomy may be permanent.

Radiation therapy and/or chemotherapy may be given before surgery to shrink the tumor, make it easier to remove the cancer, and help with bowel control after surgery. Treatment given before surgery is called neoadjuvant therapy. Even if all the cancer that can be seen at the time of the operation is removed, some patients may be given radiation therapy and/or chemotherapy after surgery to kill any cancer cells that are left. Treatment given after the surgery, to lower the risk that the cancer will come back, is called adjuvant therapy.

Radiation Therapy

Radiation therapy is a cancer treatment that uses high-energy X-rays or other types of radiation to kill cancer cells or keep them from growing. There are two types of radiation therapy:

- External radiation therapy uses a machine outside the body to send radiation toward the cancer.
- Internal radiation therapy uses a radioactive substance sealed in needles, seeds, wires, or catheters that are placed directly into or near the cancer.

The way the radiation therapy is given depends on the type and stage of the cancer being treated. External radiation therapy is used to treat rectal cancer.

Short-course preoperative radiation therapy is used in some types of rectal cancer. This treatment uses fewer and lower doses of radiation than standard treatment, followed by surgery several days after the last dose.

Chemotherapy

Chemotherapy is a cancer treatment that uses drugs to stop the growth of cancer cells, either by killing the cells or by stopping the cells from dividing. When chemotherapy is taken by mouth or injected into a vein or muscle, the drugs enter the bloodstream and can reach cancer cells throughout the body (systemic chemotherapy). When chemotherapy is placed directly in the cerebrospinal fluid, an organ, or a body cavity such as the abdomen, the drugs mainly affect cancer cells in those areas (regional chemotherapy).

Chemoembolization of the hepatic artery is a type of regional chemotherapy that may be used to treat cancer that has spread to the liver. This is done by blocking the hepatic artery (the main artery that supplies blood to the liver) and injecting anticancer drugs between the blockage and the liver. The liver's arteries then carry the drugs into the liver. Only a small amount of the drug reaches other parts of the body. The blockage may be temporary or permanent, depending on what is used to block the artery. The liver continues to receive some blood from the hepatic portal vein, which carries blood from the stomach and intestine.

The way the chemotherapy is given depends on the type and stage of the cancer being treated.

Active Surveillance

Active surveillance is closely following a patient's condition without giving any treatment unless there are changes in test results. It is used to find early signs that the condition is getting worse. In active surveillance, patients are given certain exams and tests to check if the cancer is growing. When the cancer begins to grow, treatment is given to cure the cancer. Tests include the following:

- Digital rectal exam
- MRI
- Endoscopy
- Sigmoidoscopy
- CT scan
- Carcinoembryonic antigen (CEA) assay

Targeted Therapy

Targeted therapy is a type of treatment that uses drugs or other substances to identify and attack specific cancer cells without harming normal cells. Types of targeted therapies used in the treatment of rectal cancer include the following:

- **Monoclonal antibodies:** Monoclonal antibody therapy is a type of targeted therapy being used for the treatment of rectal cancer. Monoclonal antibody therapy uses antibodies made in the laboratory from a single type of immune system cell. These antibodies can identify substances on cancer cells or normal substances that may help cancer cells grow. The antibodies attach to the substances and kill the cancer cells, block their growth, or keep them from spreading. Monoclonal antibodies are given by infusion. They may be used alone or to carry drugs, toxins, or radioactive material directly to cancer cells.
    - Bevacizumab and ramucirumab are types of monoclonal antibodies that bind to a protein called vascular endothelial

growth factor (VEGF). This may prevent the growth of new blood vessels that tumors need to grow.

- Cetuximab and panitumumab are types of monoclonal antibodies that bind to a protein called epidermal growth factor receptor (EGFR) on the surface of some types of cancer cells. This may stop cancer cells from growing and dividing.

- **Angiogenesis inhibitors:** Angiogenesis inhibitors stop the growth of new blood vessels that tumors need to grow.
  - Ziv-aflibercept is a vascular endothelial growth factor trap that blocks an enzyme needed for the growth of new blood vessels in tumors.
  - Regorafenib is used to treat colorectal cancer that has spread to other parts of the body and has not gotten better with other treatment. It blocks the action of certain proteins, including vascular endothelial growth factor. This may help keep cancer cells from growing and may kill them. It may also prevent the growth of new blood vessels that tumors need to grow.

Chapter 38

Anal Cancer

The anus is the end of the large intestine, below the rectum, through which stool (solid waste) leaves the body. The anus is formed partly from the outer skin layers of the body and partly from the intestine. Two ring-like muscles, called sphincter muscles, open and close the anal opening and let stool pass out of the body. The anal canal, the part of the anus between the rectum and the anal opening, is about 1-1½ inches long.

What Is Anal Cancer?

Anal cancer is a disease in which malignant (cancer) cells form in the tissues of the anus. The skin around the outside of the anus is called the perianal area. Tumors in this area are skin tumors, not anal cancer.

What Are the Risk Factors for Anal Cancer?

Being infected with the human papillomavirus (HPV) increases the risk of developing anal cancer. Risk factors include the following:

- Being infected with human papillomavirus (HPV)
- Having many sexual partners

This chapter includes text excerpted from "Anal Cancer Treatment (PDQ®)—Patient Version," National Cancer Institute (NCI), January 25, 2018.

- Having receptive anal intercourse (anal sex)
- Being older than 50 years
- Frequent anal redness, swelling, and soreness
- Having anal fistulas (abnormal openings)
- Smoking cigarettes

What Are the Signs and Symptoms of Anal Cancer?

Signs of anal cancer include bleeding from the anus or rectum or a lump near the anus. These and other signs and symptoms may be caused by anal cancer or by other conditions. Check with your doctor if you have any of the following:

- Bleeding from the anus or rectum
- Pain or pressure in the area around the anus
- Itching or discharge from the anus
- A lump near the anus
- A change in bowel habits

How Is Anal Cancer Diagnosed?

Tests that examine the rectum and anus are used to detect (find) and diagnose anal cancer. The following tests and procedures may be used:

- **Physical exam and history:** An exam of the body to check general signs of health, including checking for signs of disease, such as lumps or anything else that seems unusual. A history of the patient's health habits and past illnesses and treatments will also be taken.
- **Digital rectal examination (DRE):** An exam of the anus and rectum. The doctor or nurse inserts a lubricated, gloved finger into the lower part of the rectum to feel for lumps or anything else that seems unusual.
- **Anoscopy:** An exam of the anus and lower rectum using a short, lighted tube called an anoscope.
- **Proctoscopy:** An exam of the rectum using a short, lighted tube called a proctoscope.

- **Endo-anal or endorectal ultrasound:** A procedure in which an ultrasound transducer (probe) is inserted into the anus or rectum and used to bounce high-energy sound waves (ultrasound) off internal tissues or organs and make echoes. The echoes form a picture of body tissues called a sonogram.
- **Biopsy:** The removal of cells or tissues so they can be viewed under a microscope by a pathologist to check for signs of cancer. If an abnormal area is seen during the anoscopy, a biopsy may be done at that time.

What Is the Prognosis for Anal Cancer?

The prognosis (chance of recovery) depends on the following:

- The size of the tumor
- Where the tumor is in the anus
- Whether the cancer has spread to the lymph nodes

The treatment options depend on the following:

- The stage of the cancer
- Where the tumor is in the anus
- Whether the patient has human immunodeficiency virus (HIV)
- Whether cancer remains after initial treatment or has recurred

Stages of Anal Cancer

After anal cancer has been diagnosed, tests are done to find out if cancer cells have spread within the anus or to other parts of the body. The process used to find out if cancer has spread within the anus or to other parts of the body is called staging. The information gathered from the staging process determines the stage of the disease. It is important to know the stage in order to plan treatment. The following tests may be used in the staging process:

- **Computed tomography (CT)/computerized axial tomography (CAT) scan:** A procedure that makes a series of detailed pictures of areas inside the body, such as the abdomen or chest, taken from different angles. The pictures are made by a computer linked to an X-ray machine. A dye may be injected into a vein or swallowed to help the organs or tissues show up more clearly. For anal cancer, a CT scan of the pelvis and abdomen may be done.

- **Chest X-ray:** An X-ray of the organs and bones inside the chest. An X-ray is a type of energy beam that can go through the body and onto film, making a picture of areas inside the body.
- **Magnetic resonance imaging (MRI):** A procedure that uses a magnet, radio waves, and a computer to make a series of detailed pictures of areas inside the body. This procedure is also called nuclear magnetic resonance imaging (NMRI).
- **Positron emission tomography (PET) scan:** A procedure to find malignant tumor cells in the body. A small amount of radioactive glucose (sugar) is injected into a vein. The PET scanner rotates around the body and makes a picture of where glucose is being used in the body. Malignant tumor cells show up brighter in the picture because they are more active and take up more glucose than normal cells do.
- **Pelvic exam:** An exam of the vagina, cervix, uterus, fallopian tubes, ovaries, and rectum. A speculum is inserted into the vagina and the doctor or nurse looks at the vagina and cervix for signs of disease. A Pap test of the cervix is usually done. The doctor or nurse also inserts one or two lubricated, gloved fingers of one hand into the vagina and places the other hand over the lower abdomen to feel the size, shape, and position of the uterus and ovaries. The doctor or nurse also inserts a lubricated, gloved finger into the rectum to feel for lumps or abnormal areas.

The following stages are used for anal cancer:

Stage 0. In stage 0, abnormal cells are found in the mucosa (innermost layer) of the anus. These abnormal cells may become cancer and spread into nearby normal tissue. Stage 0 is also called high-grade squamous intraepithelial lesion (HSIL).

Stage I. In stage I, cancer has formed and the tumor is 2 centimeters or smaller.

Stage II. Stage II anal cancer is divided into stages IIA and IIB.

- In stage IIA, the tumor is larger than 2 centimeters but not larger than 5 centimeters.
- In stage IIB, the tumor is larger than 5 centimeters.

Stage III. Stage III anal cancer is divided into stages IIIA, IIIB, and IIIC.

- In stage IIIA, the tumor is 5 centimeters or smaller and has spread to lymph nodes near the anus or groin.
- In stage IIIB, the tumor is any size and has spread to nearby organs, such as the vagina, urethra, or bladder. Cancer has not spread to lymph nodes.
- In stage IIIC, the tumor is any size and may have spread to nearby organs. Cancer has spread to lymph nodes near the anus or groin.

Stage IV. In stage IV, the tumor is any size. Cancer may have spread to lymph nodes or nearby organs and has spread to other parts of the body, such as the liver or lungs.

Treatment Option Overview

Different types of treatments are available for patients with anal cancer. Some treatments are standard (the currently used treatment), and some are being tested in clinical trials. A treatment clinical trial is a research study meant to help improve current treatments or obtain information on new treatments for patients with cancer. When clinical trials show that a new treatment is better than the standard treatment, the new treatment may become the standard treatment. Patients may want to think about taking part in a clinical trial. Some clinical trials are open only to patients who have not started treatment.

Standard Treatment Options for Anal Cancer

Three types of standard treatment are used:

Radiation Therapy

Radiation therapy is a cancer treatment that uses high-energy X-rays or other types of radiation to kill cancer cells or keep them from growing. There are two types of radiation therapy:

- External radiation therapy uses a machine outside the body to send radiation toward the cancer.
- Internal radiation therapy uses a radioactive substance sealed in needles, seeds, wires, or catheters that are placed directly into or near the cancer.

The way the radiation therapy is given depends on the type and stage of the cancer being treated. External and internal radiation therapy are used to treat anal cancer.

Chemotherapy

Chemotherapy is a cancer treatment that uses drugs to stop the growth of cancer cells, either by killing the cells or by stopping the cells from dividing. When chemotherapy is taken by mouth or injected into a vein or muscle, the drugs enter the bloodstream and can reach cancer cells throughout the body (systemic chemotherapy). When chemotherapy is placed directly into the cerebrospinal fluid, an organ, or a body cavity such as the abdomen, the drugs mainly affect cancer cells in those areas (regional chemotherapy). The way the chemotherapy is given depends on the type and stage of the cancer being treated.

Surgery

- **Local resection:** A surgical procedure in which the tumor is cut from the anus along with some of the healthy tissue around it. Local resection may be used if the cancer is small and has not spread. This procedure may save the sphincter muscles so the patient can still control bowel movements. Tumors that form in the lower part of the anus can often be removed with local resection.
- **Abdominoperineal resection:** A surgical procedure in which the anus, the rectum, and part of the sigmoid colon are removed through an incision made in the abdomen. The doctor sews the end of the intestine to an opening, called a stoma, made in the surface of the abdomen so body waste can be collected in a disposable bag outside of the body. This is called a colostomy. Lymph nodes that contain cancer may also be removed during this operation.

Treatment for anal cancer may cause side effects. Cancer therapy can further damage the already weakened immune systems of patients who have the human immunodeficiency virus (HIV). For this reason, patients who have anal cancer and HIV are usually treated with lower doses of anticancer drugs and radiation than patients who do not have HIV.

New Types of Treatment Tested in Clinical Trials

Radiosensitizers

Radiosensitizers are drugs that make tumor cells more sensitive to radiation therapy. Combining radiation therapy with radiosensitizers may kill more tumor cells.

Follow-Up Tests

Some of the tests that were done to diagnose the cancer or to find out the stage of the cancer may be repeated. Some tests will be repeated in order to see how well the treatment is working. Decisions about whether to continue, change, or stop treatment may be based on the results of these tests.

Some of the tests will continue to be done from time to time after treatment has ended. The results of these tests can show if your condition has changed or if the cancer has recurred (come back). These tests are sometimes called follow-up tests or check-ups.

Chapter 39

Kidney Cancers

Chapter Contents

Section 39.1

Renal Cell Cancer

This section includes text excerpted from "Renal Cell Cancer Treatment (PDQ®)—Patient Version," National Cancer Institute (NCI), February 21, 2018.

There are two kidneys, one on each side of the backbone, above the waist. Tiny tubules in the kidneys filter and clean the blood. They take out waste products and make urine. The urine passes from each kidney through a long tube called a ureter into the bladder. The bladder holds the urine until it passes through the urethra and leaves the body.

General Information about Renal Cell Cancer

What Is Renal Cell Cancer?

Renal cell cancer (also called kidney cancer or renal adenocarcinoma) is a disease in which malignant (cancer) cells are found in the lining of tubules (very small tubes) in the kidney. Cancer that starts in the ureters or the renal pelvis (the part of the kidney that collects urine and drains it to the ureters) is different from renal cell cancer.

What Are the Risk Factors for Renal Cell Cancer?

Anything that increases your risk of getting a disease is called a risk factor. Having a risk factor does not mean that you will get cancer; not having risk factors doesn't mean that you will not get cancer. Talk with your doctor if you think you may be at risk.

Smoking and misuse of certain pain medicines can affect the risk of renal cell cancer. Risk factors for renal cell cancer include the following:

- Smoking
- Misusing certain pain medicines, including over-the-counter pain medicines, for a long time
- Being overweight
- Having high blood pressure

- Having a family history of renal cell cancer
- Having certain genetic conditions, such as von Hippel-Lindau disease or hereditary papillary renal cell carcinoma

What Are the Signs and Symptoms of Renal Cell Cancer?

Signs of renal cell cancer include blood in the urine and a lump in the abdomen. These and other signs and symptoms may be caused by renal cell cancer or by other conditions. There may be no signs or symptoms in the early stages. Signs and symptoms may appear as the tumor grows. Check with your doctor if you have any of the following:

- Blood in the urine
- A lump in the abdomen
- A pain in the side that doesn't go away
- Loss of appetite
- Weight loss for no known reason
- Anemia

How Is Renal Cell Cancer Diagnosed?

Tests that examine the abdomen and kidneys are used to detect (find) and diagnose renal cell cancer. The following tests and procedures may be used:

- **Physical exam and history:** An exam of the body to check general signs of health, including checking for signs of disease, such as lumps or anything else that seems unusual. A history of the patient's health habits and past illnesses and treatments will also be taken.
- **Ultrasound exam:** A procedure in which high-energy sound waves (ultrasound) are bounced off internal tissues or organs and make echoes. The echoes form a picture of body tissues called a sonogram.
- **Blood chemistry studies:** A procedure in which a blood sample is checked to measure the amounts of certain substances released into the blood by organs and tissues in the body. An

unusual (higher or lower than normal) amount of a substance can be a sign of disease.

- **Urinalysis:** A test to check the color of urine and its contents, such as sugar, protein, red blood cells, and white blood cells.
- **Liver function test:** A procedure in which a sample of blood is checked to measure the amounts of enzymes released into it by the liver. An abnormal amount of an enzyme can be a sign that cancer has spread to the liver. Certain conditions that are not cancer may also increase liver enzyme levels.
- **Intravenous pyelogram (IVP):** A series of X-rays of the kidneys, ureters, and bladder to find out if cancer is present in these organs. A contrast dye is injected into a vein. As the contrast dye moves through the kidneys, ureters, and bladder, X-rays are taken to see if there are any blockages.
- **Computed tomography(CT)/computerized axial tomography (CAT) scan:** A procedure that makes a series of detailed pictures of areas inside the body, taken from different angles. The pictures are made by a computer linked to an X-ray machine. A dye may be injected into a vein or swallowed to help the organs or tissues show up more clearly. This procedure is also called computed tomography, computerized tomography, or computerized axial tomography.
- **Magnetic resonance imaging (MRI):** A procedure that uses a magnet, radio waves, and a computer to make a series of detailed pictures of areas inside the body. This procedure is also called nuclear magnetic resonance imaging (NMRI).
- **Biopsy:** The removal of cells or tissues so they can be viewed under a microscope by a pathologist to check for signs of cancer. To do a biopsy for renal cell cancer, a thin needle is inserted into the tumor and a sample of tissue is withdrawn.

What Is the Prognosis for Renal Cell Cancer?

The prognosis (chance of recovery) and treatment options depend on the following:

- The stage of the disease
- The patient's age and general health

Stages of Renal Cell Cancer

How Is Staging Done for Renal Cell Cancer?

The process used to find out if cancer has spread within the kidney or to other parts of the body is called staging. The information gathered from the staging process determines the stage of the disease. It is important to know the stage in order to plan treatment. The following tests and procedures may be used in the staging process:

- **CT/CAT scan:** A procedure that makes a series of detailed pictures of areas inside the body, taken from different angles. The pictures are made by a computer linked to an X-ray machine. A dye may be injected into a vein or swallowed to help the organs or tissues show up more clearly.
- **Magnetic resonance imaging (MRI):** A procedure that uses a magnet, radio waves, and a computer to make a series of detailed pictures of areas inside the body. This procedure is also called nuclear magnetic resonance imaging (NMRI).
- **Chest X-ray:** An X-ray of the organs and bones inside the chest. An X-ray is a type of energy beam that can go through the body and onto film, making a picture of areas inside the body.

The following stages are used for renal cell cancer:

Stage I. In stage I, the tumor is 7 centimeters or smaller and is found only in the kidney.

Stage II. In stage II, the tumor is larger than 7 centimeters and is found only in the kidney.

Stage III. In stage III:

- the tumor is any size and cancer is found only in the kidney and in 1 or more nearby lymph nodes; or
- cancer is found in the main blood vessels of the kidney or in the layer of fatty tissue around the kidney. Cancer may be found in 1 or more nearby lymph nodes.

Stage IV. In stage IV, cancer has spread:

- beyond the layer of fatty tissue around the kidney and may be found in the adrenal gland above the kidney with cancer, or in nearby lymph nodes; or

- to other organs, such as the lungs, liver, bones, or brain, and may have spread to lymph nodes.

Treatment Option Overview

Different types of treatments are available for patients with renal cell cancer. Some treatments are standard (the currently used treatment), and some are being tested in clinical trials. A treatment clinical trial is a research study meant to help improve current treatments or obtain information on new treatments for patients with cancer. When clinical trials show that a new treatment is better than the standard treatment, the new treatment may become the standard treatment. Patients may want to think about taking part in a clinical trial. Some clinical trials are open only to patients who have not started treatment.

What Are the Standard Treatment Options Available for Patients with Renal Cell Cancer?

Five types of standard treatment are used:

Surgery

Surgery to remove part or all of the kidney is often used to treat renal cell cancer. The following types of surgery may be used:

- **Partial nephrectomy:** A surgical procedure to remove the cancer within the kidney and some of the tissue around it. A partial nephrectomy may be done to prevent loss of kidney function when the other kidney is damaged or has already been removed.
- **Simple nephrectomy:** A surgical procedure to remove the kidney only.
- **Radical nephrectomy:** A surgical procedure to remove the kidney, the adrenal gland, surrounding tissue, and, usually, nearby lymph nodes.

A person can live with part of 1 working kidney, but if both kidneys are removed or not working, the person will need dialysis (a procedure to clean the blood using a machine outside of the body) or a kidney transplant (replacement with a healthy donated kidney). A kidney transplant may be done when the disease is in the kidney only and a donated kidney can be found. If the patient has to wait for a donated kidney, other treatment is given as needed.

When surgery to remove the cancer is not possible, a treatment called arterial embolization may be used to shrink the tumor. A small incision is made and a catheter (thin tube) is inserted into the main blood vessel that flows to the kidney. Small pieces of a special gelatin sponge are injected through the catheter into the blood vessel. The sponges block the blood flow to the kidney and prevent the cancer cells from getting oxygen and other substances they need to grow.

Even if the doctor removes all the cancer that can be seen at the time of the surgery, some patients may be given chemotherapy or radiation therapy after surgery to kill any cancer cells that are left. Treatment given after the surgery, to lower the risk that the cancer will come back, is called adjuvant therapy.

Radiation Therapy

Radiation therapy is a cancer treatment that uses high-energy X-rays or other types of radiation to kill cancer cells or keep them from growing. There are two types of radiation therapy:

- External radiation therapy uses a machine outside the body to send radiation toward the cancer.
- Internal radiation therapy uses a radioactive substance sealed in needles, seeds, wires, or catheters that are placed directly into or near the cancer.

The way the radiation therapy is given depends on the type and stage of the cancer being treated. External radiation therapy is used to treat renal cell cancer, and may also be used as palliative therapy to relieve symptoms and improve quality of life.

Chemotherapy

Chemotherapy is a cancer treatment that uses drugs to stop the growth of cancer cells, either by killing the cells or by stopping them from dividing. When chemotherapy is taken by mouth or injected into a vein or muscle, the drugs enter the bloodstream and can reach cancer cells throughout the body (systemic chemotherapy). When chemotherapy is placed directly into the cerebrospinal fluid, an organ, or a body cavity such as the abdomen, the drugs mainly affect cancer cells in those areas (regional chemotherapy). The way the chemotherapy is given depends on the type and stage of the cancer being treated.

Biologic Therapy

Biologic therapy is a treatment that uses the patient's immune system to fight cancer. Substances made by the body or made in a laboratory are used to boost, direct, or restore the body's natural defenses against cancer. This type of cancer treatment is also called biotherapy or immunotherapy. The following types of biologic therapy are being used or studied in the treatment of renal cell cancer:

- **Nivolumab:** Nivolumab is a monoclonal antibody that boosts the body's immune response against renal cell cancer cells.
- **Interferon:** Interferon affects the division of cancer cells and can slow tumor growth.
- **Interleukin-2 (IL-2):** IL-2 boosts the growth and activity of many immune cells, especially lymphocytes (a type of white blood cell). Lymphocytes can attack and kill cancer cells.

Targeted Therapy

Targeted therapy uses drugs or other substances to identify and attack specific cancer cells without harming normal cells. Targeted therapy with antiangiogenic agents are used to treat advanced renal cell cancer. Antiangiogenic agents keep blood vessels from forming in a tumor, causing the tumor to starve and stop growing or to shrink. Monoclonal antibodies and kinase inhibitors are two types of antiangiogenic agents used to treat renal cell cancer.

Monoclonal antibody therapy uses antibodies made in the laboratory, from a single type of immune system cell. These antibodies can identify substances on cancer cells or normal substances that may help cancer cells grow. The antibodies attach to the substances and kill the cancer cells, block their growth, or keep them from spreading. Monoclonal antibodies are given by infusion. They may be used alone or to carry drugs, toxins, or radioactive material directly to cancer cells. Monoclonal antibodies used to treat renal cell cancer attach to and block substances that cause new blood vessels to form in tumors.

Kinase inhibitors stop cells from dividing and may prevent the growth of new blood vessels that tumors need to grow. An mTOR inhibitor is a type of kinase inhibitor. Everolimus and temsirolimus are mTOR inhibitors used to treat advanced renal cell cancer.

Is There a Need for Follow-Up Tests?

Some of the tests that were done to diagnose the cancer or to find out the stage of the cancer may be repeated. Some tests will be repeated

in order to see how well the treatment is working. Decisions about whether to continue, change, or stop treatment may be based on the results of these tests.

Some of the tests will continue to be done from time to time after treatment has ended. The results of these tests can show if your condition has changed or if the cancer has recurred (come back). These tests are sometimes called follow-up tests or check-ups.

Section 39.2

Wilms Tumor and Other Childhood Kidney Tumors

This section includes text excerpted from "Wilms Tumor and Other Childhood Kidney Tumors Treatment (PDQ®)—Patient Version," National Cancer Institute (NCI), December 12, 2017.

There are two kidneys, one on each side of the backbone, above the waist. Tiny tubules in the kidneys filter and clean the blood. They take out waste products and make urine. The urine passes from each kidney through a long tube called a ureter into the bladder. The bladder holds the urine until it passes through the urethra and leaves the body.

General Information about Childhood Kidney Tumors

What Are Childhood Kidney Tumors?

Childhood kidney tumors are diseases in which malignant (cancer) cells form in the tissues of the kidney.

The following are the types of childhood kidney tumors:

Wilms Tumor

In Wilms tumor, one or more tumors may be found in one or both kidneys. Wilms tumor may spread to the lungs, liver, bone, brain, or nearby lymph nodes. In children and adolescents younger than 15 years old, most kidney cancers are Wilms tumors.

Renal Cell Cancer

Renal cell cancer is rare in children and adolescents younger than 15 years old. It is much more common in adolescents between 15–19 years old. Children and adolescents are more likely to be diagnosed with a large renal cell tumor or cancer that has spread. Renal cell cancers may spread to the lungs, liver, or lymph nodes. Renal cell cancer may also be called renal cell carcinoma.

Rhabdoid Tumor of the Kidney

Rhabdoid tumor of the kidney is a type of kidney cancer that occurs mostly in infants and young children. It is often advanced at the time of diagnosis. Rhabdoid tumor of the kidney grows and spreads quickly, often to the lungs or brain.

- Children with a certain change in the *SMARCB1* gene are checked regularly to see if a rhabdoid tumor has formed in the kidney or has spread to the brain:
- Children younger than one year old have an ultrasound of the abdomen every 2–3 months and an ultrasound of the head every month.

Children 1–4 years old have an ultrasound of the abdomen and an magnetic resonance imaging (MRI) of the brain and spine every 3 months.

Clear Cell Sarcoma of the Kidney

Clear cell sarcoma of the kidney is a type of kidney tumor that may spread to the lung, bone, brain, or soft tissue. When it recurs (comes back) after treatment, it often recurs in the brain or lung.

Congenital Mesoblastic Nephroma

Congenital mesoblastic nephroma is a tumor of the kidney that is often diagnosed during the first year of life. It can usually be cured.

Ewing Sarcoma of the Kidney

Ewing sarcoma (previously called neuroepithelial tumor) of the kidney is rare and usually occurs in young adults. These tumors grow and spread to other parts of the body quickly.

Primary Renal Myoepithelial Carcinoma

Primary renal myoepithelial carcinoma is a rare type of cancer that usually affects soft tissues, but sometimes forms in the internal organs (such as the kidney). This type of cancer grows and spreads quickly.

Cystic Partially Differentiated Nephroblastoma

Cystic partially differentiated nephroblastoma is a very rare type of Wilms tumor made up of cysts.

Multilocular Cystic Nephroma

Multilocular cystic nephromas are benign tumors made up of cysts and are most common in infants, young children, and adult women. These tumors can occur in one or both kidneys.

Children with this type of tumor also may have pleuropulmonary blastoma, so imaging tests that check the lungs for cysts or solid tumors are done. Since multilocular cystic nephroma may be an inherited condition, genetic counseling and genetic testing may be considered.

Primary Renal Synovial Sarcoma

Primary renal synovial sarcoma is a cyst-like tumor of the kidney and is most common in young adults. These tumors grow and spread quickly.

Anaplastic Sarcoma of the Kidney

Anaplastic sarcoma of the kidney is a rare tumor that is most common in children or adolescents younger than 15 years of age. Anaplastic sarcoma of the kidney often spreads to the lungs, liver, or bones. Imaging tests that check the lungs for cysts or solid tumors may be done. Since anaplastic sarcoma may be an inherited condition, genetic counseling and genetic testing may be considered.

Nephroblastomatosis

Nephroblastomatosis is not cancer but may become Wilms tumor. Sometimes, after the kidneys form in the fetus, abnormal groups of kidney cells remain in one or both kidneys. In nephroblastomatosis (diffuse hyperplastic perilobar nephroblastomatosis), these abnormal groups of cells may grow in many places inside the kidney or make a thick layer around the kidney. When these groups of abnormal cells are found in a kidney after it was removed for Wilms tumor, the child has an increased risk of Wilms tumor in the other kidney. Frequent follow-up testing is important at least every 3 months, for at least 7 years after the child is treated.

What Are the Risk Factors for Wilms Tumor?

Anything that increases the risk of getting a disease is called a risk factor. Having a risk factor does not mean that you will get cancer; not having risk factors doesn't mean that you will not get cancer. Talk to your child's doctor if you think your child may be at risk.

Wilms tumor may be part of a genetic syndrome that affects growth or development. A genetic syndrome is a set of signs and symptoms or conditions that occur together and is caused by certain changes in the genes. Certain conditions can also increase a child's risk of developing Wilms tumor. These and other genetic syndromes and conditions have been linked to Wilms tumor:

- WAGR syndrome (Wilms tumor, aniridia, abnormal genitourinary system, and mental retardation)
- Denys-Drash syndrome (abnormal genitourinary system)
- Frasier syndrome (abnormal genitourinary system)
- Beckwith-Wiedemann syndrome (abnormally large growth of one side of the body or a body part, large tongue, umbilical hernia at birth, and abnormal genitourinary system)
- A family history of Wilms tumor
- Aniridia (the iris, the colored part of the eye, is missing)
- Isolated hemihyperplasia (abnormally large growth of one side of the body or a body part)
- Urinary tract problems such as cryptorchidism or hypospadias

Tests That Are Used to Screen Wilms Tumor

Screening tests are done in children with an increased risk of Wilms tumor. These tests may help find cancer early and decrease the chance of dying from cancer.

In general, children with an increased risk of Wilms tumor should be screened for Wilms tumor every 3 months until they are at least 8 years old. An ultrasound test of the abdomen is usually used for screening. Small Wilms tumors may be found and removed before symptoms occur.

Children with Beckwith-Wiedemann syndrome (BWS) or hemihyperplasia are also screened for liver and adrenal tumors that are linked to these genetic syndromes. A test to check the alpha-fetoprotein (AFP) level in the blood and an ultrasound of the abdomen are done until the child is 4 years old. An ultrasound of the kidneys is done after the child is 4 years old. In children with certain gene changes, a different schedule for ultrasound of the abdomen may be used.

Children with aniridia and a certain gene change are screened for Wilms tumor every 3 months until they are 8 years old. An ultrasound test of the abdomen is used for screening.

Some children develop Wilms tumor in both kidneys. These often appear when Wilms tumor is first diagnosed, but Wilms tumor may also occur in the second kidney after the child is successfully treated for Wilms tumor in one kidney. Children with an increased risk of a second Wilms tumor in the other kidney should be screened for Wilms tumor every 3 months for up to 8 years. An ultrasound test of the abdomen may be used for screening.

Genetic Counseling

Genetic counseling (a discussion with a trained professional about genetic diseases and whether genetic testing is needed) may be needed if the child has one of the following syndromes or conditions:

- A genetic syndrome or condition that increases the risk of Wilms tumor
- An inherited condition that increases the risk of renal cell cancer
- Rhabdoid tumor of the kidney
- Multilocular cystic nephroma

What Are the Signs and Symptoms of Wilms Tumor?

Signs of Wilms tumor and other childhood kidney tumors include a lump in the abdomen and blood in the urine. Sometimes childhood kidney tumors do not cause signs and symptoms and the parent finds a mass in the abdomen by chance or the mass is found during a well-child health check up. These and other signs and symptoms may be caused by kidney tumors or by other conditions. Check with your child's doctor if your child has any of the following:

- A lump, swelling, or pain in the abdomen
- Blood in the urine
- High blood pressure (headache, feeling very tired, chest pain, or trouble seeing or breathing)
- Hypercalcemia (loss of appetite, nausea and vomiting, weakness, or feeling very tired)
- Fever for no known reason
- Loss of appetite
- Weight loss for no known reason

Wilms tumor that has spread to the lungs or liver may cause the following signs and symptoms:

- Cough
- Blood in the sputum
- Trouble breathing
- Pain in the abdomen

How Is Wilms Tumor Diagnosed?

Tests that examine the kidney and the blood are used to detect (find) and diagnose Wilms tumor and other childhood kidney tumors. The following tests and procedures may be used:

- **Physical exam and history:** An exam of the body to check general signs of health, including checking for signs of disease, such as lumps or anything else that seems unusual. A history of the patient's health habits and past illnesses and treatments will also be taken.
- **Complete blood count (CBC):** A procedure in which a sample of blood is drawn and checked for the following:
    - The number of red blood cells, white blood cells, and platelets
    - The amount of hemoglobin (the protein that carries oxygen) in the red blood cells
    - The portion of the blood sample made up of red blood cells

- **Blood chemistry studies:** A procedure in which a blood sample is checked to measure the amounts of certain substances released into the blood by organs and tissues in the body. An unusual (higher or lower than normal) amount of a substance can be a sign of disease. This test is done to check how well the liver and kidneys are working.
- **Renal function test:** A procedure in which blood or urine samples are checked to measure the amounts of certain substances released into the blood or urine by the kidneys. A higher or lower than normal amount of a substance can be a sign that the kidneys are not working as they should.
- **Urinalysis:** A test to check the color of urine and its contents, such as sugar, protein, blood, and bacteria.
- **Ultrasound exam:** A procedure in which high-energy sound waves (ultrasound) are bounced off internal tissues or organs and make echoes. The echoes form a picture of body tissues called a sonogram. An ultrasound of the abdomen is done to diagnose a kidney tumor.
- **Computed tomography (CT)/computerized axial tomography (CAT) scan:** A procedure that makes a series of detailed pictures of areas inside the body, such as the chest, abdomen, and pelvis, taken from different angles. The pictures are made by a computer linked to an X-ray machine. A dye is injected into a vein or swallowed to help the organs or tissues show up more clearly.
- **MRI with gadolinium:** A procedure that uses a magnet, radio waves, and a computer to make a series of detailed pictures of areas inside the body, such as the abdomen. A substance called gadolinium is injected into a vein. The gadolinium collects around the cancer cells so they show up brighter in the picture. This procedure is also called nuclear magnetic resonance imaging (NMRI).
- **X-ray:** An X-ray is a type of energy beam that can go through the body and onto film, making a picture of areas inside the body, such as the chest and abdomen.
- **Positron emission tomography (PET)-CT scan:** A procedure that combines the pictures from a PET and a CT scan. The PET and CT scans are done at the same time on the same machine. The pictures from both scans are combined to make a more

detailed picture than either test would make by itself. A PET scan is a procedure to find malignant tumor cells in the body. A small amount of radioactive glucose (sugar) is injected into a vein. The PET scanner rotates around the body and makes a picture of where glucose is being used in the body. Malignant tumor cells show up brighter in the picture because they are more active and take up more glucose than normal cells do.

- **Biopsy:** The removal of cells or tissues so they can be viewed under a microscope by a pathologist to check for signs of cancer. The decision of whether to do a biopsy is based on the following:
    - The size of the tumor
    - The stage of the cancer
    - Whether cancer is in one or both kidneys
    - Whether imaging tests clearly show the cancer
    - Whether the tumor can be removed by surgery
    - Whether the patient is in a clinical trial

A biopsy may be done before any treatment is given, after chemotherapy to shrink the tumor, or after surgery to remove the tumor.

What Is the Prognosis for Wilms Tumor?

The prognosis (chance of recovery) and treatment options for Wilms tumor depend on the following:

- How different the tumor cells are from normal kidney cells when looked at under a microscope
- The stage of the cancer
- The type of tumor
- The age of the child
- Whether the tumor can be completely removed by surgery
- Whether there are certain changes in chromosomes or genes
- Whether the cancer has just been diagnosed or has recurred (come back)

The prognosis for renal cell cancer depends on the following:

- The stage of the cancer
- Whether the cancer has spread to the lymph nodes

The prognosis for rhabdoid tumor of the kidney depends on the following:

- The age of the child at the time of diagnosis
- The stage of the cancer
- Whether the cancer has spread to the brain or spinal cord

The prognosis for clear cell sarcoma of the kidney depends on the following:

- The age of the child at the time of diagnosis
- The stage of the cancer

Stages of Wilms Tumor

Wilms tumors are staged during surgery and with imaging tests. The process used to find out if cancer has spread outside of the kidney to other parts of the body is called staging. The information gathered from the staging process determines the stage of the disease. It is important to know the stage in order to plan treatment. The doctor will use results of the diagnostic and staging tests to help find out the stage of the disease.

The following tests may be done to see if cancer has spread to other places in the body:

- **Lymph node biopsy:** A surgical procedure in which lymph nodes in the abdomen are removed and a sample of tissue is checked under a microscope for signs of cancer. This procedure is also called lymphadenectomy or lymph node dissection.
- **Liver function test:** A procedure in which a blood sample is checked to measure the amounts of certain substances released into the blood by the liver. A higher than normal amount of a substance can be a sign that the liver is not working as it should.
- **X-ray of the chest and bones:** An X-ray is a type of energy beam that can go through the body and onto film, making a picture of areas inside the body, such as the chest.
- **CT/CAT scan:** A procedure that makes a series of detailed pictures of areas inside the body, such as the abdomen, pelvis, chest, and brain, taken from different angles. The pictures are made by a computer linked to an X-ray machine. A dye is

injected into a vein or swallowed to help the organs or tissues show up more clearly.

- **PET-CT scan:** A procedure that combines the pictures from a PET scan and a CT scan. The PET and CT scans are done at the same time on the same machine. The pictures from both scans are combined to make a more detailed picture than either test would make by itself. A PET scan is a procedure to find malignant tumor cells in the body. A small amount of radioactive glucose (sugar) is injected into a vein. The PET scanner rotates around the body and makes a picture of where glucose is being used in the body. Malignant tumor cells show up brighter in the picture because they are more active and take up more glucose than normal cells do.
- **MRI:** A procedure that uses a magnet, radio waves, and a computer to make a series of detailed pictures of areas inside the body, such as the abdomen, pelvis, and brain. This procedure is also called nuclear magnetic resonance imaging (NMRI).
- **Bone scan:** A procedure to check if there are rapidly dividing cells, such as cancer cells, in the bone. A very small amount of radioactive material is injected into a vein and travels through the bloodstream. The radioactive material collects in the bones with cancer and is detected by a scanner.
- **Ultrasound exam:** A procedure in which high-energy sound waves (ultrasound) are bounced off internal tissues or organs and make echoes. The echoes form a picture of body tissues called a sonogram. An ultrasound of the major heart vessels is done to stage Wilms tumor.
- **Cystoscopy:** A procedure to look inside the bladder and urethra to check for abnormal areas. A cystoscope is inserted through the urethra into the bladder. A cystoscope is a thin, tube-like instrument with a light and a lens for viewing. It may also have a tool to remove tissue samples, which are checked under a microscope for signs of cancer.

Histology of Wilms Tumors

In addition to the stages, Wilms tumors are described by their histology. The histology (how the cells look under a microscope) of the tumor affects the prognosis and the treatment of Wilms tumor. The histology may be favorable or anaplastic (unfavorable). Tumors with a favorable histology have a better prognosis and respond better to chemotherapy than anaplastic tumors. Tumor cells that are anaplastic divide quickly and under a microscope do not look like the type of cells they came from. Anaplastic tumors are harder to treat with chemotherapy than other Wilms tumors at the same stage.

The following stages are used for both favorable histology and anaplastic Wilms tumors:

Stage I. In stage I, the tumor was completely removed by surgery and all of the following are true:

- Cancer was found only in the kidney and had not spread to blood vessels in the renal sinus (the part of the kidney where it joins the ureter) or to the lymph nodes.
- The outer layer of the kidney did not break open.
- The tumor did not break open.
- A biopsy was not done before the tumor was removed.
- No cancer cells were found at the edges of the area where the tumor was removed.

Stage II. In stage II, the tumor was completely removed by surgery and no cancer cells were found at the edges of the area where the cancer was removed. Cancer has not spread to lymph nodes. Before the tumor was removed, one of the following was true:

- Cancer had spread to the renal sinus (the part of the kidney where it joins the ureter).
- Cancer had spread to blood vessels outside the area of the kidney where urine is made, such as the renal sinus.

Stage III. In stage III, cancer remains in the abdomen after surgery and one of the following may be true:

- Cancer has spread to lymph nodes in the abdomen or pelvis (the part of the body between the hips).
- Cancer has spread to or through the surface of the peritoneum (the layer of tissue that lines the abdominal cavity and covers most organs in the abdomen).
- A biopsy of the tumor was done before it was removed.
- The tumor broke open before or during surgery to remove it.

- The tumor was removed in more than one piece.
- Cancer cells are found at the edges of the area where the tumor was removed.
- The entire tumor could not be removed because important organs or tissues in the body would be damaged.

Stage IV. In stage IV, cancer has spread through the blood to organs such as the lungs, liver, bone, or brain, or to lymph nodes outside of the abdomen and pelvis.

Stage V. In stage V, cancer cells are found in both kidneys when the cancer is first diagnosed.

The treatment of other childhood kidney tumors depends on the tumor type.

Treatment Option Overview

Different types of treatment are available for children with Wilms and other childhood kidney tumors. Some treatments are standard (the currently used treatment), and some are being tested in clinical trials. A treatment clinical trial is a research study meant to help improve current treatments or obtain information on new treatments for patients with cancer. When clinical trials show that a new treatment is better than the standard treatment, the new treatment may become the standard treatment.

Because cancer in children is rare, taking part in a clinical trial should be considered. Some clinical trials are open only to patients who have not started treatment.

Healthcare Team for Children with Wilms Tumor

Children with Wilms tumor or other childhood kidney tumors should have their treatment planned by a team of healthcare providers who are experts in treating cancer in children.

Your child's treatment will be overseen by a pediatric oncologist, a doctor who specializes in treating children with cancer. The pediatric oncologist works with other pediatric healthcare providers who are experts in treating children with Wilms tumor or other childhood kidney tumors and who specialize in certain areas of medicine. These may include the following specialists:

- Pediatrician
- Pediatric surgeon or urologist

- Radiation oncologist
- Rehabilitation specialist
- Pediatric nurse specialist
- Social worker

Are There Any Side Effects of Cancer Treatments?

Side effects from cancer treatment that begin during or after treatment and continue for months or years are called late effects. Late effects of cancer treatment may include the following:

- Physical problems, such as heart problems, kidney problems, or problems during pregnancy
- Changes in mood, feelings, thinking, learning, or memory
- Second cancers (new types of cancer), such as cancer of the gastrointestinal tract or breast cancer

Some late effects may be treated or controlled. It is important to talk with your child's doctors about the effects cancer treatment can have on your child.

Clinical trials are being done to find out if lower doses of chemotherapy and radiation can be used to lessen the late effects of treatment without changing how well the treatment works.

What Are the Standard Treatment Options Available for Wilms Tumor?

Five types of standard treatment are used:

Surgery

Two types of surgery are used to treat kidney tumors:

- **Nephrectomy:** Wilms tumor and other childhood kidney tumors are usually treated with nephrectomy (surgery to remove the whole kidney). Nearby lymph nodes may also be removed and checked for signs of cancer. Sometimes a kidney transplant (surgery to remove the kidney and replace it with a kidney from a donor) is done when the cancer is in both kidneys and the kidneys are not working well.
- **Partial nephrectomy:** If cancer is found in both kidneys or is likely to spread to both kidneys, surgery may include a partial

nephrectomy (removal of the cancer in the kidney and a small amount of normal tissue around it). Partial nephrectomy is done to keep as much of the kidney working as possible. A partial nephrectomy is also called renal-sparing surgery.

Even if the doctor removes all the cancer that can be seen at the time of the surgery, some patients may be given chemotherapy or radiation therapy after surgery to kill any cancer cells that are left. Treatment given after the surgery, to lower the risk of the cancer coming back, is called adjuvant therapy. Sometimes, a second-look surgery is done to see if cancer remains after chemotherapy or radiation therapy.

Radiation Therapy

Radiation therapy is a cancer treatment that uses high-energy X-rays or other types of radiation to kill cancer cells or keep them from growing. There are two types of radiation therapy:

- External radiation therapy uses a machine outside the body to send radiation toward the cancer.
- Internal radiation therapy uses a radioactive substance sealed in needles, seeds, wires, or catheters that are placed directly into or near the cancer.

The way the radiation therapy is given depends on the type and stage of the cancer being treated and whether a biopsy was done before surgery to remove the tumor. External radiation therapy is used to treat Wilms tumor and other childhood kidney tumors.

Chemotherapy

Chemotherapy is a cancer treatment that uses drugs to stop the growth of cancer cells, either by killing the cells or by stopping them from dividing. When chemotherapy is taken by mouth or injected into a vein or muscle, the drugs enter the bloodstream and can reach cancer cells throughout the body (systemic chemotherapy). When chemotherapy is placed directly into the cerebrospinal fluid, an organ, or a body cavity such as the abdomen, the drugs mainly affect cancer cells in those areas (regional chemotherapy). Combination chemotherapy is treatment using two or more anticancer drugs.

The way the chemotherapy is given depends on the type and stage of the cancer being treated. Systemic chemotherapy is used to treat Wilms tumor and other childhood kidney tumors.

Sometimes the tumor cannot be removed by surgery for one of the following reasons:

- The tumor is too close to important organs or blood vessels.
- The tumor is too large to remove.
- The cancer is in both kidneys.
- There is a blood clot in the vessels near the liver.
- The patient has trouble breathing because cancer has spread to the lungs.

In this case, a biopsy is done first. Then chemotherapy is given to reduce the size of the tumor before surgery, in order to save as much healthy tissue as possible and lessen problems after surgery. This is called neoadjuvant chemotherapy. Radiation therapy is given after surgery.

Biologic Therapy

Biologic therapy is a treatment that uses the patient's immune system to fight cancer. Substances made by the body or made in a laboratory are used to boost, direct, or restore the body's natural defenses against cancer. This type of cancer treatment is also called biotherapy or immunotherapy.

Interferon and interleukin-2 (IL-2) are types of biologic therapy used to treat childhood renal cell cancer. Interferon affects the division of cancer cells and can slow tumor growth. IL-2 boosts the growth and activity of many immune cells, especially lymphocytes (a type of white blood cell). Lymphocytes can attack and kill cancer cells.

High-Dose Chemotherapy with Stem Cell Rescue

High-dose chemotherapy with stem cell rescue is a method of giving high doses of chemotherapy and replacing blood-forming cells destroyed by the cancer treatment. Stem cells (immature blood cells) are removed from the blood or bone marrow of the patient or a donor and are frozen and stored. After the chemotherapy is completed, the stored stem cells are thawed and given back to the patient through an infusion. These re-infused stem cells grow into (and restore) the body's blood cells.

High-dose chemotherapy with stem cell rescue may be used to treat recurrent Wilms tumor.

What New Types of Treatment Are Being Tested in Clinical Trials?

Targeted Therapy

Targeted therapy is a treatment that uses drugs or other substances to identify and attack specific cancer cells without harming normal cells. Targeted therapy used to treat childhood kidney tumors may include the following:

- **Monoclonal antibodies:** This targeted therapy uses antibodies made in the laboratory, from a single type of immune system cell. These antibodies can identify substances on cancer cells or normal substances that may help cancer cells grow. The antibodies attach to the substances and kill the cancer cells, block their growth, or keep them from spreading. Monoclonal antibodies are given by infusion. They may be used alone or to carry drugs, toxins, or radioactive material directly to cancer cells. Lorvotuzumab is being studied in the treatment of recurrent Wilms tumor.
- **Kinase inhibitors:** This targeted therapy blocks signals that cancer cells need to grow and divide. LOXO-101 and entrectinib are kinase inhibitors being studied to treat congenital mesoblastic nephroma. Tyrosine kinase inhibitors, such as sunitinib or cabozantinib, may be used to treat renal cell carcinoma.
- **Histone methyltransferase inhibitors:** This targeted therapy slows down the cancer cell's ability to grow and divide. Tazemetostat is being studied in the treatment of rhabdoid tumor of the kidney.

Targeted therapy is being studied for the treatment of childhood kidney tumors that have recurred (come back).

Is There a Need for Follow-Up Tests?

Some of the tests that were done to diagnose the cancer or to find out the stage of the cancer may be repeated. Some tests will be repeated in order to see how well the treatment is working. Decisions about whether to continue, change, or stop treatment may be based on the results of these tests.

Some of the tests will continue to be done from time to time after treatment has ended. The results of these tests can show if your child's condition has changed or if the cancer has recurred (come back). These tests are sometimes called follow-up tests or check-ups.

Chapter 40

Transitional Cell Cancer of the Renal Pelvis and Ureter

The renal pelvis is the top part of the ureter. The ureter is a long tube that connects the kidney to the bladder. There are two kidneys, one on each side of the backbone, above the waist. The kidneys of an adult are about 5 inches long and 3 inches wide and are shaped like a kidney bean. Tiny tubules in the kidneys filter and clean the blood. They take out waste products and make urine. The urine collects in the middle of each kidney in the renal pelvis. Urine passes from the renal pelvis through the ureter into the bladder. The bladder holds the urine until it passes through the urethra and leaves the body. The renal pelvis and ureters are lined with transitional cells. These cells can change shape and stretch without breaking apart. Transitional cell cancer starts in these cells.

What Is Transitional Cell Cancer of the Renal Pelvis and Ureter?

Transitional cell cancer of the renal pelvis and ureter is a disease in which malignant (cancer) cells form in the renal pelvis and ureter. It can form in the renal pelvis, the ureter, or both. Renal cell cancer is a more common type of kidney cancer.

This chapter includes text excerpted from "Transitional Cell Cancer of the Renal Pelvis and Ureter Treatment (PDQ®)—Patient Version," National Cancer Institute (NCI), May 22, 2015.

What Are the Risk Factors for Transitional Cell Cancer of the Renal Pelvis and Ureter?

Anything that increases your risk of getting a disease is called a risk factor. Having a risk factor does not mean that you will get cancer; not having risk factors doesn't mean that you will not get cancer. Talk with your doctor if you think you may be at risk.

A personal history of bladder cancer and smoking can affect the risk of transitional cell cancer of the renal pelvis and ureter. Risk factors for transitional cell cancer of the renal pelvis and ureter include the following:

- Having a personal history of bladder cancer
- Smoking cigarettes
- Taking a lot of certain pain medicines, such as phenacetin
- Being exposed to certain dyes and chemicals used in making leather goods, textiles, plastics, and rubber

What Are the Signs and Symptoms of Transitional Cell Cancer of the Renal Pelvis and Ureter?

Signs and symptoms of transitional cell cancer of the renal pelvis and ureter include blood in the urine and back pain. These and other signs and symptoms may be caused by transitional cell cancer of the renal pelvis and ureter or by other conditions. There may be no signs or symptoms in the early stages. Signs and symptoms may appear as the tumor grows. Check with your doctor if you have any of the following:

- Blood in the urine
- A pain in the back that doesn't go away
- Extreme tiredness
- Weight loss with no known reason
- Painful or frequent urination

How Is Transitional Cell Cancer of the Renal Pelvis and Ureter Diagnosed?

Tests that examine the abdomen and kidneys are used to detect (find) and diagnose transitional cell cancer of the renal pelvis and ureter. The following tests and procedures may be used:

- **Physical exam and history:** An exam of the body to check general signs of health, including checking for signs of disease, such as lumps or anything else that seems unusual. A history of the patient's health habits and past illnesses and treatments will also be taken.
- **Urinalysis:** A test to check the color of urine and its contents, such as sugar, protein, blood, and bacteria.
- **Ureteroscopy:** A procedure to look inside the ureter and renal pelvis to check for abnormal areas. A ureteroscope is a thin, tube-like instrument with a light and a lens for viewing. The ureteroscope is inserted through the urethra into the bladder, ureter, and renal pelvis. A tool may be inserted through the ureteroscope to take tissue samples to be checked under a microscope for signs of disease.
- **Urine cytology:** A laboratory test in which a sample of urine is checked under a microscope for abnormal cells. Cancer in the kidney, bladder, or ureter may shed cancer cells into the urine.
- **Computerized tomography (CT)/computerized axial tomography (CAT) scan:** A procedure that makes a series of detailed pictures of areas inside the body, taken from different angles. The pictures are made by a computer linked to an X-ray machine. A dye may be injected into a vein or swallowed to help the organs or tissues show up more clearly.
- **Ultrasound:** A procedure in which high-energy sound waves (ultrasound) are bounced off internal tissues or organs and make echoes. The echoes form a picture of body tissues called a sonogram. An ultrasound of the abdomen may be done to help diagnose cancer of the renal pelvis and ureter.
- **Magnetic resonance imaging (MRI):** A procedure that uses a magnet, radio waves, and a computer to make a series of detailed pictures of areas inside the body, such as the pelvis. This procedure is also called nuclear magnetic resonance imaging (NMRI).
- **Biopsy:** The removal of cells or tissues so they can be viewed under a microscope by a pathologist to check for signs of cancer. This may be done during a ureteroscopy or surgery.

What Is the Prognosis for Transitional Cell Cancer of the Renal Pelvis and Ureter?

The prognosis (chance of recovery) depends on the stage and grade of the tumor.

The treatment options depend on the following:

- The stage and grade of the tumor
- Where the tumor is
- Whether the patient's other kidney is healthy
- Whether the cancer has recurred
- Most transitional cell cancer of the renal pelvis and ureter can be cured if found early

Stages of Transitional Cell Cancer of the Renal Pelvis and Ureter

The process used to find out if cancer has spread within the renal pelvis and ureter or to other parts of the body is called staging. The information gathered from the staging process determines the stage of the disease. It is important to know the stage in order to plan treatment. The doctor will use results of the diagnostic tests to help find out the stage of the disease.

After transitional cell cancer of the renal pelvis and ureter has been diagnosed, tests are done to find out if cancer cells have spread within the renal pelvis and ureter or to other parts of the body.

The following tests and procedures may also be used in the staging process:

- **Chest X-ray:** An X-ray of the organs and bones inside the chest. An X-ray is a type of energy beam that can go through the body and onto film, making a picture of areas inside the body.
- **Positron emission tomography (PET) scan:** A procedure to find malignant tumor cells in the body. A small amount of radioactive glucose (sugar) is injected into a vein. The PET scanner rotates around the body and makes a picture of where glucose is being used in the body. Malignant tumor cells show up brighter in the picture because they are more active and take up more glucose than normal cells do.
- **Bone scan:** A procedure to check if there are rapidly dividing cells, such as cancer cells, in the bone. A very small amount of

radioactive material is injected into a vein and travels through the bloodstream. The radioactive material collects in the bones with cancer and is detected by a scanner.

The following stages are used for transitional cell cancer of the renal pelvis and/or ureter:

Stage 0 (noninvasive papillary carcinoma and carcinoma in situ). In stage 0, abnormal cells are found in tissue lining the inside of the renal pelvis or ureter. These abnormal cells may become cancer and spread into nearby normal tissue. Stage 0 is divided into stages 0a and 0 is, depending on the type of tumor:

- **Stage 0A** is also called noninvasive papillary carcinoma, which may look like long, thin growths that grow out from the tissue lining the inside of the renal pelvis or ureter.
- **Stage 0** is also called carcinoma in situ, which is a flat tumor on the tissue lining the inside of the renal pelvis or ureter.

Stage I. In stage I, cancer has formed and has spread from the tissue lining the inside of the renal pelvis or ureter to the connective tissue layer.

Stage II, In stage II, cancer has spread to the muscle layer of the renal pelvis or ureter.

Stage III, In stage III, cancer has spread:

- from the muscle layer of the renal pelvis to fat around the renal pelvis or to tissue in the kidney; or
- from the muscle layer of the ureter to fat around the ureter.

Stage IV. In stage IV, cancer has spread to at least one of the following:

- a nearby organ
- the layer of fat around the kidney
- lymph nodes
- other parts of the body, such as the lung, liver, or bone

Transitional cell cancer of the renal pelvis and ureter is also described as localized, regional, or metastatic:

Localized. The cancer is found only in the kidney.

Regional. The cancer has spread to tissues around the kidney and to nearby lymph nodes and blood vessels in the pelvis.

Metastatic. The cancer has spread to other parts of the body.

Treatment Option Overview

Different types of treatments are available for patients with transitional cell cancer of the renal pelvis and ureter. Some treatments are standard (the currently used treatment), and some are being tested in clinical trials. A treatment clinical trial is a research study meant to help improve current treatments or obtain information on new treatments for patients with cancer. When clinical trials show that a new treatment is better than the standard treatment, the new treatment may become the standard treatment. Patients may want to think about taking part in a clinical trial. Some clinical trials are open only to patients who have not started treatment.

Standard Treatment Options Available for Treating Patients with Transitional Cell Cancer of the Renal Pelvis and Ureter

One type of standard treatment is used:

Surgery

One of the following surgical procedures may be used to treat transitional cell cancer of the renal pelvis and ureter:

- **Nephroureterectomy:** Surgery to remove the entire kidney, the ureter, and the bladder cuff (tissue that connects the ureter to the bladder).
- **Segmental resection of the ureter:** A surgical procedure to remove the part of the ureter that contains cancer and some of the healthy tissue around it. The ends of the ureter are then reattached. This treatment is used when the cancer is superficial and in the lower third of the ureter only, near the bladder.

New Types of Treatment Tested in Clinical Trials

Fulguration

Fulguration is a surgical procedure that destroys tissue using an electric current. A tool with a small wire loop on the end is used to remove the cancer or to burn away the tumor with electricity.

Segmental Resection of the Renal Pelvis

This is a surgical procedure to remove localized cancer from the renal pelvis without removing the entire kidney. Segmental resection may be done to save kidney function when the other kidney is damaged or has already been removed.

Laser Surgery

A laser beam (narrow beam of intense light) is used as a knife to remove the cancer. A laser beam can also be used to kill the cancer cells. This procedure may also be called or laser fulguration.

Regional Chemotherapy and Regional Biologic Therapy

Chemotherapy is a cancer treatment that uses drugs to stop the growth of cancer cells, either by killing the cells or by stopping the cells from dividing. Biologic therapy is a treatment that uses the patient's immune system to fight cancer; substances made by the body or made in a laboratory are used to boost, direct, or restore the body's natural defenses against cancer. Regional treatment means the anticancer drugs or biologic substances are placed directly into an organ or a body cavity such as the abdomen, so the drugs will affect cancer cells in that area. Clinical trials are studying chemotherapy or biologic therapy using drugs placed directly into the renal pelvis or the ureter.

Follow-Up Tests

Some of the tests that were done to diagnose the cancer or to find out the stage of the cancer may be repeated. Some tests will be repeated in order to see how well the treatment is working. Decisions about whether to continue, change, or stop treatment may be based on the results of these tests.

Some of the tests will continue to be done from time to time after treatment has ended. The results of these tests can show if your condition has changed or if the cancer has recurred (come back). These tests are sometimes called follow-up tests or check-ups.

Chapter 41

Urethral Cancer

The urethra is the tube that carries urine from the bladder to outside the body. In women, the urethra is about 1½ inches long and is just above the vagina. In men, the urethra is about 8 inches long, and goes through the prostate gland and the penis to the outside of the body. In men, the urethra also carries semen.

What Is Urethral Cancer?

Urethral cancer is a disease in which malignant (cancer) cells form in the tissues of the urethra. It is a rare cancer that occurs more often in men than in women.

There are different types of urethral cancer that begin in cells that line the urethra. These cancers are named for the types of cells that become malignant (cancer):

- **Squamous cell carcinoma** is the most common type of urethral cancer. It forms in cells in the part of the urethra near the bladder in women, and in the lining of the urethra in the penis in men.
- **Transitional cell carcinoma** forms in the area near the urethral opening in women, and in the part of the urethra that goes through the prostate gland in men.

This chapter includes text excerpted from "Urethral Cancer Treatment (PDQ®)—Patient Version," National Cancer Institute (NCI), July 19, 2016.

- **Adenocarcinoma** forms in the glands that are around the urethra in both men and women.

Urethral cancer can metastasize (spread) quickly to tissues around the urethra and is often found in nearby lymph nodes by the time it is diagnosed.

What Are the Risk Factors for Urethral Cancer?

Anything that increases your chance of getting a disease is called a risk factor. Having a risk factor does not mean that you will get cancer; not having risk factors doesn't mean that you will not get cancer. Talk with your doctor if you think you may be at risk.

A history of bladder cancer can affect the risk of urethral cancer. Risk factors for urethral cancer include the following:

- Having a history of bladder cancer
- Having conditions that cause chronic inflammation in the urethra, including:
    - Sexually transmitted diseases (STDs), including human papillomavirus (HPV), especially HPV type 16
    - Frequent urinary tract infections (UTIs)

What Are the Signs and Symptoms of Urethral Cancer?

Signs of urethral cancer include bleeding or trouble with urination. These and other signs and symptoms may be caused by urethral cancer or by other conditions. There may be no signs or symptoms in the early stages. Check with your doctor if you have any of the following:

- Trouble starting the flow of urine
- Weak or interrupted ("stop-and-go") flow of urine
- Frequent urination, especially at night
- Incontinence
- Discharge from the urethra
- Bleeding from the urethra or blood in the urine
- A lump or thickness in the perineum or penis
- A painless lump or swelling in the groin

How Is Urethral Cancer Diagnosed?

Tests that examine the urethra and bladder are used to detect (find) and diagnose urethral cancer. The following tests and procedures may be used:

- **Physical exam and history:** An exam of the body to check general signs of health, including checking for signs of disease, such as lumps or anything else that seems unusual. A history of the patient's health habits and past illnesses and treatments will also be taken.
- **Pelvic exam:** An exam of the vagina, cervix, uterus, fallopian tubes, ovaries, and rectum. A speculum is inserted into the vagina and the doctor or nurse looks at the vagina and cervix for signs of disease. The doctor or nurse also inserts one or two lubricated, gloved fingers of one hand into the vagina and places the other hand over the lower abdomen to feel the size, shape, and position of the uterus and ovaries. The doctor or nurse also inserts a lubricated, gloved finger into the rectum to feel for lumps or abnormal areas.
- **Digital rectal exam:** An exam of the rectum. The doctor or nurse inserts a lubricated, gloved finger into the lower part of the rectum to feel for lumps or anything else that seems unusual.
- **Urine cytology:** A laboratory test in which a sample of urine is checked under a microscope for abnormal cells.
- **Urinalysis:** A test to check the color of urine and its contents, such as sugar, protein, blood, and white blood cells. If white blood cells (a sign of infection) are found, a urine culture is usually done to find out what type of infection it is.
- **Blood chemistry studies:** A procedure in which a blood sample is checked to measure the amounts of certain substances released into the blood by organs and tissues in the body. An unusual (higher or lower than normal) amount of a substance can be a sign of disease.
- **Complete blood count (CBC)**: A procedure in which a sample of blood is drawn and checked for the following:
  - The number of red blood cells, white blood cells, and platelets

- The amount of hemoglobin (the protein that carries oxygen) in the red blood cells
- The portion of the blood sample made up of red blood cells

- **Computed tomography (CT)/computerized axial tomography (CAT) scan**: A procedure that makes a series of detailed pictures of areas inside the body, such as the pelvis and abdomen, taken from different angles. The pictures are made by a computer linked to an X-ray machine. A dye may be injected into a vein or swallowed to help the organs or tissues show up more clearly.
- **Ureteroscopy:** A procedure to look inside the ureter and renal pelvis to check for abnormal areas. A ureteroscope is a thin, tube-like instrument with a light and a lens for viewing. The ureteroscope is inserted through the urethra into the bladder, ureter, and renal pelvis. A tool may be inserted through the ureteroscope to take tissue samples to be checked under a microscope for signs of disease.
- **Biopsy:** The removal of cell or tissue samples from the urethra, bladder, and, sometimes, the prostate gland. The samples are viewed under a microscope by a pathologist to check for signs of cancer.

What Is the Prognosis for Urethral Cancer?

The prognosis (chance of recovery) and treatment options depend on the following:

- Where the cancer formed in the urethra
- Whether the cancer has spread through the mucosa lining the urethra to nearby tissue, to lymph nodes, or to other parts of the body
- Whether the patient is a male or female
- The patient's general health
- Whether the cancer has just been diagnosed or has recurred (come back)

Stages of Urethral Cancer

The process used to find out if cancer has spread within the urethra or to other parts of the body is called staging. The information gathered from the staging process determines the stage of the disease. It is important to know the stage in order to plan treatment.

After urethral cancer has been diagnosed, tests are done to find out if cancer cells have spread within the urethra or to other parts of the body. The following procedures may be used in the staging process:

- **Chest X-ray:** An X-ray of the organs and bones inside the chest. An X-ray is a type of energy beam that can go through the body and onto film, making a picture of areas inside the body.
- **CT/CAT scan of the pelvis and abdomen:** A procedure that makes a series of detailed pictures of the pelvis and abdomen, taken from different angles. The pictures are made by a computer linked to an X-ray machine. A dye may be injected into a vein or swallowed to help the organs or tissues show up more clearly.
- **Magnetic resonance imaging (MRI):** A procedure that uses a magnet, radio waves, and a computer to make a series of detailed pictures of the urethra, nearby lymph nodes, and other soft tissue and bones in the pelvis. A substance called gadolinium is injected into the patient through a vein. The gadolinium collects around the cancer cells so they show up brighter in the picture. This procedure is also called nuclear magnetic resonance imaging (NMRI).
- **Urethrography:** A series of X-rays of the urethra. An X-ray is a type of energy beam that can go through the body and onto film, making a picture of areas inside the body. A dye is injected through the urethra into the bladder. The dye coats the bladder and urethra and X-rays are taken to see if the urethra is blocked and if cancer has spread to nearby tissue.

Urethral cancer is staged and treated based on the part of the urethra that is affected and how deeply the tumor has spread into tissue around the urethra. Urethral cancer can be described as distal or proximal.

Distal Urethral Cancer

In distal urethral cancer, the cancer usually has not spread deeply into the tissue. In women, the part of the urethra that is closest to the outside of the body (about ½ inch) is affected. In men, the part of the urethra that is in the penis is affected.

Proximal Urethral Cancer

Proximal urethral cancer affects the part of the urethra that is not the distal urethra. In women and men, proximal urethral cancer usually has spread deeply into tissue.

Bladder and/or Prostate Cancer May Occur at the Same Time as Urethral Cancer

In men, cancer that forms in the proximal urethra (the part of the urethra that passes through the prostate to the bladder) may occur at the same time as cancer of the bladder and/or prostate. Sometimes this occurs at diagnosis and sometimes it occurs later.

Treatment Option Overview

Different types of treatments are available for patients with urethral cancer. Some treatments are standard (the currently used treatment), and some are being tested in clinical trials. A treatment clinical trial is a research study meant to help improve current treatments or obtain information on new treatments for patients with cancer. When clinical trials show that a new treatment is better than the standard treatment, the new treatment may become the standard treatment. Patients may want to think about taking part in a clinical trial. Some clinical trials are open only to patients who have not started treatment.

Standard Treatment Options Available for Patients with Urethral Cancer

Four types of standard treatment are used:

Surgery

Surgery to remove the cancer is the most common treatment for cancer of the urethra. One of the following types of surgery may be done:

- **Open excision:** Removal of the cancer by surgery.
- **Transurethral resection (TUR):** Surgery to remove the cancer using a special tool inserted into the urethra.
- **Electroresection with fulguration:** Surgery to remove the cancer by electric current. A lighted tool with a small wire loop on the end is used to remove the cancer or to burn the tumor away with high-energy electricity.

- **Laser surgery:** A surgical procedure that uses a laser beam (a narrow beam of intense light) as a knife to make bloodless cuts in tissue or to remove or destroy tissue.
- **Lymph node dissection**: Lymph nodes in the pelvis and groin may be removed.
- **Cystourethrectomy:** Surgery to remove the bladder and the urethra.
- **Cystoprostatectomy:** Surgery to remove the bladder and the prostate.
- **Anterior exenteration:** Surgery to remove the urethra, the bladder, and the vagina. Plastic surgery may be done to rebuild the vagina.
- **Partial penectomy:** Surgery to remove the part of the penis surrounding the urethra where cancer has spread. Plastic surgery may be done to rebuild the penis.
- **Radical penectomy:** Surgery to remove the entire penis. Plastic surgery may be done to rebuild the penis.

If the urethra is removed, the surgeon will make a new way for the urine to pass from the body. This is called urinary diversion. If the bladder is removed, the surgeon will make a new way for urine to be stored and passed from the body. The surgeon may use part of the small intestine to make a tube that passes urine through an opening (stoma). This is called an ostomy or urostomy. If a patient has an ostomy, a disposable bag to collect urine is worn under clothing. The surgeon may also use part of the small intestine to make a new storage pouch (continent reservoir) inside the body where the urine can collect. A tube (catheter) is then used to drain the urine through a stoma.

Even if the doctor removes all the cancer that can be seen at the time of the surgery, some patients may be given chemotherapy or radiation therapy after surgery to kill any cancer cells that are left. Treatment given after the surgery, to lower the risk that the cancer will come back, is called adjuvant therapy.

Radiation Therapy

Radiation therapy is a cancer treatment that uses high-energy X-rays or other types of radiation to kill cancer cells or keep them from growing. There are two types of radiation therapy:

External radiation therapy uses a machine outside the body to send radiation toward the cancer.

Internal radiation therapy uses a radioactive substance sealed in needles, seeds, wires, or catheters that are placed directly into or near the cancer.

The way the radiation therapy is given depends on the type of cancer and where the cancer formed in the urethra. External and internal radiation therapy are used to treat urethral cancer.

Chemotherapy

Chemotherapy is a cancer treatment that uses drugs to stop the growth of cancer cells, either by killing the cells or by stopping the cells from dividing. When chemotherapy is taken by mouth or injected into a vein or muscle, the drugs enter the bloodstream and can reach cancer cells throughout the body (systemic chemotherapy). When chemotherapy is placed directly into the cerebrospinal fluid, an organ, or a body cavity such as the abdomen, the drugs mainly affect cancer cells in those areas (regional chemotherapy). The way the chemotherapy is given depends on the type of cancer and where the cancer formed in the urethra.

Active Surveillance

Active surveillance is following a patient's condition without giving any treatment unless there are changes in test results. It is used to find early signs that the condition is getting worse. In active surveillance, patients are given certain exams and tests, including biopsies, on a regular schedule.

Follow-Up Tests

Some of the tests that were done to diagnose the cancer or to find out the stage of the cancer may be repeated. Some tests will be repeated in order to see how well the treatment is working. Decisions about whether to continue, change, or stop treatment may be based on the results of these tests. Some of the tests will continue to be done from time to time after treatment has ended. The results of these tests can show if your condition has changed or if the cancer has recurred (come back). These tests are sometimes called follow-up tests or check-ups.

Chapter 42

Bladder Cancer

The bladder is a hollow organ in the lower part of the abdomen. It is shaped like a small balloon and has a muscular wall that allows it to get larger or smaller to store urine made by the kidneys. There are two kidneys, one on each side of the backbone, above the waist. Tiny tubules in the kidneys filter and clean the blood. They take out waste products and make urine. The urine passes from each kidney through a long tube called a ureter into the bladder. The bladder holds the urine until it passes through the urethra and leaves the body.

What Is Bladder Cancer?

Bladder cancer is a disease in which malignant (cancer) cells form in the tissues of the bladder. There are three types of bladder cancer that begin in cells in the lining of the bladder. These cancers are named for the type of cells that become malignant (cancerous):

- **Transitional cell carcinoma:** Cancer that begins in cells in the innermost tissue layer of the bladder. These cells are able to stretch when the bladder is full and shrink when it is emptied. Most bladder cancers begin in the transitional cells. Transitional cell carcinoma can be low-grade or high-grade:
    - Low-grade transitional cell carcinoma often recurs (comes back) after treatment, but rarely spreads into the muscle layer of the bladder or to other parts of the body.

This chapter includes text excerpted from "Bladder Cancer Treatment (PDQ®)—Patient Version," National Cancer Institute (NCI), January 29, 2018.

  - High-grade transitional cell carcinoma often recurs (comes back) after treatment and often spreads into the muscle layer of the bladder, to other parts of the body, and to lymph nodes. Almost all deaths from bladder cancer are due to high-grade disease.
- **Squamous cell carcinoma:** Cancer that begins in squamous cells, which are thin, flat cells that may form in the bladder after long-term infection or irritation.
- **Adenocarcinoma:** Cancer that begins in glandular (secretory) cells that are found in the lining of the bladder. This is a very rare type of bladder cancer.

Cancer that is in the lining of the bladder is called superficial bladder cancer. Cancer that has spread through the lining of the bladder and invades the muscle wall of the bladder or has spread to nearby organs and lymph nodes is called invasive bladder cancer.

What Are the Risk Factors for Bladder Cancer?

Anything that increases your chance of getting a disease is called a risk factor. Having a risk factor does not mean that you will get cancer; not having risk factors doesn't mean that you will not get cancer. Talk to your doctor if you think you may be at risk for bladder cancer.

Smoking can affect the risk of bladder cancer. Risk factors for bladder cancer include:

- Using tobacco, especially smoking cigarettes
- Having a family history of bladder cancer
- Having certain changes in the genes that are linked to bladder cancer
- Being exposed to paints, dyes, metals, or petroleum products in the workplace
- Past treatment with radiation therapy to the pelvis or with certain anticancer drugs, such as cyclophosphamide or ifosfamide
- Taking *Aristolochia fangchi*, a Chinese herb
- Drinking water from a well that has high levels of arsenic
- Drinking water that has been treated with chlorine

- Having a history of bladder infections, including bladder infections caused by *Schistosoma haematobium*
- Using urinary catheters for a long time

Older age is a risk factor for most cancers. The chance of getting cancer increases as you get older.

What Are the Signs and Symptoms of Bladder Cancer?

Signs and symptoms of bladder cancer include blood in the urine and pain during urination. These and other signs and symptoms may be caused by bladder cancer or by other conditions. Check with your doctor if you have any of the following:

- Blood in the urine (slightly rusty to bright red in color)
- Frequent urination
- Pain during urination
- Lower back pain

How Is Bladder Cancer Diagnosed?

Tests that examine the urine and bladder are used to help detect (find) and diagnose bladder cancer. The following tests and procedures may be used:

- **Physical exam and history:** An exam of the body to check general signs of health, including checking for signs of disease, such as lumps or anything else that seems unusual. A history of the patient's health habits and past illnesses and treatments will also be taken.
- **Internal exam:** An exam of the vagina and/or rectum. The doctor inserts lubricated, gloved fingers into the vagina and/or rectum to feel for lumps.
- **Urinalysis:** A test to check the color of urine and its contents, such as sugar, protein, red blood cells, and white blood cells.
- **Urine cytology:** A laboratory test in which a sample of urine is checked under a microscope for abnormal cells.
- **Cystoscopy:** A procedure to look inside the bladder and urethra to check for abnormal areas. A cystoscope is inserted through the urethra into the bladder. A cystoscope is a thin, tube-like

instrument with a light and a lens for viewing. It may also have a tool to remove tissue samples, which are checked under a microscope for signs of cancer.

- **Intravenous pyelogram (IVP):** A series of X-rays of the kidneys, ureters, and bladder to find out if cancer is present in these organs. A contrast dye is injected into a vein. As the contrast dye moves through the kidneys, ureters, and bladder, X-rays are taken to see if there are any blockages.
- **Biopsy:** The removal of cells or tissues so they can be viewed under a microscope by a pathologist to check for signs of cancer. A biopsy for bladder cancer is usually done during cystoscopy. It may be possible to remove the entire tumor during biopsy.

What Is the Prognosis for Bladder Cancer?

The prognosis (chance of recovery) depends on the following:

- The stage of the cancer (whether it is superficial or invasive bladder cancer, and whether it has spread to other places in the body). Bladder cancer in the early stages can often be cured.
- The type of bladder cancer cells and how they look under a microscope
- Whether there is carcinoma in situ in other parts of the bladder
- The patient's age and general health

If the cancer is superficial, prognosis also depends on the following:

- How many tumors there are
- The size of the tumors
- Whether the tumor has recurred (come back) after treatment
- Treatment options depend on the stage of bladder cancer

Stages of Bladder Cancer

The process used to find out if cancer has spread within the bladder lining and muscle or to other parts of the body is called staging. The information gathered from the staging process determines the stage of the disease. It is important to know the stage in order to plan treatment. After bladder cancer has been diagnosed, tests are done to find out if cancer cells have spread within the bladder or to other parts of the body. The following tests and procedures may be used in the staging process:

- **Computerized tomography (CT)/computerized axial tomography (CAT) scan:** A procedure that makes a series of detailed pictures of areas inside the body, taken from different angles. The pictures are made by a computer linked to an X-ray machine. A dye may be injected into a vein or swallowed to help the organs or tissues show up more clearly. This procedure is also called computed tomography, computerized tomography, or computerized axial tomography. To stage bladder cancer, the CT scan may take pictures of the chest, abdomen, and pelvis.
- **Magnetic resonance imaging (MRI):** A procedure that uses a magnet, radio waves, and a computer to make a series of detailed pictures of areas inside the body. This procedure is also called nuclear magnetic resonance imaging (NMRI).
- **Chest X-ray:** An X-ray of the organs and bones inside the chest. An X-ray is a type of energy beam that can go through the body and onto film, making a picture of areas inside the body.
- **Bone scan:** A procedure to check if there are rapidly dividing cells, such as cancer cells, in the bone. A very small amount of radioactive material is injected into a vein and travels through the bloodstream. The radioactive material collects in the bones with cancer and is detected by a scanner.

The following stages are used for bladder cancer:

Stage 0 (Papillary Carcinoma and Carcinoma in Situ)

In stage 0, abnormal cells are found in tissue lining the inside of the bladder. These abnormal cells may become cancer and spread into nearby normal tissue. Stage 0 is divided into stage 0a and stage 0is, depending on the type of the tumor:

- **Stage 0 A** is also called papillary carcinoma, which may look like tiny mushrooms growing from the lining of the bladder.
- **Stage 0** is also called carcinoma in situ, which is a flat tumor on the tissue lining the inside of the bladder.

Stage I. In stage I, cancer has formed and spread to the layer of connective tissue next to the inner lining of the bladder.

Stage II. In stage II, cancer has spread to the layers of muscle tissue of the bladder.

Stage III. In stage III, cancer has spread from the bladder to the layer of fat surrounding it and may have spread to the reproductive organs (prostate, seminal vesicles, uterus, or vagina).

Stage IV. In stage IV, one or more of the following is true:

- Cancer has spread from the bladder to the wall of the abdomen or pelvis.
- Cancer has spread to one or more lymph nodes.
- Cancer has spread to other parts of the body, such as the lung, bone, or liver.

Treatment Option Overview

Different types of treatment are available for patients with bladder cancer. Some treatments are standard (the currently used treatment), and some are being tested in clinical trials. A treatment clinical trial is a research study meant to help improve current treatments or obtain information on new treatments for patients with cancer. When clinical trials show that a new treatment is better than the standard treatment, the new treatment may become the standard treatment. Patients may want to think about taking part in a clinical trial. Some clinical trials are open only to patients who have not started treatment.

What Are the Standard Treatment Options Available for Bladder Cancer?

Four types of standard treatment are used:

Surgery

One of the following types of surgery may be done:

- **Transurethral resection (TUR) with fulguration:** Surgery in which a cystoscope (a thin lighted tube) is inserted into the bladder through the urethra. A tool with a small wire loop on the end is then used to remove the cancer or to burn the tumor away with high-energy electricity. This is known as fulguration.
- **Radical cystectomy:** Surgery to remove the bladder and any lymph nodes and nearby organs that contain cancer. This surgery

may be done when the bladder cancer invades the muscle wall, or when superficial cancer involves a large part of the bladder. In men, the nearby organs that are removed are the prostate and the seminal vesicles. In women, the uterus, the ovaries, and part of the vagina are removed. Sometimes, when the cancer has spread outside the bladder and cannot be completely removed, surgery to remove only the bladder may be done to reduce urinary symptoms caused by the cancer. When the bladder must be removed, the surgeon creates another way for urine to leave the body.

- **Partial cystectomy:** Surgery to remove part of the bladder. This surgery may be done for patients who have a low-grade tumor that has invaded the wall of the bladder but is limited to one area of the bladder. Because only a part of the bladder is removed, patients are able to urinate normally after recovering from this surgery. This is also called segmental cystectomy.
- **Urinary diversion:** Surgery to make a new way for the body to store and pass urine.

Even if the doctor removes all the cancer that can be seen at the time of the surgery, some patients may be given chemotherapy after surgery to kill any cancer cells that are left. Treatment given after surgery, to lower the risk that the cancer will come back, is called adjuvant therapy.

Radiation Therapy

Radiation therapy is a cancer treatment that uses high-energy X-rays or other types of radiation to kill cancer cells or keep them from growing. There are two types of radiation therapy:

- External radiation therapy uses a machine outside the body to send radiation toward the cancer.
- Internal radiation therapy uses a radioactive substance sealed in needles, seeds, wires, or catheters that are placed directly into or near the cancer.

The way the radiation therapy is given depends on the type and stage of the cancer being treated. External radiation therapy is used to treat bladder cancer.

Chemotherapy

Chemotherapy is a cancer treatment that uses drugs to stop the growth of cancer cells, either by killing the cells or by stopping them

from dividing. When chemotherapy is taken by mouth or injected into a vein or muscle, the drugs enter the bloodstream and can reach cancer cells throughout the body (systemic chemotherapy). When chemotherapy is placed directly into the cerebrospinal fluid, an organ, or a body cavity such as the abdomen, the drugs mainly affect cancer cells in those areas (regional chemotherapy). For bladder cancer, regional chemotherapy may be intravesical (put into the bladder through a tube inserted into the urethra). The way the chemotherapy is given depends on the type and stage of the cancer being treated. Combination chemotherapy is treatment using more than one anticancer drug.

Immunotherapy

Immunotherapy is a treatment that uses the patient's immune system to fight cancer. Substances made by the body or made in a laboratory are used to boost, direct, or restore the body's natural defenses against cancer. This type of cancer treatment is also called biotherapy or biologic therapy.

PD-1 inhibitors are a type of immunotherapy used in the treatment of bladder cancer. PD-1 is a protein on the surface of T cells that helps keep the body's immune responses in check. When PD-1 attaches to another protein called PDL-1 on a cancer cell, it stops the T cell from killing the cancer cell. PD-1 inhibitors attach to PDL-1 and allow the T cells to kill cancer cells.

Atezolizumab and nivolumab are types of PD-1 inhibitors.

Bladder cancer may be treated with an intravesical immunotherapy called BCG (bacillus Calmette-Guérin). The BCG is given in a solution that is placed directly into the bladder using a catheter (thin tube).

Is There a Need for Follow-Up Tests?

Some of the tests that were done to diagnose the cancer or to find out the stage of the cancer may be repeated. Some tests will be repeated in order to see how well the treatment is working. Decisions about whether to continue, change, or stop treatment may be based on the results of these tests.

Some of the tests will continue to be done from time to time after treatment has ended. The results of these tests can show if your condition has changed or if the cancer has recurred (come back). These tests are sometimes called follow-up tests or check-ups.

Bladder cancer often recurs (comes back), even when the cancer is superficial. Surveillance of the urinary tract to check for recurrence is standard after a diagnosis of bladder cancer. Surveillance is closely watching a patient's condition but not giving any treatment unless there are changes in test results that show the condition is getting worse. During active surveillance, certain exams and tests are done on a regular schedule. Surveillance may include ureteroscopy and imaging tests.

Chapter 43

Breast Cancer

Chapter Contents

Section 43.1

Breast Cancer in Women

This section includes text excerpted from "Breast Cancer Treatment (PDQ®)—Patient Version," National Cancer Institute (NCI), March 1, 2018.

The breast is made up of lobes and ducts. Each breast has 15–20 sections called lobes. Each lobe has many smaller sections called lobules. Lobules end in dozens of tiny bulbs that can make milk. The lobes, lobules, and bulbs are linked by thin tubes called ducts. Each breast also has blood vessels and lymph vessels. The lymph vessels carry an almost colorless fluid called lymph. Lymph vessels carry lymph between lymph nodes. Lymph nodes are small bean-shaped structures that are found throughout the body. They filter substances in lymph and help fight infection and disease. Clusters of lymph nodes are found near the breast in the axilla (under the arm), above the collarbone, and in the chest.

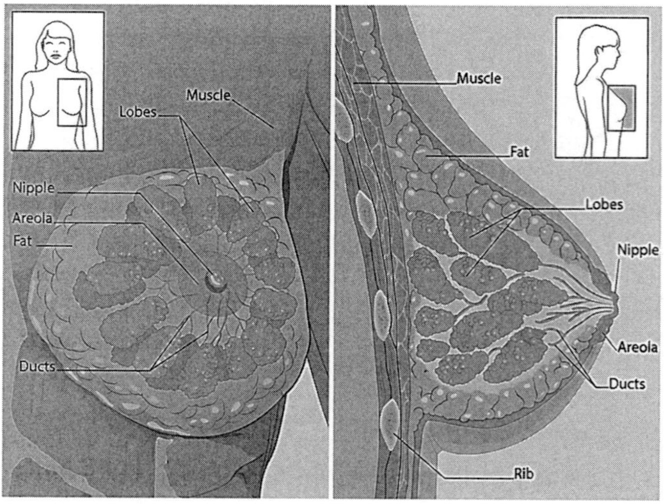

Figure 43.1. *Breasts – Anterior and Cross-Section View* (Source: "What Is Breast Cancer?" Centers for Disease Control and Prevention (CDC).)

What Is Breast Cancer?

Breast cancer is a disease in which malignant (cancer) cells form in the tissues of the breast. The most common type of breast cancer is ductal carcinoma, which begins in the cells of the ducts. Cancer that begins in the lobes or lobules is called lobular carcinoma and is more often found in both breasts than are other types of breast cancer. Inflammatory breast cancer is an uncommon type of breast cancer in which the breast is warm, red, and swollen.

What Are the Risk Factors for Breast Cancer in Women?

Anything that increases your chance of getting a disease is called a risk factor. Having a risk factor does not mean that you will get cancer; not having risk factors doesn't mean that you will not get cancer. Talk to your doctor if you think you may be at risk for breast cancer.

A family history of breast cancer and other factors increase the risk of breast cancer. Risk factors for breast cancer include the following:

- A personal history of invasive breast cancer, ductal carcinoma in situ (DCIS), or lobular carcinoma in situ (LCIS)
- A personal history of benign (noncancer) breast disease
- A family history of breast cancer in a first-degree relative (mother, daughter, or sister)
- Inherited changes in the *BRCA1* or *BRCA2* genes or in other genes that increase the risk of breast cancer
- Breast tissue that is dense on a mammogram
- Exposure of breast tissue to estrogen made by the body. This may be caused by:
    - Menstruating at an early age
    - Older age at first birth or never having given birth
    - Starting menopause at a later age
- Taking hormones such as estrogen combined with progestin for symptoms of menopause
- Treatment with radiation therapy to the breast/chest
- Drinking alcohol
- Obesity

Older age is the main risk factor for most cancers. The chance of getting cancer increases as you get older.

Is Breast Cancer Caused Due to Inherited Gene Mutations?

Breast cancer is sometimes caused by inherited gene mutations (changes). The genes in cells carry the hereditary information that is received from a person's parents. Hereditary breast cancer makes up about 5–10 percent of all breast cancer. Some mutated genes related to breast cancer are more common in certain ethnic groups.

Women who have certain gene mutations, such as a *BRCA1* or *BRCA2* mutation, have an increased risk of breast cancer. These women also have an increased risk of ovarian cancer, and may have an increased risk of other cancers. There are tests that can detect (find) mutated genes. These genetic tests are sometimes done for members of families with a high risk of cancer.

What Are the Protective Factors for Breast Cancer?

Anything that decreases your chance of getting a disease is called a protective factor. The use of certain medicines and other factors decrease the risk of breast cancer.

Protective factors for breast cancer include the following:

- Taking any of the following:
    - Estrogen-only hormone therapy after a hysterectomy
    - Selective estrogen receptor modulators (SERMs)
    - Aromatase inhibitors (AIs)
- Less exposure of breast tissue to estrogen made by the body. This can be a result of:
    - Early pregnancy
    - Breastfeeding
- Getting enough exercise
- Having any of the following procedures:
    - Mastectomy to reduce the risk of cancer
    - Oophorectomy to reduce the risk of cancer
    - Ovarian ablation

What Are the Signs and Symptoms of Breast Cancer?

Signs of breast cancer include a lump or change in the breast.

These and other signs may be caused by breast cancer or by other conditions. Check with your doctor if you have any of the following:

- A lump or thickening in or near the breast or in the underarm area
- A change in the size or shape of the breast
- A dimple or puckering in the skin of the breast
- A nipple turned inward into the breast
- Fluid, other than breast milk, from the nipple, especially if it's bloody
- Scaly, red, or swollen skin on the breast, nipple, or areola (the dark area of skin around the nipple)
- Dimples in the breast that look like the skin of an orange, called peau d'orange

How Is Breast Cancer Diagnosed?

Tests that examine the breasts are used to detect (find) and diagnose breast cancer.

Check with your doctor if you notice any changes in your breasts. The following tests and procedures may be used:

- **Physical exam and history:** An exam of the body to check general signs of health, including checking for signs of disease, such as lumps or anything else that seems unusual. A history of the patient's health habits and past illnesses and treatments will also be taken.
- **Clinical breast exam (CBE):** An exam of the breast by a doctor or other health professional. The doctor will carefully feel the breasts and under the arms for lumps or anything else that seems unusual.
- **Mammogram:** An X-ray of the breast.
- **Ultrasound exam:** A procedure in which high-energy sound waves (ultrasound) are bounced off internal tissues or organs and make echoes. The echoes form a picture of body tissues called a sonogram. The picture can be printed to be looked at later.

- **Magnetic resonance imaging (MRI):** A procedure that uses a magnet, radio waves, and a computer to make a series of detailed pictures of both breasts. This procedure is also called nuclear magnetic resonance imaging (NMRI).
- **Blood chemistry studies:** A procedure in which a blood sample is checked to measure the amounts of certain substances released into the blood by organs and tissues in the body. An unusual (higher or lower than normal) amount of a substance can be a sign of disease.
- **Biopsy:** The removal of cells or tissues so they can be viewed under a microscope by a pathologist to check for signs of cancer. If a lump in the breast is found, a biopsy may be done.

Biopsy

There are four types of biopsy used to check for breast cancer:

- **Excisional biopsy:** The removal of an entire lump of tissue.
- **Incisional biopsy:** The removal of part of a lump or a sample of tissue.
- **Core biopsy:** The removal of tissue using a wide needle.
- **Fine-needle aspiration (FNA) biopsy:** The removal of tissue or fluid, using a thin needle.

If cancer is found, tests are done to study the cancer cells.

Decisions about the best treatment are based on the results of these tests. The tests give information about:

- how quickly the cancer may grow
- how likely it is that the cancer will spread through the body
- how well certain treatments might work
- how likely the cancer is to recur (come back)

Tests include the following:

- **Estrogen receptor (ER) and progesterone receptor (PR) test:** A test to measure the amount of estrogen and progesterone (hormones) receptors in cancer tissue. If there are more estrogen and progesterone receptors than normal, the cancer is called estrogen and/or progesterone receptor positive. This type of breast cancer may grow more quickly. The test results show whether treatment to block estrogen and progesterone may stop the cancer from growing.

- **Human epidermal growth factor type 2 receptor (HER2/neu) test:** A laboratory test to measure how many *HER2/neu* genes there are and how much HER2/neu protein is made in a sample of tissue. If there are more *HER2/neu* genes or higher levels of HER2/neu protein than normal, the cancer is called HER2/neu positive. This type of breast cancer may grow more quickly and is more likely to spread to other parts of the body. The cancer may be treated with drugs that target the HER2/neu protein, such as trastuzumab and pertuzumab.
- **Multigene tests:** Tests in which samples of tissue are studied to look at the activity of many genes at the same time. These tests may help predict whether cancer will spread to other parts of the body or recur (come back).

There are many types of multigene tests. The following multigene tests have been studied in clinical trials:

- **Oncotype DX:** This test helps predict whether stage I or stage II breast cancer that is estrogen receptor positive and node negative will spread to other parts of the body. If the risk that the cancer will spread is high, chemotherapy may be given to lower the risk.
- **MammaPrint:** This test helps predict whether stage I or stage II breast cancer that is node-negative will spread to other parts of the body. If the risk that the cancer will spread is high, chemotherapy may be given to lower the risk.

Based on these tests, breast cancer is described as one of the following types:

- Hormone receptor positive (estrogen receptor positive (ER+) and progesterone receptor positive (PR+)) or hormone receptor negative (estrogen receptor negative (ER-) and progesterone receptor negative (PR-))
- HER2/neu positive or HER2/neu negative
- Triple negative (estrogen receptor, progesterone receptor, and HER2/neu negative)

This information helps the doctor decide which treatments will work best for your cancer.

How Is Staging Done for Breast Cancer?

The process used to find out whether the cancer has spread within the breast or to other parts of the body is called staging. The information gathered from the staging process determines the stage of the disease. It is important to know the stage in order to plan treatment. The results of some of the tests used to diagnose breast cancer are also used to stage the disease.

After breast cancer has been diagnosed, tests are done to find out if cancer cells have spread within the breast or to other parts of the body. The following tests and procedures also may be used in the staging process:

- **Sentinel lymph node biopsy (SLNB):** The removal of the sentinel lymph node during surgery. The sentinel lymph node is the first lymph node to receive lymphatic drainage from a tumor. It is the first lymph node the cancer is likely to spread to from the tumor. A radioactive substance and/or blue dye is injected near the tumor. The substance or dye flows through the lymph ducts to the lymph nodes. The first lymph node to receive the substance or dye is removed. A pathologist views the tissue under a microscope to look for cancer cells. If cancer cells are not found, it may not be necessary to remove more lymph nodes.
- **Chest X-ray:** An X-ray of the organs and bones inside the chest. An X-ray is a type of energy beam that can go through the body and onto film, making a picture of areas inside the body.
- **Computed tomography (CT)/computerized axial tomography (CAT) scan:** A procedure that makes a series of detailed pictures of areas inside the body, taken from different angles. The pictures are made by a computer linked to an X-ray machine. A dye may be injected into a vein or swallowed to help the organs or tissues show up more clearly.
- **Bone scan:** A procedure to check if there are rapidly dividing cells, such as cancer cells, in the bone. A very small amount of radioactive material is injected into a vein and travels through the bloodstream. The radioactive material collects in the bones with cancer and is detected by a scanner.
- **Positron emission tomography (PET) scan:** A procedure to find malignant tumor cells in the body. A small amount of radioactive glucose (sugar) is injected into a vein. The PET scanner rotates around the body and makes a picture of where glucose is

being used in the body. Malignant tumor cells show up brighter in the picture because they are more active and take up more glucose than normal cells do.

Stages of Breast Cancer

The following stages are used for breast cancer:

The breast cancer stage is based on the results of tests that are done on the tumor and lymph nodes removed during surgery and on other tests.

Stage 0 (carcinoma *in situ*). There are 3 types of breast carcinoma *in situ*:

- **Ductal carcinoma in situ (DCIS)** is a noninvasive condition in which abnormal cells are found in the lining of a breast duct. The abnormal cells have not spread outside the duct to other tissues in the breast. In some cases, DCIS may become invasive cancer and spread to other tissues. At this time, there is no way to know which lesions could become invasive.
- **Lobular carcinoma in situ (LCIS)** is a condition in which abnormal cells are found in the lobules of the breast. This condition seldom becomes invasive cancer.
- **Paget disease of the nipple** is a condition in which abnormal cells are found in the nipple only.

Stage I. In stage I, cancer has formed. Stage I is divided into stages IA and IB.

- In stage IA, the tumor is 2 centimeters or smaller. Cancer has not spread outside the breast.
- In stage IB, small clusters of breast cancer cells (larger than 0.2 millimeter but not larger than 2 millimeters) are found in the lymph nodes and either:
  - no tumor is found in the breast; or
  - the tumor is 2 centimeters or smaller.

Stage II. Stage II is divided into stages IIA and IIB.

- In stage IIA:
  - no tumor is found in the breast or the tumor is 2 centimeters or smaller. Cancer (larger than 2 millimeters) is found in 1–3

axillary lymph nodes or in the lymph nodes near the breastbone (found during a sentinel lymph node biopsy); or

- the tumor is larger than 2 centimeters but not larger than 5 centimeters. Cancer has not spread to the lymph nodes.

- In stage IIB, the tumor is:
  - larger than 2 centimeters but not larger than 5 centimeters. Small clusters of breast cancer cells (larger than 0.2 millimeter but not larger than 2 millimeters) are found in the lymph nodes; or
  - larger than 2 centimeters but not larger than 5 centimeters. Cancer has spread to 1–3 axillary lymph nodes or to the lymph nodes near the breastbone (found during a sentinel lymph node biopsy); or
  - larger than 5 centimeters. Cancer has not spread to the lymph nodes.

Stage IIIA. In stage IIIA:

- no tumor is found in the breast or the tumor may be any size. Cancer is found in 4–9 axillary lymph nodes or in the lymph nodes near the breastbone (found during imaging tests or a physical exam); or
- the tumor is larger than 5 centimeters. Small clusters of breast cancer cells (larger than 0.2 millimeter but not larger than 2 millimeters) are found in the lymph nodes; or
- the tumor is larger than 5 centimeters. Cancer has spread to 1–3 axillary lymph nodes or to the lymph nodes near the breastbone (found during a sentinel lymph node biopsy).

Stage IIIB. In stage IIIB, the tumor may be any size and cancer has spread to the chest wall and/or to the skin of the breast and caused swelling or an ulcer. Also, cancer may have spread to:

- up to 9 axillary lymph nodes; or
- the lymph nodes near the breastbone

Cancer that has spread to the skin of the breast may also be inflammatory breast cancer.

Stage IIIC. In stage IIIC, no tumor is found in the breast or the tumor may be any size. Cancer may have spread to the skin of the breast and caused swelling or an ulcer and/or has spread to the chest wall. Also, cancer has spread to:

- 10 or more axillary lymph nodes; or
- lymph nodes above or below the collarbone; or
- axillary lymph nodes and lymph nodes near the breastbone.

Cancer that has spread to the skin of the breast may also be inflammatory breast cancer.

Stage IV. In stage IV, cancer has spread to other organs of the body, most often the bones, lungs, liver, or brain.

The treatment of breast cancer depends partly on the stage of the disease.

What Are the Standard Treatments Available for Women with Breast Cancer?

Five types of standard treatment are used:

Surgery

Most patients with breast cancer have surgery to remove the cancer.

Sentinel lymph node biopsy is the removal of the sentinel lymph node during surgery. The sentinel lymph node is the first lymph node to receive lymphatic drainage from a tumor. It is the first lymph node where the cancer is likely to spread. A radioactive substance and/or blue dye is injected near the tumor. The substance or dye flows through the lymph ducts to the lymph nodes. The first lymph node to receive the substance or dye is removed. A pathologist views the tissue under a microscope to look for cancer cells. After the sentinel lymph node biopsy, the surgeon removes the tumor using breast-conserving surgery or mastectomy. If cancer cells were not found in the sentinel lymph node, it may not be necessary to remove more lymph nodes. If cancer cells were found, more lymph nodes will be removed through a separate incision. This is called a lymph node dissection.

Types of surgery include the following:

- **Breast-conserving surgery (BCS)** is an operation to remove the cancer and some normal tissue around it, but not the breast itself. Part of the chest wall lining may also be removed if the cancer is near it. This type of surgery may also be called lumpectomy, partial mastectomy, segmental mastectomy, quadrantectomy, or breast-sparing surgery.

- **Total mastectomy:** Surgery to remove the whole breast that has cancer. This procedure is also called a simple mastectomy. Some of the lymph nodes under the arm may be removed and checked for cancer. This may be done at the same time as the breast surgery or after. This is done through a separate incision.
- **Modified radical mastectomy:** Surgery to remove the whole breast that has cancer, many of the lymph nodes under the arm, the lining over the chest muscles, and sometimes, part of the chest wall muscles.

Chemotherapy may be given before surgery to remove the tumor. When given before surgery, chemotherapy will shrink the tumor and reduce the amount of tissue that needs to be removed during surgery. Treatment given before surgery is called preoperative therapy or neoadjuvant therapy.

Even if the doctor removes all the cancer that can be seen at the time of the surgery, some patients may be given radiation therapy, chemotherapy, or hormone therapy after surgery, to kill any cancer cells that are left. Treatment given after the surgery, to lower the risk that the cancer will come back, is called postoperative therapy or adjuvant therapy.

If a patient is going to have a mastectomy, breast reconstruction (surgery to rebuild a breast's shape after a mastectomy) may be considered. Breast reconstruction may be done at the time of the mastectomy or at some time after. The reconstructed breast may be made with the patient's own (nonbreast) tissue or by using implants filled with saline or silicone gel. Before the decision to get an implant is made, patients can call the U.S. Food and Drug Administration's (FDA) Center for Devices and Radiologic Health (CDRH) at 888-INFO-FDA (888-463-6332).

Radiation Therapy

Radiation therapy is a cancer treatment that uses high-energy X-rays or other types of radiation to kill cancer cells or keep them from growing. There are two types of radiation therapy:

- External radiation therapy uses a machine outside the body to send radiation toward the cancer.
- Internal radiation therapy uses a radioactive substance sealed in needles, seeds, wires, or catheters that are placed directly into or near the cancer.

The way the radiation therapy is given depends on the type and stage of the cancer being treated. External radiation therapy is used to treat breast cancer. Internal radiation therapy with strontium-89 (a radionuclide) is used to relieve bone pain caused by breast cancer that has spread to the bones. Strontium-89 is injected into a vein and travels to the surface of the bones. Radiation is released and kills cancer cells in the bones.

Chemotherapy

Chemotherapy is a cancer treatment that uses drugs to stop the growth of cancer cells, either by killing the cells or by stopping them from dividing. When chemotherapy is taken by mouth or injected into a vein or muscle, the drugs enter the bloodstream and can reach cancer cells throughout the body (systemic chemotherapy). When chemotherapy is placed directly into the cerebrospinal fluid, an organ, or a body cavity such as the abdomen, the drugs mainly affect cancer cells in those areas (regional chemotherapy).

The way the chemotherapy is given depends on the type and stage of the cancer being treated. Systemic chemotherapy is used in the treatment of breast cancer.

Hormone Therapy

Hormone therapy is a cancer treatment that removes hormones or blocks their action and stops cancer cells from growing. Hormones are substances made by glands in the body and circulated in the bloodstream. Some hormones can cause certain cancers to grow. If tests show that the cancer cells have places where hormones can attach (receptors), drugs, surgery, or radiation therapy is used to reduce the production of hormones or block them from working. The hormone estrogen, which makes some breast cancers grow, is made mainly by the ovaries. Treatment to stop the ovaries from making estrogen is called ovarian ablation.

Hormone therapy with tamoxifen is often given to patients with early localized breast cancer that can be removed by surgery and those with metastatic breast cancer (cancer that has spread to other parts of the body). Hormone therapy with tamoxifen or estrogens can act on cells all over the body and may increase the chance of developing endometrial cancer. Women taking tamoxifen should have a pelvic exam every year to look for any signs of cancer. Any vaginal bleeding, other than menstrual bleeding, should be reported to a doctor as soon as possible.

Hormone therapy with a luteinizing hormone-releasing hormone (LHRH) agonist is given to some premenopausal women who have just been diagnosed with hormone receptor positive breast cancer. LHRH agonists decrease the body's estrogen and progesterone.

Hormone therapy with an aromatase inhibitor is given to some postmenopausal women who have hormone receptor positive breast cancer. Aromatase inhibitors decrease the body's estrogen by blocking an enzyme called aromatase from turning androgen into estrogen. Anastrozole, letrozole, and exemestane are types of aromatase inhibitors.

For the treatment of early localized breast cancer that can be removed by surgery, certain aromatase inhibitors may be used as adjuvant therapy instead of tamoxifen or after 2–3 years of tamoxifen use. For the treatment of metastatic breast cancer, aromatase inhibitors are being tested in clinical trials to compare them to hormone therapy with tamoxifen.

Other types of hormone therapy include megestrol acetate or anti-estrogen therapy such as fulvestrant.

Targeted Therapy

Targeted therapy is a type of treatment that uses drugs or other substances to identify and attack specific cancer cells without harming normal cells. Monoclonal antibodies, tyrosine kinase inhibitors, cyclin-dependent kinase inhibitors, mammalian target of rapamycin (mTOR) inhibitors, and poly ADP (adenosine diphosphate) ribose polymerase (PARP) inhibitors are types of targeted therapies used in the treatment of breast cancer.

Monoclonal antibody therapy is a cancer treatment that uses antibodies made in the laboratory, from a single type of immune system cell. These antibodies can identify substances on cancer cells or normal substances that may help cancer cells grow. The antibodies attach to the substances and kill the cancer cells, block their growth, or keep them from spreading. Monoclonal antibodies are given by infusion. They may be used alone or to carry drugs, toxins, or radioactive material directly to cancer cells. Monoclonal antibodies may be used in combination with chemotherapy as adjuvant therapy.

Types of monoclonal antibody therapy include the following:

- **Trastuzumab** is a monoclonal antibody that blocks the effects of the growth factor protein HER2, which sends growth signals to breast cancer cells. It may be used with other therapies to treat HER2 positive breast cancer.

- **Pertuzumab** is a monoclonal antibody that may be combined with trastuzumab and chemotherapy to treat breast cancer. It may be used to treat certain patients with HER2 positive breast cancer that has metastasized (spread to other parts of the body). It may also be used as neoadjuvant therapy in certain patients with early stage HER2 positive breast cancer.
- **Ado-trastuzumab emtansine** is a monoclonal antibody linked to an anticancer drug. This is called an antibody-drug conjugate. It is used to treat HER2 positive breast cancer that has spread to other parts of the body or recurred (come back).

Tyrosine kinase inhibitors are targeted therapy drugs that block signals needed for tumors to grow. Tyrosine kinase inhibitors may be used with other anticancer drugs as adjuvant therapy. Tyrosine kinase inhibitors include the following:

- **Lapatinib** is a tyrosine kinase inhibitor that blocks the effects of the HER2 protein and other proteins inside tumor cells. It may be used with other drugs to treat patients with HER2 positive breast cancer that has progressed after treatment with trastuzumab.
- **Neratinib** is a tyrosine kinase inhibitor that blocks the effects of the HER2 protein and other proteins inside tumor cells. It may be used to treat patients with early stage HER2 positive breast cancer after treatment with trastuzumab.

Cyclin-dependent kinase inhibitors (CDKIs) are targeted therapy drugs that block proteins called cyclin-dependent kinases, which cause the growth of cancer cells. Cyclin-dependent kinase inhibitors include the following:

- **Palbociclib** is a cyclin-dependent kinase inhibitor used with the drug letrozole to treat breast cancer that is estrogen receptor positive and HER2 negative and has spread to other parts of the body. It is used in postmenopausal women whose cancer has not been treated with hormone therapy. Palbociclib may also be used with fulvestrant in women whose disease has gotten worse after treatment with hormone therapy.
- **Ribociclib** is a cyclin-dependent kinase inhibitor used with letrozole to treat breast cancer that is hormone receptor positive and HER2 negative and has come back or spread to other parts

of the body. It is used in postmenopausal women whose cancer has not been treated with hormone therapy.

- **Abemaciclib** is a cyclin-dependent kinase inhibitor used to treat hormone receptor positive and HER2 negative breast cancer that is advanced or has spread to other parts of the body. It may be used alone or with other drugs to treat breast cancer that has gotten worse after other treatment.

Mammalian target of rapamycin (mTOR) inhibitors block a protein called mTOR, which may keep cancer cells from growing and prevent the growth of new blood vessels that tumors need to grow. mTOR inhibitors include the following:

- **Everolimus** is an mTOR inhibitor used in postmenopausal women with advanced hormone receptor positive breast cancer that is also HER2 negative and has not gotten better with other treatment.

PARP inhibitors are a type of targeted therapy that block deoxyribonucleic acid (DNA) repair and may cause cancer cells to die. PARP inhibitor therapy is being studied for the treatment of patients with triple negative breast cancer or tumors with *BRCA1* or *BRCA2* mutations.

Side Effects of Treatment

Treatment for breast cancer may cause side effects. Some treatments for breast cancer may cause side effects that continue or appear months or years after treatment has ended. These are called late effects. Late effects of radiation therapy are not common, but may include:

- Inflammation of the lung after radiation therapy to the breast, especially when chemotherapy is given at the same time
- Arm lymphedema, especially when radiation therapy is given after lymph node dissection
- In women younger than 45 years who receive radiation therapy to the chest wall after mastectomy, there may be a higher risk of developing breast cancer in the other breast

Late effects of chemotherapy depend on the drugs used, but may include:

- Heart failure
- Blood clots

- Premature menopause
- Second cancer, such as leukemia

Late effects of targeted therapy with trastuzumab, lapatinib, or pertuzumab may include:

- Heart problems such as heart failure

What Is the Prognosis for Breast Cancer in Women?

The prognosis (chance of recovery) and treatment options depend on the following:

- The stage of the cancer (the size of the tumor and whether it is in the breast only or has spread to lymph nodes or other places in the body)
- The type of breast cancer
- Estrogen receptor and progesterone receptor levels in the tumor tissue
- Human epidermal growth factor type 2 receptor (HER2/neu) levels in the tumor tissue
- Whether the tumor tissue is triple negative (cells that do not have estrogen receptors, progesterone receptors, or high levels of HER2/neu)
- How fast the tumor is growing
- How likely the tumor is to recur (come back)
- A woman's age, general health, and menopausal status (whether a woman is still having menstrual periods)
- Whether the cancer has just been diagnosed or has recurred (come back)

Section 43.2

Breast Cancer in Men

This section includes text excerpted from "Male Breast Cancer Treatment (PDQ®)—Patient Version," National Cancer Institute (NCI), September 29, 2017.

What Is Male Breast Cancer?

Male breast cancer is a disease in which malignant (cancer) cells form in the tissues of the breast. Breast cancer may occur in men. Men at any age may develop breast cancer, but it is usually detected (found) in men between 60–70 years of age. Male breast cancer makes up less than 1 percent of all cases of breast cancer.

The following types of breast cancer are found in men:

- **Infiltrating ductal carcinoma (IDC):** Cancer that has spread beyond the cells lining ducts in the breast. Most men with breast cancer have this type of cancer.
- **Ductal carcinoma in situ (DCIS):** Abnormal cells that are found in the lining of a duct; also called intraductal carcinoma.
- **Inflammatory breast cancer:** A type of cancer in which the breast looks red and swollen and feels warm.
- **Paget disease of the nipple:** A tumor that has grown from ducts beneath the nipple onto the surface of the nipple.

Lobular carcinoma in situ (LCIS) (abnormal cells found in one of the lobes or sections of the breast), which sometimes occurs in women, has not been seen in men.

What Are the Risk Factors for Male Breast Cancer?

Anything that increases your risk of getting a disease is called a risk factor. Having a risk factor does not mean that you will get cancer; not having risk factors doesn't mean that you will not get cancer. Talk with your doctor if you think you may be at risk. A family history of breast cancer and other factors can increase a man's risk of breast cancer. Risk factors for breast cancer in men may include the following:

- Being exposed to radiation
- Having a disease linked to high levels of estrogen in the body, such as cirrhosis (liver disease) or Klinefelter syndrome (a genetic disorder)
- Having several female relatives who have had breast cancer, especially relatives who have inherited changes in the *BRCA1* or *BRCA2* genes or in other genes that increase the risk of breast cancer
- Mutations (changes) in other genes.

Is Male Breast Cancer Caused Due to Inherited Gene Mutations?

Male breast cancer is sometimes caused by inherited gene mutations (changes). The genes in cells carry the hereditary information that is received from a person's parents. Hereditary breast cancer makes up about 5–10 percent of all breast cancer. Some mutated genes related to breast cancer are more common in certain ethnic groups. Men who have a mutated gene related to breast cancer have an increased risk of this disease. There are tests that can detect (find) mutated genes. These genetic tests are sometimes done for members of families with a high risk of cancer.

Are There Any Other Signs of Male Breast Cancer?

Men with breast cancer usually have lumps that can be felt. Lumps and other signs may be caused by male breast cancer or by other conditions. Check with your doctor if you notice a change in your breasts.

How Is Male Breast Cancer Diagnosed?

Tests that examine the breasts are used to detect (find) and diagnose breast cancer in men. The following tests and procedures may be used:

- **Physical exam and history:** An exam of the body to check general signs of health, including checking for signs of disease, such as lumps or anything else that seems unusual. A history of the patient's health habits and past illnesses and treatments will also be taken.

- **Clinical breast exam (CBE):** An exam of the breast by a doctor or other health professional. The doctor will carefully feel the breasts and under the arms for lumps or anything else that seems unusual.
- **Ultrasound exam:** A procedure in which high-energy sound waves (ultrasound) are bounced off internal tissues or organs and make echoes. The echoes form a picture of body tissues called a sonogram. The picture can be printed to be looked at later.
- **Magnetic resonance imaging (MRI):** A procedure that uses a magnet, radio waves, and a computer to make a series of detailed pictures of areas inside the body. This procedure is also called nuclear magnetic resonance imaging (NMRI).
- **Blood chemistry studies:** A procedure in which a blood sample is checked to measure the amounts of certain substances released into the blood by organs and tissues in the body. An unusual (higher or lower than normal) amount of a substance can be a sign of disease.
- **Biopsy:** The removal of cells or tissues so they can be viewed under a microscope by a pathologist to check for signs of cancer. The following are different types of biopsies:
    - **Fine-needle aspiration (FNA) biopsy:** The removal of tissue or fluid using a thin needle.
    - **Core biopsy:** The removal of tissue using a wide needle.
    - **Excisional biopsy:** The removal of an entire lump of tissue.

If cancer is found, tests are done to study the cancer cells.

Decisions about the best treatment are based on the results of these tests. The tests give information about:

- How quickly the cancer may grow
- How likely it is that the cancer will spread through the body
- How well certain treatments might work
- How likely the cancer is to recur (come back)

Tests include the following:

- **Estrogen receptor (ER) and progesterone receptor (PR) test:** A test to measure the amount of estrogen and progesterone (hormones) receptors in cancer tissue. If cancer is found in the breast, tissue from the tumor is checked in the laboratory to find out whether estrogen and progesterone could affect the way cancer grows. The test results show whether hormone therapy may stop the cancer from growing.

- **HER2 test:** A test to measure the amount of HER2 in cancer tissue. HER2 is a growth factor protein that sends growth signals to cells. When cancer forms, the cells may make too much of the protein, causing more cancer cells to grow. If cancer is found in the breast, tissue from the tumor is checked in the laboratory to find out if there is too much HER2 in the cells. The test results show whether monoclonal antibody therapy may stop the cancer from growing.

What Is the Survival Percentage for Males with Breast Cancer?

Survival for men with breast cancer is similar to that for women with breast cancer when their stage at diagnosis is the same. Breast cancer in men, however, is often diagnosed at a later stage. Cancer found at a later stage may be less likely to be cured.

What Is the Prognosis for Male Breast Cancer?

The prognosis (chance of recovery) and treatment options depend on the following:

- The stage of the cancer (whether it is in the breast only or has spread to other places in the body)
- The type of breast cancer
- Estrogen-receptor and progesterone-receptor levels in the tumor tissue
- Whether the cancer is also found in the other breast
- The patient's age and general health

How Is Staging Done for Male Breast Cancer?

After breast cancer has been diagnosed, tests are done to find out if cancer cells have spread within the breast or to other parts of the body. This process is called staging. The information gathered from the staging process determines the stage of the disease. It is important to know the stage in order to plan treatment. Breast cancer in men is staged the same as it is in women. The spread of cancer from the breast to lymph nodes and other parts of the body appears to be similar in men and women.

The following tests and procedures may be used in the staging process:

- **Sentinel lymph node biopsy (SLNB):** The removal of the sentinel lymph node during surgery. The sentinel lymph node is the first lymph node to receive lymphatic drainage from a tumor. It is the first lymph node the cancer is likely to spread to from the tumor. A radioactive substance and/or blue dye is injected near the tumor. The substance or dye flows through the lymph ducts to the lymph nodes. The first lymph node to receive the substance or dye is removed. A pathologist views the tissue under a microscope to look for cancer cells. If cancer cells are not found, it may not be necessary to remove more lymph nodes.
- **Chest X-ray:** An X-ray of the organs and bones inside the chest. An X-ray is a type of energy beam that can go through the body and onto film, making a picture of areas inside the body.
- **Computed tomography (CT)/computerized axial tomography (CAT) scan:** A procedure that makes a series of detailed pictures of areas inside the body, taken from different angles. The pictures are made by a computer linked to an X-ray machine. A dye may be injected into a vein or swallowed to help the organs or tissues show up more clearly. This procedure is also called computed tomography, computerized tomography, or computerized axial tomography.
- **Bone scan:** A procedure to check if there are rapidly dividing cells, such as cancer cells, in the bone. A very small amount of radioactive material is injected into a vein and travels through the bloodstream. The radioactive material collects in the bones and is detected by a scanner.
- **Positron emission tomography (PET) scan:** A procedure to find malignant tumor cells in the body. A small amount of radioactive glucose (sugar) is injected into a vein. The PET scanner rotates around the body and makes a picture of where glucose is being used in the body. Malignant tumor cells show up brighter in the picture because they are more active and take up more glucose than normal cells do.

Stages of Male Breast Cancer

The following stages are used for male breast cancer:

The breast cancer stage is based on the results of testing that is done on the tumor and lymph nodes removed during surgery and other tests.

Stage 0 (carcinoma *in situ*). There are 3 types of breast carcinoma *in situ*:

- **Ductal carcinoma in situ (DCIS)** is a noninvasive condition in which abnormal cells are found in the lining of a breast duct. The abnormal cells have not spread outside the duct to other tissues in the breast. In some cases, DCIS may become invasive cancer and spread to other tissues. At this time, there is no way to know which lesions could become invasive.
- **Paget disease of the nipple** is a condition in which abnormal cells are found in the nipple only.
- **Lobular carcinoma in situ (LCIS)** is a condition in which abnormal cells are found in the lobules of the breast. This condition has not been seen in men.

Stage I. In stage I, cancer has formed. Stage I is divided into stages IA and IB.

- In stage IA, the tumor is 2 centimeters or smaller. Cancer has not spread outside the breast.
- In stage IB, small clusters of breast cancer cells (larger than 0.2 millimeter but not larger than 2 millimeters) are found in the lymph nodes and either:
    - no tumor is found in the breast; or
    - the tumor is 2 centimeters or smaller.

Stage II. Stage II is divided into stages IIA and IIB.

- In stage IIA
    - no tumor is found in the breast or the tumor is 2 centimeters or smaller. Cancer (larger than 2 millimeters) is found in 1–3 axillary lymph nodes or in the lymph nodes near the breastbone (found during a sentinel lymph node biopsy); or
    - the tumor is larger than 2 centimeters but not larger than 5 centimeters. Cancer has not spread to the lymph nodes.

- In stage IIB, the tumor is:
    - larger than 2 centimeters but not larger than 5 centimeters. Small clusters of breast cancer cells (larger than 0.2 millimeter but not larger than 2 millimeters) are found in the lymph nodes; or
    - larger than 2 centimeters but not larger than 5 centimeters. Cancer has spread to 1–3 axillary lymph nodes or to the lymph nodes near the breastbone (found during a sentinel lymph node biopsy); or
    - larger than 5 centimeters. Cancer has not spread to the lymph nodes.

Stage IIIA. In stage IIIA:

- no tumor is found in the breast or the tumor may be any size. Cancer is found in 4–9 axillary lymph nodes or in the lymph nodes near the breastbone (found during imaging tests or a physical exam); or
- the tumor is larger than 5 centimeters. Small clusters of breast cancer cells (larger than 0.2 millimeter but not larger than 2 millimeters) are found in the lymph nodes; or
- the tumor is larger than 5 centimeters. Cancer has spread to 1–3 axillary lymph nodes or to the lymph nodes near the breastbone (found during a sentinel lymph node biopsy).

Stage IIIB. In stage IIIB, the tumor may be any size and cancer has spread to the chest wall and/or to the skin of the breast and caused swelling or an ulcer. Also, cancer may have spread to:

- up to 9 axillary lymph nodes; or
- the lymph nodes near the breastbone.

Cancer that has spread to the skin of the breast may also be inflammatory breast cancer.

Stage IIIC. In stage IIIC, no tumor is found in the breast or the tumor may be any size. Cancer may have spread to the skin of the breast and caused swelling or an ulcer and/or has spread to the chest wall. Also, cancer has spread to:

- 10 or more axillary lymph nodes; or
- lymph nodes above or below the collarbone; or

- axillary lymph nodes and lymph nodes near the breastbone.

Cancer that has spread to the skin of the breast may also be inflammatory breast cancer. For treatment, stage IIIC breast cancer is divided into operable and inoperable stage IIIC.

Stage IV. In stage IV, cancer has spread to other organs of the body, most often the bones, lungs, liver, or brain.

What Is Inflammatory Male Breast Cancer?

In inflammatory breast cancer, cancer has spread to the skin of the breast and the breast looks red and swollen and feels warm. The redness and warmth occur because the cancer cells block the lymph vessels in the skin. The skin of the breast may also show the dimpled appearance called peau d'orange (like the skin of an orange). There may not be any lumps in the breast that can be felt. Inflammatory breast cancer may be stage IIIB, stage IIIC, or stage IV.

What Are the Standard Treatment Options Available for Males with Breast Cancer?

Five types of standard treatment are used to treat men with breast cancer:

Surgery

Surgery for men with breast cancer is usually a modified radical mastectomy (removal of the breast, many of the lymph nodes under the arm, the lining over the chest muscles, and sometimes part of the chest wall muscles).

Breast-conserving surgery, an operation to remove the cancer but not the breast itself, is also used for some men with breast cancer. A lumpectomy is done to remove the tumor (lump) and a small amount of normal tissue around it. Radiation therapy is given after surgery to kill any cancer cells that are left.

Chemotherapy

Chemotherapy is a cancer treatment that uses drugs to stop the growth of cancer cells, either by killing the cells or by stopping them from dividing. When chemotherapy is taken by mouth or injected into a vein or muscle, the drugs enter the bloodstream and can reach cancer cells throughout the body (systemic chemotherapy). When chemotherapy is placed directly into the cerebrospinal fluid, an organ, or a body cavity such as the abdomen, the drugs mainly affect cancer cells in those areas (regional chemotherapy). The way the chemotherapy is given depends on the type and stage of the cancer being treated.

Hormone Therapy

Hormone therapy is a cancer treatment that removes hormones or blocks their action and stops cancer cells from growing. Hormones are substances made by glands in the body and circulated in the bloodstream. Some hormones can cause certain cancers to grow. If tests show that the cancer cells have places where hormones can attach (receptors), drugs, surgery, or radiation therapy is used to reduce the production of hormones or block them from working.

Hormone therapy with tamoxifen is often given to patients with early localized breast cancer that can be removed by surgery and those with metastatic breast cancer (cancer that has spread to other parts of the body).

Radiation Therapy

Radiation therapy is a cancer treatment that uses high-energy X-rays or other types of radiation to kill cancer cells or keep them from growing. There are two types of radiation therapy:

- External radiation therapy uses a machine outside the body to send radiation toward the cancer.
- Internal radiation therapy uses a radioactive substance sealed in needles, seeds, wires, or catheters that are placed directly into or near the cancer.

The way the radiation therapy is given depends on the type and stage of the cancer being treated. External radiation therapy is used to treat male breast cancer.

Targeted Therapy

Targeted therapy is a type of treatment that uses drugs or other substances to identify and attack specific cancer cells without harming normal cells. Monoclonal antibody therapy is a type of targeted therapy used to treat men with breast cancer.

Monoclonal antibody therapy uses antibodies made in the laboratory from a single type of immune system cell. These antibodies can identify substances on cancer cells or normal substances that may help cancer cells grow. The antibodies attach to the substances and kill the cancer cells, block their growth, or keep them from spreading. Monoclonal antibodies are given by infusion. They may be used alone or to carry drugs, toxins, or radioactive material directly to cancer cells. Monoclonal antibodies are also used with chemotherapy as adjuvant therapy (treatment given after surgery to lower the risk that the cancer will come back).

Trastuzumab is a monoclonal antibody that blocks the effects of the growth factor protein HER2. Treatment for male breast cancer may cause side effects.

Chapter 44

Gynecological Cancers

Chapter Contents

Section 44.1

Overview of Gynecological Cancers

This section includes text excerpted from "Gynecologic Cancers," Centers for Disease Control and Prevention (CDC), January 2, 2018.

All women are at risk for gynecologic cancers, and risk increases with age. You can lower your risk for some of these cancers. When gynecologic cancers are found early, treatment works best.

What Is Gynecologic Cancer?

Gynecologic cancer is any cancer that starts in a woman's reproductive organs. Cancer is always named for the part of the body where it starts. Gynecologic cancers begin in different places within a woman's pelvis, which is the area below the stomach and in between the hip bones.

- **Cervical cancer** begins in the cervix, which is the lower, narrow end of the uterus. (The uterus is also called the womb.)
- **Ovarian cancer** begins in the ovaries, which are located on each side of the uterus.
- **Uterine cancer** begins in the uterus, the pear-shaped organ in a woman's pelvis where the baby grows when a woman is pregnant.
- **Vaginal cancer** begins in the vagina, which is the hollow, tube-like channel between the bottom of the uterus and the outside of the body.
- **Vulvar cancer** begins in the vulva, the outer part of the female genital organs.

Each gynecologic cancer is unique, with different signs and symptoms, different risk factors (things that may increase your chance of getting a disease), and different prevention strategies. All women are at risk for gynecologic cancers, and risk increases with age. When gynecologic cancers are found early, treatment is most effective.

What Are the Symptoms?

There is no way to know for sure if you will get a gynecologic cancer. That's why it is important to pay attention to your body and know what is normal for you, so you can recognize the warning signs or symptoms of gynecologic cancer. If you have vaginal bleeding that is unusual for you, talk to a doctor right away. You should also see a doctor if you have any other warning signs that last for two weeks or longer and are not normal for you. Symptoms may be caused by something other than cancer, but the only way to know is to see a doctor. Signs and symptoms are not the same for everyone and each gynecologic cancer (cervical, ovarian, uterine, vaginal, and vulvar cancers) has its own signs and symptoms.

What Can I Do to Reduce My Risk?

Human Papillomavirus (HPV) Vaccine

Some gynecologic cancers are caused by the human papillomavirus (HPV), a very common sexually transmitted infection.

The HPV vaccine protects against the types of HPV that most often cause cervical, vaginal, and vulvar cancers. It is recommended for preteens (both boys and girls) aged 11–12 years, but can be given as early as age 9 and until age 26. The vaccine is given in a series of either two or three shots, depending on age. If vaccination is started before age 15, a two-dose schedule is recommended, with the doses given 6–12 months apart. For teens and young adults who start the series at age 15 through 26, the vaccine is given in a series of three shots.

Screening Tests

Screening is when a test is used to look for a disease before there are any symptoms. Cancer screening tests are effective when they can find disease early, which can lead to more effective treatment. (Diagnostic tests are used when a person has symptoms. The purpose of diagnostic tests is to find out, or diagnose, what is causing the symptoms. Diagnostic tests also may be used to check a person who is considered at high risk for cancer.)

Of all the gynecologic cancers, only cervical cancer has a screening test—the Pap test—that can find this cancer early, when treatment works best. The Pap test also helps prevent cervical cancer by finding precancers, cell changes on the cervix that might become cervical cancer if they are not treated appropriately. In addition to the Pap test, which is the main screening test for cervical cancer, a test called the HPV test looks for HPV infection. It can be used along with the Pap test for screening women aged 30 years and older. It also is used to provide more information when Pap test results are unclear for women aged 21 and older.

Since there is no simple and reliable way to screen for any gynecologic cancers except cervical cancer, it is especially important to recognize warning signs and learn if there are things you can do to reduce your risk. Talk with your doctor if you believe that you are at increased risk for gynecologic cancer. Ask what you might do to lower your risk and whether there are tests that you should have.

How Are Gynecologic Cancers Treated?

If your doctor says that you have a gynecologic cancer, ask to be referred to a gynecologic oncologist—a doctor who has been trained to treat cancers of a woman's reproductive system. This doctor will work with you to create a treatment plan.

Types of Treatment

Gynecologic cancers are treated in several ways. It depends on the kind of cancer and how far it has spread. Treatments include surgery, chemotherapy, and radiation. Women with a gynecologic cancer often get more than one kind of treatment.

- **Surgery:** Doctors remove cancer tissue in an operation.
- **Chemotherapy:** Using special medicines to shrink or kill the cancer. The drugs can be pills you take or medicines given in your veins, or sometimes both.
- **Radiation:** Using high-energy rays (similar to X-rays) to kill the cancer.

Different treatments may be provided by different doctors on your medical team.

- Gynecologic oncologists are doctors who are trained to treat cancers of a woman's reproductive system
- Surgeons are doctors who perform operations
- Medical oncologists are doctors who treat cancer with medicine
- Radiation oncologists are doctors who treat cancer with radiation

Clinical Trials

Clinical trials use new treatment options to see if they are safe and effective.

Complementary and Alternative Medicine

Complementary and alternative medicine are medicines and health practices that are not standard cancer treatments. Complementary medicine is used in addition to standard treatments, and alternative medicine is used instead of standard treatments. Meditation, yoga, and supplements like vitamins and herbs are some examples.

Many kinds of complementary and alternative medicine have not been tested scientifically and may not be safe. Talk to your doctor about the risks and benefits before you start any kind of complementary or alternative medicine.

Which Treatment Is Right for Me?

Choosing the treatment that is right for you may be hard. Talk to your cancer doctor about the treatment options available for your type and stage of cancer. Your doctor can explain the risks and benefits of each treatment and their side effects. Side effects are how your body reacts to drugs or other treatments.

Sometimes people get an opinion from more than one cancer doctor. This is called a "second opinion." Getting a second opinion may help you choose the treatment that is right for you.

Section 44.2

Cervical Cancer

This section includes text excerpted from "Gynecologic Cancers—Cervical Cancer," Centers for Disease Control and Prevention (CDC), February 8, 2018.

The cervix is the lower, narrow end of the uterus. The cervix connects the vagina (birth canal) to the upper part of the uterus. The uterus (or womb) is where a baby grows when a woman is pregnant.

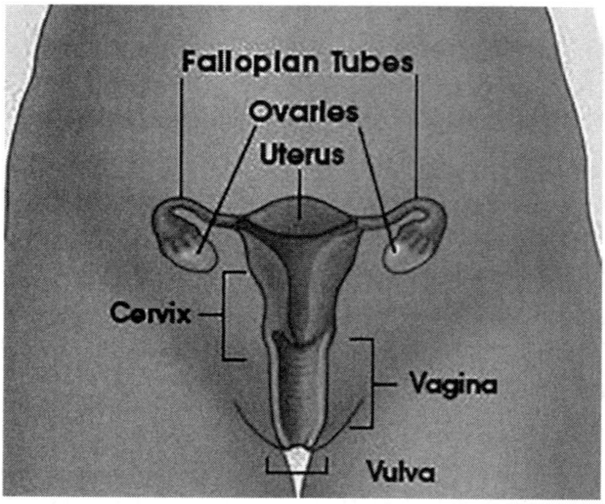

Figure 44.1. *Cervix*

What Is Cervical Cancer?

When cancer starts in the cervix, it is called cervical cancer. All women are at risk for cervical cancer. It occurs most often in women over age 30. Each year, about 12,000 women in the United States get cervical cancer and about 4,000 women die from it. Human papillomavirus (HPV) is the main cause of cervical cancer. HPV is a common virus that is passed from one person to another during sex. At least half of sexually active people will have HPV at some point in their lives, but few women will get cervical cancer. It is highly preventable in most Western countries because screening tests and a vaccine to prevent HPV infections are available. When cervical cancer is found early, it is highly treatable and associated with long survival and good quality of life.

What Are the Risk Factors for Cervical Cancer?

Almost all cervical cancers are caused by human papillomavirus (HPV), a common virus that can be passed from one person to another during sex. There are many types of HPV. Some HPV types can cause changes on a woman's cervix that can lead to cervical cancer over time, while other types can cause genital or skin warts.

HPV is so common that most people get it at some time in their lives. HPV usually causes no symptoms so you can't tell that you have it. For most women, HPV will go away on its own; however, if it does not, there is a chance that over time it may cause cervical cancer.

Other things can increase your risk of cervical cancer:

- Smoking
- Having human immunodeficiency virus (HIV), the virus that causes acquired immunodeficiency syndrome (AIDS), or another condition that makes it hard for your body to fight off health problems
- Using birth control pills for a long time (five or more years)
- Having given birth to three or more children
- Having several sexual partners

What Are the Symptoms of Cervical Cancer?

Early on, cervical cancer may not cause signs and symptoms. Advanced cervical cancer may cause bleeding or discharge from the vagina that is not normal for you, such as bleeding after sex. If you have any of these signs, see your doctor. They may be caused by something other than cancer, but the only way to know is to see your doctor.

What Can I Do to Reduce My Risk of Cervical Cancer?

Two tests can help prevent cervical cancer:

1. The Pap test (or Pap smear) looks for precancers, cell changes on the cervix that may become cervical cancer if they are not treated appropriately. You should start getting Pap tests at age 21.
2. The HPV test looks for the virus that can cause these cell changes.

The most important thing you can do to help prevent cervical cancer is to have regular screening tests starting at age 21.

If your Pap test results are normal, your chance of getting cervical cancer in the next few years is very low. For that reason, your doctor may tell you that you will not need another Pap test for as long as three years. If you are 30 years old or older, you may choose to have an HPV test along with the Pap test. If both test results are normal, your doctor may tell you that you can wait five years to have your next Pap test. But you should still go to the doctor regularly for a checkup.

For women aged 21–65, it is important to continue getting a Pap test as directed by your doctor—even if you think you are too old to have a child or are not having sex anymore. However, if you are older than 65 and have had normal Pap test results for several years, or if you have had your cervix removed as part of a total hysterectomy for a noncancerous condition, like fibroids, your doctor may tell you that you do not need to have a Pap test anymore.

Getting an HPV Vaccine

The HPV vaccine protects against the types of HPV that most often cause cervical, vaginal, and vulvar cancers. It is recommended for preteens (both boys and girls) aged 11–12 years, but can be given as early as age 9 and until age 26. The vaccine is given in a series of either two or three shots, depending on age. It is important to note that even women who are vaccinated against HPV need to have regular Pap tests to screen for cervical cancer.

More Steps to Help Prevent Cervical Cancer

These things may also help lower your risk for cervical cancer:

- Don't smoke
- Use condoms during sex*
- Limit your number of sexual partners

**HPV infection can occur in both male and female genital areas that are covered or protected by a latex condom, as well as in areas that are not covered. While the effect of condoms in preventing HPV infection is unknown, condom use has been associated with a lower rate of cervical cancer.*

What Should I Know about Screening?

Cervical cancer is the easiest gynecologic cancer to prevent, with regular screening tests and follow-up. Two screening tests can help prevent cervical cancer or find it early:

- The **Pap test** (or Pap smear) looks for precancers, cell changes on the cervix that might become cervical cancer if they are not treated appropriately.
- The **HPV test** looks for the virus (human papillomavirus) that can cause these cell changes.

The Pap test is recommended for all women between the ages of 21–65 years old, and can be done in a doctor's office or clinic. During the Pap test, the doctor will use a plastic or metal instrument, called a speculum, to widen your vagina. This helps the doctor examine the vagina and the cervix, and collect a few cells and mucus from the cervix and the area around it. The cells are then placed on a slide or in a bottle of liquid and sent to a laboratory. The laboratory will check to be sure that the cells are normal.

If you get the HPV test along with the Pap test, the cells collected during the Pap test will be tested for HPV at the laboratory. Talk with your doctor, nurse, or other healthcare professional about whether the HPV test is right for you.

When you have a Pap test, the doctor may also perform a pelvic exam, checking your uterus, ovaries, and other organs to make sure there are no problems. There are times when your doctor may perform a pelvic exam without giving you a Pap test. Ask your doctor which tests you are having, if you are unsure.

If you have a low income or do not have health insurance, you may be able to get a free or low-cost Pap test through the National Breast and Cervical Cancer Early Detection Program (NBCCEDP).

How to Prepare for Your Pap Test

You should not schedule your Pap test for a time when you are having your period. If you are going to have a Pap test in the next two days:

- You should not douche (rinse the vagina with water or another fluid).
- You should not use a tampon.
- You should not have sex.
- You should not use a birth control foam, cream, or jelly.
- You should not use a medicine or cream in your vagina.

When to Get Screened

You should start getting regular Pap tests at age 21. The Pap test, which screens for cervical cancer, is one of the most reliable and effective cancer screening tests available. The only cancer for which the Pap test screens is cervical cancer. It does **not** screen for ovarian, uterine, vaginal, or vulvar cancers. So even if you have a Pap test regularly, if you notice any signs or symptoms that are unusual for you, see a doctor to find out why you're having them. If your Pap test results are normal, your doctor may tell you that you can wait three years until your next Pap test.

If you are 30 years old or older, you may choose to have an HPV test along with the Pap test. Both tests can be performed by your doctor at the same time. When both tests are performed together, it is called co-testing. If your test results are normal, your chance of getting cervical cancer in the next few years is very low. Your doctor may then tell you that you can wait as long as five years for your next screening. But you should still go to the doctor regularly for a checkup.

If you are 21–65 years old, it is important for you to continue getting a Pap test as directed by your doctor—even if you think you are too old to have a child or are not having sex anymore. If you are older than 65 and have had normal Pap test results for several years, or if you have had your cervix removed as part of a total hysterectomy for noncancerous conditions, like fibroids, your doctor may tell you that you do not need to have a Pap test anymore.

Test Results

It can take as long as three weeks to receive your test results. If your test shows that something might not be normal, your doctor will contact you and figure out how best to follow up. There are many reasons why test results might not be normal. It usually does not mean you have cancer.

If your test results show cells that are not normal and may become cancer, your doctor will let you know if you need to be treated. In most cases, treatment prevents cervical cancer from developing. It is important to follow-up with your doctor right away to learn more about your test results and receive any treatment that may be needed.

Cervical Cancer Screening Guidelines

The Cervical Cancer Screening Guidelines compares recommendations from the American Cancer Society (ACS), U.S. Preventive Services Task Force (USPSTF), and the American College of Obstetricians and Gynecologists (ACOG) regarding:

- When to start screening
- Screening methods and intervals
- When to stop screening
- Screening after a total hysterectomy

- Pelvic exams
- Screening among women who have been vaccinated against human papillomavirus (HPV)

How Is Cervical Cancer Diagnosed and Treated?

If your doctor says that you have cervical cancer, ask to be referred to a gynecologic oncologist—a doctor who has been trained to treat cancers of a woman's reproductive system. This doctor will work with you to create a treatment plan.

The extent of disease is referred to as the stage. Information about the size of the cancer or how far it has spread is often used to determine the stage. Doctors use this information to plan treatment and to monitor progress.

Types of Treatment

Cervical cancer is treated in several ways. It depends on the kind of cervical cancer and how far it has spread. Treatments include surgery, chemotherapy, and radiation therapy.

- **Surgery:** Doctors remove cancer tissue in an operation.
- **Chemotherapy:** Using special medicines to shrink or kill the cancer. The drugs can be pills you take or medicines given in your veins, or sometimes both.
- **Radiation:** Using high-energy rays (similar to X-rays) to kill the cancer.

Different treatments may be provided by different doctors on your medical team.

- Gynecologic oncologists are doctors who have been trained to treat cancers of a woman's reproductive system.
- Surgeons are doctors who perform operations.
- Medical oncologists are doctors who treat cancer with medicine.
- Radiation oncologists are doctors who treat cancer with radiation.

Clinical Trials

Clinical trials use new treatment options to see if they are safe and effective. If you have cancer, you may want to take part.

Complementary and Alternative Medicine

Complementary and alternative medicine are medicines and health practices that are not standard cancer treatments. Complementary medicine is used in addition to standard treatments, and alternative medicine is used instead of standard treatments. Meditation, yoga, and supplements like vitamins and herbs are some examples.

Many kinds of complementary and alternative medicine have not been tested scientifically and may not be safe. Talk to your doctor about the risks and benefits before you start any kind of complementary or alternative medicine.

Which Treatment Is Right for Me?

Choosing the treatment that is right for you may be hard. Talk to your cancer doctor about the treatment options available for your type and stage of cancer. Your doctor can explain the risks and benefits of each treatment and their side effects. Side effects are how your body reacts to drugs or other treatments.

Sometimes people get an opinion from more than one cancer doctor. This is called a "second opinion." Getting a second opinion may help you choose the treatment that is right for you.

Section 44.3

Endometrial Cancer

This section includes text excerpted from "Endometrial Cancer Treatment (PDQ®)—Patient Version," National Cancer Institute (NCI), January 24, 2018.

The endometrium is the lining of the uterus, a hollow, muscular organ in a woman's pelvis. The uterus is where a fetus grows. In most nonpregnant women, the uterus is about 3 inches long. The lower, narrow end of the uterus is the cervix, which leads to the vagina.

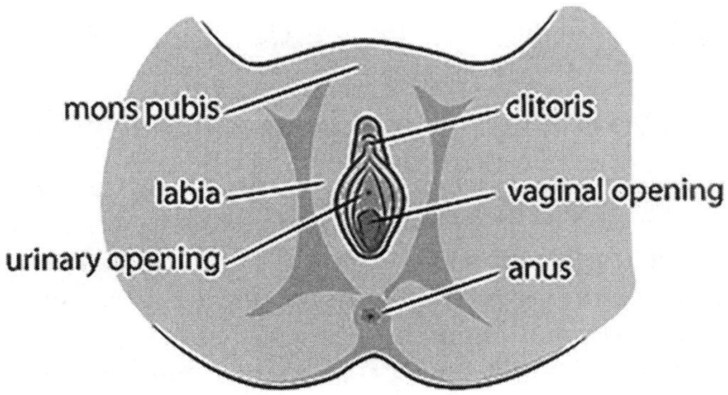

Figure 44.2. *Female Reproductive System (Exterior)* (Source: "How the Female Reproductive System Works," girlshealth.gov, Office on Women's Health (OWH).)

What Is Endometrial Cancer?

Endometrial cancer is a disease in which malignant (cancer) cells form in the tissues of the endometrium. Cancer of the endometrium is different from cancer of the muscle of the uterus, which is called sarcoma of the uterus.

What Are the Risk Factors for Endometrial Cancer?

Obesity and having metabolic syndrome may increase the risk of endometrial cancer. Risk factors for endometrial cancer include the following:

- Having endometrial hyperplasia
- Being obese
- Having metabolic syndrome, a set of conditions that occur together, including extra fat around the abdomen, high blood sugar, high blood pressure, high levels of triglycerides, and low levels of high-density lipoproteins in the blood
- Never giving birth
- Beginning menstruation at an early age
- Reaching menopause at an older age
- Having polycystic ovarian syndrome (PCOS)
- Having a mother, sister, or daughter with uterine cancer

- Having a certain gene change that is linked to Lynch syndrome (hereditary nonpolyposis colon cancer)
- Having hyperinsulinemia (high levels of insulin in the blood)

Talk with your doctor if you think you may be at risk. Endometrial cancer may develop in breast cancer patients who have been treated with tamoxifen. A patient who takes this drug and has abnormal vaginal bleeding should have a follow-up exam and a biopsy of the endometrial lining if needed. Women taking estrogen (a hormone that can affect the growth of some cancers) alone also have an increased risk of endometrial cancer. Taking estrogen combined with progesterone (another hormone) does not increase a woman's risk of endometrial cancer.

What Are the Signs and Symptoms of Endometrial Cancer?

Signs and symptoms of endometrial cancer include unusual vaginal bleeding or pain in the pelvis. These and other signs and symptoms may be caused by endometrial cancer or by other conditions. Check with your doctor if you have any of the following:

- Vaginal bleeding or discharge not related to menstruation (periods)
- Vaginal bleeding after menopause
- Difficult or painful urination
- Pain during sexual intercourse
- Pain in the pelvic area

How Is Endometrial Cancer Diagnosed?

Tests that examine the endometrium are used to detect (find) and diagnose endometrial cancer. Because endometrial cancer begins inside the uterus, it does not usually show up in the results of a Pap test. For this reason, a sample of endometrial tissue must be removed and checked under a microscope to look for cancer cells. One of the following procedures may be used:

- **Endometrial biopsy:** The removal of tissue from the endometrium (inner lining of the uterus) by inserting a thin, flexible tube through the cervix and into the uterus. The tube is used to gently scrape a small amount of tissue from the endometrium and then remove the tissue samples. A pathologist views the tissue under a microscope to look for cancer cells.

- **Dilatation and curettage:** A procedure to remove samples of tissue from the inner lining of the uterus. The cervix is dilated and a curette (spoon-shaped instrument) is inserted into the uterus to remove tissue. The tissue samples are checked under a microscope for signs of disease. This procedure is also called a D&C.
- **Hysteroscopy:** A procedure to look inside the uterus for abnormal areas. A hysteroscope is inserted through the vagina and cervix into the uterus. A hysteroscope is a thin, tube-like instrument with a light and a lens for viewing. It may also have a tool to remove tissue samples, which are checked under a microscope for signs of cancer.

Other tests and procedures used to diagnose endometrial cancer include the following:

- **Physical exam and history:** An exam of the body to check general signs of health, including checking for signs of disease, such as lumps or anything else that seems unusual. A history of the patient's health habits and past illnesses and treatments will also be taken.
- **Transvaginal ultrasound exam:** A procedure used to examine the vagina, uterus, fallopian tubes, and bladder. An ultrasound transducer (probe) is inserted into the vagina and used to bounce high energy sound waves (ultrasound) off internal tissues or organs and make echoes. The echoes form a picture of body tissues called a sonogram. The doctor can identify tumors by looking at the sonogram.

What Is the Prognosis for Endometrial Cancer?

The prognosis (chance of recovery) and treatment options depend on the following:

- The stage of the cancer (whether it is in the endometrium only, involves the uterus wall, or has spread to other places in the body)
- How the cancer cells look under a microscope
- Whether the cancer cells are affected by progesterone

Endometrial cancer can usually be cured because it is usually diagnosed early.

How Is Staging of Endometrial Cancer Done?

After endometrial cancer has been diagnosed, tests are done to find out if cancer cells have spread within the uterus or to other parts of the body.

The process used to find out whether the cancer has spread within the uterus or to other parts of the body is called staging. The information gathered from the staging process determines the stage of the disease. It is important to know the stage in order to plan treatment. Certain tests and procedures are used in the staging process. A hysterectomy (an operation in which the uterus is removed) will usually be done to treat endometrial cancer. Tissue samples are taken from the area around the uterus and checked under a microscope for signs of cancer to help find out whether the cancer has spread.

The following procedures may be used in the staging process:

- **Pelvic exam:** An exam of the vagina, cervix, uterus, fallopian tubes, ovaries, and rectum. A speculum is inserted into the vagina and the doctor or nurse looks at the vagina and cervix for signs of disease. A Pap test of the cervix is usually done. The doctor or nurse also inserts one or two lubricated, gloved fingers of one hand into the vagina and places the other hand over the lower abdomen to feel the size, shape, and position of the uterus and ovaries. The doctor or nurse also inserts a lubricated, gloved finger into the rectum to feel for lumps or abnormal areas.
- **Chest X-ray:** An X-ray of the organs and bones inside the chest. An X-ray is a type of energy beam that can go through the body and onto film, making a picture of areas inside the body.
- **Computed tomography (CT)/computerized axial tomography (CAT) scan:** A procedure that makes a series of detailed pictures of areas inside the body, taken from different angles. The pictures are made by a computer linked to an X-ray machine. A dye may be injected into a vein or swallowed to help the organs or tissues show up more clearly.
- **Magnetic resonance imaging (MRI):** A procedure that uses a magnet, radio waves, and a computer to make a series of detailed pictures of areas inside the body. This procedure is also called nuclear magnetic resonance imaging (NMRI).

- **Positron emission tomography (PET) scan:** A procedure to find malignant tumor cells in the body. A small amount of radioactive glucose (sugar) is injected into a vein. The PET scanner rotates around the body and makes a picture of where glucose is being used in the body. Malignant tumor cells show up brighter in the picture because they are more active and take up more glucose than normal cells do.
- **Lymph node dissection:** A surgical procedure in which the lymph nodes are removed from the pelvic area and a sample of tissue is checked under a microscope for signs of cancer. This procedure is also called lymphadenectomy.

The following stages are used for endometrial cancer:

Stage I. In stage I, cancer is found in the uterus only. Stage I is divided into stages IA and IB, based on how far the cancer has spread.

- **Stage IA:** Cancer is in the endometrium only or less than halfway through the myometrium (muscle layer of the uterus).
- **Stage IB:** Cancer has spread halfway or more into the myometrium.

Stage II. In stage II, cancer has spread into connective tissue of the cervix, but has not spread outside the uterus.

Stage III. In stage III, cancer has spread beyond the uterus and cervix, but has not spread beyond the pelvis. Stage III is divided into stages IIIA, IIIB, and IIIC, based on how far the cancer has spread within the pelvis.

- **Stage IIIA:** Cancer has spread to the outer layer of the uterus and/or to the fallopian tubes, ovaries, and ligaments of the uterus.
- **Stage IIIB:** Cancer has spread to the vagina and/or to the parametrium (connective tissue and fat around the uterus).
- **Stage IIIC:** Cancer has spread to lymph nodes in the pelvis and/or around the aorta (largest artery in the body, which carries blood away from the heart).

Stage IV. In stage IV, cancer has spread beyond the pelvis. Stage IV is divided into stages IVA and IVB, based on how far the cancer has spread.

- **Stage IVA:** Cancer has spread to the bladder and/or bowel wall.
- **Stage IVB:** Cancer has spread to other parts of the body beyond the pelvis, including the abdomen and/or lymph nodes in the groin.

Grouping Endometrial Cancer

Endometrial cancer may be grouped for treatment as follows:

Low-Risk Endometrial Cancer

Grades 1 and 2 tumors are usually considered low-risk. They usually do not spread to other parts of the body.

High-Risk Endometrial Cancer

Grade 3 tumors are considered high risk. They often spread to other parts of the body. Uterine papillary serous, clear cell, and carcinosarcoma are three subtypes of endometrial cancer that are considered grade 3.

What Standard Treatment Options Are Available for Endometrial Cancer?

Five types of standard treatment are used:

Surgery

Surgery (removing the cancer in an operation) is the most common treatment for endometrial cancer. The following surgical procedures may be used:

- **Total hysterectomy:** Surgery to remove the uterus, including the cervix. If the uterus and cervix are taken out through the vagina, the operation is called a vaginal hysterectomy. If the uterus and cervix are taken out through a large incision (cut) in the abdomen, the operation is called a total abdominal hysterectomy. If the uterus and cervix are taken out through a small incision (cut) in the abdomen using a laparoscope, the operation is called a total laparoscopic hysterectomy.
- **Bilateral salpingo-oophorectomy:** Surgery to remove both ovaries and both fallopian tubes.

- **Radical hysterectomy:** Surgery to remove the uterus, cervix, and part of the vagina. The ovaries, fallopian tubes, or nearby lymph nodes may also be removed.
- **Lymph node dissection:** A surgical procedure in which the lymph nodes are removed from the pelvic area and a sample of tissue is checked under a microscope for signs of cancer. This procedure is also called lymphadenectomy.

Even if the doctor removes all the cancer that can be seen at the time of the surgery, some patients may be given radiation therapy or hormone treatment after surgery to kill any cancer cells that are left. Treatment given after the surgery, to lower the risk that the cancer will come back, is called adjuvant therapy.

Radiation Therapy

Radiation therapy is a cancer treatment that uses high-energy X-rays or other types of radiation to kill cancer cells or keep them from growing. There are two types of radiation therapy:

- External radiation therapy uses a machine outside the body to send radiation toward the cancer.
- Internal radiation therapy uses a radioactive substance sealed in needles, seeds, wires, or catheters that are placed directly into or near the cancer.

The way the radiation therapy is given depends on the type and stage of the cancer being treated. External and internal radiation therapy are used to treat endometrial cancer, and may also be used as palliative therapy to relieve symptoms and improve quality of life.

Chemotherapy

Chemotherapy is a cancer treatment that uses drugs to stop the growth of cancer cells, either by killing the cells or by stopping the cells from dividing. When chemotherapy is taken by mouth or injected into a vein or muscle, the drugs enter the bloodstream and can reach cancer cells throughout the body (systemic chemotherapy). When chemotherapy is placed directly into the cerebrospinal fluid, an organ, or a body cavity such as the abdomen, the drugs mainly affect cancer cells in those areas (regional chemotherapy).

The way the chemotherapy is given depends on the type and stage of the cancer being treated.

Hormone Therapy

Hormone therapy is a cancer treatment that removes hormones or blocks their action and stops cancer cells from growing. Hormones are substances made by glands in the body and circulated in the bloodstream. Some hormones can cause certain cancers to grow. If tests show that the cancer cells have places where hormones can attach (receptors), drugs, surgery, or radiation therapy is used to reduce the production of hormones or block them from working.

Targeted Therapy

Targeted therapy is a type of treatment that uses drugs or other substances to identify and attack specific cancer cells without harming normal cells. Monoclonal antibodies, mTOR inhibitors, and signal transduction inhibitors are three types of targeted therapy used to treat endometrial cancer.

- **Monoclonal antibody therapy** is a cancer treatment that uses antibodies made in the laboratory from a single type of immune system cell. These antibodies can identify substances on cancer cells or normal substances that may help cancer cells grow. The antibodies attach to the substances and kill the cancer cells, block their growth, or keep them from spreading. Monoclonal antibodies are given by infusion. They may be used alone or to carry drugs, toxins, or radioactive material directly to cancer cells. Bevacizumab is used to treat stage III, stage IV, and recurrent endometrial cancer.
- **mTOR inhibitors** block a protein called mTOR, which helps control cell division. mTOR inhibitors may keep cancer cells from growing and prevent the growth of new blood vessels that tumors need to grow. Everolimus and ridaforalimus are used to treat stage III, stage IV, and recurrent endometrial cancer.
- **Signal transduction inhibitors** block signals that are passed from one molecule to another inside a cell. Blocking these signals may kill cancer cells. Metformin is being studied to treat stage III, stage IV, and recurrent endometrial cancer.

Is There a Need for Follow-Up Tests?

Some of the tests that were done to diagnose the cancer or to find out the stage of the cancer may be repeated. Some tests will be repeated

in order to see how well the treatment is working. Decisions about whether to continue, change, or stop treatment may be based on the results of these tests.

Some of the tests will continue to be done from time to time after treatment has ended. The results of these tests can show if your condition has changed or if the cancer has recurred (come back). These tests are sometimes called follow-up tests or check-ups.

Section 44.4

Gestational Trophoblastic Tumors

This section includes text excerpted from "Gestational Trophoblastic Disease Treatment (PDQ®)—Patient Version," National Cancer Institute (NCI), October 13, 2017.

What Is Gestational Trophoblastic Disease (GTD)?

Gestational trophoblastic disease (GTD) is a group of rare diseases in which abnormal trophoblast cells grow inside the uterus after conception. In GTD, a tumor develops inside the uterus from tissue that forms after conception (the joining of sperm and egg). This tissue is made of trophoblast cells and normally surrounds the fertilized egg in the uterus. Trophoblast cells help connect the fertilized egg to the wall of the uterus and form part of the placenta (the organ that passes nutrients from the mother to the fetus).

Sometimes there is a problem with the fertilized egg and trophoblast cells. Instead of a healthy fetus developing, a tumor forms. Until there are signs or symptoms of the tumor, the pregnancy will seem like a normal pregnancy. Most GTD is benign (not cancer) and does not spread, but some types become malignant (cancer) and spread to nearby tissues or distant parts of the body. It includes different types of disease:

- Hydatidiform Moles (HM)
    - Complete HM
    - Partial HM

- Gestational Trophoblastic Neoplasia (GTN)
    - Invasive moles
    - Choriocarcinomas
    - Placental-site trophoblastic tumors (PSTT; very rare)
    - Epithelioid trophoblastic tumors (ETT; even more rare)

What Is Hydatidiform Mole (HM)?

Hydatidiform mole (HM) is the most common type of GTD. HMs are slow-growing tumors that look like sacs of fluid. An HM is also called a molar pregnancy. The cause of hydatidiform moles is not known.

HMs may be complete or partial:

- A **complete HM** forms when sperm fertilizes an egg that does not contain the mother's deoxyribonucleic acid (DNA). The egg has DNA from the father and the cells that were meant to become the placenta are abnormal.
- A **partial HM** forms when sperm fertilizes a normal egg and there are two sets of DNA from the father in the fertilized egg. Only part of the fetus forms and the cells that were meant to become the placenta are abnormal.

Most HMs are benign, but they sometimes become cancer. Having one or more of the following risk factors increases the risk that a hydatidiform mole will become cancer:

A pregnancy before 20 or after 35 years of age.

- A very high level of beta-human chorionic gonadotropin (β-hCG), a hormone made by the body during pregnancy
- A large tumor in the uterus
- An ovarian cyst larger than 6 centimeters
- High blood pressure during pregnancy
- An overactive thyroid gland (extra thyroid hormone is made)
- Severe nausea and vomiting during pregnancy
- Trophoblastic cells in the blood, which may block small blood vessels
- Serious blood clotting problems caused by the HM

What Is Gestational Trophoblastic Neoplasia (GTN)?

It is a type of gestational trophoblastic disease (GTD) that is almost always malignant.

Gestational trophoblastic neoplasia (GTN) includes the following:

Invasive Moles

Invasive moles are made up of trophoblast cells that grow into the muscle layer of the uterus. Invasive moles are more likely to grow and spread than a hydatidiform mole. Rarely, a complete or partial HM may become an invasive mole. Sometimes an invasive mole will disappear without treatment.

Choriocarcinomas

A choriocarcinoma is a malignant tumor that forms from trophoblast cells and spreads to the muscle layer of the uterus and nearby blood vessels. It may also spread to other parts of the body, such as the brain, lungs, liver, kidney, spleen, intestines, pelvis, or vagina. A choriocarcinoma is more likely to form in women who have had any of the following:

- Molar pregnancy, especially with a complete hydatidiform mole
- Normal pregnancy
- Tubal pregnancy (the fertilized egg implants in the fallopian tube rather than the uterus)
- Miscarriage

Placental Site Trophoblastic Tumors (PSTT)

A placental site trophoblastic tumor (PSTT) is a rare type of gestational trophoblastic neoplasia that forms where the placenta attaches to the uterus. The tumor forms from trophoblast cells and spreads into the muscle of the uterus and into blood vessels. It may also spread to the lungs, pelvis, or lymph nodes. A PSTT grows very slowly and signs or symptoms may appear months or years after a normal pregnancy.

Epithelioid Trophoblastic Tumors (ETT)

An epithelioid trophoblastic tumor (ETT) is a very rare type of gestational trophoblastic neoplasia that may be benign or malignant. When the tumor is malignant, it may spread to the lungs.

What Are the Risk Factors for GTD?

Anything that increases your risk of getting a disease is called a risk factor. Having a risk factor does not mean that you will get cancer; not having risk factors doesn't mean that you will not get cancer. Talk to your doctor if you think you may be at risk. Age and a previous molar pregnancy affect the risk of GTD. Risk factors for GTD include the following:

- Being pregnant when you are younger than 20 or older than 35 years of age
- Having a personal history of hydatidiform mole

What Are the Signs and Symptoms of GTD?

Signs of GTD include abnormal vaginal bleeding and a uterus that is larger than normal.

These and other signs and symptoms may be caused by gestational trophoblastic disease or by other conditions. Check with your doctor if you have any of the following:

- Vaginal bleeding not related to menstruation
- A uterus that is larger than expected during pregnancy
- Pain or pressure in the pelvis
- Severe nausea and vomiting during pregnancy
- High blood pressure with headache and swelling of feet and hands early in the pregnancy
- Vaginal bleeding that continues for longer than normal after delivery
- Fatigue, shortness of breath, dizziness, and a fast or irregular heartbeat caused by anemia

GTD sometimes causes an overactive thyroid. Signs and symptoms of an overactive thyroid include the following:

- Fast or irregular heartbeat
- Shakiness
- Sweating
- Frequent bowel movements
- Trouble sleeping

- Feeling anxious or irritable
- Weight loss

How Is GTD Diagnosed?

Tests that examine the uterus are used to detect (find) and diagnose gestational trophoblastic disease. The following tests and procedures may be used:

- **Physical exam and history:** An exam of the body to check general signs of health, including checking for signs of disease, such as lumps or anything else that seems unusual. A history of the patient's health habits and past illnesses and treatments will also be taken.
- **Pelvic exam:** An exam of the vagina, cervix, uterus, fallopian tubes, ovaries, and rectum. A speculum is inserted into the vagina and the doctor or nurse looks at the vagina and cervix for signs of disease. A Pap test of the cervix is usually done. The doctor or nurse also inserts one or two lubricated, gloved fingers of one hand into the vagina and places the other hand over the lower abdomen to feel the size, shape, and position of the uterus and ovaries. The doctor or nurse also inserts a lubricated, gloved finger into the rectum to feel for lumps or abnormal areas.
- **Ultrasound exam of the pelvis:** A procedure in which high-energy sound waves (ultrasound) are bounced off internal tissues or organs in the pelvis and make echoes. The echoes form a picture of body tissues called a sonogram. Sometimes a transvaginal ultrasound (TVUS) will be done. For TVUS, an ultrasound transducer (probe) is inserted into the vagina to make the sonogram.
- **Blood chemistry studies:** A procedure in which a blood sample is checked to measure the amounts of certain substances released into the blood by organs and tissues in the body. An unusual (higher or lower than normal) amount of a substance can be a sign of disease. Blood is also tested to check the liver, kidney, and bone marrow.
- **Serum tumor marker test:** A procedure in which a sample of blood is checked to measure the amounts of certain substances made by organs, tissues, or tumor cells in the body. Certain substances are linked to specific types of cancer when found in

increased levels in the body. These are called tumor markers. For GTD, the blood is checked for the level of beta-human chorionic gonadotropin (β-hCG), a hormone that is made by the body during pregnancy. β-hCG in the blood of a woman who is not pregnant may be a sign of GTD.

- **Urinalysis:** A test to check the color of urine and its contents, such as sugar, protein, blood, bacteria, and the level of β-hCG.

What Is the Prognosis for GTD?

Gestational trophoblastic disease usually can be cured. Treatment and prognosis depend on the following:

- The type of GTD
- Whether the tumor has spread to the uterus, lymph nodes, or distant parts of the body
- The number of tumors and where they are in the body
- The size of the largest tumor
- The level of β-hCG in the blood
- How soon the tumor was diagnosed after the pregnancy began
- Whether GTD occurred after a molar pregnancy, miscarriage, or normal pregnancy
- Previous treatment for gestational trophoblastic neoplasia

Treatment options also depend on whether the woman wishes to become pregnant in the future.

What Are the Stages of Gestational Trophoblastic Tumors and Neoplasia (GTN)?

After gestational trophoblastic neoplasia has been diagnosed, tests are done to find out if cancer has spread from where it started to other parts of the body.

The process used to find out the extent or spread of cancer is called staging, The information gathered from the staging process helps determine the stage of disease. For GTN, stage is one of the factors used to plan treatment.

The following tests and procedures may be done to help find out the stage of the disease:

- **Chest X-ray:** An X-ray of the organs and bones inside the chest. An X-ray is a type of energy beam that can go through the body onto filmmaking pictures of areas inside the body.
- **Computed tomography (CT)/computerized axial tomography (CAT) scan:** A procedure that makes a series of detailed pictures of areas inside the body, taken from different angles. The pictures are made by a computer linked to an X-ray machine. A dye may be injected into a vein or swallowed to help the organs or tissues show up more clearly.
- **Magnetic resonance imaging (MRI) with gadolinium:** A procedure that uses a magnet, radio waves, and a computer to make a series of detailed pictures of areas inside the body, such as brain and spinal cord. A substance called gadolinium is injected into a vein. The gadolinium collects around the cancer cells so they show up brighter in the picture. This procedure is also called nuclear magnetic resonance imaging (NMRI).
- **Lumbar puncture (LP):** A procedure used to collect cerebrospinal fluid (CSF) from the spinal column. This is done by placing a needle between two bones in the spine and into the CSF around the spinal cord and removing a sample of the fluid. The sample of CSF is checked under a microscope for signs that the cancer has spread to the brain and spinal cord. This procedure is also called spinal tap.

The following stages are used for GTN:

Stage I. In stage I, the tumor is in the uterus only.

Stage II. In stage II, cancer has spread outside of the uterus to the ovary, fallopian tube, vagina, and/or the ligaments that support the uterus.

Stage III. In stage III, cancer has spread to the lung.

Stage IV. In stage IV, cancer has spread to distant parts of the body other than the lungs.

What Treatment Options Are Available for Patients with GTN?

The treatment of gestational trophoblastic neoplasia is based on the type of disease, stage, or risk group. Invasive moles and choriocarcinomas are treated based on risk groups. The stage of the invasive mole or choriocarcinoma is one factor used to determine risk group. Other factors include the following:

- The age of the patient when the diagnosis is made
- Whether the GTN occurred after a molar pregnancy, miscarriage, or normal pregnancy
- How soon the tumor was diagnosed after the pregnancy began
- The level of beta-human chorionic gonadotropin (β-hCG) in the blood
- The size of the largest tumor
- Where the tumor has spread to and the number of tumors in the body
- How many chemotherapy drugs the tumor has been treated with (for recurrent or resistant tumors)

There are two risk groups for invasive moles and choriocarcinomas: low risk and high risk. Patients with low-risk disease usually receive less aggressive treatment than patients with high-risk disease.

Placental site trophoblastic tumor (PSTT) and epithelioid trophoblastic tumor (ETT) treatments depend on the stage of disease.

What Are the Treatment Options Available for Patients with GTD?

Different types of treatment are available for patients with GTD. Some treatments are standard (the currently used treatment), and some are being tested in clinical trials. Before starting treatment, patients may want to think about taking part in a clinical trial. A treatment clinical trial is a research study meant to help improve current treatments or obtain information on new treatments for patients with cancer. When clinical trials show that a new treatment is better than the standard treatment, the new treatment may become the standard treatment.

Three types of standard treatment are used:

Surgery

The doctor may remove the cancer using one of the following operations:

- **Dilatation and curettage (D&C) with suction evacuation:** A surgical procedure to remove abnormal tissue and parts of the inner lining of the uterus. The cervix is dilated and the material inside the uterus is removed with a small vacuum like device. The walls of the uterus are then gently scraped with a curette (spoon-shaped instrument) to remove any material that may remain in the uterus. This procedure may be used for molar pregnancies.
- **Hysterectomy:** Surgery to remove the uterus, and sometimes the cervix. If the uterus and cervix are taken out through the vagina, the operation is called a vaginal hysterectomy. If the uterus and cervix are taken out through a large incision (cut) in the abdomen, the operation is called a total abdominal hysterectomy. If the uterus and cervix are taken out through a small incision (cut) in the abdomen using a laparoscope, the operation is called a total laparoscopic hysterectomy.

Chemotherapy

Chemotherapy is a cancer treatment that uses drugs to stop the growth of cancer cells, either by killing the cells or by stopping them from dividing. When chemotherapy is taken by mouth or injected into a vein or muscle, the drugs enter the bloodstream and can reach cancer cells throughout the body (systemic chemotherapy). When chemotherapy is placed directly into the cerebrospinal fluid, an organ, or a body cavity such as the abdomen, the drugs mainly affect cancer cells in those areas (regional chemotherapy). The way the chemotherapy is given depends on the type and stage of the cancer being treated, or whether the tumor is low risk or high risk.

Combination chemotherapy is treatment using more than one anticancer drug.

Even if the doctor removes all the cancer that can be seen at the time of the surgery, some patients may be given chemotherapy after surgery to kill any tumor cells that are left. Treatment given after the surgery, to lower the risk that the cancer will come back, is called adjuvant therapy.

Radiation Therapy

Radiation therapy is a cancer treatment that uses high-energy X-rays or other types of radiation to kill cancer cells or keep them from growing. There are two types of radiation therapy:

- External radiation therapy uses a machine outside the body to send radiation toward the cancer.

- Internal radiation therapy uses a radioactive substance sealed in needles, seeds, wires, or catheters that are placed directly into or near the cancer.

The way the radiation therapy is given depends on the type of gestational trophoblastic disease being treated. External radiation therapy is used to treat gestational trophoblastic disease.

Is There a Need for Follow-Up Tests?

Some of the tests that were done to diagnose the cancer or to find out the stage of the cancer may be repeated. Some tests will be repeated in order to see how well the treatment is working. Decisions about whether to continue, change, or stop treatment may be based on the results of these tests. Some of the tests will continue to be done from time to time after treatment has ended. The results of these tests can show if your condition has changed or if the cancer has recurred (come back). These tests are sometimes called follow-up tests or check-ups. Blood levels of beta-human chorionic gonadotropin (β-hCG) will be checked for up to 6 months after treatment has ended. This is because a β-hCG level that is higher than normal may mean that the tumor has not responded to treatment or it has become cancer.

Section 44.5

Ovarian Epithelial Cancer

This section includes text excerpted from "Ovarian Epithelial, Fallopian Tube, and Primary Peritoneal Cancer Treatment (PDQ®)—Patient Version," National Cancer Institute (NCI), February 20, 2018.

The ovaries are a pair of organs in the female reproductive system. They are in the pelvis, one on each side of the uterus (the hollow, pear-shaped organ where a fetus grows). Each ovary is about the size and shape of an almond. The ovaries make eggs and female hormones (chemicals that control the way certain cells or organs work). The lead fallopian tubes are a pair of long, slender tubes, one on each side of the uterus. Eggs pass from the ovaries, through the fallopian tubes, to the uterus. Cancer sometimes begins at the end of the fallopian tube near the ovary and spreads to the ovary. The peritoneum is the tissue that lines the abdominal wall and covers organs in the abdomen.

What Is Ovarian Epithelial Cancer?

Ovarian epithelial cancer, fallopian tube cancer, and primary peritoneal cancer are diseases in which malignant (cancer) cells form in the tissue covering the ovary or lining the fallopian tube or peritoneum. Primary peritoneal cancer is cancer that forms in the peritoneum and has not spread there from another part of the body. Cancer sometimes begins in the peritoneum and spreads to the ovary. Ovarian epithelial cancer, fallopian tube cancer, and primary peritoneal cancer form in the same type of tissue and are treated the same way.

What Are the Risk Factors for Ovarian Epithelial Cancer?

Anything that increases your risk of getting a disease is called a risk factor. Having a risk factor does not mean that you will get cancer; not having risk factors doesn't mean that you will not get cancer. Talk with your doctor if you think you may be at risk. Women who have a family history of ovarian cancer are at an increased risk of ovarian cancer. Women who have one first degree relative (mother, daughter, or sister) with a history of ovarian cancer have an increased risk of ovarian cancer. This risk is higher in women who have one first degree relative and one second degree relative (grandmother or aunt) with a history of ovarian cancer. This risk is even higher in women who have two or more first degree relatives with a history of ovarian cancer.

Can Inherited Gene Mutation Lead to Ovarian Epithelial Cancer?

Some ovarian, fallopian tube, and primary peritoneal cancers are caused by inherited gene mutations (changes). Hereditary ovarian cancer makes up about 20 percent of all cases of ovarian cancer. There are three hereditary patterns: ovarian cancer alone, ovarian and breast cancers, and ovarian and colon cancers. Fallopian tube cancer and peritoneal cancer may also be caused by certain inherited gene mutations. There are tests that can detect gene mutations.

These genetic tests are sometimes done for members of families with a high risk of cancer.

How Can Surgery Protect Women with an Increased Risk of Ovarian Cancer?

Some women who have an increased risk of ovarian cancer may choose to have a risk reducing oophorectomy (the removal of healthy ovaries so that cancer cannot grow in them). In high-risk women, this procedure has been shown to greatly decrease the risk of ovarian cancer.

What Are the Signs and Symptoms of Ovarian, Fallopian Tube, or Peritoneal Cancer?

Signs and symptoms of ovarian, fallopian tube, or peritoneal cancer include pain or swelling in the abdomen. They may not cause early signs or symptoms. When signs or symptoms do appear, the cancer is often advanced. Signs and symptoms may include the following:

- Pain, swelling, or a feeling of pressure in the abdomen or pelvis
- Vaginal bleeding that is heavy or irregular, especially after menopause
- Vaginal discharge that is clear, white, or colored with blood.
- A lump in the pelvic area
- Gastrointestinal problems, such as gas, bloating, or constipation

These signs and symptoms also may be caused by other conditions and not by ovarian, fallopian tube, or peritoneal cancer. If the signs or symptoms get worse or do not go away on their own, check with your doctor so that any problem can be diagnosed and treated as early as possible.

How Is Ovarian, Fallopian Tube, or Peritoneal Cancer Diagnosed?

Tests that examine the ovaries and pelvic area are used to detect (find) and diagnose ovarian, fallopian tube, and peritoneal cancer. The following tests and procedures may be used:

- **Physical exam and history:** An exam of the body to check general signs of health, including checking for signs of disease,

such as lumps or anything else that seems unusual. A history of the patient's health habits and past illnesses and treatments will also be taken.

- **Pelvic exam:** An exam of the vagina, cervix, uterus, fallopian tubes, ovaries, and rectum. A speculum is inserted into the vagina and the doctor or nurse looks at the vagina and cervix for signs of disease. A Pap test of the cervix is usually done. The doctor or nurse also inserts one or two lubricated, gloved fingers of one hand into the vagina and places the other hand over the lower abdomen to feel the size, shape, and position of the uterus and ovaries. The doctor or nurse also inserts a lubricated, gloved finger into the rectum to feel for lumps or abnormal areas.
- **CA 125 assay:** A test that measures the level of CA 125 in the blood. CA 125 is a substance released by cells into the bloodstream. An increased CA 125 level can be a sign of cancer or another condition such as endometriosis.
- **Ultrasound exam:** A procedure in which high energy sound waves (ultrasound) are bounced off internal tissues or organs in the abdomen, and make echoes. The echoes form a picture of body tissues called a sonogram. The picture can be printed to be looked at later.
- **Computed tomography (CT)/computerized axial tomography (CAT) scan:** A procedure that makes a series of detailed pictures of areas inside the body, taken from different angles. The pictures are made by a computer linked to an X-ray machine. A dye may be injected into a vein or swallowed to help the organs or tissues show up more clearly.
- **Positron emission tomography (PET):** A procedure to find malignant tumor cells in the body. A very small amount of radioactive glucose (sugar) is injected into a vein. The PET scanner rotates around the body and makes a picture of where glucose is being used in the body. Malignant tumor cells show up brighter in the picture because they are more active and take up more glucose than normal cells do.
- **Magnetic resonance imaging (MRI):** A procedure that uses a magnet, radio waves, and a computer to make a series of detailed pictures of areas inside the body. This procedure is also called nuclear magnetic resonance imaging (NMRI).

- **Chest X-ray:** An X-ray of the organs and bones inside the chest. An X-ray is a type of energy beam that can go through the body and onto film, making a picture of areas inside the body.
- **Biopsy:** The removal of cells or tissues so they can be viewed under a microscope by a pathologist to check for signs of cancer. The tissue is usually removed during surgery to remove the tumor.

What Is the Prognosis for Ovarian Cancer?

The prognosis (chance of recovery) and treatment options depend on the following:

- The type of ovarian cancer and how much cancer there is
- The stage and grade of the cancer
- Whether the patient has extra fluid in the abdomen that causes swelling
- Whether all of the tumor can be removed by surgery
- Whether there are changes in the *BRCA1* or *BRCA2* genes
- The patient's age and general health
- Whether the cancer has just been diagnosed or has recurred (come back)

What Are the Stages of Ovarian Epithelial, Fallopian Tube, and Primary Peritoneal Cancer?

After ovarian, fallopian tube, or peritoneal cancer has been diagnosed, tests are done to find out if cancer cells have spread within the ovaries or to other parts of the body.

The process used to find out whether cancer has spread within the organ or to other parts of the body is called staging. The information gathered from the staging process determines the stage of the disease. It is important to know the stage in order to plan treatment. The results of the tests used to diagnose cancer are often also used to stage the disease.

The following stages are used for ovarian epithelial, fallopian tube, and primary peritoneal cancer:

Stage I. In stage I, cancer is found in one or both ovaries or fallopian tubes. Stage I is divided into stage IA, stage IB, and stage IC.

- **Stage IA:** Cancer is found inside a single ovary or fallopian tube.
- **Stage IB:** Cancer is found inside both ovaries or fallopian tubes.
- **Stage IC:** Cancer is found inside one or both ovaries or fallopian tubes and one of the following is true:
  - cancer is also found on the outside surface of one or both ovaries or fallopian tubes; or
  - the capsule (outer covering) of the ovary ruptured (broke open) before or during surgery; or
  - cancer cells are found in the fluid of the peritoneal cavity (the body cavity that contains most of the organs in the abdomen) or in washings of the peritoneum (tissue lining the peritoneal cavity).

Stage II. In stage II, cancer is found in one or both ovaries or fallopian tubes and has spread into other areas of the pelvis, or primary peritoneal cancer is found within the pelvis. Stage II ovarian epithelial and fallopian tube cancers are divided into stage IIA and stage IIB.

- **Stage IIA:** Cancer has spread from where it first formed to the uterus and/or the fallopian tubes and/or the ovaries.
- **Stage IIB:** Cancer has spread from the ovary or fallopian tube to organs in the peritoneal cavity (the space that contains the abdominal organs).

Stage III. In stage III, cancer is found in one or both ovaries or fallopian tubes, or is primary peritoneal cancer, and has spread outside the pelvis to other parts of the abdomen and/or to nearby lymph nodes. Stage III is divided into stage IIIA, stage IIIB, and stage IIIC.

- In **stage IIIA**, one of the following is true:
  - Cancer has spread to lymph nodes in the area outside or behind the peritoneum only; or
  - Cancer cells that can be seen only with a microscope have spread to the surface of the peritoneum outside the pelvis. Cancer may have spread to nearby lymph nodes.
- **Stage IIIB:** Cancer has spread to the peritoneum outside the pelvis and the cancer in the peritoneum is 2 centimeters or smaller. Cancer may have spread to lymph nodes behind the peritoneum.

- **Stage IIIC:** Cancer has spread to the peritoneum outside the pelvis and the cancer in the peritoneum is larger than 2 centimeters. Cancer may have spread to lymph nodes behind the peritoneum or to the surface of the liver or spleen.

Stage IV. In stage IV, cancer has spread beyond the abdomen to other parts of the body. Stage IV is divided into stage IVA and stage IVB.

- **Stage IVA:** Cancer cells are found in extra fluid that builds up around the lungs.
- **Stage IVB:** Cancer has spread to organs and tissues outside the abdomen, including lymph nodes in the groin.

Stage I ovarian epithelial and fallopian tube cancers are treated as early cancers. Stages II, III, and IV ovarian epithelial, fallopian tube, and primary peritoneal cancers are treated as advanced cancers.

What Treatment Options Are Available for Patients with Ovarian Epithelial Cancer?

Different types of treatment are available for patients with ovarian epithelial cancer. Some treatments are standard, and some are being tested in clinical trials. A treatment clinical trial is a research study meant to help improve current treatments or obtain information on new treatments for patients with cancer. When clinical trials show that a new treatment is better than the treatment currently used as standard treatment, the new treatment may become the standard treatment. Patients with any stage of ovarian cancer may want to think about taking part in a clinical trial. Some clinical trials are open only to patients who have not started treatment.

Three kinds of standard treatment are used:

Surgery

Most patients have surgery to remove as much of the tumor as possible. Different types of surgery may include:

- **Hysterectomy:** Surgery to remove the uterus and, sometimes, the cervix. When only the uterus is removed, it is called a partial hysterectomy. When both the uterus and the cervix are removed, it is called a total hysterectomy. If the uterus and cervix are taken out through the vagina, the operation is called a vaginal hysterectomy. If the uterus and cervix are taken out through a large incision (cut) in the abdomen, the operation is called a total abdominal hysterectomy. If the uterus and cervix are taken out through a small incision (cut) in the abdomen using a laparoscope, the operation is called a total laparoscopic hysterectomy.

- **Unilateral salpingo-oophorectomy:** A surgical procedure to remove one ovary and one fallopian tube.
- **Bilateral salpingo-oophorectomy:** A surgical procedure to remove both ovaries and both fallopian tubes.
- **Omentectomy:** A surgical procedure to remove the omentum (tissue in the peritoneum that contains blood vessels, nerves, lymph vessels, and lymph nodes).
- **Lymph node biopsy:** The removal of all or part of a lymph node. A pathologist views the tissue under a microscope to look for cancer cells.

Chemotherapy

Chemotherapy is a cancer treatment that uses drugs to stop the growth of cancer cells, either by killing the cells or by stopping them from dividing. When chemotherapy is taken by mouth or injected into a vein or muscle, the drugs enter the bloodstream and can reach cancer cells throughout the body (systemic chemotherapy). When chemotherapy is placed directly into the cerebrospinal fluid, an organ, or a body cavity such as the abdomen, the drugs mainly affect cancer cells in those areas (regional chemotherapy).

A type of regional chemotherapy used to treat ovarian cancer is intraperitoneal (IP) chemotherapy. In IP chemotherapy, the anticancer drugs are carried directly into the peritoneal cavity (the space that contains the abdominal organs) through a thin tube.

Treatment with more than one anticancer drug is called combination chemotherapy.

The way the chemotherapy is given depends on the type and stage of the cancer being treated.

Targeted Therapy

Targeted therapy is a type of treatment that uses drugs or other substances to identify and attack specific cancer cells without harming normal cells.

Monoclonal antibody therapy is a type of targeted therapy that uses antibodies made in the laboratory, from a single type of immune system cell. These antibodies can identify substances on cancer cells or normal substances that may help cancer cells grow. The antibodies attach to the substances and kill the cancer cells, block their growth, or keep them from spreading. Monoclonal antibodies are given by infusion. They may be used alone or to carry drugs, toxins, or radioactive material directly to cancer cells.

Bevacizumab is a monoclonal antibody that may be used with chemotherapy to treat ovarian epithelial cancer, fallopian tube cancer, or primary peritoneal cancer that has recurred (come back).

Poly (ADP-ribose) polymerase inhibitors (PARP inhibitors) are targeted therapy drugs that block deoxyribonucleic acid (DNA) repair and may cause cancer cells to die. Olaparib and niraparib are PARP inhibitors that may be used to treat advanced ovarian cancer.

Treatment for ovarian epithelial, fallopian tube, and primary peritoneal cancer may cause side effects.

What New Types of Treatment Are Being Tested in Clinical Trials?

Radiation Therapy

Radiation therapy is a cancer treatment that uses high-energy X-rays or other types of radiation to kill cancer cells or keep them from growing. Some women receive a treatment called intraperitoneal radiation therapy, in which radioactive liquid is put directly in the abdomen through a catheter. Intraperitoneal radiation therapy is being studied to treat advanced ovarian cancer.

Immunotherapy

Immunotherapy is a treatment that uses the patient's immune system to fight cancer. Substances made by the body or made in a laboratory are used to boost, direct, or restore the body's natural defenses against cancer. This type of cancer treatment is also called biotherapy or immunotherapy.

Vaccine therapy uses a substance to stimulate the immune system to destroy a tumor. Vaccine therapy is being studied to treat advanced ovarian cancer.

Section 44.6

Uterine Sarcoma

This section includes text excerpted from "Uterine Sarcoma," National Cancer Institute (NCI), October 13, 2017.

The uterus is part of the female reproductive system. The uterus is the hollow, pear-shaped organ in the pelvis, where a fetus grows. The cervix is at the lower, narrow end of the uterus, and leads to the vagina.

What Is Uterine Sarcoma?

Uterine sarcoma is a disease in which malignant (cancer) cells form in the muscles of the uterus or other tissues that support the uterus. It is a very rare kind of cancer. It is different from cancer of the endometrium, a disease in which cancer cells start growing inside the lining of the uterus.

What Are the Risk Factors for Uterine Sarcoma?

Anything that increases your risk of getting a disease is called a risk factor. Having a risk factor does not mean that you will get cancer; not having risk factors doesn't mean that you will not get cancer. Talk with your doctor if you think you may be at risk.

Being exposed to X-rays can increase the risk of uterine sarcoma. Risk factors for uterine sarcoma include the following:

- Past treatment with radiation therapy to the pelvis
- Treatment with tamoxifen for breast cancer. If you are taking this drug, have a pelvic exam every year and report any vaginal bleeding (other than menstrual bleeding) as soon as possible

What Are the Signs and Symptoms of Uterine Sarcoma?

Abnormal bleeding from the vagina and other signs and symptoms may be caused by uterine sarcoma or by other conditions. Check with your doctor if you have any of the following:

- Bleeding that is not part of menstrual periods
- Bleeding after menopause
- A mass in the vagina
- Pain or a feeling of fullness in the abdomen
- Frequent urination

How Is Uterine Sarcoma Diagnosed?

Tests that examine the uterus are used to detect (find) and diagnose uterine sarcoma. The following tests and procedures may be used:

- **Physical exam and history:** An exam of the body to check general signs of health, including checking for signs of disease, such as lumps or anything else that seems unusual. A history of the patient's health habits and past illnesses and treatments will also be taken.
- **Pelvic exam:** An exam of the vagina, cervix, uterus, fallopian tubes, ovaries, and rectum. A speculum is inserted into the vagina and the doctor or nurse looks at the vagina and cervix for signs of disease. A Pap test of the cervix is usually done. The doctor or nurse also inserts one or two lubricated, gloved fingers of one hand into the vagina and places the other hand over the lower abdomen to feel the size, shape, and position of the uterus and ovaries. The doctor or nurse also inserts a lubricated, gloved finger into the rectum to feel for lumps or abnormal areas.
- **Pap test**: A procedure to collect cells from the surface of the cervix and vagina. A piece of cotton, a brush, or a small wooden stick is used to gently scrape cells from the cervix and vagina. The cells are viewed under a microscope to find out if they are abnormal. This procedure is also called a Pap smear. Because uterine sarcoma begins inside the uterus, this cancer may not show up on the Pap test.
- **Transvaginal ultrasound exam:** A procedure used to examine the vagina, uterus, fallopian tubes, and bladder. An ultrasound

transducer (probe) is inserted into the vagina and used to bounce high-energy sound waves (ultrasound) off internal tissues or organs and make echoes. The echoes form a picture of body tissues called a sonogram. The doctor can identify tumors by looking at the sonogram.

- **Dilatation and curettage:** A procedure to remove samples of tissue from the inner lining of the uterus. The cervix is dilated and a curette (spoon-shaped instrument) is inserted into the uterus to remove tissue. The tissue samples are checked under a microscope for signs of disease. This procedure is also called a D&C.
- **Endometrial biopsy:** The removal of tissue from the endometrium (inner lining of the uterus) by inserting a thin, flexible tube through the cervix and into the uterus. The tube is used to gently scrape a small amount of tissue from the endometrium and then remove the tissue samples. A pathologist views the tissue under a microscope to look for cancer cells.

What Is the Prognosis for Uterine Sarcoma?

The prognosis (chance of recovery) and treatment options depend on the following:

- The stage of the cancer
- The type and size of the tumor
- The patient's general health
- Whether the cancer has just been diagnosed or has recurred (come back)

How Is Uterine Sarcoma Staged?

After uterine sarcoma has been diagnosed, tests are done to find out if cancer cells have spread within the uterus or to other parts of the body.

The process used to find out if cancer has spread within the uterus or to other parts of the body is called staging. The information gathered from the staging process determines the stage of the disease. It is important to know the stage in order to plan treatment. The following procedures may be used in the staging process:

- **Blood chemistry studies:** A procedure in which a blood sample is checked to measure the amounts of certain substances released into the blood by organs and tissues in the body. An unusual (higher or lower than normal) amount of a substance can be a sign of disease.

- **CA 125 assay:** A test that measures the level of CA 125 in the blood. CA 125 is a substance released by cells into the bloodstream. An increased CA 125 level is sometimes a sign of cancer or other condition.
- **Chest X-ray:** An X-ray of the organs and bones inside the chest. An X-ray is a type of energy beam that can go through the body and onto film, making a picture of areas inside the body.
- **Transvaginal ultrasound exam:** A procedure used to examine the vagina, uterus, fallopian tubes, and bladder. An ultrasound transducer (probe) is inserted into the vagina and used to bounce high energy sound waves (ultrasound) off internal tissues or organs and make echoes. The echoes form a picture of body tissues called a sonogram. The doctor can identify tumors by looking at the sonogram.
- **Computed tomography (CT)/computerized axial tomography (CAT) scan:** A procedure that makes a series of detailed pictures of areas inside the body, such as the abdomen and pelvis, taken from different angles. The pictures are made by a computer linked to an X-ray machine. A dye may be injected into a vein or swallowed to help the organs or tissues to show up more clearly.
- **Cystoscopy:** A procedure to look inside the bladder and urethra to check for abnormal areas. A cystoscope is inserted through the urethra into the bladder. A cystoscope is a thin, tube-like instrument with a light and a lens for viewing. It may also have a tool to remove tissue samples, which are checked under a microscope for signs of cancer.

The following stages are used for uterine sarcoma:

Stage I. In stage I, cancer is found in the uterus only. Stage I is divided into stages IA and IB, based on how far the cancer has spread.

- **Stage IA:** Cancer is in the endometrium only or less than halfway through the myometrium (muscle layer of the uterus).
- **Stage IB:** Cancer has spread halfway or more into the myometrium.

Stage II. In stage II, cancer has spread into connective tissue of the cervix, but has not spread outside the uterus.

Stage III. In stage III, cancer has spread beyond the uterus and cervix, but has not spread beyond the pelvis. Stage III is divided into stages IIIA, IIIB, and IIIC, based on how far the cancer has spread within the pelvis.

- **Stage IIIA:** Cancer has spread to the outer layer of the uterus and/or to the fallopian tubes, ovaries, and ligaments of the uterus.
- **Stage IIIB:** Cancer has spread to the vagina or to the parametrium (connective tissue and fat around the uterus).
- **Stage IIIC:** Cancer has spread to lymph nodes in the pelvis and/or around the aorta (largest artery in the body, which carries blood away from the heart).

Stage IV

In stage IV, cancer has spread beyond the pelvis. Stage IV is divided into stages IVA and IVB, based on how far the cancer has spread.

- **Stage IVA:** Cancer has spread to the bladder and/or bowel wall.
- **Stage IVB:** Cancer has spread to other parts of the body beyond the pelvis, including the abdomen and/or lymph nodes in the groin.

How Is Surgery Used for Diagnosing, Staging, and Treating Uterine Sarcoma?

Surgery is used to diagnose, stage, and treat uterine sarcoma. During this surgery, the doctor removes as much of the cancer as possible. The following procedures may be used to diagnose, stage, and treat uterine sarcoma:

- **Laparotomy:** A surgical procedure in which an incision (cut) is made in the wall of the abdomen to check the inside of the abdomen for signs of disease. The size of the incision depends on the reason the laparotomy is being done. Sometimes organs are removed or tissue samples are taken and checked under a microscope for signs of disease.
- **Abdominal and pelvic washings:** A procedure in which a saline solution is placed into the abdominal and pelvic body

cavities. After a short time, the fluid is removed and viewed under a microscope to check for cancer cells.

- **Total abdominal hysterectomy:** A surgical procedure to remove the uterus and cervix through a large incision (cut) in the abdomen.
- **Bilateral salpingo-oophorectomy:** Surgery to remove both ovaries and both fallopian tubes.
- **Lymphadenectomy:** A surgical procedure in which lymph nodes are removed and checked under a microscope for signs of cancer. For a regional lymphadenectomy, some of the lymph nodes in the tumor area are removed. For a radical lymphadenectomy, most or all of the lymph nodes in the tumor area are removed. This procedure is also called lymph node dissection.

What Treatment Options Are Available for Treating Uterine Sarcoma?

Different types of treatments are available for patients with uterine sarcoma. Some treatments are standard (the currently used treatment), and some are being tested in clinical trials. A treatment clinical trial is a research study meant to help improve current treatments or obtain information on new treatments for patients with cancer. When clinical trials show that a new treatment is better than the standard treatment, the new treatment may become the standard treatment. Patients may want to think about taking part in a clinical trial. Some clinical trials are open only to patients who have not started treatment.

What Are the Standard Treatment Options Are Available for the Patients with Uterine Sarcoma?

Four types of standard treatment are used:

Surgery

Surgery is the most common treatment for uterine sarcoma, as described in the Stages of Uterine Sarcoma section of this summary.

Even if the doctor removes all the cancer that can be seen at the time of the surgery, some patients may be given chemotherapy or radiation therapy after surgery to kill any cancer cells that are left.

Treatment given after the surgery, to lower the risk that the cancer will come back, is called adjuvant therapy.

Radiation Therapy

Radiation therapy is a cancer treatment that uses high energy X-rays or other types of radiation to kill cancer cells or keep them from growing. There are two types of radiation therapy:

- External radiation therapy uses a machine outside the body to send radiation toward the cancer.
- Internal radiation therapy uses a radioactive substance sealed in needles, seeds, wires, or catheters that are placed directly into or near the cancer.

The way the radiation therapy is given depends on the type and stage of the cancer being treated. External and internal radiation therapy are used to treat uterine sarcoma, and may also be used as palliative therapy to relieve symptoms and improve quality of life.

Chemotherapy

Chemotherapy is a cancer treatment that uses drugs to stop the growth of cancer cells, either by killing the cells or by stopping them from dividing. When chemotherapy is taken by mouth or injected into a vein or muscle, the drugs enter the bloodstream and can reach cancer cells throughout the body (systemic chemotherapy). When chemotherapy is placed directly into the cerebrospinal fluid, an organ, or a body cavity such as the abdomen, the drugs mainly affect cancer cells in those areas (regional chemotherapy). The way the chemotherapy is given depends on the type and stage of the cancer being treated.

Hormone Therapy

Hormone therapy is a cancer treatment that removes hormones or blocks their action and stops cancer cells from growing. Hormones are substances produced by glands in the body and circulated in the bloodstream. Some hormones can cause certain cancers to grow. If tests show the cancer cells have places where hormones can attach (receptors), drugs, surgery, or radiation therapy is used to reduce the production of hormones or block them from working.

Treatment for uterine sarcoma may cause side effects.

Is There a Need for Follow-Up Tests?

Some of the tests that were done to diagnose the cancer or to find out the stage of the cancer may be repeated. Some tests will be repeated in order to see how well the treatment is working. Decisions about whether to continue, change, or stop treatment may be based on the results of these tests.

Some of the tests will continue to be done from time to time after treatment has ended. The results of these tests can show if your condition has changed or if the cancer has recurred (come back). These tests are sometimes called follow-up tests or check-ups.

Section 44.7

Vaginal Cancer

This section includes text excerpted from "Vaginal Cancer Treatment (PDQ®)—Patient Version," National Cancer Institute (NCI), October 13, 2017.

The vagina is the canal leading from the cervix (the opening of uterus) to the outside of the body. At birth, a baby passes out of the body through the vagina (also called the birth canal).

What Is Vaginal Cancer?

Vaginal cancer is a disease in which malignant (cancer) cells form in the vagina.

Vaginal cancer is not common. There are two main types of vaginal cancer:

- **Squamous cell carcinoma:** Cancer that forms in squamous cells, the thin, flat cells lining the vagina. Squamous cell vaginal cancer spreads slowly and usually stays near the vagina, but may spread to the lungs, liver, or bone. This is the most common type of vaginal cancer.
- **Adenocarcinoma:** Cancer that begins in glandular (secretory) cells. Glandular cells in the lining of the vagina make and

release fluids such as mucus. Adenocarcinoma is more likely than squamous cell cancer to spread to the lungs and lymph nodes. A rare type of adenocarcinoma is linked to being exposed to diethylstilbestrol (DES) before birth. Adenocarcinomas that are not linked with being exposed to DES are most common in women after menopause.

What Are the Risk Factors for Vaginal Cancer?

Anything that increases your risk of getting a disease is called a risk factor. Having a risk factor does not mean that you will get cancer; not having risk factors doesn't mean that you will not get cancer. Talk with your doctor if you think you may be at risk.

Age and being exposed to the drug DES (diethylstilbestrol) before birth affect a woman's risk of vaginal cancer. Risk factors for vaginal cancer include the following:

- Being aged 60 or older
- Being exposed to DES while in the mother's womb. In the 1950s, the drug DES was given to some pregnant women to prevent miscarriage (premature birth of a fetus that cannot survive). Women who were exposed to DES before birth have an increased risk of vaginal cancer. Some of these women develop a rare form of vaginal cancer called clear cell adenocarcinoma.
- Having human papillomavirus (HPV) infection
- Having a history of abnormal cells in the cervix or cervical cancer
- Having a history of abnormal cells in the uterus or cancer of the uterus
- Having had a hysterectomy for health problems that affect the uterus

What Are the Signs and Symptoms of Vaginal Cancer?

Vaginal cancer often does not cause early signs or symptoms. It may be found during a routine pelvic exam and Pap test. Signs and symptoms of vaginal cancer include pain or abnormal vaginal bleeding. They may be caused by vaginal cancer or by other conditions. Check with your doctor if you have any of the following:

- Bleeding or discharge not related to menstrual periods

- Pain during sexual intercourse
- Pain in the pelvic area
- A lump in the vagina
- Pain when urinating
- Constipation

How Is Vaginal Cancer Diagnosed?

Tests that examine the vagina and other organs in the pelvis are used to detect (find) and diagnose vaginal cancer.

The following tests and procedures may be used:

- **Physical exam and history:** An exam of the body to check general signs of health, including checking for signs of disease, such as lumps or anything else that seems unusual. A history of the patient's health habits and past illnesses and treatments will also be taken.
- **Pelvic exam:** An exam of the vagina, cervix, uterus, fallopian tubes, ovaries, and rectum. A speculum is inserted into the vagina and the doctor or nurse looks at the vagina and cervix for signs of disease. A Pap test of the cervix is usually done. The doctor or nurse also inserts one or two lubricated, gloved fingers of one hand into the vagina and places the other hand over the lower abdomen to feel the size, shape, and position of the uterus and ovaries. The doctor or nurse also inserts a lubricated, gloved finger into the rectum to feel for lumps or abnormal areas.
- **Pap test:** A procedure to collect cells from the surface of the cervix and vagina. A piece of cotton, a brush, or a small wooden stick is used to gently scrape cells from the cervix and vagina. The cells are viewed under a microscope to find out if they are abnormal. This procedure is also called a Pap smear.
- **Colposcopy:** A procedure in which a colposcope (a lighted, magnifying instrument) is used to check the vagina and cervix for abnormal areas. Tissue samples may be taken using a curette (spoon-shaped instrument) or a brush and checked under a microscope for signs of disease.
- **Biopsy:** The removal of cells or tissues from the vagina and cervix so they can be viewed under a microscope by a pathologist to

check for signs of cancer. If a Pap test shows abnormal cells in the vagina, a biopsy may be done during a colposcopy.

What Is the Prognosis for Vaginal Cancer?

The prognosis (chance of recovery) depends on the following:

- The stage of the cancer (whether it is in the vagina only or has spread to other areas)
- The size of the tumor
- The grade of tumor cells (how different they look from normal cells under a microscope)
- Where the cancer is within the vagina
- Whether there are signs or symptoms at diagnosis
- The patient's age and general health
- Whether the cancer has just been diagnosed or has recurred (come back)

When found in early stages, vaginal cancer can often be cured.

How Is Staging Done for Vaginal Cancer?

After vaginal cancer has been diagnosed, tests are done to find out if cancer cells have spread within the vagina or to other parts of the body.

The process used to find out if cancer has spread within the vagina or to other parts of the body is called staging. The information gathered from the staging process determines the stage of the disease. It is important to know the stage in order to plan treatment. The following procedures may be used in the staging process:

- **Chest X-ray:** An X-ray of the organs and bones inside the chest. An X-ray is a type of energy beam that can go through the body and onto film, making a picture of areas inside the body.
- **Computed tomography (CT)/computerized axial tomography (CAT) scan:** A procedure that makes a series of detailed pictures of areas inside the body, taken from different angles. The pictures are made by a computer linked to an X-ray machine. A dye may be injected into a vein or swallowed to help the organs or tissues show up more clearly.
- **Magnetic resonance imaging (MRI):** A procedure that uses a magnet, radio waves, and a computer to make a series of

detailed pictures of areas inside the body. This procedure is also called nuclear magnetic resonance imaging (NMRI).

- **Positron emission tomography (PET) scan:** A procedure to find malignant tumor cells in the body. A small amount of radioactive glucose (sugar) is injected into a vein. The PET scanner rotates around the body and makes a picture of where glucose is being used in the body. Malignant tumor cells show up brighter in the picture because they are more active and take up more glucose than normal cells do.
- **Cystoscopy:** A procedure to look inside the bladder and urethra to check for abnormal areas. A cystoscope is inserted through the urethra into the bladder. A cystoscope is a thin, tube-like instrument with a light and a lens for viewing. It may also have a tool to remove tissue samples, which are checked under a microscope for signs of cancer.
- **Ureteroscopy:** A procedure to look inside the ureters to check for abnormal areas. A ureteroscope is inserted through the bladder and into the ureters. A ureteroscope is a thin, tube-like instrument with a light and a lens for viewing. It may also have a tool to remove tissue to be checked under a microscope for signs of disease. A ureteroscopy and cystoscopy may be done during the same procedure.
- **Proctoscopy:** A procedure to look inside the rectum to check for abnormal areas. A proctoscope is inserted through the rectum. A proctoscope is a thin, tube-like instrument with a light and a lens for viewing. It may also have a tool to remove tissue to be checked under a microscope for signs of disease.
- **Biopsy:** A biopsy may be done to find out if cancer has spread to the cervix. A sample of tissue is removed from the cervix and viewed under a microscope. A biopsy that removes only a small amount of tissue is usually done in the doctor's office. A cone biopsy (removal of a larger, cone-shaped piece of tissue from the cervix and cervical canal) is usually done in the hospital. A biopsy of the vulva may also be done to see if cancer has spread there.

Vaginal Intraepithelial Neoplasia (VAIN)

In vaginal intraepithelial neoplasia (VAIN), abnormal cells are found in tissue lining the inside of the vagina.

These abnormal cells are not cancer. Vaginal intraepithelial neoplasia (VAIN) is grouped based on how deep the abnormal cells are in the tissue lining the vagina:

- **VAIN 1:** Abnormal cells are found in the outermost one-third of the tissue lining the vagina.
- **VAIN 2:** Abnormal cells are found in the outermost two-thirds of the tissue lining the vagina.
- **VAIN 3:** Abnormal cells are found in more than two-thirds of the tissue lining the vagina. When abnormal cells are found throughout the tissue lining, it is called carcinoma in situ.

VAIN may become cancer and spread into the vaginal wall. VAIN is sometimes called stage 0.

The following stages are used for vaginal cancer:

Stage I. In stage I, cancer is found in the vaginal wall only.

Stage II. In stage II, cancer has spread through the wall of the vagina to the tissue around the vagina. Cancer has not spread to the wall of the pelvis.

Stage III. In stage III, cancer has spread to the wall of the pelvis.

Stage IV. Stage IV is divided into stage IVA and stage IVB:

- **Stage IVA:** Cancer may have spread to one or more of the following areas:
    - The lining of the bladder
    - The lining of the rectum
    - Beyond the area of the pelvis that has the bladder, uterus, ovaries, and cervix
- **Stage IVB:** Cancer has spread to parts of the body that are not near the vagina, such as the lung or bone.

What Factors Are Taken into Account for Deciding on Treatment Options?

Treatment options depend on the following:

- The stage and size of the cancer

- Whether the cancer is close to other organs that may be damaged by treatment
- Whether the tumor is made up of squamous cells or is an adenocarcinoma
- Whether the patient has a uterus or has had a hysterectomy
- Whether the patient has had past radiation treatment to the pelvis

What Are the Standard Treatment Options for Patients with Vaginal Cancer?

Three types of standard treatment are used:

Surgery

Surgery is the most common treatment of vaginal cancer. The following surgical procedures may be used:

- **Laser surgery:** A surgical procedure that uses a laser beam (a narrow beam of intense light) as a knife to make bloodless cuts in tissue or to remove a surface lesion such as a tumor.
- **Wide local excision:** A surgical procedure that takes out the cancer and some of the healthy tissue around it.
- **Vaginectomy:** Surgery to remove all or part of the vagina.
- **Total hysterectomy:** Surgery to remove the uterus, including the cervix. If the uterus and cervix are taken out through the vagina, the operation is called a vaginal hysterectomy. If the uterus and cervix are taken out through a large incision (cut) in the abdomen, the operation is called a total abdominal hysterectomy. If the uterus and cervix are taken out through a small incision in the abdomen using a laparoscope, the operation is called a total laparoscopic hysterectomy.
- **Lymph node dissection:** A surgical procedure in which lymph nodes are removed and a sample of tissue is checked under a microscope for signs of cancer. This procedure is also called lymphadenectomy. If the cancer is in the upper vagina, the pelvic lymph nodes may be removed. If the cancer is in the lower vagina, lymph nodes in the groin may be removed.

- **Pelvic exenteration:** Surgery to remove the lower colon, rectum, bladder, cervix, vagina, and ovaries. Nearby lymph nodes are also removed. Artificial openings (stoma) are made for urine and stool to flow from the body into a collection bag.

Skin grafting may follow surgery, to repair or reconstruct the vagina. Skin grafting is a surgical procedure in which skin is moved from one part of the body to another. A piece of healthy skin is taken from a part of the body that is usually hidden, such as the buttock or thigh, and used to repair or rebuild the area treated with surgery.

Even if the doctor removes all the cancer that can be seen at the time of the surgery, some patients may be given radiation therapy after surgery to kill any cancer cells that are left. Treatment given after the surgery, to lower the risk that the cancer will come back, is called adjuvant therapy.

Radiation Therapy

Radiation therapy is a cancer treatment that uses high-energy X-rays or other types of radiation to kill cancer cells or keep them from growing. There are two types of radiation therapy:

- External radiation therapy uses a machine outside the body to send radiation toward the cancer.
- Internal radiation therapy uses a radioactive substance sealed in needles, seeds, wires, or catheters that are placed directly into or near the cancer.

The way the radiation therapy is given depends on the type and stage of the cancer being treated. External and internal radiation therapy are used to treat vaginal cancer, and may also be used as palliative therapy to relieve symptoms and improve quality of life.

Chemotherapy

Chemotherapy is a cancer treatment that uses drugs to stop the growth of cancer cells, either by killing the cells or by stopping them from dividing. When chemotherapy is taken by mouth or injected into a vein or muscle, the drugs enter the bloodstream and can affect cancer cells throughout the body (systemic chemotherapy). When chemotherapy is placed directly into the cerebrospinal fluid, an organ, or a body cavity such as the abdomen, the drugs mainly affect cancer cells in those areas (regional chemotherapy). The way the chemotherapy is given depends on the type and stage of the cancer being treated.

Topical chemotherapy for squamous cell vaginal cancer may be applied to the vagina in a cream or lotion.

Treatment for vaginal cancer may cause side effects.

What New Types of Treatment Are Being Tested in Clinical Trials?

Radiosensitizers

Radiosensitizers are drugs that make tumor cells more sensitive to radiation therapy. Combining radiation therapy with radiosensitizers may kill more tumor cells.

Is There a Need for Follow-Up Tests?

Some of the tests that were done to diagnose the cancer or to find out the stage of the cancer may be repeated. Some tests will be repeated in order to see how well the treatment is working. Decisions about whether to continue, change, or stop treatment may be based on the results of these tests.

Section 44.8

Vulvar Cancer

This section includes text excerpted from "Vulvar Cancer Treatment (PDQ®)—Patient Version," National Cancer Institute (NCI), October 13, 2017.

The vulva includes:

- Inner and outer lips of the vagina
- Clitoris (sensitive tissue between the lips)
- Opening of the vagina and its glands

- Mons pubis (the rounded area in front of the pubic bones that becomes covered with hair at puberty)
- Perineum (the area between the vulva and the anus)

What Is Vulvar Cancer?

Vulvar cancer is a rare disease in which malignant (cancer) cells form in the tissues of the vulva. It most often affects the outer vaginal lips. Less often, cancer affects the inner vaginal lips, clitoris, or vaginal glands. Vulvar cancer usually forms slowly over a number of years. Abnormal cells can grow on the surface of the vulvar skin for a long time. This condition is called vulvar intraepithelial neoplasia (VIN). Because it is possible for VIN to become vulvar cancer, it is very important to get treatment.

What Are the Risk Factors for Vulvar Cancer?

Having vulvar intraepithelial neoplasia or HPV infection can affect the risk of vulvar cancer. Anything that increases your risk of getting a disease is called a risk factor. Having a risk factor does not mean that you will get cancer; not having risk factors doesn't mean that you will not get cancer. Talk with your doctor if you think you may be at risk. Risk factors for vulvar cancer include the following:

- Having vulvar intraepithelial neoplasia (VIN)
- Having human papillomavirus (HPV) infection
- Having a history of genital warts

Other possible risk factors include the following:

- Having many sexual partners
- Having first sexual intercourse at a young age
- Having a history of abnormal Pap tests (Pap smears)

What Are the Signs and Symptoms of Vulvar Cancer?

Vulvar cancer often does not cause early signs or symptoms. Signs of vulvar cancer include bleeding or itching. It may be caused by vulvar cancer or by other conditions. Check with your doctor if you have any of the following:

- A lump or growth on the vulva

- Changes in the vulvar skin, such as color changes or growths that look like a wart or ulcer
- Itching in the vulvar area, that does not go away
- Bleeding not related to menstruation (periods)
- Tenderness in the vulvar area

How Is Vulvar Cancer Diagnosed?

Tests that examine the vulva are used to detect (find) and diagnose vulvar cancer. The following tests and procedures may be used:

- **Physical exam and history:** An exam of the body to check general signs of health, including checking the vulva for signs of disease, such as lumps or anything else that seems unusual. A history of the patient's health habits and past illnesses and treatments will also be taken.
- **Biopsy:** The removal of samples of cells or tissues from the vulva so they can be viewed under a microscope by a pathologist to check for signs of cancer.

What Is the Prognosis for Vulvar Cancer?

The prognosis (chance of recovery) and treatment options depend on the following:

- The stage of the cancer
- The patient's age and general health
- Whether the cancer has just been diagnosed or has recurred (come back)

How Is Staging Done for Vulvar Cancer?

After vulvar cancer has been diagnosed, tests are done to find out if cancer cells have spread within the vulva or to other parts of the body.

The process used to find out if cancer has spread within the vulva or to other parts of the body is called staging. The information gathered from the staging process determines the stage of the disease. It is important to know the stage in order to plan treatment. The following tests and procedures may be used in the staging process:

- **Pelvic exam:** An exam of the vagina, cervix, uterus, fallopian tubes, ovaries, and rectum. A speculum is inserted into the vagina and the doctor or nurse looks at the vagina and cervix for signs of disease. A Pap test of the cervix is usually done. The doctor or nurse also inserts one or two lubricated, gloved fingers of one hand into the vagina and places the other hand over the lower abdomen to feel the size, shape, and position of the uterus and ovaries. The doctor or nurse also inserts a lubricated, gloved finger into the rectum to feel for lumps or abnormal areas.
- **Colposcopy:** A procedure in which a colposcope (a lighted, magnifying instrument) is used to check the vagina and cervix for abnormal areas. Tissue samples may be taken using a curette (spoon-shaped instrument) or a brush and checked under a microscope for signs of disease.
- **Cystoscopy:** A procedure to look inside the bladder and urethra to check for abnormal areas. A cystoscope is inserted through the urethra into the bladder. A cystoscope is a thin, tube-like instrument with a light and a lens for viewing. It may also have a tool to remove tissue samples, which are checked under a microscope for signs of cancer.
- **Proctoscopy:** A procedure to look inside the rectum and anus to check for abnormal areas. A proctoscope is inserted into the anus and rectum. A proctoscope is a thin, tube-like instrument with a light and a lens for viewing. It may also have a tool to remove tissue samples, which are checked under a microscope for signs of cancer.
- **X-rays:** An X-ray is a type of energy beam that can go through the body and onto filmmaking a picture of areas inside the body. To stage vulvar cancer, X-rays may be taken of the organs and bones inside the chest, and the pelvic bones.
- **Intravenous pyelogram (IVP):** A series of X-rays of the kidneys, ureters, and bladder to find out if cancer has spread to these organs. A contrast dye is injected into a vein. As the contrast dye moves through the kidneys, ureters and bladder, X-rays are taken to see if there are any blockages. This procedure is also called intravenous urography.
- **Computed tomography (CT)/computerized axial tomography (CAT) scan:** A procedure that makes a series of detailed pictures of areas inside the body, taken from different angles.

The pictures are made by a computer linked to an X-ray machine. A dye may be injected into a vein or swallowed to help the organs or tissues show up more clearly.

- **Magnetic resonance imaging (MRI):** A procedure that uses a magnet, radio waves, and a computer to make a series of detailed pictures of areas inside the body. This procedure is also called nuclear magnetic resonance imaging (NMRI).
- **Positron emission tomography (PET) scan:** A procedure to find malignant tumor cells in the body. A small amount of radioactive glucose (sugar) is injected into a vein. The PET scanner rotates around the body and makes a picture of where glucose is being used in the body. Malignant tumor cells show up brighter in the picture because they are more active and take up more glucose than normal cells do.
- **Sentinel lymph node biopsy:** The removal of the sentinel lymph node during surgery. The sentinel lymph node is the first lymph node to receive lymphatic drainage from a tumor. It is the first lymph node the cancer is likely to spread to from the tumor. A radioactive substance and/or blue dye is injected near the tumor. The substance or dye flows through the lymph ducts to the lymph nodes. The first lymph node to receive the substance or dye is removed. A pathologist views the tissue under a microscope to look for cancer cells. If cancer cells are not found, it may not be necessary to remove more lymph nodes. Sentinel lymph node biopsy may be done during surgery to remove the tumor for early-stage vulvar cancer.

Vulvar Intraepithelial Neoplasia (VIN)

In vulvar intraepithelial neoplasia (VIN), abnormal cells are found on the surface of the vulvar skin. These abnormal cells are not cancer. Vulvar intraepithelial neoplasia (VIN) may become cancer and spread into nearby tissue. VIN is sometimes called stage 0 or carcinoma in situ.

The following stages are used for vulvar cancer:

Stage I. In stage I, cancer has formed. The tumor is found only in the vulva or perineum (area between the rectum and the vagina). Stage I is divided into stages IA and IB.

- In stage IA, the tumor is 2 centimeters or smaller and has spread 1 millimeter or less into the tissue of the vulva. Cancer has not spread to the lymph nodes.

- In stage IB, the tumor is larger than 2 centimeters or has spread more than 1 millimeter into the tissue of the vulva. Cancer has not spread to the lymph nodes.

Stage II. In stage II, the tumor is any size and has spread into the lower part of the urethra, the lower part of the vagina, or the anus. Cancer has not spread to the lymph nodes.

Stage III. In stage III, the tumor is any size and may have spread into the lower part of the urethra, the lower part of the vagina, or the anus. Cancer has spread to one or more nearby lymph nodes. Stage III is divided into stages IIIA, IIIB, and IIIC.

- In stage IIIA, cancer is found in 1 or 2 lymph nodes that are smaller than 5 millimeters or in one lymph node that is 5 millimeters or larger.
- In stage IIIB, cancer is found in 2 or more lymph nodes that are 5 millimeters or larger, or in 3 or more lymph nodes that are smaller than 5 millimeters.
- In stage IIIC, cancer is found in lymph nodes and has spread to the outside surface of the lymph nodes.

Stage IV. In stage IV, the tumor has spread into the upper part of the urethra, the upper part of the vagina, or to other parts of the body. Stage IV is divided into stages IVA and IVB.

- In stage IVA:
  - cancer has spread into the lining of the upper urethra, the upper vagina, the bladder, or the rectum, or has attached to the pelvic bone; or
  - cancer has spread to nearby lymph nodes and the lymph nodes are not moveable or have formed an ulcer.
- In stage IVB, cancer has spread to lymph nodes in the pelvis or to other parts of the body.

What Are the Standard Treatments Available for Patients with Vulvar Cancer?

Four types of standard treatment are used:

Surgery

Surgery is the most common treatment for vulvar cancer. The goal of surgery is to remove all the cancer without any loss of the woman's sexual function. One of the following types of surgery may be done:

- **Laser surgery:** A surgical procedure that uses a laser beam (a narrow beam of intense light) as a knife to make bloodless cuts in tissue or to remove a surface lesion such as a tumor.
- **Wide local excision:** A surgical procedure to remove the cancer and some of the normal tissue around the cancer.
- **Radical local excision:** A surgical procedure to remove the cancer and a large amount of normal tissue around it. Nearby lymph nodes in the groin may also be removed.
- **Ultrasound surgical aspiration (USA):** A surgical procedure to break the tumor up into small pieces using very fine vibrations. The small pieces of tumor are washed away and removed by suction. This procedure causes less damage to nearby tissue.
- **Vulvectomy:** A surgical procedure to remove part or all of the vulva:
    - **Skinning vulvectomy:** The top layer of vulvar skin where the cancer is found is removed. Skin grafts from other parts of the body may be needed to cover the area where the skin was removed.
    - **Modified radical vulvectomy:** Surgery to remove part of the vulva. Nearby lymph nodes may also be removed.
    - **Radical vulvectomy:** Surgery to remove the entire vulva. Nearby lymph nodes are also removed.
- **Pelvic exenteration:** A surgical procedure to remove the lower colon, rectum, and bladder. The cervix, vagina, ovaries, and nearby lymph nodes are also removed. Artificial openings (stoma) are made for urine and stool to flow from the body into a collection bag.

Even if the doctor removes all the cancer that can be seen at the time of the surgery, some patients may have chemotherapy or radiation therapy after surgery to kill any cancer cells that are left. Treatment given after the surgery, to lower the risk that the cancer will come back, is called adjuvant therapy.

Radiation Therapy

Radiation therapy is a cancer treatment that uses high-energy X-rays or other types of radiation to kill cancer cells or keep them from growing. There are two types of radiation therapy:

- External radiation therapy uses a machine outside the body to send radiation toward the cancer.
- Internal radiation therapy uses a radioactive substance sealed in needles, seeds, wires, or catheters that are placed directly into or near the cancer.

The way the radiation therapy is given depends on the type and stage of the cancer being treated. External and internal radiation therapy are used to treat vulvar cancer, and external radiation therapy may also be used as palliative therapy to relieve symptoms and improve quality of life.

Chemotherapy

Chemotherapy is a cancer treatment that uses drugs to stop the growth of cancer cells, either by killing the cells or by stopping the cells from dividing. When chemotherapy is taken by mouth or injected into a vein or muscle, the drugs enter the bloodstream and can reach cancer cells throughout the body (systemic chemotherapy). When chemotherapy is placed directly into the cerebrospinal fluid, an organ, a body cavity such as the abdomen, or onto the skin, the drugs mainly affect cancer cells in those areas (regional chemotherapy). The way the chemotherapy is given depends on the type and stage of the cancer being treated.

Biologic Therapy

Biologic therapy is a treatment that uses the patient's immune system to fight cancer. Substances made by the body or made in a laboratory are used to boost, direct, or restore the body's natural defenses against cancer. This type of cancer treatment is also called biotherapy or immunotherapy.

Imiquimod is a biologic therapy that may be used to treat vulvar lesions and is applied to the skin in a cream.

Treatment for vulvar cancer may cause side effects.

Is There a Need for Follow-Up Tests?

Some of the tests that were done to diagnose the cancer or to find out the stage of the cancer may be repeated. Some tests will be repeated in order to see how well the treatment is working. Decisions about whether to continue, change, or stop treatment may be based on the results of these tests. Some of the tests will continue to be done from time to time after treatment has ended. The results of these tests can show if your condition has changed or if the cancer has recurred (come back). These tests are sometimes called follow-up tests or check-ups. It is important to have regular follow-up exams to check for recurrent vulvar cancer.

Chapter 45

Andrological Cancers

Chapter Contents

Section 45.1

Penile Cancer

This section includes text excerpted from "Penile Cancer Treatment (PDQ®)—Patient Version," National Cancer Institute (NCI), April 14, 2017.

The penis is a rod-shaped male reproductive organ that passes sperm and urine from the body. It contains two types of erectile tissue (spongy tissue with blood vessels that fill with blood to make an erection):

- **Corpora cavernosa:** The two columns of erectile tissue that form most of the penis.
- **Corpus spongiosum:** The single column of erectile tissue that forms a small portion of the penis. The corpus spongiosum surrounds the urethra (the tube through which urine and sperm pass from the body).

The erectile tissue is wrapped in connective tissue and covered with skin. The glans (head of the penis) is covered with loose skin called the foreskin.

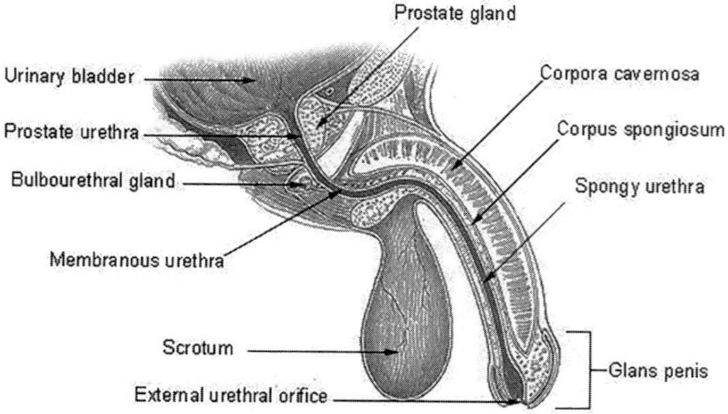

Figure 45.1. *Penis* (Source: "Penis," Surveillance, Epidemiology and End Results Program (SEER), National Cancer Institute (NCI).)

What Is Penile Cancer?

Penile cancer is a disease in which malignant (cancer) cells form in the tissues of the penis.

What Are the Risk Factors for Penile Cancer?

Anything that increases your chance of getting a disease is called a risk factor. Having a risk factor does not mean that you will get cancer; not having risk factors doesn't mean that you will not get cancer. Talk with your doctor if you think you may be at risk.

Risk factors for penile cancer include the following:

Human papillomavirus (HPV) infection may increase the risk of developing penile cancer. Circumcision may help prevent infection with the HPV. A circumcision is an operation in which the doctor removes part or all of the foreskin from the penis. Many boys are circumcised shortly after birth. Men who were not circumcised at birth may have a higher risk of developing penile cancer.

Other risk factors for penile cancer include the following:

- Being age 60 or older
- Having phimosis (a condition in which the foreskin of the penis cannot be pulled back over the glans)
- Having poor personal hygiene
- Having many sexual partners
- Using tobacco products

What Are the Signs and Symptoms of Penile Cancer?

Signs of penile cancer include sores, discharge, and bleeding. These and other signs may be caused by penile cancer or by other conditions. Check with your doctor if you have any of the following:

- Redness, irritation, or a sore on the penis
- A lump on the penis

How Is Penile Cancer Diagnosed?

Tests that examine the penis are used to detect (find) and diagnose penile cancer. The following tests and procedures may be used:

- **Physical exam and history:** An exam of the body to check general signs of health, including checking the penis for signs of disease, such as lumps or anything else that seems unusual. A history of the patient's health habits and past illnesses and treatments will also be taken.

- **Biopsy:** The removal of cells or tissues so they can be viewed under a microscope by a pathologist to check for signs of cancer. The tissue sample is removed during one of the following procedures:
    - **Fine-needle aspiration (FNA) biopsy:** The removal of tissue or fluid using a thin needle.
    - **Incisional biopsy:** The removal of part of a lump or a sample of tissue that doesn't look normal.
    - **Excisional biopsy:** The removal of an entire lump or area of tissue that doesn't look normal.

What Is the Prognosis for Penile Cancer?

The prognosis (chance of recovery) and treatment options depend on the following:

- The stage of the cancer
- The location and size of the tumor
- Whether the cancer has just been diagnosed or has recurred (come back)

How Is Staging Done for Penile Cancer?

After penile cancer has been diagnosed, tests are done to find out if cancer cells have spread within the penis or to other parts of the body.

The process used to find out if cancer has spread within the penis or to other parts of the body is called staging. The information gathered from the staging process determines the stage of the disease. It is important to know the stage in order to plan treatment.

The following tests and procedures may be used in the staging process:

- **Computed tomography (CT)/computerized axial tomography (CAT scan):** A procedure that makes a series of detailed pictures of areas inside the body, taken from different angles. The pictures are made by a computer linked to an X-ray machine. A dye may be injected into a vein or swallowed to help the organs or tissues show up more clearly.

- **Magnetic resonance imaging (MRI):** A procedure that uses a magnet, radio waves, and a computer to make a series of detailed pictures of areas inside the body. A substance called gadolinium is injected into a vein. The gadolinium collects around the cancer cells so they show up brighter in the picture. This procedure is also called nuclear magnetic resonance imaging (NMRI).
- **Ultrasound exam:** A procedure in which high-energy sound waves (ultrasound) are bounced off internal tissues or organs and make echoes. The echoes form a picture of body tissues called a sonogram.
- **Chest X-ray:** An X-ray of the organs and bones inside the chest. An X-ray is a type of energy beam that can go through the body and onto film, making a picture of areas inside the body.
- **Biopsy:** The removal of cells or tissues so they can be viewed under a microscope by a pathologist to check for signs of cancer. The tissue sample is removed during one of the following procedures:
    - **Sentinel lymph node biopsy:** The removal of the sentinel lymph node during surgery. The sentinel lymph node is the first lymph node to receive lymphatic drainage from a tumor. It is the first lymph node the cancer is likely to spread to from the tumor. A radioactive substance and/or blue dye is injected near the tumor. The substance or dye flows through the lymph ducts to the lymph nodes. The first lymph node to receive the substance or dye is removed. A pathologist views the tissue under a microscope to look for cancer cells. If cancer cells are not found, it may not be necessary to remove more lymph nodes.
    - **Lymph node dissection:** A procedure to remove one or more lymph nodes during surgery. A sample of tissue is checked under a microscope for signs of cancer. This procedure is also called a lymphadenectomy.

The following stages are used for penile cancer:

Stage 0 (carcinoma in situ). In stage 0, abnormal cells or growths that look like warts are found on the surface of the skin of the penis. These abnormal cells or growths may become cancer and spread into nearby normal tissue. Stage 0 is also called carcinoma in situ.

Stage I. In stage I, cancer has formed and spread to connective tissue just under the skin of the penis. Cancer has not spread to lymph vessels or blood vessels. The tumor cells look a lot like normal cells under a microscope.

Stage II. In stage II, cancer has spread:

- to connective tissue just under the skin of the penis. Also, cancer has spread to lymph vessels or blood vessels or the tumor cells may look very different from normal cells under a microscope; or
- through connective tissue to erectile tissue (spongy tissue that fills with blood to make an erection); or
- beyond erectile tissue to the urethra.

Stage III. Stage III is divided into stage IIIA and stage IIIB.

In stage IIIA, cancer has spread to one lymph node in the groin. Cancer has also spread:

- to connective tissue just under the skin of the penis. Also, cancer may have spread to lymph vessels or blood vessels or the tumor cells may look very different from normal cells under a microscope; or
- through connective tissue to erectile tissue (spongy tissue that fills with blood to make an erection); or
- beyond erectile tissue to the urethra.

In stage IIIB, cancer has spread to more than one lymph node on one side of the groin or to lymph nodes on both sides of the groin. Cancer has also spread:

- to connective tissue just under the skin of the penis. Also, cancer may have spread to lymph vessels or blood vessels or the tumor cells may look very different from normal cells under a microscope; or
- through connective tissue to erectile tissue (spongy tissue that fills with blood to make an erection); or
- beyond erectile tissue to the urethra.

Stage IV. In stage IV, cancer has spread:

- to tissues near the penis such as the prostate, and may have spread to lymph nodes in the groin or pelvis; or

- to one or more lymph nodes in the pelvis, or cancer has spread from the lymph nodes to the tissues around the lymph nodes; or
- to distant parts of the body.

What Are the Standard Treatment Options for People with Penile Cancer?

Four types of standard treatment are used:

Surgery

Surgery is the most common treatment for all stages of penile cancer. A doctor may remove the cancer using one of the following operations:

- **Mohs microsurgery:** A procedure in which the tumor is cut from the skin in thin layers. During the surgery, the edges of the tumor and each layer of tumor removed are viewed through a microscope to check for cancer cells. Layers continue to be removed until no more cancer cells are seen. This type of surgery removes as little normal tissue as possible and is often used to remove cancer on the skin.
- **Laser surgery:** A surgical procedure that uses a laser beam (a narrow beam of intense light) as a knife to make bloodless cuts in tissue or to remove a surface lesion such as a tumor.
- **Cryosurgery:** A treatment that uses an instrument to freeze and destroy abnormal tissue. This type of treatment is also called cryotherapy.
- **Circumcision:** Surgery to remove part or all of the foreskin of the penis.
- **Wide local excision:** Surgery to remove only the cancer and some normal tissue around it.
- **Amputation of the penis:** Surgery to remove part or all of the penis. If part of the penis is removed, it is a partial penectomy. If all of the penis is removed, it is a total penectomy.

Lymph nodes in the groin may be taken out during surgery.

Even if the doctor removes all the cancer that can be seen at the time of the surgery, some patients may be given chemotherapy or radiation therapy after surgery to kill any cancer cells that are left. Treatment given after the surgery, to lower the risk that the cancer will come back, is called adjuvant therapy.

Radiation Therapy

Radiation therapy is a cancer treatment that uses high-energy X-rays or other types of radiation to kill cancer cells or keep them from growing. There are two types of radiation therapy:

- External radiation therapy uses a machine outside the body to send radiation toward the cancer.
- Internal radiation therapy uses a radioactive substance sealed in needles, seeds, wires, or catheters that are placed directly into or near the cancer.

The way the radiation therapy is given depends on the type and stage of the cancer being treated. External and internal radiation therapy are used to treat penile cancer.

Chemotherapy

Chemotherapy is a cancer treatment that uses drugs to stop the growth of cancer cells, either by killing the cells or by stopping them from dividing. When chemotherapy is taken by mouth or injected into a vein or muscle, the drugs enter the bloodstream and can reach cancer cells throughout the body (systemic chemotherapy). When chemotherapy is placed directly onto the skin (topical chemotherapy) or into the cerebrospinal fluid, an organ, or a body cavity such as the abdomen, the drugs mainly affect cancer cells in those areas (regional chemotherapy). The way the chemotherapy is given depends on the type and stage of the cancer being treated.

Topical chemotherapy may be used to treat stage 0 penile cancer.

Biologic Therapy

Biologic therapy is a treatment that uses the patient's immune system to fight cancer. Substances made by the body or made in a laboratory are used to boost, direct, or restore the body's natural defenses against cancer. This type of cancer treatment is also called biotherapy or immunotherapy. Topical biologic therapy with imiquimod may be used to treat stage 0 penile cancer.

What New Types of Treatment Are Being Tested in Clinical Trials?

New types of treatment are being tested in clinical trials.

Radiosensitizers

Radiosensitizers are drugs that make tumor cells more sensitive to radiation therapy. Combining radiation therapy with radiosensitizers helps kill more tumor cells.

Sentinel Lymph Node Biopsy Followed by Surgery

Sentinel lymph node biopsy is the removal of the sentinel lymph node during surgery. The sentinel lymph node is the first lymph node to receive lymphatic drainage from a tumor. It is the first lymph node the cancer is likely to spread to from the tumor. A radioactive substance and/or blue dye is injected near the tumor. The substance or dye flows through the lymph ducts to the lymph nodes. The first lymph node to receive the substance or dye is removed. A pathologist views the tissue under a microscope to look for cancer cells. If cancer cells are not found, it may not be necessary to remove more lymph nodes. After the sentinel lymph node biopsy, the surgeon removes the cancer.

Is There a Need for Follow-Up Tests?

Some of the tests that were done to diagnose the cancer or to find out the stage of the cancer may be repeated. Some tests will be repeated in order to see how well the treatment is working. Decisions about whether to continue, change, or stop treatment may be based on the results of these tests. Some of the tests will continue to be done from time to time after treatment has ended. The results of these tests can show if your condition has changed or if the cancer has recurred (come back). These tests are sometimes called follow-up tests or check-ups.

Section 45.2

Prostate Cancer

This section includes text excerpted from "Prostate Cancer," Centers for Disease Control and Prevention (CDC), February 15, 2018.

The prostate is a part of the male reproductive system, which includes the penis, prostate, and testicles. The prostate is located just below the bladder and in front of the rectum. It is about the size of a walnut and surrounds the urethra (the tube that empties urine from the bladder). It produces fluid that makes up a part of semen.

As a man ages, the prostate tends to increase in size. This can cause the urethra to narrow and decrease urine flow. This is called benign prostatic hyperplasia, and it is not the same as prostate cancer. Men may also have other prostate changes that are not cancer.

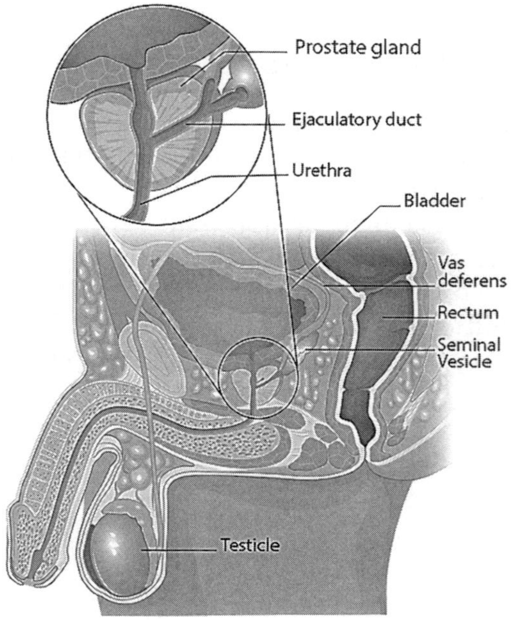

Figure 45.2. *Prostate*

What Is Prostate Cancer?

Cancer is a disease in which cells in the body grow out of control. When cancer starts in the prostate, it is called prostate cancer. Many men with prostate cancer—especially those with tumors that have not spread beyond the prostate—die of other causes without ever having any symptoms from the cancer. Except for skin cancer, prostate cancer is the most common cancer in American men. It is the second most common cause of death from cancer among white, African American, American Indian/Alaska Native, and Hispanic men, and the fourth most common cause of death from cancer among Asian/Pacific Islander men.

What Are the Risk Factors?

Research has found risk factors that increase your chances of getting prostate cancer. These risk factors include:

- **Age:** The older a man is, the greater his risk for getting prostate cancer.
- **Family history:** Certain genes (passed from parent to child) that you inherited from your parents may affect your prostate cancer risk. Currently, no single gene is sure to raise or lower your risk of getting prostate cancer. However, a man with a father, brother, or son who has had prostate cancer is 2–3 times more likely to develop the disease himself.
- **Race:** Prostate cancer is more common in African-American men. It tends to start at younger ages and grow faster than in other racial or ethnic groups, but medical experts do not know why.

Researchers are trying to determine the causes of prostate cancer and whether it can be prevented. They do not yet agree on the factors that can influence a man's risk of developing the disease, either positively or negatively.

What Are the Symptoms of Prostate Cancer?

Different people have different symptoms for prostate cancer. Some men do not have symptoms at all.

Some symptoms of prostate cancer are:

- Difficulty starting urination

- Weak or interrupted flow of urine
- Frequent urination, especially at night
- Difficulty emptying the bladder completely
- Pain or burning during urination
- Blood in the urine or semen
- Pain in the back, hips, or pelvis that doesn't go away
- Painful ejaculation

If you have any symptoms that worry you, be sure to see your doctor right away. Keep in mind that these symptoms may be caused by conditions other than prostate cancer.

What Screening Tests Are There for Prostate Cancer?

Cancer screening means looking for cancer before it causes symptoms. However, most prostate cancers grow slowly or not at all.

Two tests are commonly used to screen for prostate cancer:

- **Digital rectal exam (DRE):** A doctor or nurse inserts a gloved, lubricated finger into the rectum to estimate the size of the prostate and feel for lumps or other abnormalities.
- **Prostate-specific antigen (PSA) test:** Measures the level of PSA in the blood. PSA is a substance made by the prostate. The levels of PSA in the blood can be higher in men who have prostate cancer. The PSA level may also be elevated in other conditions that affect the prostate.

As a rule, the higher the PSA level in the blood, the more likely a prostate problem is present. But many factors, such as age and race, can affect PSA levels. Some prostate glands make more PSA than others. PSA levels also can be affected by:

- Certain medical procedures
- Certain medications
- An enlarged prostate
- A prostate infection

Because many factors can affect PSA levels, your doctor is the best person to interpret your PSA test results. Only a biopsy can diagnose prostate cancer for sure.

Should I Get Screened for Prostate Cancer?

Centers for Disease Control and Prevention (CDC) and other federal agencies follow the prostate cancer screening recommendations set forth by the U.S. Preventive Services Task Force (USPSTF), which recommends against PSA-based screening for men who do not have symptoms. Other organizations, like the American Urological Association (AUA), the American Cancer Society (ACS), and the American College of Physicians (ACP) may have other recommendations.

A PSA test can find prostate cancer earlier than no screening at all. However, the PSA test may have false positive or false negative results. This can mean that men without cancer may have abnormal results and get tests that are not necessary. It could also mean that the test could miss cancer in men who may need to be treated.

Abnormal results can cause anxiety. The test that comes after an abnormal result on a PSA test is a biopsy (a minor surgery to get small samples of prostate cells or tissues), which can cause pain, infection, bleeding, and may even miss cancer that needs to be treated.

Talk to your doctor about the right decision for you.

Informed Decision Making

Informed decision making occurs when a man:

- Understands the nature and risk of prostate cancer
- Understands the risks of, benefits of, and alternatives to screening
- Participates in the decision to be screened or not at a level he desires
- Makes a decision consistent with his preferences and values

What Are the Benefits and Harms of Screening?

The USPSTF is an organization made up of doctors and disease experts who look at research on the best way to prevent diseases and make recommendations on how doctors can help patients avoid diseases or find them early. The USPSTF recommends that men do not get a PSA blood test to screen for prostate cancer. Every screening test has benefits and risks, and the USPSTF says that the risks of PSA testing tend to outweigh the potential benefits.

Most prostate cancers found by screening are small and slow-growing, and may not cause problems at all over a man's lifetime. Some men screened with a PSA test will have the test show that they have prostate cancer when they really don't, which is called a false positive. Doctors may want to check to see if there really is cancer, so they may do a test called a biopsy to remove a sample of prostate cells or tissue for a pathologist to look at under a microscope. A biopsy can cause infection, pain, and bleeding, and the test may not show that there is cancer of the prostate at all.

If the biopsy shows cancer, the cancer may not grow quickly enough to cause problems for a man. Still, these cancers are sometimes treated with radiation or surgery when they may not need to be. This is called overtreatment. Surgery and radiation can cause side effects like infections, impotence (inability to get an erection), or problems with the bladder or the bowels. Still, sometimes screening does show doctors a fast-growing cancer that might pose a danger to a man's life. Not all medical groups agree about whether men should be screened with a PSA test. Men should talk their doctor about their risk factors and whether screening for prostate cancer is right for them.

How Is Prostate Cancer Diagnosed?

If your PSA test or DRE is abnormal, doctors may do more tests to find or diagnose prostate cancer. A biopsy is when a small piece of tissue is removed from the prostate and looked at under a microscope to see if there are cancer cells. A Gleason score is determined when the biopsy is looked at under the microscope. If there is a cancer, the score indicates how likely it is to spread. The score ranges from 2–10. The lower the score, the less likely it is that the cancer will spread.

A biopsy is the main tool for diagnosing prostate cancer, but a doctor can use other tools to help make sure the biopsy is made in the right place. For example, doctors may use a transrectal ultrasound, when a probe the size of a finger is inserted into the rectum and high-energy sound waves (ultrasound) are bounced off the prostate to create a picture of the prostate called a sonogram. Doctors also may use magnetic resonance imaging (MRI) to guide the biopsy.

Staging

If prostate cancer is diagnosed, other tests are done to find out if cancer cells have spread within the prostate or to other parts of the body. This process is called staging. Whether the cancer is only in the prostate, or has spread outside the prostate, determines your stage of prostate cancer. The stage of prostate cancer tells doctors what kind of treatment you need.

How Is Prostate Cancer Treated?

Different types of treatment are available for prostate cancer. You and your doctor will decide which treatment is right for you. Some common treatments are:

- **Active surveillance.** Closely monitoring the prostate cancer by PSA and DRE tests regularly, and treating the cancer only if it grows or causes symptoms.
- **Surgery.** A prostatectomy is an operation where doctors remove the prostate. Radical prostatectomy removes the prostate as well as the surrounding tissue.
- **Radiation therapy.** Using high-energy rays (similar to X-rays) to kill the cancer. There are two types of radiation therapy:
    - **External radiation therapy.** A machine outside the body directs radiation at the cancer cells.
    - **Internal radiation therapy (brachytherapy).** Radioactive seeds or pellets are surgically placed into or near the cancer to destroy the cancer cells.

Hormone therapy. Blocks cancer cells from getting the hormones they need to grow.

Other therapies used in the treatment of prostate cancer that are still under investigation include:

- **Cryotherapy.** Placing a special probe inside or near the prostate cancer to freeze and kill the cancer cells.
- **Chemotherapy.** Using special drugs to shrink or kill the cancer. The drugs can be pills you take or medicines given through your veins, or, sometimes, both.
- **Biological therapy.** Works with your body's immune system to help it fight cancer or to control side effects from other cancer treatments. Side effects are how your body reacts to drugs or other treatments.

- **High-intensity focused ultrasound.** This therapy directs high-energy sound waves (ultrasound) at the cancer to kill cancer cells.

Complementary and Alternative Medicine

Complementary and alternative medicine are medicines and health practices that are not standard cancer treatments. Complementary medicine is used in addition to standard treatments, and alternative medicine is used instead of standard treatments. Meditation, yoga, and supplements like vitamins and herbs are some examples.

Many kinds of complementary and alternative medicine have not been tested scientifically and may not be safe. Talk to your doctor about the risks and benefits before you start any kind of complementary or alternative medicine.

Which Treatment Is Right for Me?

Choosing the treatment that is right for you may be hard. Talk to your cancer doctor about the treatment options available for your type and stage of cancer. Your doctor can explain the risks and benefits of each treatment and their side effects. Side effects are how your body reacts to drugs or other treatments.

Sometimes people get an opinion from more than one cancer doctor. This is called a "second opinion." Getting a second opinion may help you choose the treatment that is right for you.

Section 45.3

Testicular Cancer

This section includes text excerpted from "Testicular Cancer Treatment (PDQ®)—Patient Version," National Cancer Institute (NCI), July 7, 2016.

The testicles are 2 egg-shaped glands located inside the scrotum (a sac of loose skin that lies directly below the penis). The testicles are held within the scrotum by the spermatic cord, which also contains the vas deferens and vessels and nerves of the testicles.

The testicles are the male sex glands and produce testosterone and sperm. Germ cells within the testicles produce immature sperm that travel through a network of tubules (tiny tubes) and larger tubes into the epididymis (a long coiled tube next to the testicles) where the sperm mature and are stored.

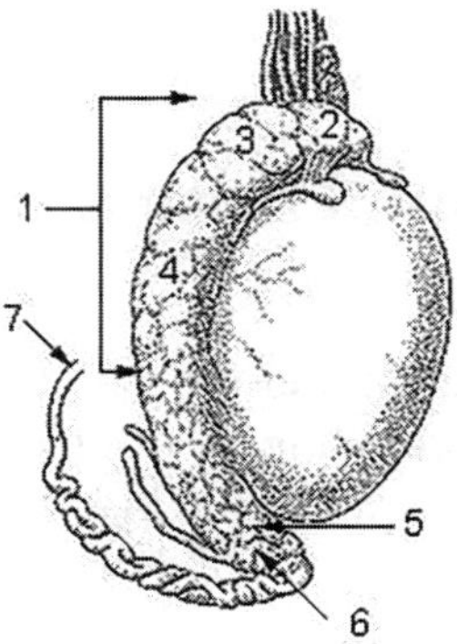

1. **Epididymis**
2. **Head of epididymis**
3. **Lobules of epididymis**
4. **Body of epididymis**
5. **Tail of epididymis**
6. **Duct of epididymis**
7. **Deferent duct (ductus deferens or vas deferens)**

Figure 45.3. *Testicle and Epididymis* (Source: "Anatomy of the Testis," Surveillance, Epidemiology and End Results Program (SEER), National Cancer Institute (NCI).)

What Is Testicular Cancer?

Testicular cancer is a disease in which malignant (cancer) cells form in the tissues of one or both testicles. Almost all testicular cancers start in the germ cells. The two main types of testicular germ cell tumors are seminomas and nonseminomas. These 2 types grow and spread differently and are treated differently. Nonseminomas tend to grow and spread more quickly than seminomas. Seminomas are more sensitive to radiation. A testicular tumor that contains both seminoma and nonseminoma cells is treated as a nonseminoma. Testicular cancer is the most common cancer in men 20–35 years old.

What Are the Risk Factors for Testicular Cancer?

Anything that increases the chance of getting a disease is called a risk factor. Having a risk factor does not mean that you will get cancer; not having risk factors doesn't mean that you will not get cancer. Talk with your doctor if you think you may be at risk.

Health history can affect the risk of testicular cancer. Risk factors for testicular cancer include:

- Having had an undescended testicle
- Having had abnormal development of the testicles
- Having a personal history of testicular cancer
- Having a family history of testicular cancer (especially in a father or brother)
- Being white

What Are the Signs and Symptoms of Testicular Cancer?

Signs and symptoms of testicular cancer include swelling or discomfort in the scrotum. These and other signs and symptoms may be caused by testicular cancer or by other conditions. Check with your doctor if you have any of the following:

- A painless lump or swelling in either testicle
- A change in how the testicle feels
- A dull ache in the lower abdomen or the groin
- A sudden buildup of fluid in the scrotum
- Pain or discomfort in a testicle or in the scrotum

How Is Testicular Cancer Diagnosed?

Tests that examine the testicles and blood are used to detect (find) and diagnose testicular cancer. The following tests and procedures may be used:

- **Physical exam and history:** An exam of the body to check general signs of health, including checking for signs of disease, such as lumps or anything else that seems unusual. The testicles will be examined to check for lumps, swelling, or pain. A history of the patient's health habits and past illnesses and treatments will also be taken.
- **Ultrasound exam:** A procedure in which high-energy sound waves (ultrasound) are bounced off internal tissues or organs and make echoes. The echoes form a picture of body tissues called a sonogram.

- **Serum tumor marker test:** A procedure in which a sample of blood is examined to measure the amounts of certain substances released into the blood by organs, tissues, or tumor cells in the body. Certain substances are linked to specific types of cancer when found in increased levels in the blood. These are called tumor markers. The following tumor markers are used to detect testicular cancer:
  - Alpha-fetoprotein (AFP).
  - Beta-human chorionic gonadotropin (β-hCG).

Tumor marker levels are measured before inguinal orchiectomy and biopsy, to help diagnose testicular cancer.

- **Inguinal orchiectomy:** A procedure to remove the entire testicle through an incision in the groin. A tissue sample from the testicle is then viewed under a microscope to check for cancer cells. (The surgeon does not cut through the scrotum into the testicle to remove a sample of tissue for biopsy, because if cancer is present, this procedure could cause it to spread into the scrotum and lymph nodes. It's important to choose a surgeon who has experience with this kind of surgery.) If cancer is found, the cell type (seminoma or nonseminoma) is determined in order to help plan treatment.

What Is the Prognosis for Testicular Cancer?

The prognosis (chance of recovery) and treatment options depend on the following:

- Stage of the cancer (whether it is in or near the testicle or has spread to other places in the body, and blood levels of AFP, β-hCG, and LDH)
- Type of cancer
- Size of the tumor
- Number and size of retroperitoneal lymph nodes

Testicular cancer can usually be cured in patients who receive adjuvant chemotherapy or radiation therapy after their primary treatment.

How Is Staging Done for Testicular Cancer?

After testicular cancer has been diagnosed, tests are done to find out if cancer cells have spread within the testicles or to other parts of the body.

The process used to find out if cancer has spread within the testicles or to other parts of the body is called staging. The information gathered from the staging process determines the stage of the disease. It is important to know the stage in order to plan treatment.

The following tests and procedures may be used in the staging process:

- **Chest X-ray:** An X-ray of the organs and bones inside the chest. An X-ray is a type of energy beam that can go through the body and onto film, making a picture of areas inside the body.
- **Computed tomography (CT)/computerized axial tomography (CAT) scan:** A procedure that makes a series of detailed pictures of areas inside the body, taken from different angles. The pictures are made by a computer linked to an X-ray machine. A dye may be injected into a vein or swallowed to help the organs or tissues show up more clearly.
- **Positron emission tomography (PET) scan:** A procedure to find malignant tumor cells in the body. A small amount of radioactive glucose (sugar) is injected into a vein. The PET scanner rotates around the body and makes a picture of where glucose is being used in the body. Malignant tumor cells show up brighter in the picture because they are more active and take up more glucose than normal cells do.
- **Magnetic resonance imaging (MRI):** A procedure that uses a magnet, radio waves, and a computer to make a series of detailed pictures of areas inside the body. This procedure is also called nuclear magnetic resonance imaging (NMRI).
- **Abdominal lymph node dissection:** A surgical procedure in which lymph nodes in the abdomen are removed and a sample of tissue is checked under a microscope for signs of cancer. This procedure is also called lymphadenectomy. For patients with nonseminoma, removing the lymph nodes may help stop the spread of disease. Cancer cells in the lymph nodes of seminoma patients can be treated with radiation therapy.
- **Serum tumor marker test:** A procedure in which a sample of blood is examined to measure the amounts of certain substances released into the blood by organs, tissues, or tumor cells in the body. Certain substances are linked to specific types of cancer when found in increased levels in the blood. These are called

tumor markers. The following 3 tumor markers are used in staging testicular cancer:

- Alpha-fetoprotein (AFP)
- Beta-human chorionic gonadotropin (β-hCG)
- Lactate dehydrogenase (LDH)

Tumor marker levels are measured again, after inguinal orchiectomy and biopsy, in order to determine the stage of the cancer. This helps to show if all of the cancer has been removed or if more treatment is needed. Tumor marker levels are also measured during follow-up as a way of checking if the cancer has come back.

The following stages are used for testicular cancer:

Stage 0 (Testicular intraepithelial neoplasia). In stage 0, abnormal cells are found in the tiny tubules where the sperm cells begin to develop. These abnormal cells may become cancer and spread into nearby normal tissue. All tumor marker levels are normal. Stage 0 is also called testicular intraepithelial neoplasia and testicular intratubular germ cell neoplasia.

Stage I. In stage I, cancer has formed. Stage I is divided into stage IA, stage IB, and stage IS and is determined after an inguinal orchiectomy is done.

- In stage IA, cancer is in the testicle and epididymis and may have spread to the inner layer of the membrane surrounding the testicle. All tumor marker levels are normal.
- In stage IB, cancer:
    - is in the testicle and the epididymis and has spread to the blood vessels or lymph vessels in the testicle; or
    - has spread to the outer layer of the membrane surrounding the testicle; or
    - is in the spermatic cord or the scrotum and may be in the blood vessels or lymph vessels of the testicle.

  All tumor marker levels are normal.
- In stage IS, cancer is found anywhere within the testicle, spermatic cord, or the scrotum and either:
    - all tumor marker levels are slightly above normal; or

- one or more tumor marker levels are moderately above normal or high.

Stage II. Stage II is divided into stage IIA, stage IIB, and stage IIC and is determined after an inguinal orchiectomy is done.

- In stage IIA, cancer:
  - is anywhere within the testicle, spermatic cord, or scrotum; and
  - has spread to up to 5 lymph nodes in the abdomen, none larger than 2 centimeters.

  All tumor marker levels are normal or slightly above normal.

- In stage IIB, cancer is anywhere within the testicle, spermatic cord, or scrotum; and either:
  - has spread to up to 5 lymph nodes in the abdomen; at least one of the lymph nodes is larger than 2 centimeters, but none are larger than 5 centimeters; or
  - has spread to more than 5 lymph nodes; the lymph nodes are not larger than 5 centimeters.

  All tumor marker levels are normal or slightly above normal.

- In stage IIC, cancer:
  - is anywhere within the testicle, spermatic cord, or scrotum; and
  - has spread to a lymph node in the abdomen that is larger than 5 centimeters.

  All tumor marker levels are normal or slightly above normal.

Stage III. Stage III is divided into stage IIIA, stage IIIB, and stage IIIC and is determined after an inguinal orchiectomy is done.

- In stage IIIA, cancer:
  - is anywhere within the testicle, spermatic cord, or scrotum; and
  - may have spread to one or more lymph nodes in the abdomen; and
  - has spread to distant lymph nodes or to the lungs.

Tumor marker levels may range from normal to slightly above normal.

- In stage IIIB, cancer:
  - is anywhere within the testicle, spermatic cord, or scrotum; and
  - may have spread to one or more lymph nodes in the abdomen, to distant lymph nodes, or to the lungs.

  The level of one or more tumor markers is moderately above normal.
- In stage IIIC, cancer:
  - is anywhere within the testicle, spermatic cord, or scrotum; and
  - may have spread to one or more lymph nodes in the abdomen, to distant lymph nodes, or to the lungs.

  The level of one or more tumor markers is high.
  or
  Cancer:

- is anywhere within the testicle, spermatic cord, or scrotum; and
- may have spread to one or more lymph nodes in the abdomen; and
- has not spread to distant lymph nodes or the lung but has spread to other parts of the body.

Tumor marker levels may range from normal to high.

Testicular Tumors Classification Based on Response to Treatment

Testicular tumors are divided into 3 groups, based on how well the tumors are expected to respond to treatment.

Good Prognosis

For nonseminoma, all of the following must be true:

- The tumor is found only in the testicle or in the retroperitoneum (area outside or behind the abdominal wall); and
- The tumor has not spread to organs other than the lungs; and

- The levels of all the tumor markers are slightly above normal.

For seminoma, all of the following must be true:

- The tumor has not spread to organs other than the lungs; and
- The level of alpha-fetoprotein (AFP) is normal. Beta-human chorionic gonadotropin (β-hCG) and lactate dehydrogenase (LDH) may be at any level.

Intermediate Prognosis

For nonseminoma, all of the following must be true:

- The tumor is found in one testicle only or in the retroperitoneum (area outside or behind the abdominal wall); and
- The tumor has not spread to organs other than the lungs; and
- The level of any one of the tumor markers is more than slightly above normal.

For seminoma, all of the following must be true:

- The tumor has spread to organs other than the lungs; and
- The level of AFP is normal. β-hCG and LDH may be at any level.

Poor Prognosis

For nonseminoma, at least one of the following must be true:

- The tumor is in the center of the chest between the lungs; or
- The tumor has spread to organs other than the lungs; or
- The level of any one of the tumor markers is high.

There is no poor prognosis grouping for seminoma testicular tumors.

What Are the Standard Treatment Available for People with Testicular Cancer?

Five types of standard treatment are used:

Surgery

Surgery to remove the testicle (inguinal orchiectomy) and some of the lymph nodes may be done at diagnosis and staging. Tumors that have spread to other places in the body may be partly or entirely removed by surgery.

Even if the doctor removes all the cancer that can be seen at the time of the surgery, some patients may be given chemotherapy or radiation therapy after surgery to kill any cancer cells that are left. Treatment given after the surgery, to lower the risk that the cancer will come back, is called adjuvant therapy.

Radiation Therapy

Radiation therapy is a cancer treatment that uses high-energy X-rays or other types of radiation to kill cancer cells or keep them from growing. There are two types of radiation therapy:

- External radiation therapy uses a machine outside the body to send radiation toward the cancer.
- Internal radiation therapy uses a radioactive substance sealed in needles, seeds, wires, or catheters that are placed directly into or near the cancer.

The way the radiation therapy is given depends on the type and stage of the cancer being treated. External radiation therapy is used to treat testicular cancer.

Chemotherapy

Chemotherapy is a cancer treatment that uses drugs to stop the growth of cancer cells, either by killing the cells or by stopping the cells from dividing. When chemotherapy is taken by mouth or injected into a vein or muscle, the drugs enter the bloodstream and can reach cancer cells throughout the body (systemic chemotherapy). When chemotherapy is placed directly into the cerebrospinal fluid, an organ, or a body cavity such as the abdomen, the drugs mainly affect cancer cells in those areas (regional chemotherapy). The way the chemotherapy is given depends on the type and stage of the cancer being treated.

Surveillance

Surveillance is closely following a patient's condition without giving any treatment unless there are changes in test results. It is used to find early signs that the cancer has recurred (come back). In surveillance, patients are given certain exams and tests on a regular schedule.

High-Dose Chemotherapy with Stem Cell Transplant

High-dose chemotherapy with stem cell transplant is a method of giving high doses of chemotherapy and replacing blood-forming cells destroyed by the cancer treatment. Stem cells (immature blood cells) are removed from the blood or bone marrow of the patient or a donor and are frozen and stored. After the chemotherapy is completed, the stored stem cells are thawed and given back to the patient through an infusion. These reinfused stem cells grow into (and restore) the body's blood cells.

Can Treatment for Testicular Cancer Cause Infertility?

Certain treatments for testicular cancer can cause infertility that may be permanent. Patients who may wish to have children should consider sperm banking before having treatment. Sperm banking is the process of freezing sperm and storing it for later use.

Is There a Need for Follow-Up Tests?

Some of the tests that were done to diagnose the cancer or to find out the stage of the cancer may be repeated. Some tests will be repeated in order to see how well the treatment is working. Decisions about whether to continue, change, or stop treatment may be based on the results of these tests.

Some of the tests will continue to be done from time to time after treatment has ended. The results of these tests can show if your condition has changed or if the cancer has recurred (come back). These tests are sometimes called follow-up tests or check-ups.

Men who have had testicular cancer have an increased risk of developing cancer in the other testicle. A patient is advised to regularly check the other testicle and report any unusual symptoms to a doctor right away. Long-term clinical exams are very important. The patient will probably have check-ups frequently during the first year after surgery and less often after that.

Chapter 46

Leukemia

Chapter Contents

Section 46.1

Overview of Leukemia

This section includes text excerpted from "Leukemia," Centers for Disease Control and Prevention (CDC), February 8, 2018.

What Is Leukemia?

Leukemia is a cancer of the bone marrow (the soft, sponge-like tissue in the center of most bones that makes blood cells) and blood. The two main kinds of leukemia are:

- **Lymphocytic leukemia** (also known as lymphoblastic leukemia), is when the body makes too many of a certain kind of white blood cells, called lymphocytes.
- **Myelogenous leukemia** (also known as myeloid or myelocytic leukemia), is when the body makes too many of a certain kind of white blood cells, called granulocytes.

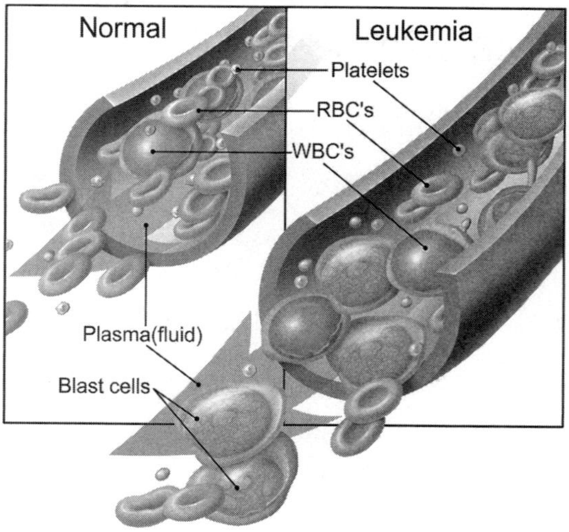

Figure 46.1. *Normal Blood Cells and Blood Cells with Leukemia*

Leukemia can be acute or chronic. Acute types of leukemia progress quickly, while chronic types of leukemia progress slowly, leading to different treatments.

Leukemia is the most common kind of cancer among children and teens. Acute lymphocytic leukemia is more common among children and teens than among adults. However, because other types of leukemia become more common with age, most leukemia is found in among adults.

What Causes Leukemia?

Scientists do not fully understand all of the causes of leukemia, but research has found many links. For example:

- Being exposed to benzene or large doses of ionizing radiation have caused leukemia in some people.
- Tobacco smoke contains cancer-causing chemicals (including benzene), which are linked to acute myeloid leukemia in adults.
- Family history also has been linked with higher risk of some kinds of leukemia, such as chronic lymphocytic leukemia.
- Some people with Down syndrome or blood disorders such as polycythemia vera (a disease in which there are too many red blood cells in the bone marrow and blood, causing the blood to thicken) may be more likely to develop leukemia.
- Most people with chronic myelogenous leukemia have a gene mutation (change) called the Philadelphia chromosome. It results in the bone marrow making an enzyme that causes too many stem cells to become white blood cells. The Philadelphia chromosome is not passed from parent to child.
- White people are more likely than black people to develop lymphocytic leukemia, but scientists do not know why. Scientists also do not know why men are more likely than women to develop leukemia.

What Are the Symptoms of Leukemia?

Chronic lymphocytic leukemia usually does not cause any symptoms and is usually found during a routine blood test. If it does cause symptoms, they can include swollen lymph nodes and feeling tired. Symptoms of chronic myelogenous leukemia include fever, night sweats, and feeling tired. Sometimes chronic myelogenous leukemia does not cause any symptoms. The early symptoms of acute myelogenous leukemia and acute lymphocytic leukemia may be like those caused by the flu or other common diseases. Symptoms include fever, night sweats, feeling tired, feeling out of breath, and bruising or bleeding easily. These symptoms can also come from other conditions. If you have any of them, talk to your doctor.

Statistics

In the United States in 2014:

- 47,135 people (27,489 men and 19,646 women) were diagnosed with leukemia, and 23,564 people (13,542 men and 10,022 women) died from it.
- Among men, white men had the highest rate of developing leukemia (17.5 per 100,000 men), followed by black men (13.0), Hispanic† men (12.3), Asian/Pacific Islander men (9.4), and American Indian/Alaska Native men (9.2).
- Among women, white women had the highest rate of developing leukemia (10.6 per 100,000 women), followed by Hispanic† women (8.9), black women (8.4), Asian/Pacific Islander women (6.2), and American Indian/Alaska Native women (5.3).

†*Hispanic origin is not mutually exclusive from race categories (white, black, Asian / Pacific Islander, American Indian / Alaska Native).*

Section 46.2

Adult Acute Lymphoblastic Leukemia

This section includes text excerpted from "Adult Acute Lymphoblastic Leukemia Treatment (PDQ®)—Patient Version," National Cancer Institute (NCI), October 26, 2017.

What Is Adult Acute Lymphoblastic Leukemia (ALL)?

Adult acute lymphoblastic leukemia (ALL) is a type of cancer in which the bone marrow makes too many lymphocytes (a type of white blood cell). It is also called acute lymphocytic leukemia. It is a cancer of the blood and bone marrow. This type of cancer usually gets worse quickly if it is not treated.

What Are the Risk Factors for ALL?

Anything that increases your risk of getting a disease is called a risk factor. Having a risk factor does not mean that you will get cancer; not having risk factors doesn't mean that you will not get cancer. Talk with your doctor if you think you may be at risk. Previous chemotherapy and exposure to radiation may increase the risk of developing ALL. Possible risk factors for ALL include the following:

- Being male
- Being white
- Being older than 70
- Past treatment with chemotherapy or radiation therapy
- Being exposed to high levels of radiation in the environment (such as nuclear radiation)
- Having certain genetic disorders, such as Down syndrome

What Are the Signs and Symptoms of ALL?

Signs and symptoms of adult ALL include fever, feeling tired, and easy bruising or bleeding. The early signs and symptoms of ALL may be like the flu or other common diseases. Check with your doctor if you have any of the following:

- Weakness or feeling tired
- Fever or night sweats
- Easy bruising or bleeding
- Petechiae (flat, pinpoint spots under the skin, caused by bleeding)
- Shortness of breath
- Weight loss or loss of appetite
- Pain in the bones or stomach
- Pain or feeling of fullness below the ribs
- Painless lumps in the neck, underarm, stomach, or groin
- Having many infections

These and other signs and symptoms may be caused by adult acute lymphoblastic leukemia or by other conditions.

How Is ALL Diagnosed?

Tests that examine the blood and bone marrow are used to detect (find) and diagnose adult ALL. The following tests and procedures may be used:

- **Physical exam and history:** An exam of the body to check general signs of health, including checking for signs of disease, such as infection or anything else that seems unusual. A history of the patient's health habits and past illnesses and treatments will also be taken.
- **Complete blood count (CBC) with differential:** A procedure in which a sample of blood is drawn and checked for the following:
  - The number of red blood cells and platelets
  - The number and type of white blood cells
  - The amount of hemoglobin (the protein that carries oxygen) in the red blood cells
  - The portion of the blood sample made up of red blood cells

- **Blood chemistry studies:** A procedure in which a blood sample is checked to measure the amounts of certain substances released into the blood by organs and tissues in the body. An unusual (higher or lower than normal) amount of a substance can be a sign of disease.
- **Peripheral blood smear:** A procedure in which a sample of blood is checked for blast cells, the number and kinds of white blood cells, the number of platelets, and changes in the shape of blood cells.
- **Bone marrow aspiration and biopsy:** The removal of bone marrow, blood, and a small piece of bone by inserting a hollow needle into the hipbone or breastbone. A pathologist views the bone marrow, blood, and bone under a microscope to look for abnormal cells.

The following tests may be done on the samples of blood or bone marrow tissue that are removed:

- **Cytogenetic analysis:** A laboratory test in which the cells in a sample of blood or bone marrow are looked at under a microscope to find out if there are certain changes in the chromosomes of lymphocytes. For example, in Philadelphia chromosome–positive ALL, part of one chromosome switches places with part of another chromosome. This is called the "Philadelphia chromosome."
- **Immunophenotyping:** A process used to identify cells, based on the types of antigens or markers on the surface of the cell. This process is used to diagnose the subtype of ALL by comparing the cancer cells to normal cells of the immune system. For example, a cytochemistry study may test the cells in a sample of tissue using chemicals (dyes) to look for certain changes in the sample. A chemical may cause a color change in one type of leukemia cell but not in another type of leukemia cell.

What Is the Prognosis for ALL?

The prognosis (chance of recovery) and treatment options depend on the following:

- The age of the patient
- Whether the cancer has spread to the brain or spinal cord

- Whether there are certain changes in the genes, including the Philadelphia chromosome
- Whether the cancer has been treated before or has recurred (come back)

How Is Staging Done for ALL?

Once adult All has been diagnosed, tests are done to find out if the cancer has spread to the central nervous system (brain and spinal cord) or to other parts of the body. The extent or spread of cancer is usually described as stages. It is important to know whether the leukemia has spread outside the blood and bone marrow in order to plan treatment. The following tests and procedures may be used to determine if the leukemia has spread:

- **Chest X-ray:** An X-ray of the organs and bones inside the chest. An X-ray is a type of energy beam that can go through the body and onto film, making a picture of areas inside the body.
- **Lumbar puncture (LP):** A procedure used to collect a sample of cerebrospinal fluid (CSF) from the spinal column. This is done by placing a needle between two bones in the spine and into the CSF around the spinal cord and removing a sample of the fluid. The sample of CSF is checked under a microscope for signs that leukemia cells have spread to the brain and spinal cord. This procedure is also called spinal tap.
- **Computed tomography (CT)/computerized axial tomography (CAT) scan:** A procedure that makes a series of detailed pictures of the abdomen, taken from different angles. The pictures are made by a computer linked to an X-ray machine. A dye may be injected into a vein or swallowed to help the organs or tissues show up more clearly.
- **Magnetic resonance imaging (MRI):** A procedure that uses a magnet, radio waves, and a computer to make a series of detailed pictures of areas inside the body. This procedure is also called nuclear magnetic resonance imaging (NMRI).

What Standard Treatment Options Are Available for People with ALL?

Four types of standard treatment are used:

Chemotherapy

Chemotherapy is a cancer treatment that uses drugs to stop the growth of cancer cells, either by killing the cells or by stopping them from dividing. When chemotherapy is taken by mouth or injected into a vein or muscle, the drugs enter the bloodstream and can reach cancer cells throughout the body (systemic chemotherapy). When chemotherapy is placed directly into the cerebrospinal fluid (intrathecal chemotherapy), an organ, or a body cavity such as the abdomen, the drugs mainly affect cancer cells in those areas (regional chemotherapy). Combination chemotherapy is treatment using more than one anticancer drug. The way the chemotherapy is given depends on the type and stage of the cancer being treated.

Intrathecal chemotherapy may be used to treat adult ALL that has spread, or may spread, to the brain and spinal cord. When used to lessen the chance leukemia cells will spread to the brain and spinal cord, it is called CNS sanctuary therapy or CNS prophylaxis.

Radiation Therapy

Radiation therapy is a cancer treatment that uses high-energy X-rays or other types of radiation to kill cancer cells or keep them from growing. There are two types of radiation therapy:

- External radiation therapy uses a machine outside the body to send radiation toward the cancer.
- Internal radiation therapy uses a radioactive substance sealed in needles, seeds, wires, or catheters that are placed directly into or near the cancer.

The way the radiation therapy is given depends on the type of cancer. External radiation therapy may be used to treat adult ALL that has spread, or may spread, to the brain and spinal cord. When used this way, it is called CNS sanctuary therapy or CNS prophylaxis. External radiation therapy may also be used as palliative therapy to relieve symptoms and improve quality of life.

Chemotherapy with Stem Cell Transplant

Stem cell transplant is a method of giving chemotherapy and replacing blood-forming cells destroyed by the cancer treatment. Stem cells (immature blood cells) are removed from the blood or bone marrow of the patient or a donor and are frozen and stored. After the chemotherapy is completed, the stored stem cells are thawed and given back to the patient through an infusion. These reinfused stem cells grow into (and restore) the body's blood cells.

Targeted Therapy

Targeted therapy is a type of treatment that uses drugs or other substances to identify and attack specific cancer cells without harming normal cells. Monoclonal antibody therapy and tyrosine kinase inhibitor therapy are types of targeted therapy used to treat adult ALL.

Monoclonal antibody therapy is a cancer treatment that uses antibodies made in the laboratory, from a single type of immune system cell. These antibodies can identify substances on cancer cells or normal substances that may help cancer cells grow. The antibodies attach to the substances and kill the cancer cells, block their growth, or keep them from spreading. Monoclonal antibodies are given by infusion. They may be used alone or to carry drugs, toxins, or radioactive material directly to cancer cells. Blinatumomab is a monoclonal antibody used with stem cell transplant to treat adult ALL.

Tyrosine kinase inhibitor therapy blocks the enzyme, tyrosine kinase, that causes stem cells to develop into more white blood cells (blasts) than the body needs. Imatinib mesylate (Gleevec), dasatinib, and nilotinib are tyrosine kinase inhibitors used to treat adult ALL.

What New Types of Treatment Are Being Tested in Clinical Trials?

Biologic Therapy

Biologic therapy is a treatment that uses the patient's immune system to fight cancer. Substances made by the body or made in a laboratory are used to boost, direct, or restore the body's natural defenses against cancer. This type of cancer treatment is also called biotherapy or immunotherapy.

Chimeric Antigen Receptor (CAR) T-Cell Therapy

CAR T-cell therapy is a type of immunotherapy that changes the patient's T cells (a type of immune system cell) so they will attack certain proteins on the surface of cancer cells. T cells are taken from the patient and special receptors are added to their surface in the laboratory. The changed cells are called chimeric antigen receptor (CAR) T cells. The CAR T cells are grown in the laboratory and given to the patient by infusion. The CAR T cells multiply in the patient's blood and attack cancer cells. CAR T-cell therapy is being studied in the treatment of adult ALL that has recurred (come back).

Is There a Need for Follow-Up Tests?

Some of the tests that were done to diagnose the cancer or to find out the stage of the cancer may be repeated. Some tests will be repeated in order to see how well the treatment is working. Decisions about whether to continue, change, or stop treatment may be based on the results of these tests.

Some of the tests will continue to be done from time to time after treatment has ended. The results of these tests can show if your condition has changed or if the cancer has recurred (come back). These tests are sometimes called follow-up tests or check-ups.

Section 46.3

Adult Acute Myeloid Leukemia

This section includes text excerpted from "Adult Acute Myeloid Leukemia Treatment (PDQ®)—Patient Version," National Cancer Institute (NCI), March 6, 2017.

What Is Adult Acute Myeloid Leukemia (AML)?

Adult acute myeloid leukemia (AML) is a type of cancer in which the bone marrow makes abnormal myeloblasts (a type of white blood cell), red blood cells, or platelets.

AML is a cancer of the blood and bone marrow. This type of cancer usually gets worse quickly if it is not treated. It is the most common type of acute leukemia in adults. AML is also called acute myelogenous leukemia, acute myeloblastic leukemia, acute granulocytic leukemia, and acute nonlymphocytic leukemia.

How Does Leukemia Affect Red Blood Cells, White Blood Cells, and Platelets?

Leukemia may affect red blood cells, white blood cells, and platelets. Normally, the bone marrow makes blood stem cells (immature cells) that become mature blood cells over time. A blood stem cell may become a myeloid stem cell or a lymphoid stem cell. A lymphoid stem cell becomes a white blood cell.

A myeloid stem cell becomes one of three types of mature blood cells:

- Red blood cells that carry oxygen and other substances to all tissues of the body
- White blood cells that fight infection and disease
- Platelets that form blood clots to stop bleeding

In AML, the myeloid stem cells usually become a type of immature white blood cell called myeloblasts (or myeloid blasts). The myeloblasts in AML are abnormal and do not become healthy white blood cells. Sometimes in AML, too many stem cells become abnormal red blood cells or platelets. These abnormal white blood cells, red blood cells, or platelets are also called leukemia cells or blasts. Leukemia cells can build up in the bone marrow and blood so there is less room for healthy white blood cells, red blood cells, and platelets. When this happens, infection, anemia, or easy bleeding may occur. The leukemia cells can spread outside the blood to other parts of the body, including the central nervous system (brain and spinal cord), skin, and gums.

What Are the Subtypes of Adult AML?

There are different subtypes of adult AML. Most AML subtypes are based on how mature (developed) the cancer cells are at the time of diagnosis and how different they are from normal cells. Acute promyelocytic leukemia (APL) is a subtype of AML that occurs when parts of two genes stick together. APL usually occurs in middle-aged adults. Signs of APL may include both bleeding and forming blood clots.

What Are the Risk Factors for Adult AML?

Anything that increases your risk of getting a disease is called a risk factor. Having a risk factor does not mean that you will get cancer; not having risk factors doesn't mean that you will not get cancer. Talk with your doctor if you think you may be at risk.

Smoking, previous chemotherapy treatment, and exposure to radiation may affect the risk of adult AML. Possible risk factors for AML include the following:

- Being male
- Smoking, especially after age 60
- Having had treatment with chemotherapy or radiation therapy in the past
- Having had treatment for childhood acute lymphoblastic leukemia (ALL) in the past
- Being exposed to radiation from an atomic bomb or to the chemical benzene
- Having a history of a blood disorder such as myelodysplastic syndrome

What Are the Signs and Symptoms of Adult AML?

Signs and symptoms of adult AML include fever, feeling tired, and easy bruising or bleeding. The early signs and symptoms of AML may be like those caused by the flu or other common diseases. Check with your doctor if you have any of the following:

- Fever
- Shortness of breath
- Easy bruising or bleeding
- Petechiae (flat, pinpoint spots under the skin caused by bleeding)
- Weakness or feeling tired
- Weight loss or loss of appetite

How Is Adult AML Diagnosed?

Tests that examine the blood and bone marrow are used to detect (find) and diagnose adult AML.

Physical exam and history: An exam of the body to check general signs of health, including checking for signs of disease, such as lumps or anything else that seems unusual. A history of the patient's health habits and past illnesses and treatments will also be taken.

Complete blood count (CBC): A procedure in which a sample of blood is drawn and checked for the following:

- The number of red blood cells, white blood cells, and platelets
- The amount of hemoglobin (the protein that carries oxygen) in the red blood cells
- The portion of the sample made up of red blood cells

Peripheral blood smear: A procedure in which a sample of blood is checked for blast cells, the number and kinds of white blood cells, the number of platelets, and changes in the shape of blood cells.

Bone marrow aspiration and biopsy: The removal of bone marrow, blood, and a small piece of bone by inserting a hollow needle into the hipbone or breastbone. A pathologist views the bone marrow, blood, and bone under a microscope to look for signs of cancer.

Cytogenetic analysis: A laboratory test in which the cells in a sample of blood or bone marrow are viewed under a microscope to look for certain changes in the chromosomes. Other tests, such as fluorescence in situ hybridization (FISH), may also be done to look for certain changes in the chromosomes.

Immunophenotyping: A process used to identify cells, based on the types of antigens or markers on the surface of the cell. This process is used to diagnose the subtype of AML by comparing the cancer cells to normal cells of the immune system. For example, a cytochemistry study may test the cells in a sample of tissue using chemicals (dyes) to look for certain changes in the sample. A chemical may cause a color change in one type of leukemia cell but not in another type of leukemia cell.

Reverse transcription–polymerase chain reaction test (RT–PCR): A laboratory test in which cells in a sample of tissue are studied using chemicals to look for certain changes in the structure or function of genes. This test is used to diagnose certain types of AML including APL.

What Is the Prognosis for Adult ALL?

The prognosis (chance of recovery) and treatment options depend on:

- The age of the patient
- The subtype of AML

- Whether the patient received chemotherapy in the past to treat a different cancer
- Whether there is a history of a blood disorder such as myelodysplastic syndrome
- Whether the cancer has spread to the central nervous system
- Whether the cancer has been treated before or recurred (come back)

It is important that acute leukemia be treated right away.

How Is Staging Done for Adult AML?

Once adult AML has been diagnosed, tests are done to find out if the cancer has spread to other parts of the body.

The extent or spread of cancer is usually described as stages. In adult AML, the subtype of AML and whether the leukemia has spread outside the blood and bone marrow are used instead of the stage to plan treatment. The following tests and procedures may be used to determine if the leukemia has spread:

- **Lumbar puncture (LP):** A procedure used to collect a sample of cerebrospinal fluid (CSF) from the spinal column. This is done by placing a needle between two bones in the spine and into the CSF around the spinal cord and removing a sample of the fluid. The sample of CSF is checked under a microscope for signs that leukemia cells have spread to the brain and spinal cord. This procedure is also called spinal tap.
- **Computed tomography (CT)/computerized axial tomography (CAT) scan:** A procedure that makes a series of detailed pictures of the abdomen, taken from different angles. The pictures are made by a computer linked to an X-ray machine. A dye may be injected into a vein or swallowed to help the organs or tissues show up more clearly.

What Standard Treatment Options Are Available for People with Adult AML?

Four types of standard treatment are used:

Chemotherapy

Chemotherapy is a cancer treatment that uses drugs to stop the growth of cancer cells, either by killing the cells or by stopping them

from dividing. When chemotherapy is taken by mouth or injected into a vein or muscle, the drugs enter the bloodstream and can reach cancer cells throughout the body (systemic chemotherapy). When chemotherapy is placed directly into the cerebrospinal fluid (intrathecal chemotherapy), an organ, or a body cavity such as the abdomen, the drugs mainly affect cancer cells in those areas (regional chemotherapy). Intrathecal chemotherapy may be used to treat adult AML that has spread to the brain and spinal cord. Combination chemotherapy is treatment using more than one anticancer drug.

The way the chemotherapy is given depends on the subtype of AML being treated and whether leukemia cells have spread to the brain and spinal cord.

Radiation Therapy

Radiation therapy is a cancer treatment that uses high-energy X-rays or other types of radiation to kill cancer cells or keep them from growing. There are two types of radiation therapy:

- External radiation therapy uses a machine outside the body to send radiation toward the cancer.
- Internal radiation therapy uses a radioactive substance sealed in needles, seeds, wires, or catheters that are placed directly into or near the cancer.

The way the radiation therapy is given depends on the type of cancer being treated and whether leukemia cells have spread to the brain and spinal cord. External radiation therapy is used to treat adult AML.

Stem Cell Transplant

Stem cell transplant is a method of giving chemotherapy and replacing blood-forming cells that are abnormal or destroyed by the cancer treatment. Stem cells (immature blood cells) are removed from the blood or bone marrow of the patient or a donor and are frozen and stored. After the chemotherapy is completed, the stored stem cells are thawed and given back to the patient through an infusion. These reinfused stem cells grow into (and restore) the body's blood cells.

Other Drug Therapy

Arsenic trioxide and all-trans retinoic acid (ATRA) are anticancer drugs that kill leukemia cells, stop the leukemia cells from dividing, or help the leukemia cells mature into white blood cells. These drugs are used in the treatment of a subtype of AML called acute promyelocytic leukemia.

What New Types of Treatment Are Being Tested in Clinical Trials?

Targeted Therapy

Targeted therapy is a type of treatment that uses drugs or other substances to identify and attack specific cancer cells without harming normal cells. Monoclonal antibody therapy is one type of targeted therapy being studied in the treatment of adult AML.

Monoclonal antibody therapy is a cancer treatment that uses antibodies made in the laboratory from a single type of immune system cell. These antibodies can identify substances on cancer cells or normal substances that may help cancer cells grow. The antibodies attach to the substances and kill the cancer cells, block their growth, or keep them from spreading. Monoclonal antibodies are given by infusion. They may be used alone or to carry drugs, toxins, or radioactive material directly to cancer cells.

Is There a Need for Follow-Up Tests?

Some of the tests that were done to diagnose the cancer or to find out the stage of the cancer may be repeated. Some tests will be repeated in order to see how well the treatment is working. Decisions about whether to continue, change, or stop treatment may be based on the results of these tests. Some of the tests will continue to be done from time to time after treatment has ended. The results of these tests can show if your condition has changed or if the cancer has recurred (come back). These tests are sometimes called follow-up tests or check-ups.

Section 46.4

Chronic Lymphocytic Leukemia

This section includes text excerpted from "Chronic Lymphocytic Leukemia Treatment (PDQ®)—Patient Version," National Cancer Institute (NCI), October 26, 2017.

What Is Chronic Lymphocytic Leukemia (CLL)?

Chronic lymphocytic leukemia (CLL) is a type of cancer in which the bone marrow makes too many lymphocytes (a type of white blood cell (WBC)). It is a blood and bone marrow disease that usually gets worse slowly. CLL is one of the most common types of leukemia in adults. It often occurs during or after middle age; it rarely occurs in children.

How Does Leukemia Affect Red Blood Cells (RBCs), White Blood Cells (WBCs), and Platelets?

Leukemia may affect red blood cells, white blood cells, and platelets. Normally, the body makes blood stem cells (immature cells) that become mature blood cells over time. A blood stem cell may become a myeloid stem cell or a lymphoid stem cell.

A myeloid stem cell becomes one of three types of mature blood cells:

- Red blood cells that carry oxygen and other substances to all tissues of the body
- White blood cells that fight infection and disease
- Platelets that form blood clots to stop bleeding

A lymphoid stem cell becomes a lymphoblast cell and then one of three types of lymphocytes (white blood cells):

- B lymphocytes that make antibodies to help fight infection
- T lymphocytes that help B lymphocytes make antibodies to fight infection
- Natural killer cells that attack cancer cells and viruses

In CLL, too many blood stem cells become abnormal lymphocytes and do not become healthy white blood cells. The abnormal lymphocytes may also be called leukemia cells. The lymphocytes are not able to fight infection very well. Also, as the number of lymphocytes increases in the blood and bone marrow, there is less room for healthy white blood cells, red blood cells, and platelets. This may cause infection, anemia, and easy bleeding.

What Are the Risk Factors for CLL?

Anything that increases your risk of getting a disease is called a risk factor. Having a risk factor does not mean that you will get cancer; not having risk factors doesn't mean that you will not get cancer. Talk with your doctor if you think you may be at risk.

Older age can affect the risk of developing CLL. Risk factors for CLL include the following:

- Being middle-aged or older, male, or white
- A family history of CLL or cancer of the lymph system
- Having relatives who are Russian Jews or Eastern European Jews

What Are the Signs and Symptoms of CLL?

Signs and symptoms of chronic lymphocytic leukemia include swollen lymph nodes and tiredness. Usually, CLL does not cause any signs or symptoms and is found during a routine blood test. Signs and symptoms may be caused by CLL or by other conditions. Check with your doctor if you have any of the following:

- Painless swelling of the lymph nodes in the neck, underarm, stomach, or groin
- Feeling very tired
- Pain or fullness below the ribs
- Fever and infection
- Weight loss for no known reason

How Is CLL Diagnosed?

Tests that examine the blood, bone marrow, and lymph nodes are used to detect (find) and diagnose chronic lymphocytic leukemia.

The following tests and procedures may be used:

- **Physical exam and history:** An exam of the body to check general signs of health, including checking for signs of disease, such as lumps or anything else that seems unusual. A history of the patient's health habits and past illnesses and treatments will also be taken.
- **Complete blood count (CBC) with differential:** A procedure in which a sample of blood is drawn and checked for the following:
    - The number of red blood cells and platelets
    - The number and type of white blood cells
    - The amount of hemoglobin (the protein that carries oxygen) in the red blood cells
    - The portion of the blood sample made up of red blood cells
- **Immunophenotyping:** A laboratory test in which the antigens or markers on the surface of a blood or bone marrow cell are checked to see if they are lymphocytes or myeloid cells. If the cells are malignant lymphocytes (cancer), they are checked to see if they are B lymphocytes or T lymphocytes.
- **Fluorescence in situ hybridization (FISH):** A laboratory technique used to look at genes or chromosomes in cells and tissues. Pieces of deoxyribonucleic acid (DNA) that contain a fluorescent dye are made in the laboratory and added to cells or tissues on a glass slide. When these pieces of DNA bind to specific genes or areas of chromosomes on the slide, they light up when viewed under a microscope with a special light.
- **Flow cytometry:** A laboratory test that measures the number of cells in a sample, the percentage of live cells in a sample, and certain characteristics of cells, such as size, shape, and the presence of tumor markers on the cell surface. The cells are stained with a light-sensitive dye, placed in a fluid, and passed in a stream before a laser or other type of light. The measurements are based on how the light-sensitive dye reacts to the light.
- ***IgVH* gene mutation test:** A laboratory test done on a bone marrow or blood sample to check for an *IgVH* gene mutation. Patients with an *IgVH* gene mutation have a better prognosis.

- **Bone marrow aspiration and biopsy:** The removal of bone marrow, blood, and a small piece of bone by inserting a hollow needle into the hipbone or breastbone. A pathologist views the bone marrow, blood, and bone under a microscope to look for abnormal cells.

What Is the Prognosis for CLL?

Treatment options depend on:

- The stage of the disease
- Red blood cell, white blood cell, and platelet blood counts
- Whether there are signs or symptoms, such as fever, chills, or weight loss
- Whether the liver, spleen, or lymph nodes are larger than normal
- The response to initial treatment
- Whether the CLL has recurred (come back)

The prognosis (chance of recovery) depends on:

- Whether there is a change in the DNA and the type of change, if there is one
- Whether lymphocytes are spread throughout the bone marrow.
- The stage of the disease
- Whether the CLL gets better with treatment or has recurred (come back)
- Whether the CLL progresses to lymphoma or prolymphocytic leukemia
- The patient's general health

How Is Staging Done for CLL?

After CLL has been diagnosed, tests are done to find out how far the cancer has spread in the blood and bone marrow.

Staging is the process used to find out how far the cancer has spread. It is important to know the stage of the disease in order to plan the best treatment. The following tests may be used in the staging process:

- **Chest X-ray:** An X-ray of the organs and bones inside the chest. An X-ray is a type of energy beam that can go through the body and onto film, making a picture of areas inside the body, such as the lymph nodes.

- **Magnetic resonance imaging (MRI):** A procedure that uses a magnet, radio waves, and a computer to make a series of detailed pictures of areas inside the body, such as the brain and spinal cord. This procedure is also called nuclear magnetic resonance imaging (NMRI).
- **Computed tomography (CT)/computerized axial tomography (CAT) scan:** A procedure that makes a series of detailed pictures of areas inside the body, taken from different angles. The pictures are made by a computer linked to an X-ray machine. A dye may be injected into a vein or swallowed to help the organs or tissues show up more clearly.
- **Positron emission tomography (PET)-CT scan:** A procedure that combines the pictures from a PET scan and a CT scan. The PET and CT scans are done at the same time with the same machine. The combined scans give more detailed pictures of areas inside the body than either scan gives by itself. A PET scan is a procedure to find malignant tumor cells in the body. A small amount of radioactive glucose (sugar) is injected into a vein. The PET scanner rotates around the body and makes a picture of where glucose is being used in the body. Malignant tumor cells show up brighter in the picture because they are more active and take up more glucose than normal cells do.
- **Blood chemistry studies:** A procedure in which a blood sample is checked to measure the amounts of certain substances released into the blood by organs and tissues in the body. An unusual (higher or lower than normal) amount of a substance can be a sign of disease.
- **Antiglobulin test:** A test in which a sample of blood is looked at under a microscope to find out if there are any antibodies on the surface of red blood cells or platelets. These antibodies may react with and destroy the red blood cells and platelets. This test is also called a Coombs test.

The following stages are used for CLL:

Stage 0. In stage 0 chronic lymphocytic leukemia, there are too many lymphocytes in the blood, but there are no other signs or symptoms of leukemia. Stage 0 chronic lymphocytic leukemia is indolent (slow growing).

Stage I. In stage I chronic lymphocytic leukemia, there are too many lymphocytes in the blood and the lymph nodes are larger than normal.

Stage II. In stage II chronic lymphocytic leukemia, there are too many lymphocytes in the blood, the liver or spleen is larger than normal, and the lymph nodes may be larger than normal.

Stage III. In stage III chronic lymphocytic leukemia, there are too many lymphocytes in the blood and there are too few red blood cells. The lymph nodes, liver, or spleen may be larger than normal.

Stage IV. In stage IV chronic lymphocytic leukemia, there are too many lymphocytes in the blood and too few platelets. The lymph nodes, liver, or spleen may be larger than normal and there may be too few red blood cells.

What Standard Treatments Are Available for Patients with CLL?

Five types of standard treatment are used:

Watchful Waiting

Watchful waiting is closely monitoring a patient's condition without giving any treatment until signs or symptoms appear or change. This is also called observation. During this time, problems caused by the disease, such as infection, are treated.

Radiation Therapy

Radiation therapy is a cancer treatment that uses high-energy X-rays or other types of radiation to kill cancer cells or keep them from growing. There are two types of radiation therapy:

- External radiation therapy uses a machine outside the body to send radiation toward the cancer.
- Internal radiation therapy uses a radioactive substance sealed in needles, seeds, wires, or catheters that are placed directly into or near the cancer.

The way the radiation therapy is given depends on the type of cancer being treated. External radiation therapy is used to treat chronic lymphocytic leukemia.

Chemotherapy

Chemotherapy is a cancer treatment that uses drugs to stop the growth of cancer cells, either by killing the cells or by stopping them from dividing. When chemotherapy is taken by mouth or injected into a vein or muscle, the drugs enter the bloodstream and can reach cancer cells throughout the body (systemic chemotherapy). When chemotherapy is placed directly into the cerebrospinal fluid, an organ, or a body cavity such as the abdomen, or the drugs mainly affect cancer cells in those areas (regional chemotherapy). The way the chemotherapy is given depends on the type and stage of the cancer being treated.

Surgery

Splenectomy is surgery to remove the spleen.

Targeted therapy

Targeted therapy is a type of treatment that uses drugs or other substances to identify and attack specific cancer cells without harming normal cells. Monoclonal antibody therapy, tyrosine kinase inhibitor therapy, and BCL2 inhibitor therapy are types of targeted therapy used in the treatment of chronic lymphocytic leukemia.

Monoclonal antibody therapy is a cancer treatment that uses antibodies made in the laboratory from a single type of immune system cell. These antibodies can identify substances on cancer cells or normal substances in the body that may help cancer cells grow. The antibodies attach to the substances and kill the cancer cells, block their growth, or keep them from spreading. Monoclonal antibodies are given by infusion. They may be used alone or to carry drugs, toxins, or radioactive material directly to cancer cells.

Tyrosine kinase inhibitor therapy is a cancer treatment that blocks signals needed for tumors to grow.

BCL2 inhibitor therapy is a cancer treatment that blocks a protein called BCL2. BCL2 inhibitor therapy may kill cancer cells and may make them more sensitive to other anticancer drugs.

What Therapies Are Available for Patients with CLL?

Chemotherapy with Stem Cell Transplant

Chemotherapy with stem cell transplant is a method of giving chemotherapy and replacing blood-forming cells destroyed by the cancer treatment. Stem cells (immature blood cells) are removed from the blood or bone marrow of the patient or a donor and are frozen and stored. After the chemotherapy is completed, the stored stem cells are thawed and given back to the patient through an infusion. These reinfused stem cells grow into (and restore) the body's blood cells.

Biologic Therapy

Biologic therapy is a treatment that uses the patient's immune system to fight cancer. Substances made by the body or made in a laboratory are used to boost, direct, or restore the body's natural defenses against cancer. This type of cancer treatment is also called biotherapy or immunotherapy.

Chimeric Antigen Receptor (CAR) T-Cell Therapy

CAR T-cell therapy is a type of immunotherapy that changes the patient's T cells (a type of immune system cell) so they will attack certain proteins on the surface of cancer cells. T cells are taken from the patient and special receptors are added to their surface in the laboratory. The changed cells are called chimeric antigen receptor (CAR) T cells. The CAR T cells are grown in the laboratory and given to the patient by infusion. The CAR T cells multiply in the patient's blood and attack cancer cells. CAR T-cell therapy is being studied in the treatment of chronic lymphocytic leukemia.

Is There a Need for Follow-Up Tests?

Some of the tests that were done to diagnose the cancer or to find out the stage of the cancer may be repeated. Some tests will be repeated in order to see how well the treatment is working. Decisions about whether to continue, change, or stop treatment may be based on the results of these tests.

Some of the tests will continue to be done from time to time after treatment has ended. The results of these tests can show if your condition has changed or if the cancer has recurred (come back). These tests are sometimes called follow-up tests or check-ups.

Section 46.5

Chronic Myelogenous Leukemia

This section includes text excerpted from "Chronic Myelogenous Leukemia Treatment (PDQ®)—Patient Version," National Cancer Institute (NCI), March 6, 2017.

What Is Chronic Myelogenous Leukemia (CML)?

Chronic myelogenous leukemia (CML) is a disease in which the bone marrow makes too many white blood cells (WBCs). It is also called chronic granulocytic leukemia and is a slowly progressing blood and bone marrow disease that usually occurs during or after middle age, and rarely occurs in children.

How Does Leukemia Affect Red Blood Cells, White Blood Cells, and Platelets?

Leukemia may affect red blood cells, white blood cells, and platelets. Normally, the bone marrow makes blood stem cells (immature cells) that become mature blood cells over time. A blood stem cell may become a myeloid stem cell or a lymphoid stem cell. A lymphoid stem cell becomes a white blood cell.

A myeloid stem cell becomes one of three types of mature blood cells:

- Red blood cells that carry oxygen and other substances to all tissues of the body
- Platelets that form blood clots to stop bleeding
- Granulocytes (white blood cells) that fight infection and disease

In CML, too many blood stem cells become a type of white blood cell called granulocytes. These granulocytes are abnormal and do not become healthy white blood cells. They are also called leukemia cells. The leukemia cells can build up in the blood and bone marrow so there is less room for healthy white blood cells, red blood cells, and platelets. When this happens, infection, anemia, or easy bleeding may occur.

What Are the Signs and Symptoms for CML?

Signs and symptoms of chronic myelogenous leukemia include fever, night sweats, and tiredness. These and other signs and symptoms may be caused by CML or by other conditions. Check with your doctor if you have any of the following:

- Feeling very tired
- Weight loss for no known reason
- Night sweats
- Fever
- Pain or a feeling of fullness below the ribs on the left side
- Sometimes CML does not cause any symptoms at all

What Is Philadelphia Chromosome?

Every cell in the body contains deoxyribonucleic acid (DNA), genetic material, that determines how the cell looks and acts. DNA is contained inside chromosomes. In CML, part of the DNA from one chromosome moves to another chromosome. This change is called the " Philadelphia chromosome." It results in the bone marrow making an enzyme, called tyrosine kinase, that causes too many stem cells to become white blood cells (granulocytes or blasts). The Philadelphia chromosome is not passed from parent to child.

How Is CML Diagnosed?

Tests that examine the blood and bone marrow are used to detect (find) and diagnose CML. The following tests and procedures may be used:

- **Physical exam and history:** An exam of the body to check general signs of health, including checking for signs of disease such as an enlarged spleen. A history of the patient's health habits and past illnesses and treatments will also be taken.

- **Complete blood count (CBC) with differential:** A procedure in which a sample of blood is drawn and checked for the following:
  - The number of red blood cells and platelets
  - The number and type of white blood cells
  - The amount of hemoglobin (the protein that carries oxygen) in the red blood cells
  - The portion of the blood sample made up of red blood cells
- **Blood chemistry studies:** A procedure in which a blood sample is checked to measure the amounts of certain substances released into the blood by organs and tissues in the body. An unusual (higher or lower than normal) amount of a substance can be a sign of disease.
- **Bone marrow aspiration and biopsy:** The removal of bone marrow, blood, and a small piece of bone by inserting a needle into the hipbone or breastbone. A pathologist views the bone marrow, blood, and bone under a microscope to look for abnormal cells.

One of the following tests may be done on the samples of blood or bone marrow tissue that are removed:

- **Cytogenetic analysis:** A test in which cells in a sample of blood or bone marrow are viewed under a microscope to look for certain changes in the chromosomes, such as the Philadelphia chromosome.
- **Fluorescence in situ hybridization (FISH):** A laboratory technique used to look at genes or chromosomes in cells and tissues. Pieces of DNA that contain a fluorescent dye are made in the laboratory and added to cells or tissues on a glass slide. When these pieces of DNA bind to specific genes or areas of chromosomes on the slide, they light up when viewed under a microscope with a special light.
- **Reverse transcription–polymerase chain reaction (RT–PCR):** A laboratory test in which cells in a sample of tissue are studied using chemicals to look for certain changes in the structure or function of genes.

What Is the Prognosis for CML?

The prognosis (chance of recovery) and treatment options depend on the following:

- The patient's age
- The phase of CML
- The amount of blasts in the blood or bone marrow
- The size of the spleen at diagnosis
- The patient's general health

How Is Staging Done for CML?

After CML has been diagnosed, tests are done to find out if the cancer has spread. Staging is the process used to find out how far the cancer has spread. There is no standard staging system for CML. Instead, the disease is classified by phase: chronic phase, accelerated phase, or blastic phase. It is important to know the phase in order to plan treatment. The information from tests and procedures done to detect (find) and diagnose chronic myelogenous leukemia is also used to plan treatment.

Three Phases of CML

As the amount of blast cells increases in the blood and bone marrow, there is less room for healthy white blood cells, red blood cells, and platelets. This may result in infections, anemia, and easy bleeding, as well as bone pain and pain or a feeling of fullness below the ribs on the left side. The number of blast cells in the blood and bone marrow and the severity of signs or symptoms determine the phase of the disease.

Chronic Phase

In chronic phase CML, fewer than 10 percent of the cells in the blood and bone marrow are blast cells.

Accelerated Phase

In accelerated phase CML, 10–19 percent of the cells in the blood and bone marrow are blast cells.

Blastic Phase

In blastic phase CML, 20 percent or more of the cells in the blood or bone marrow are blast cells. When tiredness, fever, and an enlarged spleen occur during the blastic phase, it is called blast crisis.

What Standard Treatments Are Available for People with CML?

Six types of standard treatment are used for treating people with CML. They are:

Targeted Therapy

Targeted therapy is a type of treatment that uses drugs or other substances to identify and attack specific cancer cells without harming normal cells. Tyrosine kinase inhibitors are targeted therapy drugs used to treat chronic myelogenous leukemia.

Imatinib mesylate, nilotinib, dasatinib, and ponatinib are tyrosine kinase inhibitors that are used to treat CML.

Chemotherapy

Chemotherapy is a cancer treatment that uses drugs to stop the growth of cancer cells, either by killing the cells or by stopping them from dividing. When chemotherapy is taken by mouth or injected into a vein or muscle, the drugs enter the bloodstream and can reach cancer cells throughout the body (systemic chemotherapy). When chemotherapy is placed directly into the cerebrospinal fluid, an organ, or a body cavity such as the abdomen, the drugs mainly affect cancer cells in those areas (regional chemotherapy). The way the chemotherapy is given depends on the type and stage of the cancer being treated.

Biologic Therapy

Biologic therapy is a treatment that uses the patient's immune system to fight cancer. Substances made by the body or made in a laboratory are used to boost, direct, or restore the body's natural defenses against cancer. This type of cancer treatment is also called biotherapy or immunotherapy.

High-Dose Chemotherapy with Stem Cell Transplant

High-dose chemotherapy with stem cell transplant is a method of giving high doses of chemotherapy and replacing blood-forming cells destroyed by the cancer treatment. Stem cells (immature blood cells) are removed from the blood or bone marrow of the patient or a donor and are frozen and stored. After the chemotherapy is completed, the stored stem cells are thawed and given back to the patient through an infusion. These reinfused stem cells grow into (and restore) the body's blood cells.

Donor Lymphocyte Infusion (DLI)

Donor lymphocyte infusion (DLI) is a cancer treatment that may be used after stem cell transplant. Lymphocytes (a type of white blood cell) from the stem cell transplant donor are removed from the donor's blood and may be frozen for storage. The donor's lymphocytes are thawed if they were frozen and then given to the patient through one or more infusions. The lymphocytes see the patient's cancer cells as not belonging to the body and attack them.

Surgery

Splenectomy is surgery to remove the spleen.

Is There a Need for Follow-Up Tests?

Some of the tests that were done to diagnose the cancer or to find out the stage of the cancer may be repeated. Some tests will be repeated in order to see how well the treatment is working. Decisions about whether to continue, change, or stop treatment may be based on the results of these tests.

Some of the tests will continue to be done from time to time after treatment has ended. The results of these tests can show if your condition has changed or if the cancer has recurred (come back). These tests are sometimes called follow-up tests or check-ups.

Section 46.6

Hairy Cell Leukemia

This section includes text excerpted from "Hairy Cell Leukemia Treatment (PDQ®)—Patient Version," National Cancer Institute (NCI), April 6, 2016.

What Is Hairy Cell Leukemia?

Hairy cell leukemia is a cancer of the blood and bone marrow. It is a type of cancer in which the bone marrow makes too many lymphocytes (a type of white blood cell). This rare type of leukemia gets worse slowly or does not get worse at all. The disease is called hairy cell leukemia because the leukemia cells look "hairy" when viewed under a microscope.

How Does Leukemia Affect Red Blood Cells, White Blood Cells, and Platelets?

Leukemia may affect red blood cells, white blood cells, and platelets. Normally, the bone marrow makes blood stem cells (immature cells) that become mature blood cells over time. A blood stem cell may become a myeloid stem cell or a lymphoid stem cell.

A myeloid stem cell becomes one of three types of mature blood cells:

- Red blood cells that carry oxygen and other substances to all tissues of the body
- White blood cells that fight infection and disease
- Platelets that form blood clots to stop bleeding

A lymphoid stem cell becomes a lymphoblast cell and then into one of three types of lymphocytes (white blood cells):

- B lymphocytes that make antibodies to help fight infection
- T lymphocytes that help B lymphocytes make antibodies to help fight infection
- Natural killer cells that attack cancer cells and viruses

In hairy cell leukemia, too many blood stem cells become lymphocytes. These lymphocytes are abnormal and do not become healthy white blood cells. They are also called leukemia cells. The leukemia cells can build up in the blood and bone marrow so there is less room for healthy white blood cells, red blood cells, and platelets. This may cause infection, anemia, and easy bleeding. Some of the leukemia cells may collect in the spleen and cause it to swell.

What Are the Risk Factors for Hairy Cell Leukemia?

Anything that increases your chance of getting a disease is called a risk factor. Having a risk factor does not mean that you will get cancer; not having risk factors doesn't mean that you will not get cancer. Talk with your doctor if you think you may be at risk. The cause of hairy cell leukemia is unknown. Gender and age may affect the risk of hairy cell leukemia. It occurs more often in older men.

What Are Signs and Symptoms of Hairy Cell Leukemia?

Signs and symptoms of hairy cell leukemia include infections, tiredness, and pain below the ribs. These and other signs and symptoms may be caused by hairy cell leukemia or by other conditions. Check with your doctor if you have any of the following:

- Weakness or feeling tired
- Fever or frequent infections
- Easy bruising or bleeding
- Shortness of breath
- Weight loss for no known reason
- Pain or a feeling of fullness below the ribs
- Painless lumps in the neck, underarm, stomach, or groin

How Is Hairy Cell Leukemia Diagnosed?

Tests that examine the blood and bone marrow are used to detect (find) and diagnose hairy cell leukemia. The following tests and procedures may be used:

- **Physical exam and history:** An exam of the body to check general signs of health, including checking for signs of disease, such as a swollen spleen, lumps, or anything else that seems unusual. A history of the patient's health habits and past illnesses and treatments will also be taken.

- **Complete blood count (CBC):** A procedure in which a sample of blood is drawn and checked for the following:
  - The number of red blood cells, white blood cells, and platelets
  - The amount of hemoglobin (the protein that carries oxygen) in the red blood cells
  - The portion of the sample made up of red blood cells
- **Peripheral blood smear:** A procedure in which a sample of blood is checked for cells that look "hairy," the number and kinds of white blood cells, the number of platelets, and changes in the shape of blood cells.
- **Blood chemistry studies:** A procedure in which a blood sample is checked to measure the amounts of certain substances released into the blood by organs and tissues in the body. An unusual (higher or lower than normal) amount of a substance can be a sign of disease.
- **Bone marrow aspiration and biopsy:** The removal of bone marrow, blood, and a small piece of bone by inserting a hollow needle into the hipbone or breastbone. A pathologist views the bone marrow, blood, and bone under a microscope to look for signs of cancer.
- **Immunophenotyping:** A laboratory test in which the antigens or markers on the surface of a blood or bone marrow cell are checked to see what type of cell it is. This test is done to diagnose the specific type of leukemia by comparing the cancer cells to normal cells of the immune system.
- **Flow cytometry:** A laboratory test that measures the number of cells in a sample, the percentage of live cells in a sample, and certain characteristics of cells, such as size, shape, and the presence of tumor markers on the cell surface. The cells are stained with a light-sensitive dye, placed in a fluid, and passed in a stream before a laser or other type of light. The measurements are based on how the light-sensitive dye reacts to the light.

- **Cytogenetic analysis:** A laboratory test in which cells in a sample of tissue are viewed under a microscope to look for certain changes in the chromosomes.
- **Gene mutation test:** A laboratory test done on a bone marrow or blood sample to check for mutations in the *BRAF* gene. A *BRAF* gene mutation is often found in patients with hairy cell leukemia.
- **Computed tomography (CT)/computerized axial tomography (CAT) scan:** A procedure that makes a series of detailed pictures of areas inside the body, taken from different angles. The pictures are made by a computer linked to an X-ray machine. A dye may be injected into a vein or swallowed to help the organs or tissues show up more clearly. A CT scan of the abdomen may be done to check for swollen lymph nodes or a swollen spleen.

What is the Prognosis for Hairy Cell Leukemia?

The prognosis (chance of recovery) depends on the following:

- Whether the hairy cell leukemia does not grow or grows so slowly it does not need treatment
- Whether the hairy cell leukemia responds to treatment

Treatment often results in a long-lasting remission (a period during which some or all of the signs and symptoms of the leukemia are gone). If leukemia returns after it has been in remission, retreatment often causes another remission.

How Is Staging Done for Hairy Cell Leukemia?

There is no standard staging system for hairy cell leukemia. Staging is the process used to find out how far the cancer has spread. Groups are used in place of stages for hairy cell leukemia. The disease is grouped as untreated, progressive, or refractory.

Untreated Hairy Cell Leukemia

The hairy cell leukemia is newly diagnosed and has not been treated except to relieve signs or symptoms such as weight loss and infections. In untreated hairy cell leukemia, some or all of the following conditions occur:

- Hairy (leukemia) cells are found in the blood and bone marrow.
- The number of red blood cells, white blood cells, or platelets may be lower than normal.
- The spleen may be larger than normal.

Progressive Hairy Cell Leukemia

In progressive hairy cell leukemia, the leukemia has been treated with either chemotherapy or splenectomy (removal of the spleen) and one or both of the following conditions occur:

- There is an increase in the number of hairy cells in the blood or bone marrow.
- The number of red blood cells, white blood cells, or platelets in the blood is lower than normal.

What Standard Treatment Options Are Available for People with Hairy Cell Leukemia?

Five types of standard treatment are used for people with hairy cell leukemia. They are:

Watchful Waiting

Watchful waiting is closely monitoring a patient's condition, without giving any treatment until signs or symptoms appear or change.

Chemotherapy

Chemotherapy is a cancer treatment that uses drugs to stop the growth of cancer cells, either by killing the cells or by stopping them from dividing. When chemotherapy is taken by mouth or injected into a vein or muscle, the drugs enter the bloodstream and can reach cancer cells throughout the body (systemic chemotherapy). When chemotherapy is placed directly into the cerebrospinal fluid, an organ, or a body cavity such as the abdomen, the drugs mainly affect cancer cells in those areas (regional chemotherapy). The way the chemotherapy is given depends on the type and stage of the cancer being treated. Cladribine and pentostatin are anticancer drugs commonly used to treat hairy cell leukemia. These drugs may increase the risk of other types of cancer, especially Hodgkin lymphoma and non-Hodgkin lymphoma. Long-term follow-up for second cancers is very important.

Biologic therapy

Biologic therapy is a cancer treatment that uses the patient's immune system to fight cancer. Substances made by the body or made in a laboratory are used to boost, direct, or restore the body's natural defenses against cancer. This type of cancer treatment is also called biotherapy or immunotherapy. Interferon alfa is a biologic agent commonly used to treat hairy cell leukemia.

Surgery

Splenectomy is a surgical procedure to remove the spleen.

Targeted therapy

Targeted therapy is a treatment that uses drugs or other substances to identify and attack specific cancer cells without harming normal cells. Monoclonal antibody therapy is a type of targeted therapy used to treat hairy cell leukemia.

Monoclonal antibody therapy uses antibodies made in the laboratory from a single type of immune system cell. These antibodies can identify substances on cancer cells or normal substances that may help cancer cells grow. The antibodies attach to the substances and kill the cancer cells, block their growth, or keep them from spreading. Monoclonal antibodies are given by infusion. They may be used alone or to carry drugs, toxins, or radioactive material directly to cancer cells.

A monoclonal antibody called rituximab may be used for certain patients with hairy cell leukemia.

Other types of targeted therapies are being studied.

Is There a Need for Follow-Up Tests?

Some of the tests that were done to diagnose the cancer or to find out the stage of the cancer may be repeated. Some tests will be repeated in order to see how well the treatment is working. Decisions about whether to continue, change, or stop treatment may be based on the results of these tests.

Some of the tests will continue to be done from time to time after treatment has ended. The results of these tests can show if your condition has changed or if the cancer has recurred (come back). These tests are sometimes called follow-up tests or check-ups.

Chapter 47

Lymphoma

Chapter Contents

Section 47.1

Overview of Lymphoma

This section includes text excerpted from "Kidney Cancer—Lymphoma," Centers for Disease Control and Prevention (CDC), September 20, 2017.

Lymphoma is a general term for a group of cancers that originate in the lymph system (the tissues and organs that produce, store, and carry white blood cells that fight infections and other diseases). The two main kinds of lymphoma are:

- Hodgkin lymphoma, which spreads in an orderly manner from one group of lymph nodes to another
- Non-Hodgkin lymphoma, which spreads through the lymphatic system in a nonorderly manner

Hodgkin lymphoma and non-Hodgkin lymphoma can occur in children, teens, and adults.

Causes of Lymphoma

Non-Hodgkin lymphoma becomes more common as people get older. Unlike most cancers, rates of Hodgkin lymphoma are highest among teens and young adults (ages 15–39 years) and again among older adults (ages 75 years or older). White people are more likely than black people to develop non-Hodgkin lymphoma, and men are more likely than women to develop lymphoma.

Scientists do not fully understand all of the causes of lymphoma, but research has found many links. For example:

- Research has shown that people who are infected with the human immunodeficiency virus (HIV) are at much higher risk of developing lymphoma.
- Other viruses, such as human T-cell lymphotropic virus and Epstein Barr virus, also have been linked with certain kinds of lymphoma.

- People exposed to high levels of ionizing radiation have a higher risk of developing non-Hodgkin lymphoma.
- Family history has been linked with a higher risk of Hodgkin lymphoma.
- Some studies suggest that specific ingredients in herbicides and pesticides may be linked with lymphoma, but scientists don't know how much is needed to raise the risk of developing lymphoma.

Symptoms of Lymphoma

Symptoms of Hodgkin lymphoma and non-Hodgkin lymphoma include swollen lymph nodes, especially in the part of the body where the lymphoma starts to grow. Other symptoms include fever, night sweats, feeling tired, and weight loss.

These symptoms can also come from other conditions. If you have any of them, talk to your doctor.

Section 47.2

Adult Hodgkin Lymphoma

This section includes text excerpted from "Adult Hodgkin Lymphoma Treatment (PDQ®)—Patient Version," National Cancer Institute (NCI), April 20, 2017.

The immune system protects the body from foreign substances, infection, and diseases. The lymph system is made up of the following:

- **Lymph:** Colorless, watery fluid that carries white blood cells called lymphocytes through the lymph system. Lymphocytes protect the body against infections and the growth of tumors.
- **Lymph vessels:** A network of thin tubes that collect lymph from different parts of the body and return it to the bloodstream.
- **Lymph nodes:** Small, bean-shaped structures that filter lymph and store white blood cells that help fight infection and disease.

Lymph nodes are located along the network of lymph vessels found throughout the body. Clusters of lymph nodes are found in the neck, underarm, abdomen, pelvis, and groin.

- **Spleen:** An organ that makes lymphocytes, filters the blood, stores blood cells, and destroys old blood cells. It is located on the left side of the abdomen near the stomach.
- **Thymus:** An organ in which lymphocytes grow and multiply. The thymus is in the chest behind the breastbone.
- **Tonsils:** Two small masses of lymph tissue at the back of the throat. The tonsils make lymphocytes.
- **Bone marrow:** The soft, spongy tissue in the center of large bones. Bone marrow makes white blood cells, red blood cells, and platelets.

Lymph tissue is also found in other parts of the body such as the stomach, thyroid gland, brain, and skin.

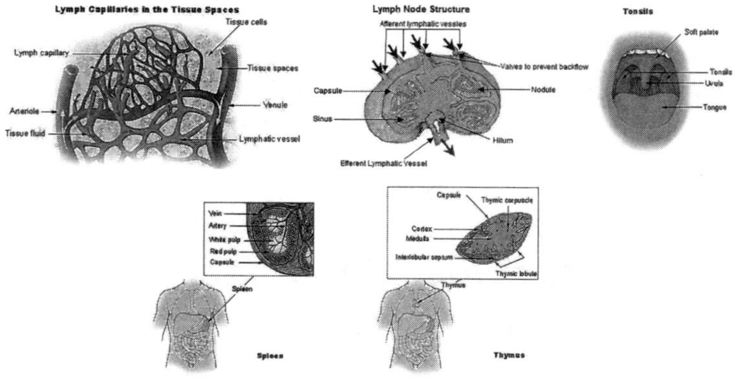

Figure 47.1. *Lymphatic System* (Source: "Lymphatic System," Surveillance, Epidemiology, and End Results Program (SEER), National Cancer Institute (NCI).)

What Is Adult Hodgkin Lymphoma?

Adult Hodgkin lymphoma is a type of cancer that develops in the lymph system, part of the body's immune system.

Lymphomas are divided into two general types: Hodgkin lymphoma and non-Hodgkin lymphoma.

Hodgkin lymphoma can occur in both adults and children. Treatment for adults is different than treatment for children. Hodgkin lymphoma may also occur in patients who have acquired immunodeficiency syndrome (AIDS); these patients require special treatment.

Hodgkin lymphoma in pregnant women is the same as the disease in nonpregnant women of childbearing age. However, treatment is different for pregnant women.

There are two main types of Hodgkin lymphoma: Classical and nodular lymphocyte-predominant.

Most Hodgkin lymphomas are the classical type. The classical type is broken down into the following four subtypes:

- Nodular sclerosing Hodgkin lymphoma
- Mixed cellularity Hodgkin lymphoma
- Lymphocyte depletion Hodgkin lymphoma
- Lymphocyte-rich classical Hodgkin lymphoma

What Are the Risk Factors for Adult Hodgkin Lymphoma?

Anything that increases your risk of getting a disease is called a risk factor. Having a risk factor does not mean that you will get cancer; not having risk factors doesn't mean that you will not get cancer. Talk with your doctor if you think you may be at risk.

Age, gender, and Epstein-Barr infection can affect the risk of adult Hodgkin lymphoma. Risk factors for adult Hodgkin lymphoma include the following:

- Being in young or late adulthood
- Being male
- Being infected with the Epstein-Barr virus
- Having a first-degree relative (parent, brother, or sister) with Hodgkin lymphoma

Pregnancy is not a risk factor for Hodgkin lymphoma.

What Are the Signs of Adult Hodgkin Lymphoma?

Signs of adult Hodgkin lymphoma include swollen lymph nodes, fever, night sweats, and weight loss. These and other signs and symptoms may be caused by adult Hodgkin lymphoma or by other conditions. Check with your doctor if any of the following do not go away:

- Painless, swollen lymph nodes in the neck, underarm, or groin
- Fever for no known reason
- Drenching night sweats
- Weight loss for no known reason
- Itchy skin
- Feeling very tired

How Is Adult Hodgkin Lymphoma Diagnosed?

Tests that examine the lymph nodes are used to detect (find) and diagnose adult Hodgkin lymphoma. The following tests and procedures may be used:

- **Physical exam and history:** An exam of the body to check general signs of health, including checking for signs of disease, such as lumps or anything else that seems unusual. A history of the patient's past illnesses and treatments will also be taken.
- **Complete blood count (CBC):** A procedure in which a sample of blood is drawn and checked for the following:
    - The number of red blood cells, white blood cells, and platelets.
    - The amount of hemoglobin (the protein that carries oxygen) in the red blood cells.
    - The portion of the sample made up of red blood cells.
- **Blood chemistry studies:** A procedure in which a blood sample is checked to measure the amounts of certain substances released into the blood by organs and tissues in the body. An unusual (higher or lower than normal) amount of a substance can be a sign of disease.
- **Sedimentation rate:** A procedure in which a sample of blood is drawn and checked for the rate at which the red blood cells settle to the bottom of the test tube. The sedimentation rate is a measure of how much inflammation is in the body. A higher than normal sedimentation rate may be a sign of lymphoma or another condition. Also called erythrocyte sedimentation rate, sed rate, or ESR.

- **Lymph node biopsy:** The removal of all or part of a lymph node. One of the following types of biopsies may be done:
  - **Excisional biopsy:** The removal of an entire lymph node.
  - **Incisional biopsy:** The removal of part of a lymph node.
  - **Core biopsy:** The removal of part of a lymph node using a wide needle.

A pathologist views the tissue under a microscope to look for cancer cells, especially Reed-Sternberg cells. Reed-Sternberg cells are common in classical Hodgkin lymphoma.

The following test may be done on tissue that was removed:

- **Immunophenotyping:** A laboratory test used to identify cells, based on the types of antigens or markers on the surface of the cell. This test is used to diagnose the specific type of lymphoma by comparing the cancer cells to normal cells of the immune system.

How Is Staging Done for Adult Hodgkin Lymphoma?

After adult Hodgkin lymphoma has been diagnosed, tests are done to find out if cancer cells have spread within the lymph system or to other parts of the body.

The process used to find out if cancer has spread within the lymph system or to other parts of the body is called staging. The information gathered from the staging process determines the stage of the disease. It is important to know the stage in order to plan treatment. The following tests and procedures may be used in the staging process:

- **Computed tomography (CT)/computerized axial tomography (CAT) scan:** A procedure that makes a series of detailed pictures of areas inside the body, taken from different angles. The pictures are made by a computer linked to an X-ray machine. A dye may be injected into a vein or swallowed to help the organs or tissues show up more clearly. For adult Hodgkin lymphoma, CT scans of the neck, chest, abdomen, and pelvis are taken.
- **Positron emission tomography (PET)-CT scan:** A procedure that combines the pictures from a PET and a CT scan. The PET and CT scans are done at the same time on the same machine. The pictures from both scans are combined to make a more

detailed picture than either test would make by itself. A PET scan is a procedure to find malignant tumor cells in the body. A small amount of radioactive glucose (sugar) is injected into a vein. The PET scanner rotates around the body and makes a picture of where glucose is being used in the body. Malignant tumor cells show up brighter in the picture because they are more active and take up more glucose than normal cells do.

- **Bone marrow aspiration and biopsy:** The removal of bone marrow, blood, and a small piece of bone by inserting a hollow needle into the hipbone or breastbone. A pathologist views the bone marrow, blood, and bone under a microscope to look for signs of cancer.

For pregnant women with Hodgkin lymphoma, staging tests that protect the fetus from the harms of radiation are used. These include:

- **Magnetic resonance imaging (MRI):** A procedure that uses a magnet, radio waves, and a computer to make a series of detailed pictures of areas inside the body. This procedure is also called nuclear magnetic resonance imaging (NMRI).
- **Ultrasound exam:** A procedure in which high-energy sound waves (ultrasound) are bounced off internal tissues or organs and make echoes. The echoes form a picture of body tissues called a sonogram.

Stages of Adult Hodgkin Lymphoma May Include A, B, E, and S

Adult Hodgkin lymphoma may be described as follows:

- **A:** The patient does not have B symptoms (fever, weight loss, or night sweats).
- **B:** The patient has B symptoms.
- **E:** Cancer is found in an organ or tissue that is not part of the lymph system but which may be next to an involved area of the lymph system.
- **S:** Cancer is found in the spleen.

The following stages are used for adult Hodgkin lymphoma:

Stage I. Stage I is divided into stage I and stage IE.

- **Stage I:** Cancer is found in one of the following places in the lymph system:
  - One or more lymph nodes in one lymph node group
  - Waldeyer's ring
  - Thymus
  - Spleen
- Stage IE: Cancer is found outside the lymph system in one organ or area.

Stage II. Stage II is divided into stage II and stage IIE.

- **Stage II:** Cancer is found in two or more lymph node groups either above or below the diaphragm (the thin muscle below the lungs that helps breathing and separates the chest from the abdomen).
- **Stage IIE:** Cancer is found in one or more lymph node groups either above or below the diaphragm and outside the lymph nodes in a nearby organ or area.

Stage III. Stage III is divided into stage III, stage IIIE, stage IIIS, and stage IIIE, S.

- **Stage III:** Cancer is found in lymph node groups above and below the diaphragm (the thin muscle below the lungs that helps breathing and separates the chest from the abdomen).
- **Stage IIIE:** Cancer is found in lymph node groups above and below the diaphragm and outside the lymph nodes in a nearby organ or area.
- **Stage IIIS:** Cancer is found in lymph node groups above and below the diaphragm, and in the spleen.
- **Stage IIIE, S:** Cancer is found in lymph node groups above and below the diaphragm, outside the lymph nodes in a nearby organ or area, and in the spleen.

Stage IV. In stage IV, the cancer:

- is found outside the lymph nodes throughout one or more organs, and may be in lymph nodes near those organs; or
- is found outside the lymph nodes in one organ and has spread to areas far away from that organ; or

- is found in the lung, liver, bone marrow, or cerebrospinal fluid (CSF). The cancer has not spread to the lung, liver, bone marrow, or CSF from nearby areas.

Adult Hodgkin lymphoma may be grouped for treatment as follows:

Early favorable. Early favorable adult Hodgkin lymphoma is stage I or stage II, without risk factors.

Early unfavorable. Early unfavorable adult Hodgkin lymphoma is stage I or stage II with one or more of the following risk factors:

- A tumor in the chest that is larger than 1/3 of the width of the chest or at least 10 centimeters
- Cancer in an organ other than the lymph nodes
- A high sedimentation rate (in a sample of blood, the red blood cells settle to the bottom of the test tube more quickly than normal)
- Three or more lymph nodes with cancer
- Symptoms such as fever, weight loss, or night sweats

Advanced. Advanced Hodgkin lymphoma includes some or all of the following risk factors:

- Being male
- Being aged 45 years or older
- Having stage IV disease
- Having a low blood albumin (protein) level (below 4)
- Having a low hemoglobin level (below 10.5)
- Having a high white blood cell count (15,000 or higher)
- Having a low lymphocyte count (below 600 or less than 8 percent of the white blood cell count)

What Treatment Options Are Available for People with Adult Hodgkin Lymphoma?

Different types of treatment are available for patients with adult Hodgkin lymphoma. Some treatments are standard (the currently used treatment), and some are being tested in clinical trials. A treatment clinical trial is a research study meant to help improve current treatments or obtain information on new treatments for patients with cancer. When clinical trials show that a new treatment is better than the standard treatment, the new treatment may become the standard treatment. Patients may want to think about taking part in a clinical trial. Some clinical trials are open only to patients who have not started treatment.

Treatment Options for Pregnant Women

For pregnant women with Hodgkin lymphoma, treatment is carefully chosen to protect the fetus. Treatment decisions are based on the mother's wishes, the stage of the Hodgkin lymphoma, and the age of the fetus. The treatment plan may change as the signs and symptoms, cancer, and pregnancy change. Choosing the most appropriate cancer treatment is a decision that ideally involves the patient, family, and healthcare team.

Healthcare Team for Patients with Hodgkin Lymphoma

Treatment will be overseen by a medical oncologist, a doctor who specializes in treating cancer. The medical oncologist may refer you to other healthcare providers who have experience and expertise in treating adult Hodgkin lymphoma and who specialize in certain areas of medicine. These may include the following specialists:

- Neurosurgeon
- Neurologist
- Rehabilitation specialist
- Radiation oncologist
- Endocrinologist
- Hematologist
- Other oncology specialists

Late Effects of Treatment

Treatment with chemotherapy and/or radiation therapy for Hodgkin lymphoma may increase the risk of second cancers and other health problems for many months or years after treatment. These late effects depend on the type of treatment and the patient's age when treated, and may include:

- Acute myelogenous leukemia
- Cancer of the breast, bone, cervix, gastrointestinal tract, head and neck, lung, soft tissue, and thyroid
- Heart, lung, and thyroid disease
- Avascular necrosis of bone (death of bone cells caused by lack of blood flow)
- Herpes zoster (shingles) or severe infection
- Depression and fatigue
- Infertility
- Hypogonadism (low levels of testosterone and estrogen)

Regular follow-up by doctors who are expert in finding and treating late effects is important for the long-term health of patients treated for Hodgkin lymphoma.

Types of Standard Treatments

Three types of standard treatment are used:

Chemotherapy

Chemotherapy is a cancer treatment that uses drugs to stop the growth of cancer cells, either by killing the cells or by stopping them from dividing. When chemotherapy is taken by mouth or injected into a vein or muscle, the drugs enter the bloodstream and can reach cancer cells throughout the body (systemic chemotherapy). When chemotherapy is placed directly into the cerebrospinal fluid, an organ, or a body cavity such as the abdomen, the drugs mainly affect cancer cells in those areas (regional chemotherapy). The way the chemotherapy is given depends on the type and stage of the cancer being treated. Combination chemotherapy is treatment with more than one anticancer drug.

When a pregnant woman is treated with chemotherapy for Hodgkin lymphoma, it isn't possible to protect the fetus from being exposed to the chemotherapy. Some chemotherapy regimens may cause birth defects if given in the first trimester. Vinblastine is an anticancer drug that has not been linked with birth defects when given in the second half of pregnancy.

Radiation Therapy

Radiation therapy is a cancer treatment that uses high-energy X-rays or other types of radiation to kill cancer cells or keep them from growing. There are two types of radiation therapy:

- External radiation therapy uses a machine outside the body to send radiation toward the cancer.
- Internal radiation therapy uses a radioactive substance sealed in needles, seeds, wires, or catheters that are placed directly into or near the cancer.

The way the radiation therapy is given depends on the type and stage of the cancer being treated. External radiation therapy is used to treat adult Hodgkin lymphoma.

For a pregnant woman with Hodgkin lymphoma, radiation therapy should be postponed until after delivery, if possible, to avoid any risk to the fetus. If immediate treatment is needed, the woman may decide to continue the pregnancy and receive radiation therapy. However, lead used to shield the fetus may not protect it from scattered radiation that could possibly cause cancer in the future.

Surgery

Laparotomy is a procedure in which an incision (cut) is made in the wall of the abdomen to check the inside of the abdomen for signs of disease. The size of the incision depends on the reason the laparotomy is being done. Sometimes organs are removed or tissue samples are taken and checked under a microscope for signs of disease. If cancer is found, the tissue or organ is removed during the laparotomy.

For pregnant patients with Hodgkin lymphoma, treatment options also include:

Watchful Waiting

Watchful waiting is closely monitoring a patient's condition without giving any treatment unless signs or symptoms appear or change. Delivery may be induced when the fetus is 32 to 36 weeks old, so that the mother can begin treatment.

Steroid Therapy

Steroids are hormones made naturally in the body by the adrenal glands and by reproductive organs. Some types of steroids are made in a laboratory. Certain steroid drugs have been found to help chemotherapy work better and help stop the growth of cancer cells. Steroids can also help the lungs of the fetus develop faster than normal. This is important when delivery is induced early.

What Is the Prognosis for Adult Hodgkin Lymphoma?

The prognosis (chance of recovery) and treatment options depend on the following:

- The patient's signs and symptoms
- The stage of the cancer
- The type of Hodgkin lymphoma
- Blood test results
- The patient's age, gender, and general health
- Whether the cancer is recurrent or progressive

For Hodgkin lymphoma during pregnancy, treatment options also depend on:

- The wishes of the patient
- The age of the fetus

Adult Hodgkin lymphoma can usually be cured if found and treated early.

What New Types of Treatment Are Being Tested in Clinical Trials?

Chemotherapy and Radiation Therapy with Stem Cell Transplant

High-dose chemotherapy and radiation therapy with stem cell transplant is a way of giving high doses of chemotherapy and radiation therapy and replacing blood-forming cells destroyed by the cancer treatment. Stem cells (immature blood cells) are removed from the blood or bone marrow of the patient or a donor and are frozen and stored. After therapy is completed, the stored stem cells are thawed and given back to the patient through an infusion. These reinfused stem cells grow into (and restore) the body's blood cells. The use of lower-dose chemotherapy and radiation therapy with stem cell transplant is also being studied.

Monoclonal Antibody Therapy

Monoclonal antibody therapy is a cancer treatment that uses antibodies made in the laboratory, from a single type of immune system cell. These antibodies can identify substances on cancer cells or normal substances that may help cancer cells grow. The antibodies attach to the substances and kill the cancer cells, block their growth, or keep them from spreading. Monoclonal antibodies are given by infusion. They may be used alone or to carry drugs, toxins, or radioactive material directly to cancer cells.

Is There a Need for Follow-Up Tests?

Some of the tests that were done to diagnose the cancer or to find out the stage of the cancer may be repeated. Some tests will be repeated in order to see how well the treatment is working. Decisions about whether to continue, change, or stop treatment may be based on the results of these tests.

Some of the tests will continue to be done from time to time after treatment has ended. The results of these tests can show if your condition has changed or if the cancer has recurred (come back). These tests are sometimes called follow-up tests or check-ups.

Section 47.3

Adult Non-Hodgkin Lymphoma

This section includes text excerpted from "Adult Non-Hodgkin Lymphoma Treatment (PDQ®)—Patient Version," National Cancer Institute (NCI), December 8, 2017.

What Is Adult Non-Hodgkin Lymphoma?

Adult non-Hodgkin lymphoma is a disease in which malignant (cancer) cells form in the lymph system, which is part of the body's immune system. The immune system protects the body from foreign substances, infection, and diseases.

Non-Hodgkin lymphoma during pregnancy is rare. Non-Hodgkin lymphoma in pregnant women is the same as the disease in nonpregnant women of childbearing age. However, treatment is different for pregnant women.

Non-Hodgkin lymphoma can occur in both adults and children. Treatment for adults is different than treatment for children.

The major types of lymphoma are Hodgkin lymphoma and non-Hodgkin lymphoma.

Non-Hodgkin Lymphoma Can Be Indolent or Aggressive

Non-Hodgkin lymphoma grows and spreads at different rates and can be indolent or aggressive. Indolent lymphoma tends to grow and spread slowly, and has few signs and symptoms. Aggressive lymphoma grows and spreads quickly, and has signs and symptoms that can be severe. The treatments for indolent and aggressive lymphoma are different.

Indolent Non-Hodgkin Lymphomas

Follicular lymphoma. Follicular lymphoma is the most common type of indolent non-Hodgkin lymphoma. It is a very slow-growing type of non-Hodgkin lymphoma that begins in B lymphocytes. It affects the lymph nodes and may spread to the bone marrow or spleen. Most patients with follicular lymphoma are age 50 years and older when they are diagnosed. Follicular lymphoma may go away without treatment. The patient is closely watched for signs or symptoms that the disease has come back. Treatment is needed if signs or symptoms occur after the cancer disappeared or after initial cancer treatment. Sometimes follicular lymphoma can become a more aggressive type of lymphoma, such as diffuse large B-cell lymphoma.

Lymphoplasmacytic lymphoma. In most cases of lymphoplasmacytic lymphoma, B lymphocytes that are turning into plasma cells make large amounts of a protein called monoclonal immunoglobulin M (IgM) antibody. High levels of IgM antibody in the blood cause the blood plasma to thicken. This may cause signs or symptoms such as trouble seeing or hearing, heart problems, shortness of breath, headache, dizziness, and numbness or tingling of the hands and feet. Sometimes there are no signs or symptoms of lymphoplasmacytic lymphoma. It may be found when a blood test is done for another reason. Lymphoplasmacytic lymphoma often spreads to the bone marrow, lymph nodes, and spleen. It is also called Waldenström macroglobulinemia.

Marginal zone lymphoma. This type of non-Hodgkin lymphoma begins in B lymphocytes in a part of lymph tissue called the marginal zone. There are five different types of marginal zone lymphoma. They are grouped by the type of tissue where the lymphoma formed:

- **Nodal marginal zone lymphoma.** Nodal marginal zone lymphoma forms in lymph nodes. This type of non-Hodgkin lymphoma is rare. It is also called monocytoid B-cell lymphoma.
- **Gastric mucosa-associated lymphoid tissue (MALT) lymphoma.** Gastric MALT lymphoma usually begins in the stomach. This type of marginal zone lymphoma forms in cells in the mucosa that help make antibodies. Patients with gastric MALT lymphoma may also have Helicobacter gastritis or an autoimmune disease, such as Hashimoto thyroiditis or Sjögren syndrome.
- **Extragastric MALT lymphoma.** Extragastric MALT lymphoma begins outside of the stomach in almost every part of the body including other parts of the gastrointestinal tract, salivary glands, thyroid, lung, skin, and around the eye. This type of marginal zone lymphoma forms in cells in the mucosa that help make antibodies. Extragastric MALT lymphoma may come back many years after treatment.
- **Mediterranean abdominal lymphoma.** This is a type of MALT lymphoma that occurs in young adults in eastern Mediterranean countries. It often forms in the abdomen and patients may also be infected with bacteria called Campylobacter jejuni. This type of lymphoma is also called immunoproliferative small intestinal disease.
- **Splenic marginal zone lymphoma.** This type of marginal zone lymphoma begins in the spleen and may spread to the peripheral blood and bone marrow. The most common sign of this type of splenic marginal zone lymphoma is a spleen that is larger than normal.
- **Primary cutaneous anaplastic large cell lymphoma.** This type of non-Hodgkin lymphoma is in the skin only. It can be a benign (not cancer) nodule that may go away on its own or it can spread to many places on the skin and need treatment.

Aggressive Non-Hodgkin Lymphomas

Diffuse large B-cell lymphoma. Diffuse large B-cell lymphoma is the most common type of non-Hodgkin lymphoma. It grows quickly in the lymph nodes and often the spleen, liver, bone marrow, or other organs are also affected. Signs and symptoms of diffuse large B-cell lymphoma may include fever, recurring night sweats, and weight loss. These are also called B symptoms.

Primary mediastinal large B-cell lymphoma is a type of diffuse large B-cell lymphoma.

- **Primary mediastinal large B-cell lymphoma.** This type of non-Hodgkin lymphoma is marked by the overgrowth of fibrous (scar-like) lymph tissue. A tumor most often forms behind the breastbone. It may press on the airways and cause coughing and trouble breathing. Most patients with primary mediastinal large B-cell lymphoma are women who are age 30–40 years.

Follicular large cell lymphoma, stage III. Follicular large cell lymphoma, stage III, is a very rare type of non-Hodgkin lymphoma. It is more like diffuse large B-cell lymphoma than other types of follicular lymphoma.

Anaplastic large cell lymphoma. Anaplastic large cell lymphoma is a type of non-Hodgkin lymphoma that usually begins in T lymphocytes. The cancer cells also have a marker called CD30 on the surface of the cell.

There are two types of anaplastic large cell lymphoma:

- **Cutaneous anaplastic large cell lymphoma.** This type of anaplastic large cell lymphoma mostly affects the skin, but other parts of the body may also be affected. Signs of cutaneous anaplastic large cell lymphoma include one or more bumps or ulcers on the skin.
- **Systemic anaplastic large cell lymphoma.** This type of anaplastic large cell lymphoma begins in the lymph nodes and may affect other parts of the body. Patients may have a lot of anaplastic lymphoma kinase (ALK) protein inside the lymphoma cells. These patients have a better prognosis than patients who do not have extra ALK protein. Systemic anaplastic large cell lymphoma is more common in children than adults.

Extranodal NK-/T-cell lymphoma. Extranodal NK-/T-cell lymphoma usually begins in the area around the nose. It may also affect the paranasal sinus (hollow spaces in the bones around the nose), roof of the mouth, trachea, skin, stomach, and intestines. Most cases of extranodal NK-/T-cell lymphoma have Epstein-Barr virus in the tumor cells. Sometimes hemophagocytic syndrome occurs (a serious condition in which there are too many active histiocytes and T cells that cause severe inflammation in the body). Treatment to suppress the immune system is needed. This type of non-Hodgkin lymphoma is not common in the United States.

Lymphomatoid granulomatosis. Lymphomatoid granulomatosis mostly affects the lungs. It may also affect the paranasal sinuses (hollow spaces in the bones around the nose), skin, kidneys, and central nervous system (CNS). In lymphomatoid granulomatosis, cancer invades the blood vessels and kills tissue. Because the cancer may spread to the brain, intrathecal chemotherapy or radiation therapy to the brain is given.

Angioimmunoblastic T-cell lymphoma. This type of non-Hodgkin lymphoma begins in T cells. Swollen lymph nodes are a common sign. Other signs may include a skin rash, fever, weight loss, or night sweats. There may also be high levels of gamma globulin (antibodies) in the blood. Patients may also have opportunistic infections because their immune systems are weakened.

Peripheral T-cell lymphoma. Peripheral T-cell lymphoma begins in mature T lymphocytes. This type of T lymphocyte matures in the thymus gland and travels to other lymphatic sites in the body such as the lymph nodes, bone marrow, and spleen. There are three subtypes of peripheral T-cell lymphoma:

- **Hepatosplenic T-cell lymphoma.** This is an uncommon type of peripheral T-cell lymphoma that occurs mostly in young men. It begins in the liver and spleen and the cancer cells also have a T-cell receptor called gamma/delta on the surface of the cell.
- **Subcutaneous panniculitis-like T-cell lymphoma.** Subcutaneous panniculitis-like T-cell lymphoma begins in the skin or mucosa. It may occur with hemophagocytic syndrome (a serious condition in which there are too many active histiocytes and T cells that cause severe inflammation in the body). Treatment to suppress the immune system is needed.
- **Enteropathy-type intestinal T-cell lymphoma.** This type of peripheral T-cell lymphoma occurs in the small bowel of patients with untreated celiac disease (an immune response to gluten that causes malnutrition). Patients who are diagnosed with celiac disease in childhood and stay on a gluten-free diet rarely develop enteropathy-type intestinal T-cell lymphoma.

Intravascular large B-cell lymphoma. This type of non-Hodgkin lymphoma affects blood vessels, especially the small blood vessels in the brain, kidney, lung, and skin. Signs and symptoms of intravascular large B-cell lymphoma are caused by blocked blood vessels. It is also called intravascular lymphomatosis.

Burkitt lymphoma. Burkitt lymphoma is a type of B-cell non-Hodgkin lymphoma that grows and spreads very quickly. It may affect the jaw, bones of the face, bowel, kidneys, ovaries, or other organs. There are three main types of Burkitt lymphoma (endemic, sporadic, and immunodeficiency related). Endemic Burkitt lymphoma commonly occurs in Africa and is linked to the Epstein-Barr virus, and sporadic Burkitt lymphoma occurs throughout the world. Immunodeficiency-related Burkitt lymphoma is most often seen in patients who have acquired immunodeficiency syndrome (AIDS). Burkitt lymphoma may spread to the brain and spinal cord and treatment to prevent its spread may be given. Burkitt lymphoma occurs most often in children and young adults. Burkitt lymphoma is also called diffuse small noncleaved-cell lymphoma.

Lymphoblastic lymphoma. Lymphoblastic lymphoma may begin in T cells or B cells, but it usually begins in T cells. In this type of non-Hodgkin lymphoma, there are too many lymphoblasts (immature white blood cells) in the lymph nodes and the thymus gland. These lymphoblasts may spread to other places in the body, such as the bone marrow, brain, and spinal cord. Lymphoblastic lymphoma is most common in teenagers and young adults. It is a lot like acute lymphoblastic leukemia (lymphoblasts are mostly found in the bone marrow and blood).

Adult T-cell leukemia/lymphoma. Adult T-cell leukemia/lymphoma is caused by the human T-cell leukemia virus type 1 (HTLV-1). Signs include bone and skin lesions, high blood calcium levels, and lymph nodes, spleen, and liver that are larger than normal.

Mantle cell lymphoma. Mantle cell lymphoma is a type of B-cell non-Hodgkin lymphoma that usually occurs in middle-aged or older adults. It begins in the lymph nodes and spreads to the spleen, bone marrow, blood, and sometimes the esophagus, stomach, and intestines. Patients with mantle cell lymphoma have too much of a protein called cyclin-D1 or a certain gene change in the lymphoma cells. In some patients who do not have signs or symptoms of lymphoma delaying the start of treatment does not affect the prognosis.

Posttransplant lymphoproliferative disorder (PTLD). This disease occurs in patients who have had a heart, lung, liver, kidney, or pancreas transplant and need lifelong immunosuppressive therapy. Most posttransplant lymphoproliferative disorders affect the B cells and have Epstein-Barr virus in the cells. Lymphoproliferative disorders are often treated like cancer.

True histiocytic lymphoma. This is a rare, very aggressive type of lymphoma. It is not known whether it begins in B cells or T cells. It does not respond well to treatment with standard chemotherapy.

Primary effusion lymphoma. Primary effusion lymphoma begins in B cells that are found in an area where there is a large buildup of fluid, such as the areas between the lining of the lung and chest wall (pleural effusion), the sac around the heart and the heart (pericardial effusion), or in the abdominal cavity. There is usually no tumor that can be seen. This type of lymphoma often occurs in patients who have AIDS.

Plasmablastic lymphoma. Plasmablastic lymphoma is a type of large B-cell non-Hodgkin lymphoma that is very aggressive. It is most often seen in patients with human immunodeficiency virus (HIV) infection.

What Are the Risk Factors for Adult Non-Hodgkin Lymphoma?

Anything that increases your risk of getting a disease is called a risk factor. Having a risk factor does not mean that you will get cancer; not having risk factors doesn't mean that you will not get cancer. Talk with your doctor if you think you may be at risk.

Age, gender, and a weakened immune system can affect the risk of adult non-Hodgkin lymphoma. These and other risk factors may increase the risk of certain types of adult non-Hodgkin lymphoma:

- Being older, male, or white
- Having one of the following medical conditions:
    - An inherited immune disorder (such as hypogammaglobulinemia or Wiskott–Aldrich syndrome (WAS))
    - An autoimmune disease (such as rheumatoid arthritis (RA), psoriasis, or Sjögren syndrome)
    - HIV/AIDS

    - *Human T-cell lymphotropic* virus type I or Epstein-Barr virus infection
    - *Helicobacter pylori* infection
- Taking immunosuppressant drugs after an organ transplant

What Are the Signs and Symptoms of Adult Non-Hodgkin Lymphoma?

Signs and symptoms of adult non-Hodgkin lymphoma include swelling in the lymph nodes, fever, night sweats, weight loss, and fatigue. These signs and symptoms may be caused by adult non-Hodgkin lymphoma or by other conditions. Check with your doctor if you have any of the following:

- Swelling in the lymph nodes in the neck, underarm, groin, or stomach
- Fever for no known reason
- Recurring night sweats
- Feeling very tired
- Weight loss for no known reason
- Skin rash or itchy skin
- Pain in the chest, abdomen, or bones for no known reason

When fever, night sweats, and weight loss occur together, this group of symptoms is called B symptoms.

Other signs and symptoms of adult non-Hodgkin lymphoma may occur and depend on the following:

- Where the cancer forms in the body
- The size of the tumor
- How fast the tumor grows

How Is Adult Non-Hodgkin Lymphoma Diagnosed?

Tests that examine the body and lymph system are used to help detect (find) and diagnose adult non-Hodgkin lymphoma. The following tests and procedures may be used:

- **Physical exam and history:** An exam of the body to check general signs of health, including checking for signs of disease,

such as lumps or anything else that seems unusual. A history of the patient's health habits and past illnesses and treatments will also be taken.

- **Flow cytometry:** A laboratory test that measures the number of cells in a sample, the percentage of live cells in a sample, and certain characteristics of cells, such as size, shape, and the presence of tumor markers on the cell surface. The cells are stained with a light-sensitive dye, placed in a fluid, and passed in a stream before a laser or other type of light. The measurements are based on how the light-sensitive dye reacts to the light. This test is used to diagnose lymphoplasmacytic lymphoma.
- **Bone marrow aspiration and biopsy:** The removal of bone marrow and a small piece of bone by inserting a needle into the hipbone or breastbone. A pathologist views the bone marrow and bone under a microscope to look for signs of cancer.
- **Lymph node biopsy:** The removal of all or part of a lymph node. A pathologist views the tissue under a microscope to look for cancer cells. One of the following types of biopsies may be done:
    - **Excisional biopsy:** The removal of an entire lymph node.
    - **Incisional biopsy:** The removal of part of a lymph node.
    - **Core biopsy:** The removal of part of a lymph node using a wide needle.
    - **Fine-needle aspiration (FNA) biopsy:** The removal of tissue or fluid using a thin needle.
    - **Laparoscopy:** A surgical procedure to look at the organs inside the abdomen to check for signs of disease. Small incisions (cuts) are made in the wall of the abdomen and a laparoscope (a thin, lighted tube) is inserted into one of the incisions. Other instruments may be inserted through the same or other incisions to take tissue samples to be checked under a microscope for signs of disease.
    - **Laparotomy:** A surgical procedure in which an incision (cut) is made in the wall of the abdomen to check the inside of the abdomen for signs of disease. Tissue samples are taken and checked under a microscope for signs of disease.

If cancer is found, the following tests may be done to study the cancer cells:

- **Immunohistochemistry:** A test that uses antibodies to check for certain antigens in a sample of tissue. The antibody is usually linked to a radioactive substance or a dye that causes the tissue to light up under a microscope. This type of test may be used to tell the difference between different types of cancer.
- **Cytogenetic analysis:** A laboratory test in which cells in a sample of tissue are viewed under a microscope to look for certain changes in the chromosomes.
- **Fluorescence in situ hybridization (FISH):** A laboratory test used to look at genes or chromosomes in cells and tissues. Pieces of deoxyribonucleic acid (DNA) that contain a fluorescent dye are made in the laboratory and added to cells or tissues on a glass slide. When these pieces of DNA attach to certain genes or areas of chromosomes on the slide, they light up when viewed under a microscope with a special light. This type of test is used to look for certain genetic markers.
- **Immunophenotyping:** A process used to identify cells, based on the types of antigens or markers on the surface of the cell. This process is used to diagnose specific types of leukemia and lymphoma by comparing the cancer cells to normal cells of the immune system.

Other tests and procedures may be done depending on the signs and symptoms seen and where the cancer forms in the body.

How Is Staging Done for Adult Non-Hodgkin Lymphoma?

After adult non-Hodgkin lymphoma has been diagnosed, tests are done to find out if cancer cells have spread within the lymph system or to other parts of the body.

The process used to find out the type of cancer and if cancer cells have spread within the lymph system or to other parts of the body is called staging. The information gathered from the staging process determines the stage of the disease. It is important to know the stage of the disease in order to plan treatment. The results of the tests and procedures done to diagnose non-Hodgkin lymphoma are used to help make decisions about treatment.

The following tests and procedures may also be used in the staging process:

- **Complete blood count (CBC) with differential:** A procedure in which a sample of blood is drawn and checked for the following:
  - The number of red blood cells and platelets
  - The number and type of white blood cells
  - The amount of hemoglobin (the protein that carries oxygen) in the red blood cells
  - The portion of the blood sample made up of red blood cells
- **Blood chemistry studies:** A procedure in which a blood sample is checked to measure the amounts of certain substances released into the blood by organs and tissues in the body. An unusual (higher or lower than normal) amount of a substance can be a sign of disease.
- **Computed tomography (CT)/computerized axial tomography (CAT) scan:** A procedure that makes a series of detailed pictures of areas inside the body, such as the lung, lymph nodes, and liver, taken from different angles. The pictures are made by a computer linked to an X-ray machine. A dye may be injected into a vein or swallowed to help the organs or tissues show up more clearly.
- **Positron emission tomography (PET) scan:** A procedure to find malignant tumor cells in the body. A small amount of radioactive glucose (sugar) is injected into a vein. The PET scanner rotates around the body and makes a picture of where glucose is being used in the body. Malignant tumor cells show up brighter in the picture because they are more active and take up more glucose than normal cells do.
- **Magnetic resonance imaging (MRI):** A procedure that uses a magnet, radio waves, and a computer to make a series of detailed pictures of areas inside the body. This procedure is also called nuclear magnetic resonance imaging (NMRI).
- **Bone marrow aspiration and biopsy:** The removal of bone marrow and a small piece of bone by inserting a needle into the hipbone or breastbone. A pathologist views the bone marrow and bone under a microscope to look for signs of cancer.

- **Lumbar puncture (LP):** A procedure used to collect cerebrospinal fluid (CSF) from the spinal column. This is done by placing a needle between two bones in the spine and into the CSF around the spinal cord and removing a sample of the fluid. The sample of CSF is checked under a microscope for signs that the cancer has spread to the brain and spinal cord. This procedure is also called spinal tap.

For pregnant women with non-Hodgkin lymphoma, staging tests and procedures that protect the baby from the harms of radiation are used. These tests and procedures include MRI, bone marrow aspiration and biopsy, lumbar puncture, and ultrasound. An ultrasound exam is a procedure in which high-energy sound waves (ultrasound) are bounced off internal tissues or organs and make echoes. The echoes form a picture of body tissues called a sonogram.

Stages of Adult Non-Hodgkin Lymphoma May Include E and S

Adult non-Hodgkin lymphoma may be described as follows:

- **E:** "E" stands for extranodal and means the cancer is found in an area or organ other than the lymph nodes or has spread to tissues beyond, but near, the major lymphatic areas.
- **S:** "S" stands for spleen and means the cancer is found in the spleen.

The following stages are used for adult non-Hodgkin lymphoma:

Stage I. Stage I adult non-Hodgkin lymphoma is divided into stage I and stage IE.

- **Stage I:** Cancer is found in one lymphatic area (lymph node group, tonsils and nearby tissue, thymus, or spleen).
- **Stage IE:** Cancer is found in one organ or area outside the lymph nodes.

Stage II. Stage II adult non-Hodgkin lymphoma is divided into stage II and stage IIE.

- **Stage II:** Cancer is found in two or more lymph node groups either above or below the diaphragm (the thin muscle below the lungs that helps breathing and separates the chest from the abdomen).

- **Stage IIE:** Cancer is found in one or more lymph node groups either above or below the diaphragm. Cancer is also found outside the lymph nodes in one organ or area on the same side of the diaphragm as the affected lymph nodes.

Stage III. Stage III adult non-Hodgkin lymphoma is divided into stage III, stage IIIE, stage IIIS, and stage IIIE+S.

- **Stage III:** Cancer is found in lymph node groups above and below the diaphragm (the thin muscle below the lungs that helps breathing and separates the chest from the abdomen).
- **Stage IIIE:** Cancer is found in lymph node groups above and below the diaphragm and outside the lymph nodes in a nearby organ or area.
- **Stage IIIS:** Cancer is found in lymph node groups above and below the diaphragm, and in the spleen.
- **Stage IIIE+S:** Cancer is found in lymph node groups above and below the diaphragm, outside the lymph nodes in a nearby organ or area, and in the spleen.

Stage IV. In stage IV adult non-Hodgkin lymphoma, the cancer:

- is found throughout one or more organs that are not part of a lymphatic area (lymph node group, tonsils and nearby tissue, thymus, or spleen), and may be in lymph nodes near those organs; or
- is found in one organ that is not part of a lymphatic area and has spread to organs or lymph nodes far away from that organ; or
- is found in the liver, bone marrow, cerebrospinal fluid (CSF), or lungs (other than cancer that has spread to the lungs from nearby areas).

Adult non-Hodgkin lymphomas may be grouped for treatment according to whether the cancer is indolent or aggressive and whether affected lymph nodes are next to each other in the body.

Non-Hodgkin lymphoma can also be described as contiguous or noncontiguous:

- **Contiguous lymphomas:** Lymphomas in which the lymph nodes with cancer are next to each other.
- **Noncontiguous lymphomas:** Lymphomas in which the lymph nodes with cancer are not next to each other, but are on the same side of the diaphragm.

What Treatment Options Are Available for People with Adult Non-Hodgkin Lymphoma?

Different types of treatment are available for patients with non-Hodgkin lymphoma. Some treatments are standard (the currently used treatment), and some are being tested in clinical trials. A treatment clinical trial is a research study meant to help improve current treatments or obtain information on new treatments for patients with cancer. When clinical trials show that a new treatment is better than the standard treatment, the new treatment may become the standard treatment. Patients may want to think about taking part in a clinical trial. Some clinical trials are open only to patients who have not started treatment.

Treatment Options for Pregnant Women

For pregnant women with non-Hodgkin lymphoma, treatment is carefully chosen to protect the baby. Treatment decisions are based on the mother's wishes, the stage of the non-Hodgkin lymphoma, and the age of the baby. The treatment plan may change as the signs and symptoms, cancer, and pregnancy change. Choosing the most appropriate cancer treatment is a decision that ideally involves the patient, family, and healthcare team.

Healthcare Team for Patients with Non-Hodgkin lymphoma

Patients with non-Hodgkin lymphoma should have their treatment planned by a team of healthcare providers who are experts in treating lymphomas.

Treatment will be overseen by a medical oncologist, a doctor who specializes in treating cancer, or a hematologist, a doctor who specializes in treating blood cancers. The medical oncologist may refer you to other healthcare providers who have experience and are experts in treating adult non-Hodgkin lymphoma and who specialize in certain areas of medicine. These may include the following specialists:

- Neurosurgeon
- Neurologist
- Radiation oncologist
- Endocrinologist
- Rehabilitation specialist
- Other oncology specialists

Late Effects of Treatment

Patients may develop late effects that appear months or years after their treatment for non-Hodgkin lymphoma. Side effects from cancer treatment that begin during or after treatment and continue for months or years are called late effects. Treatment with chemotherapy, radiation therapy, or stem cell transplant for non-Hodgkin lymphoma may increase the risk of late effects.

Late effects of cancer treatment may include the following:

- Heart problems
- Infertility (inability to have children)
- Loss of bone density
- Neuropathy (nerve damage that causes numbness or trouble walking)
- A second cancer, such as:
    - Lung cancer
    - Brain cancer
    - Kidney cancer
    - Bladder cancer
    - Melanoma
    - Hodgkin lymphoma
    - Myelodysplastic syndrome
    - Acute myeloid leukemia

Some late effects may be treated or controlled. It is important to talk with your doctor about the effects cancer treatment can have on you. Regular follow-up to check for late effects is important.

Types of Standard Treatments

Radiation Therapy

Radiation therapy is a cancer treatment that uses high-energy X-rays or other types of radiation to kill cancer cells or keep them from growing. There are two types of radiation therapy:

- External radiation therapy uses a machine outside the body to send radiation toward the cancer.

- Internal radiation therapy uses a radioactive substance sealed in needles, seeds, wires, or catheters that are placed directly into or near the cancer.

Total-body irradiation is a type of external radiation therapy that is given to the entire body. It may be given before a stem cell transplant.

The way the radiation therapy is given depends on the type and stage of the cancer being treated. External radiation therapy is used to treat adult non-Hodgkin lymphoma, and may also be used as palliative therapy to relieve symptoms and improve quality of life.

For pregnant women with non-Hodgkin lymphoma, radiation therapy should be given after delivery, if possible, to avoid any risk to the baby. If treatment is needed right away, pregnant women may decide to continue the pregnancy and receive radiation therapy. However, lead used to shield the baby may not protect it from scattered radiation that could possibly cause cancer in the future.

Chemotherapy

Chemotherapy is a cancer treatment that uses drugs to stop the growth of cancer cells, either by killing the cells or by stopping them from dividing. When chemotherapy is taken by mouth or injected into a vein or muscle, the drugs enter the bloodstream and can reach cancer cells throughout the body (systemic chemotherapy). When chemotherapy is placed directly into the cerebrospinal fluid (intrathecal chemotherapy), an organ, or a body cavity such as the abdomen, the drugs mainly affect cancer cells in those areas (regional chemotherapy). Combination chemotherapy is treatment using two or more anticancer drugs. Steroid drugs may be added, to lessen inflammation and lower the body's immune response.

The way the chemotherapy is given depends on the type and stage of the cancer being treated.

Intrathecal chemotherapy may also be used in the treatment of lymphoma that first forms in the testicles or sinuses (hollow areas) around the nose, diffuse large B-cell lymphoma, Burkitt lymphoma, lymphoblastic lymphoma, and some aggressive T-cell lymphomas. It is given to lessen the chance that lymphoma cells will spread to the brain and spinal cord. This is called CNS prophylaxis.

In pregnant women, the baby is exposed to chemotherapy when the mother is treated, and some anticancer drugs cause birth defects. Because anticancer drugs are passed to the baby through the mother, both must be watched closely when chemotherapy is given.

Immunotherapy

Immunotherapy is a treatment that uses the patient's immune system to fight cancer. Substances made by the body or made in a laboratory are used to boost, direct, or restore the body's natural defenses against cancer.

Immunomodulators are a type of immunotherapy. Lenalidomide is an immunomodulator used to treat adult non-Hodgkin lymphoma.

Targeted Therapy

Targeted therapy is a type of treatment that uses drugs or other substances to identify and attack specific cancer cells without harming normal cells. Monoclonal antibody therapy, proteasome inhibitor therapy, and kinase inhibitor therapy are types of targeted therapy used to treat adult non-Hodgkin lymphoma.

Monoclonal antibody therapy is a cancer treatment that uses antibodies made in the laboratory from a single type of immune system cell. These antibodies can identify substances on cancer cells or normal substances that may help cancer cells grow. The antibodies attach to the substances and kill the cancer cells, block their growth, or keep them from spreading. They may be used alone or to carry drugs, toxins, or radioactive material directly to cancer cells. Rituximab is a monoclonal antibody used to treat many types of non-Hodgkin lymphoma. Monoclonal antibodies that have been joined to radioactive material are called radiolabeled monoclonal antibodies. Yttrium Y 90-ibritumomab tiuxetan is an example of a radiolabeled monoclonal antibody. Monoclonal antibodies are given by infusion.

Proteasome inhibitor therapy blocks the action of proteasomes in cancer cells. Proteasomes remove proteins no longer needed by the cell. When the proteasomes are blocked, the proteins build up in the cell and may cause the cancer cell to die. Bortezomib is used to decrease how much immunoglobulin M is in the blood after cancer treatment for lymphoplasmacytic lymphoma. It is also being studied to treat relapsed mantle cell lymphoma.

Kinase inhibitor therapy, such as idelalisib, blocks certain proteins, which may help keep lymphoma cells from growing and may kill them. It is used to treat indolent lymphoma. Ibrutinib, a type of Bruton's tyrosine kinase inhibitor therapy, is used to treat lymphoplasmacytic lymphoma and mantle cell lymphoma.

Plasmapheresis

If the blood becomes thick with extra antibody proteins and affects circulation, plasmapheresis is done to remove extra plasma and antibody proteins from the blood. In this procedure, blood is removed from the patient and sent through a machine that separates the plasma (the liquid part of the blood) from the blood cells. The patient's plasma contains the unneeded antibodies and is not returned to the patient. The normal blood cells are returned to the bloodstream along with donated plasma or a plasma replacement. Plasmapheresis does not keep new antibodies from forming.

Watchful Waiting

Watchful waiting is closely monitoring a patient's condition without giving any treatment until signs or symptoms appear or change.

Antibiotic Therapy

Antibiotic therapy is a treatment that uses drugs to treat infections and cancer caused by bacteria and other microorganisms.

Surgery

Surgery may be used to remove the lymphoma in certain patients with indolent or aggressive non-Hodgkin lymphoma.

The type of surgery used depends on where the lymphoma formed in the body:

- **Local excision** for certain patients with mucosa-associated lymphoid tissue (MALT) lymphoma, PTLD, and small bowel T-cell lymphoma.
- **Splenectomy** for patients with marginal zone lymphoma of the spleen.

Patients who have a heart, lung, liver, kidney, or pancreas transplant usually need to take drugs to suppress their immune system for the rest of their lives. Long-term immunosuppression after an organ transplant can cause a certain type of non-Hodgkin lymphoma called posttransplant lymphoproliferative disorder (PTLD).

Small bowel surgery is often needed to diagnose celiac disease in adults who develop a type of T-cell lymphoma.

Stem Cell Transplant

Stem cell transplant is a method of giving high doses of chemotherapy and/or total-body irradiation and then replacing blood-forming cells destroyed by the cancer treatment. Stem cells (immature blood cells) are removed from the blood or bone marrow of the patient (autologous transplant) or a donor (allogeneic transplant) and are frozen and stored. After the chemotherapy and/or radiation therapy is completed, the stored stem cells are thawed and given back to the patient through an infusion. These reinfused stem cells grow into (and restore) the body's blood cells.

What Is the Prognosis for Adult Non-Hodgkin Lymphoma?

The prognosis (chance of recovery) and treatment options depend on the following:

- The stage of the cancer
- The type of non-Hodgkin lymphoma
- The amount of lactate dehydrogenase (LDH) in the blood
- Whether there are certain changes in the genes
- The patient's age and general health
- Whether the lymphoma has just been diagnosed or has recurred (come back)

For non-Hodgkin lymphoma during pregnancy, the treatment options also depend on:

- The wishes of the patient
- Which trimester of pregnancy the patient is in
- Whether the baby can be delivered early

Some types of non-Hodgkin lymphoma spread more quickly than others do. Most non-Hodgkin lymphomas that occur during pregnancy are aggressive. Delaying treatment of aggressive lymphoma until after the baby is born may lessen the mother's chance of survival. Immediate treatment is often recommended, even during pregnancy.

What New Types of Treatment Are Being Tested in Clinical Trials

Vaccine Therapy

Vaccine therapy is a type of biologic therapy. Biologic therapy is a treatment that uses the patient's immune system to fight cancer. Substances made by the body or made in a laboratory are used to boost, direct, or restore the body's natural defenses against cancer. This type of cancer treatment is also called biotherapy or immunotherapy. Vaccine therapy can also be a type of targeted therapy.

Is There a Need for Follow-Up Tests?

Some of the tests that were done to diagnose the cancer or to find out the stage of the cancer may be repeated. Some tests will be repeated in order to see how well the treatment is working. Decisions about whether to continue, change, or stop treatment may be based on the results of these tests.

Some of the tests will continue to be done from time to time after treatment has ended. The results of these tests can show if your condition has changed or if the cancer has recurred (come back). These tests are sometimes called follow-up tests or check-ups.

Chapter 48

Plasma Cell Neoplasms

Plasma cells develop from B lymphocytes (B cells), a type of white blood cell that is made in the bone marrow. Normally, when bacteria or viruses enter the body, some of the B cells will change into plasma cells. The plasma cells make antibodies to fight bacteria and viruses, to stop infection and disease.

What Is Plasma Cell Neoplasms?

Plasma cell neoplasms are diseases in which the body makes too many plasma cells. Plasma cell neoplasms are diseases in which abnormal plasma cells or myeloma cells form tumors in the bones or soft tissues of the body. The plasma cells also make an antibody protein, called M protein, that is not needed by the body and does not help fight infection. These antibody proteins build up in the bone marrow and can cause the blood to thicken or can damage the kidneys.

Plasma Cell Neoplasms Can Be Benign (Not Cancer) or Malignant (Cancer)

Monoclonal gammopathy of undetermined significance (MGUS) is not cancer but can become cancer. The following types of plasma cell neoplasms are cancer:

- Lymphoplasmacytic lymphoma

This chapter includes text excerpted from "Plasma Cell Neoplasms (including Multiple Myeloma) Treatment (PDQ®)—Patient Version," National Cancer Institute (NCI), December 8, 2017.

- Plasmacytoma
- Multiple myeloma

Types of Plasma Cell Neoplasms

Plasma cell neoplasms include the following:

Monoclonal Gammopathy of Undetermined Significance (MGUS)

In this type of plasma cell neoplasm, less than 10 percent of the bone marrow is made up of abnormal plasma cells and there is no cancer. The abnormal plasma cells make M protein, which is sometimes found during a routine blood or urine test. In most patients, the amount of M protein stays the same and there are no signs, symptoms, or health problems.

In some patients, MGUS may later become a more serious condition, such as amyloidosis, or cause problems with the kidneys, heart, or nerves. MGUS can also become cancer, such as multiple myeloma, lymphoplasmacytic lymphoma, or chronic lymphocytic leukemia.

Plasmacytoma

In this type of plasma cell neoplasm, the abnormal plasma cells (myeloma cells) are in one place and form one tumor, called a plasmacytoma. Sometimes plasmacytoma can be cured. There are two types of plasmacytoma.

- In **isolated plasmacytoma** of bone, one plasma cell tumor is found in the bone, less than 10 percent of the bone marrow is made up of plasma cells, and there are no other signs of cancer. Plasmacytoma of the bone often becomes multiple myeloma.
- In **extramedullary plasmacytoma,** one plasma cell tumor is found in soft tissue but not in the bone or the bone marrow. Extramedullary plasmacytomas commonly form in tissues of the throat, tonsil, and paranasal sinuses.

Signs and symptoms depend on where the tumor is:

- In bone, the plasmacytoma may cause pain or broken bones.
- In soft tissue, the tumor may press on nearby areas and cause pain or other problems. For example, a plasmacytoma in the throat can make it hard to swallow.

Multiple Myeloma

In multiple myeloma, abnormal plasma cells (myeloma cells) build up in the bone marrow and form tumors in many bones of the body. These tumors may keep the bone marrow from making enough healthy blood cells. Normally, the bone marrow makes stem cells (immature cells) that become three types of mature blood cells:

- Red blood cells that carry oxygen and other substances to all tissues of the body
- White blood cells that fight infection and disease
- Platelets that form blood clots to help prevent bleeding

As the number of myeloma cells increases, fewer red blood cells, white blood cells, and platelets are made. The myeloma cells also damage and weaken the bone.

Sometimes multiple myeloma does not cause any signs or symptoms. This is called smoldering multiple myeloma. It may be found when a blood or urine test is done for another condition.

Signs and symptoms may be caused by multiple myeloma or other conditions. Check with your doctor if you have any of the following:

- Bone pain, especially in the back or ribs
- Bones that break easily
- Fever for no known reason or frequent infections
- Easy bruising or bleeding
- Trouble breathing
- Weakness of the arms or legs
- Feeling very tired

A tumor can damage the bone and cause hypercalcemia (too much calcium in the blood). This can affect many organs in the body, including the kidneys, nerves, heart, muscles, and digestive tract, and cause serious health problems.

Hypercalcemia may cause the following signs and symptoms:

- Loss of appetite
- Nausea or vomiting
- Feeling thirsty
- Frequent urination

- Constipation
- Feeling very tired
- Muscle weakness
- Restlessness
- Confusion or trouble thinking

What Is Amyloidosis?

In rare cases, multiple myeloma can cause peripheral nerves (nerves that are not in the brain or spinal cord) and organs to fail. This may be caused by a condition called amyloidosis. Antibody proteins build up and stick together in peripheral nerves and organs, such as the kidney and heart. This can cause the nerves and organs to become stiff and unable to work the way they should.

Amyloidosis may cause the following signs and symptoms:

- Feeling very tired
- Purple spots on the skin
- Enlarged tongue
- Diarrhea
- Swelling caused by fluid in your body's tissues
- Tingling or numbness in your legs and feet

What Are the Risk Factors for Plasma Cell Neoplasms?

Anything that increases your risk of getting a disease is called a risk factor. Having a risk factor does not mean that you will get cancer; not having risk factors doesn't mean that you will not get cancer. Talk with your doctor if you think you may be at risk.

Age can affect the risk of plasma cell neoplasms. They are most common in people who are middle-aged or older. For multiple myeloma and plasmacytoma, other risk factors include the following:

- Being black
- Being male
- Having a personal history of MGUS or plasmacytoma
- Being exposed to radiation or certain chemicals

How Is Plasma Cell Neoplasms Diagnosed?

Tests that examine the blood, bone marrow, and urine are used to detect (find) and diagnose multiple myeloma and other plasma cell neoplasms. The following tests and procedures may be used:

- **Physical exam and history:** An exam of the body to check general signs of health, including checking for signs of disease, such as lumps or anything else that seems unusual. A history of the patient's health habits and past illnesses and treatments will also be taken.
- **Blood and urine immunoglobulin studies:** A procedure in which a blood or urine sample is checked to measure the amounts of certain antibodies (immunoglobulins). For multiple myeloma, beta-2-microglobulin, M protein, free light chains, and other proteins made by the myeloma cells are measured. A higher-than-normal amount of these substances can be a sign of disease.
- **Bone marrow aspiration and biopsy:** The removal of bone marrow, blood, and a small piece of bone by inserting a hollow needle into the hipbone or breastbone. A pathologist views the bone marrow, blood, and bone under a microscope to look for abnormal cells.

The following test may be done on the sample of tissue removed during the bone marrow aspiration and biopsy:

- **Cytogenetic analysis:** A test in which cells in a sample of bone marrow are viewed under a microscope to look for certain changes in the chromosomes. Other tests, such as fluorescence in situ hybridization (FISH) and flow cytometry, may also be done to look for certain changes in the chromosomes.
- **Skeletal bone survey:** In a skeletal bone survey, X-rays of all the bones in the body are taken. The X-rays are used to find areas where the bone is damaged. An X-ray is a type of energy beam that can go through the body and onto film, making a picture of areas inside the body.
- **Complete blood count (CBC) with differential:** A procedure in which a sample of blood is drawn and checked for the following:
    - The number of red blood cells and platelets
    - The number and type of white blood cells

- The amount of hemoglobin (the protein that carries oxygen) in the red blood cells
- The portion of the blood sample made up of red blood cells

- **Blood chemistry studies:** A procedure in which a blood sample is checked to measure the amounts of certain substances, such as calcium or albumin, released into the blood by organs and tissues in the body. An unusual (higher or lower than normal) amount of a substance can be a sign of disease.
- **24-hour urine test:** A test in which urine is collected for 24 hours to measure the amounts of certain substances. An unusual (higher or lower than normal) amount of a substance can be a sign of disease in the organ or tissue that makes it. A higher than normal amount of protein may be a sign of multiple myeloma.
- **Magnetic resonance imaging (MRI):** A procedure that uses a magnet, radio waves, and a computer to make a series of detailed pictures of areas inside the body. This procedure is also called nuclear magnetic resonance imaging (NMRI). An MRI of the spine and pelvis may be used to find areas where the bone is damaged.
- **Computed tomography (CT)/computerized axial tomography (CAT) scan:** A procedure that makes a series of detailed pictures of areas inside the body, such as the spine, taken from different angles. The pictures are made by a computer linked to an X-ray machine. A dye may be injected into a vein or swallowed to help the organs or tissues show up more clearly.
- **Positron emission tomography (PET)-CT scan:** A procedure that combines the pictures from a PET scan and a CT scan. The PET and CT scans are done at the same time with the same machine. The combined scans give more detailed pictures of areas inside the body, such as the spine, than either scan gives by itself.

Stages of Plasma Cell Neoplasms

There are no standard staging systems for monoclonal gammopathy of undetermined significance (MGUS), macroglobulinemia, and plasmacytoma.

After multiple myeloma has been diagnosed, tests are done to find out the amount of cancer in the body. The process used to find out the amount of cancer in the body is called staging. It is important to know the stage in order to plan treatment. The following tests and procedures may be used in the staging process:

- **Skeletal bone survey:** In a skeletal bone survey, X-rays of all the bones in the body are taken. The X-rays are used to find areas where the bone is damaged. An X-ray is a type of energy beam that can go through the body and onto film, making a picture of areas inside the body.
- **MRI:** A procedure that uses a magnet, radio waves, and a computer to make a series of detailed pictures of areas inside the body, such as the bone marrow. This procedure is also called nuclear magnetic resonance imaging (NMRI).
- **Bone densitometry:** A procedure that uses a special type of X-ray to measure bone density.

Beta-2-Microglobulin and Albumin

Beta-2-microglobulin and albumin are found in the blood. Beta-2-microglobulin is a protein found on plasma cells. Albumin makes up the biggest part of the blood plasma. It keeps fluid from leaking out of blood vessels. It also brings nutrients to tissues, and carries hormones, vitamins, drugs, and other substances, such as calcium, all through the body. In the blood of patients with multiple myeloma, the amount of beta-2-microglobulin is increased and the amount of albumin is decreased.

Stages That Are Used for Multiple Myeloma

Stage I multiple myeloma. In stage I multiple myeloma, the blood levels are as follows:

- beta-2-microglobulin level is lower than 3.5 mg/L; and
- albumin level is 3.5 g/dL or higher

Stage II multiple myeloma. In stage II multiple myeloma, the blood levels are in between the levels for stage I and stage III.

Stage III multiple myeloma. In stage III multiple myeloma, the blood level of beta-2-microglobulin is 5.5 mg/L or higher and the patient also has one of the following:

- high levels of lactate dehydrogenase (LDH); or
- certain changes in the chromosomes

Treatment Options

Eight types of treatment are used:

Chemotherapy

Chemotherapy is a cancer treatment that uses drugs to stop the growth of cancer cells, either by killing the cells or by stopping them from dividing. When chemotherapy is taken by mouth or injected into a vein or muscle, the drugs enter the bloodstream and can reach cancer cells throughout the body (systemic chemotherapy). When chemotherapy is placed directly into the cerebrospinal fluid, an organ, or a body cavity such as the abdomen, the drugs mainly affect cancer cells in those areas (regional chemotherapy). The way the chemotherapy is given depends on the type and stage of the cancer being treated.

Other Drug Therapy

Corticosteroids are steroids that have antitumor effects in multiple myeloma.

Targeted Therapy

Targeted therapy is a treatment that uses drugs or other substances to identify and attack specific cancer cells without harming normal cells. Several types of targeted therapy may be used to treat multiple myeloma and other plasma cell neoplasms.

Proteasome inhibitor therapy is a cancer treatment that blocks the action of proteasomes in cancer cells. A proteasome is a protein that removes other proteins no longer needed by the cell. When the proteins are not removed from the cell, they build up and may cause the cancer cell to die. Bortezomib, carfilzomib, and ixazomib are proteasome inhibitors used in the treatment of multiple myeloma and other plasma cell neoplasms.

Monoclonal antibody therapy is a cancer treatment that uses antibodies made in the laboratory, from a single type of immune system cell. These antibodies can identify substances on cancer cells or normal substances that may help cancer cells grow. The antibodies attach to the substances and kill the cancer cells, block their growth, or keep them from spreading. Monoclonal antibodies are given by infusion. They may be used alone or to carry drugs, toxins, or radioactive material directly to cancer cells. Daratumumab and elotuzumab are monoclonal antibodies used in the treatment of multiple myeloma and other plasma cell neoplasms.

Histone deacetylase (HDAC) inhibitor therapy is a type of targeted therapy that blocks enzymes needed for cell division and may stop the growth of cancer cells. Panobinostat is an HDAC inhibitor used in the treatment of multiple myeloma and other plasma cell neoplasms.

High-Dose Chemotherapy with Stem Cell Transplant

This treatment is a way of giving high doses of chemotherapy and replacing blood-forming cells destroyed by the cancer treatment. Stem cells (immature blood cells) are removed from the blood or bone marrow of the patient (autologous transplant) or a donor (allogeneic transplant) and are frozen and stored. After the chemotherapy is completed, the stored stem cells are thawed and given back to the patient through an infusion. These reinfused stem cells grow into (and restore) the body's blood cells.

Biologic Therapy

Biologic therapy is a treatment that uses the patient's immune system to fight cancer. Substances made by the body or made in a laboratory are used to boost, direct, or restore the body's natural defenses against cancer. This type of cancer treatment is also called biotherapy or immunotherapy.

Immunomodulators are a type of biologic therapy. Thalidomide, lenalidomide, and pomalidomide are immunomodulators used to treat multiple myeloma and other plasma cell neoplasms.

Interferon is a type of biologic therapy. It affects the division of cancer cells and can slow tumor growth.

Radiation Therapy

Radiation therapy is a cancer treatment that uses high-energy X-rays or other types of radiation to kill cancer cells or keep them from growing. There are two types of radiation therapy:

- External radiation therapy uses a machine outside the body to send radiation toward the cancer.

- Internal radiation therapy uses a radioactive substance sealed in needles, seeds, wires, or catheters that are placed directly into or near the cancer.

The way the radiation therapy is given depends on the type and stage of the cancer being treated. External radiation therapy is used to treat plasma cell neoplasms.

Surgery

Surgery to remove the tumor may be done and is usually followed by radiation therapy. Treatment given after the surgery, to lower the risk that the cancer will come back, is called adjuvant therapy.

Watchful Waiting

Watchful waiting is closely monitoring a patient's condition without giving any treatment until signs or symptoms appear or change.

What Is the Role of Supportive Care in Treatment?

Supportive care is given to lessen the problems caused by the disease or its treatment. This therapy controls problems or side effects caused by the disease or its treatment, and improves quality of life. Supportive care is given to treat problems caused by multiple myeloma and other plasma cell neoplasms.

Supportive care may include the following:

- **Plasmapheresis:** If the blood becomes thick with extra antibody proteins and interferes with circulation, plasmapheresis is done to remove extra plasma and antibody proteins from the blood. In this procedure blood is removed from the patient and sent through a machine that separates the plasma (the liquid part of the blood) from the blood cells. The patient's plasma contains the unneeded antibodies and is not returned to the patient. The normal blood cells are returned to the bloodstream along with donated plasma or a plasma replacement. Plasmapheresis does not keep new antibodies from forming.
- **High-dose chemotherapy with stem cell transplant:** If amyloidosis occurs, treatment may include high-dose chemotherapy followed by stem cell transplant using the patient's own stem cells.

- **Biologic therapy:** Biologic therapy with thalidomide, lenalidomide, or pomalidomide is given to treat amyloidosis.
- **Targeted therapy:** Targeted therapy with proteasome inhibitors is given to decrease how much immunoglobulin M is in the blood and treat amyloidosis.
- **Radiation therapy:** Radiation therapy is given for bone lesions of the spine.
- **Chemotherapy:** Chemotherapy is given to reduce back pain from osteoporosis or compression fractures of the spine.

Is There a Need for Follow-Up Tests?

Some of the tests that were done to diagnose the cancer or to find out the stage of the cancer may be repeated. Some tests will be repeated in order to see how well the treatment is working. Decisions about whether to continue, change, or stop treatment may be based on the results of these tests.

Some of the tests will continue to be done from time to time after treatment has ended. The results of these tests can show if your condition has changed or if the cancer has recurred (come back). These tests are sometimes called follow-up tests or check-ups.

What Is the Prognosis for Plasma Cell Neoplasms?

The prognosis (chance of recovery) depends on the following:

- The type of plasma cell neoplasm
- The stage of the disease
- Whether a certain immunoglobulin (antibody) is present
- Whether there are certain genetic changes
- Whether the kidney is damaged
- Whether the cancer responds to initial treatment or recurs (comes back)

Chapter 49

Myelodysplastic and Myeloproliferative Diseases

General Information about Myelodysplastic and Myeloproliferative Diseases

What Are Myelodysplastic and Myeloproliferative Diseases?

Myelodysplastic/myeloproliferative neoplasms are diseases of the blood and bone marrow. They are a group of diseases in which the bone marrow makes too many white blood cells.

Normally, the bone marrow makes blood stem cells (immature cells) that become mature blood cells over time. A blood stem cell may become a myeloid stem cell or a lymphoid stem cell. A lymphoid stem cell becomes a white blood cell. A myeloid stem cell becomes one of three types of mature blood cells:

- Red blood cells that carry oxygen and other substances to all tissues of the body
- White blood cells that fight infection and disease
- Platelets that form blood clots to stop bleeding

This chapter includes text excerpted from "Myelodysplastic/Myeloproliferative Neoplasms Treatment (PDQ®)—Patient Version," National Cancer Institute (NCI), August 12, 2015.

What Are the Characteristic Features of Myelodysplastic and Myeloproliferative Diseases?

Myelodysplastic/myeloproliferative neoplasms have features of both myelodysplastic syndromes and myeloproliferative neoplasms.

In myelodysplastic diseases, the blood stem cells do not mature into healthy red blood cells, white blood cells, or platelets. The immature blood cells, called blasts, do not work the way they should and die in the bone marrow or soon after they enter the blood. As a result, there are fewer healthy red blood cells, white blood cells, and platelets.

In myeloproliferative diseases, a greater than normal number of blood stem cells become one or more types of blood cells and the total number of blood cells slowly increases.

How Many Types of Myelodysplastic / Myeloproliferative Neoplasms Are There?

There are different types of myelodysplastic/myeloproliferative neoplasms. The 3 main types of myelodysplastic/myeloproliferative neoplasms include the following:

- Chronic myelomonocytic leukemia (CMML)
- Juvenile myelomonocytic leukemia (JMML)
- Atypical chronic myelogenous leukemia (aCML)

When a myelodysplastic/myeloproliferative neoplasm does not match any of these types, it is called myelodysplastic/myeloproliferative neoplasm, unclassifiable (MDS/MPN-UC).

Myelodysplastic/myeloproliferative neoplasms may progress to acute leukemia.

How Is Myelodysplastic / Myeloproliferative Neoplasms Diagnosed?

Tests that examine the blood and bone marrow are used to detect (find) and diagnose myelodysplastic/myeloproliferative neoplasms. The following tests and procedures may be used:

- **Physical exam and history:** An exam of the body to check general signs of health, including checking for signs of disease such as an enlarged spleen and liver. A history of the patient's health habits and past illnesses and treatments will also be taken.

- **Complete blood count (CBC) with differential:** A procedure in which a sample of blood is drawn and checked for the following:
    - The number of red blood cells and platelets
    - The number and type of white blood cells
    - The amount of hemoglobin (the protein that carries oxygen) in the red blood cells
    - The portion of the sample made up of red blood cells
- **Peripheral blood smear:** A procedure in which a sample of blood is checked for blast cells, the number and kinds of white blood cells, the number of platelets, and changes in the shape of blood cells.
- **Blood chemistry studies:** A procedure in which a blood sample is checked to measure the amounts of certain substances released into the blood by organs and tissues in the body. An unusual (higher or lower than normal) amount of a substance can be a sign of disease.
- **Bone marrow aspiration and biopsy:** The removal of a small piece of bone and bone marrow by inserting a needle into the hipbone or breastbone. A pathologist views both the bone and bone marrow samples under a microscope to look for abnormal cells.

The following tests may be done on the sample of tissue that is removed:

- **Cytogenetic analysis:** A test in which cells in a sample of blood or bone marrow are viewed under a microscope to look for certain changes in the chromosomes. The cancer cells in myelodysplastic/myeloproliferative neoplasms do not contain the Philadelphia chromosome that is present in chronic myelogenous leukemia.
- **Immunocytochemistry:** A test that uses antibodies to check for certain antigens in a sample of bone marrow. The antibody is usually linked to a radioactive substance or a dye that causes the cells in the sample to light up under a microscope. This type of test is used to tell the difference between myelodysplastic/myeloproliferative neoplasms, leukemia, and other conditions.

Chronic Myelomonocytic Leukemia (CMML)

What Is Chronic Myelomonocytic Leukemia (CMML)?

Chronic myelomonocytic leukemia (CMML) is a disease in which too many myelocytes and monocytes (immature white blood cells) are made in the bone marrow.

In CMML, the body tells too many blood stem cells to become two types of white blood cells called myelocytes and monocytes. Some of these blood stem cells never become mature white blood cells. These immature white blood cells are called blasts. Over time, the myelocytes, monocytes, and blasts crowd out the red blood cells and platelets in the bone marrow. When this happens, infection, anemia, or easy bleeding may occur.

What Are the Risk Factors for CMML?

Anything that increases your chance of getting a disease is called a risk factor. Older age and being male increase the risk of chronic myelomonocytic leukemia. Possible risk factors for CMML include the following:

- Older age
- Being male
- Being exposed to certain substances at work or in the environment
- Being exposed to radiation
- Past treatment with certain anticancer drugs

What Are the Signs and Symptoms of CMML?

Signs and symptoms of chronic myelomonocytic leukemia include fever, weight loss, and feeling very tired. These and other signs and symptoms may be caused by CMML or by other conditions. Check with your doctor if you have any of the following:

- Fever for no known reason
- Infection
- Feeling very tired
- Weight loss for no known reason
- Easy bruising or bleeding
- Pain or a feeling of fullness below the ribs

What Is the Prognosis for CMML?

The prognosis (chance of recovery) and treatment options for CMML depend on the following:

- The number of white blood cells or platelets in the blood or bone marrow
- Whether the patient is anemic
- The amount of blasts in the blood or bone marrow
- The amount of hemoglobin in red blood cells
- Whether there are certain changes in the chromosomes

Juvenile Myelomonocytic Leukemia (JMML)

What Is Juvenile Myelomonocytic Leukemia (JMML)?

Juvenile myelomonocytic leukemia is a childhood disease in which too many myelocytes and monocytes (immature white blood cells) are made in the bone marrow. It is a rare childhood cancer that occurs more often in children younger than 2 years. Children who have neurofibromatosis type 1 and males have an increased risk of juvenile myelomonocytic leukemia.

In JMML, the body tells too many blood stem cells to become two types of white blood cells called myelocytes and monocytes. Some of these blood stem cells never become mature white blood cells. These immature white blood cells are called blasts. Over time, the myelocytes, monocytes, and blasts crowd out the red blood cells and platelets in the bone marrow. When this happens, infection, anemia, or easy bleeding may occur.

What Are the Signs and Symptoms of JMML?

Signs and symptoms of JMML include fever, weight loss, and feeling very tired.

These and other signs and symptoms may be caused by JMML or by other conditions. Check with your doctor if you have any of the following:

- Fever for no known reason
- Having infections, such as bronchitis or tonsillitis
- Feeling very tired

- Easy bruising or bleeding
- Skin rash
- Painless swelling of the lymph nodes in the neck, underarm, stomach, or groin
- Pain or a feeling of fullness below the ribs

What Is the Prognosis for JMML?

The prognosis (chance of recovery) and treatment options for JMML depend on the following:

- The age of the child at diagnosis
- The number of platelets in the blood
- The amount of a certain type of hemoglobin in red blood cells

Atypical Chronic Myelogenous Leukemia (CML)

What Is Chronic Myelogenous Leukemia (CML)?

Atypical chronic myelogenous leukemia (CML) is a disease in which too many granulocytes (immature white blood cells) are made in the bone marrow.

In atypical CML, the body tells too many blood stem cells to become a type of white blood cell called granulocytes. Some of these blood stem cells never become mature white blood cells. These immature white blood cells are called blasts. Over time, the granulocytes and blasts crowd out the red blood cells and platelets in the bone marrow.

The leukemia cells in atypical CML and CML look alike under a microscope. However, in atypical CML a certain chromosome change, called the "Philadelphia chromosome" is not there.

What Are the Signs and Symptoms of CML?

Signs and symptoms of atypical CML include easy bruising or bleeding and feeling tired and weak. These and other signs and symptoms may be caused by atypical CML or by other conditions. Check with your doctor if you have any of the following:

- Shortness of breath
- Pale skin
- Feeling very tired and weak

- Easy bruising or bleeding
- Petechiae (flat, pinpoint spots under the skin caused by bleeding)
- Pain or a feeling of fullness below the ribs on the left side

What Is the Prognosis for CML?

The prognosis (chance of recovery) for atypical CML depends on the number of red blood cells and platelets in the blood.

Myelodysplastic/Myeloproliferative Neoplasm, Unclassifiable (MDS/MPD-UC)

What Is Myelodysplastic / Myeloproliferative Neoplasm, Unclassifiable (MDS / MPD-UC)?

Myelodysplastic/myeloproliferative neoplasm, unclassifiable (MDS/MPD-UC), is a disease that has features of both myelodysplastic and myeloproliferative diseases but is not chronic myelomonocytic leukemia, juvenile myelomonocytic leukemia, or atypical chronic myelogenous leukemia. In MDS/MPD-UC, the body tells too many blood stem cells to become red blood cells, white blood cells, or platelets. Some of these blood stem cells never become mature blood cells. These immature blood cells are called blasts. Over time, the abnormal blood cells and blasts in the bone marrow crowd out the healthy red blood cells, white blood cells, and platelets.

MDS/MPN-UC is a very rare disease. Because it is so rare, the factors that affect risk and prognosis are not known.

What Are the Signs and Symptoms of MDS / MPD-UC?

Signs and symptoms of myelodysplastic/myeloproliferative neoplasm, unclassifiable, include fever, weight loss, and feeling very tired. These and other signs and symptoms may be caused by MDS/MPN-UC or by other conditions. Check with your doctor if you have any of the following:

- Fever or frequent infections
- Shortness of breath
- Feeling very tired and weak
- Pale skin

- Easy bruising or bleeding
- Petechiae (flat, pinpoint spots under the skin caused by bleeding)
- Pain or a feeling of fullness below the ribs

Stages of Myelodysplastic/Myeloproliferative Neoplasms

Staging is the process used to find out how far the cancer has spread. There is no standard staging system for myelodysplastic/myeloproliferative neoplasms. Treatment is based on the type of myelodysplastic/myeloproliferative neoplasm the patient has. It is important to know the type in order to plan treatment.

Treatment Option Overview

Different types of treatments are available for patients with myelodysplastic/myeloproliferative neoplasms. Some treatments are standard (the currently used treatment), and some are being tested in clinical trials. A treatment clinical trial is a research study meant to help improve current treatments or obtain information on new treatments for patients with cancer. When clinical trials show that a new treatment is better than the standard treatment, the new treatment may become the standard treatment. Patients may want to think about taking part in a clinical trial. Some clinical trials are open only to patients who have not started treatment.

What Are the Standard Treatment Options Available for People with Myelodysplastic / Myeloproliferative Neoplasms?

Five types of standard treatment are used:

Chemotherapy

Chemotherapy is a cancer treatment that uses drugs to stop the growth of cancer cells, either by killing the cells or by stopping them from dividing. When chemotherapy is taken by mouth or injected into a vein or muscle, the drugs enter the bloodstream and can reach cancer cells throughout the body (systemic chemotherapy). When chemotherapy is placed directly into the cerebrospinal fluid, an organ, or a body cavity such as the abdomen, the drugs mainly affect cancer cells in those areas (regional chemotherapy). The way the chemotherapy is given depends on the type and stage of the cancer being treated. Combination chemotherapy is treatment using more than one anticancer drug.

Other Drug Therapy

13-cis retinoic acid is a vitamin like drug that slows the cancer's ability to make more cancer cells and changes the way these cells look and act.

Stem Cell Transplant

Stem cell transplant is a method of replacing blood-forming cells that are destroyed by chemotherapy. Stem cells (immature blood cells) are removed from the blood or bone marrow of the patient or a donor and are frozen and stored. After the chemotherapy is completed, the stored stem cells are thawed and given back to the patient through an infusion. These reinfused stem cells grow into (and restore) the body's blood cells.

Supportive Care

Supportive care is given to lessen the problems caused by the disease or its treatment. Supportive care may include transfusion therapy or drug therapy, such as antibiotics to fight infection.

Targeted Therapy

Targeted therapy is a cancer treatment that uses drugs or other substances to attack cancer cells without harming normal cells. Targeted therapy drugs called tyrosine kinase inhibitors (TKIs) are used to treat myelodysplastic/myeloproliferative neoplasm, unclassifiable. TKIs block the enzyme, tyrosine kinase, that causes stem cells to become more blood cells (blasts) than the body needs. Imatinib mesylate (Gleevec) is a TKI that may be used. Other targeted therapy drugs are being studied in the treatment of JMML.

Is There a Need for Follow-Up Tests?

Some of the tests that were done to diagnose the cancer or to find out the stage of the cancer may be repeated. Some tests will be repeated in order to see how well the treatment is working. Decisions about whether to continue, change, or stop treatment may be based on the results of these tests.

Some of the tests will continue to be done from time to time after treatment has ended. The results of these tests can show if your condition has changed or if the cancer has recurred (come back). These tests are sometimes called follow-up tests or check-ups.

Chapter 50

Thymoma and Thymic Carcinoma

The thymus, a small organ that lies in the upper chest under the breastbone, is part of the lymph system. It makes white blood cells, called lymphocytes, that protect the body against infections.

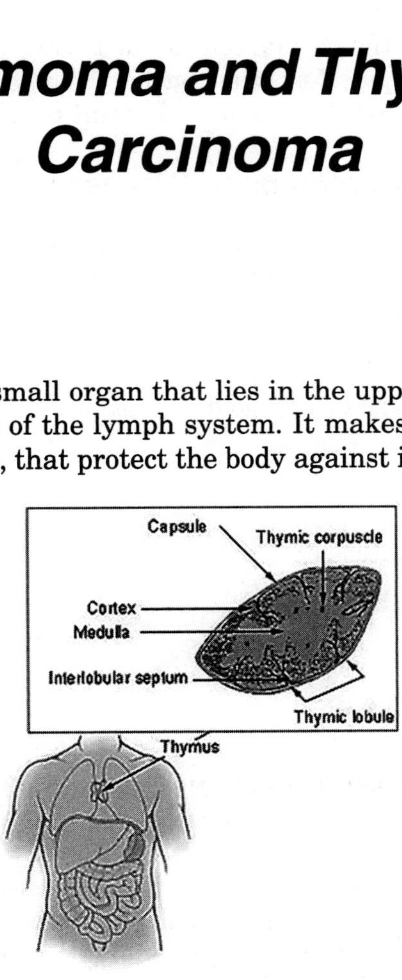

Figure 50.1. *Thymus* (Source: "Thymus," Surveillance, Epidemiology, and End Results Program (SEER), National Cancer Institute (NCI).)

This chapter includes text excerpted from "Thymoma and Thymic Carcinoma Treatment (PDQ®)—Patient Version," National Cancer Institute (NCI), November 9, 2017.

What Are Thymoma and Thymic Carcinoma?

Thymoma and thymic carcinoma are diseases in which malignant (cancer) cells form on the outside surface of the thymus.

There are different types of tumors of the thymus. Thymomas and thymic carcinomas are rare tumors of the cells that are on the outside surface of the thymus. The tumor cells in a thymoma look similar to the normal cells of the thymus, grow slowly, and rarely spread beyond the thymus. On the other hand, the tumor cells in a thymic carcinoma look very different from the normal cells of the thymus, grow more quickly, and have usually spread to other parts of the body when the cancer is found. Thymic carcinoma is more difficult to treat than thymoma.

Thymoma and Autoimmune Diseases

People with thymoma often have autoimmune diseases as well. These diseases cause the immune system to attack healthy tissue and organs. They include:

- Myasthenia gravis
- Acquired pure red cell aplasia
- Hypogammaglobulinemia
- Polymyositis
- Lupus erythematosus
- Rheumatoid arthritis (RA)
- Thyroiditis
- Sjögren syndrome

What Are the Signs and Symptoms of Thymoma and Thymic Carcinoma?

Thymoma and thymic carcinoma may not cause early signs or symptoms. The cancer may be found during a routine chest X-ray. Signs and symptoms of thymoma and thymic carcinoma include a cough and chest pain. Check with your doctor if you have any of the following:

- A cough that doesn't go away
- Chest pain
- Trouble breathing

How Is Thymoma and Thymic Carcinoma Diagnosed?

Tests that examine the thymus are used to detect (find) thymoma or thymic carcinoma. The following tests and procedures may be used:

- **Physical exam and history:** An exam of the body to check general signs of health, including checking for signs of disease, such as lumps or anything else that seems unusual. A history of the patient's health habits and past illnesses and treatments will also be taken.
- **Chest X-ray:** An X-ray of the organs and bones inside the chest. An X-ray is a type of energy beam that can go through the body and onto film, making a picture of areas inside the body.
- **Computed tomography (CT)/computerized axial tomography (CAT) scan:** A procedure that makes a series of detailed pictures of areas inside the body, such as the chest, taken from different angles. The pictures are made by a computer linked to an X-ray machine. A dye may be injected into a vein or swallowed to help the organs or tissues show up more clearly.
- **Magnetic resonance imaging (MRI):** A procedure that uses a magnet, radio waves, and a computer to make a series of detailed pictures of areas inside the body, such as the chest. This procedure is also called nuclear magnetic resonance imaging (NMRI).
- **Positron emission tomography (PET):** A procedure to find malignant tumor cells in the body. A small amount of radioactive glucose (sugar) is injected into a vein. The PET scanner rotates around the body and makes a picture of where glucose is being used in the body. Malignant tumor cells show up brighter in the picture because they are more active and take up more glucose than normal cells do.

Thymoma and thymic carcinoma are usually diagnosed, staged, and treated during surgery. A biopsy of the tumor is done to diagnose the disease. The biopsy may be done before or during surgery (a mediastinoscopy or mediastinotomy), using a thin needle to remove a sample of cells. This is called a fine needle aspiration (FNA) biopsy. Sometimes a wide needle is used to remove a sample of cells and this is called a core biopsy. A pathologist will view the sample under a microscope to check for cancer. If thymoma or thymic carcinoma is diagnosed, the pathologist will determine the type of cancer cell in the tumor. There may be more than one type of cancer cell in a thymoma. The surgeon will decide if all or part of the tumor can be removed by surgery. In some cases, lymph nodes and other tissues may be removed as well.

Stages of Thymoma and Thymic Carcinoma

Tests done to detect thymoma or thymic carcinoma are also used to stage the disease. Staging is the process used to find out if cancer has spread from the thymus to other parts of the body. The findings made during surgery and the results of tests and procedures are used to determine the stage of the disease. It is important to know the stage in order to plan treatment.

The following stages are used for thymoma:

- **Stage I.** In stage I, cancer is found only within the thymus. All cancer cells are inside the capsule (sac) that surrounds the thymus.
- **Stage II.** In stage II, cancer has spread through the capsule and into the fat around the thymus or into the lining of the chest cavity.
- **Stage III.** In stage III, cancer has spread to nearby organs in the chest, including the lung, the sac around the heart, or large blood vessels that carry blood to the heart.
- **Stage IV.**Stage IV is divided into stage IVA and stage IVB, depending on where the cancer has spread.
    - In stage IVA, cancer has spread widely around the lungs and heart.
    - In stage IVB, cancer has spread to the blood or lymph system.

The staging system used for thymomas is sometimes used for thymic carcinomas.

Treatment Options

Four types of standard treatment are used:

Surgery

Surgery to remove the tumor is the most common treatment of thymoma.

Even if the doctor removes all the cancer that can be seen at the time of the surgery, some patients may be given radiation therapy after surgery to kill any cancer cells that are left. Treatment given after the surgery, to lower the risk that the cancer will come back, is called adjuvant therapy.

Radiation Therapy

Radiation therapy is a cancer treatment that uses high-energy X-rays or other types of radiation to kill cancer cells or keep them from growing. There are two types of radiation therapy:

- External radiation therapy uses a machine outside the body to send radiation toward the cancer.
- Internal radiation therapy uses a radioactive substance sealed in needles, seeds, wires, or catheters that are placed directly into or near the cancer.

The way the radiation therapy is given depends on the type and stage of the cancer being treated. External radiation therapy is used to treat thymoma and thymic carcinoma.

Chemotherapy

Chemotherapy is a cancer treatment that uses drugs to stop the growth of cancer cells, either by killing the cells or by stopping them from dividing. When chemotherapy is taken by mouth or injected into a vein or muscle, the drugs enter the bloodstream and can reach cancer cells throughout the body (systemic chemotherapy). When chemotherapy is placed directly into the cerebrospinal fluid, an organ, or a body cavity such as the abdomen, the drugs mainly affect cancer cells in those areas (regional chemotherapy). The way the chemotherapy is given depends on the type and stage of the cancer being treated.

Chemotherapy may be used to shrink the tumor before surgery or radiation therapy. This is called neoadjuvant chemotherapy.

Hormone Therapy

Hormone therapy is a cancer treatment that removes hormones or blocks their action and stops cancer cells from growing. Hormones are substances produced by glands in the body and circulated in the bloodstream. Some hormones can cause certain cancers to grow. If tests show that the cancer cells have places where hormones can attach (receptors), drugs, surgery, or radiation therapy is used to reduce the production of hormones or block them from working.

Hormone therapy with drugs called corticosteroids may be used to treat thymoma or thymic carcinoma.

Is There a Need for Follow-Up Tests?

Some of the tests that were done to diagnose the cancer or to find out the stage of the cancer may be repeated. Some tests will be repeated in order to see how well the treatment is working. Decisions about whether to continue, change, or stop treatment may be based on the results of these tests.

Some of the tests will continue to be done from time to time after treatment has ended. The results of these tests can show if your condition has changed or if the cancer has recurred (come back). These tests are sometimes called follow-up tests or check-ups.

What Is the Prognosis for Thymic Carcinoma?

The prognosis (chance of recovery) and treatment options depend on the following:

- The stage of the cancer
- The type of cancer cell
- Whether the tumor can be removed completely by surgery.
- The patient's general health
- Whether the cancer has just been diagnosed or has recurred (come back)

Chapter 51

Skin Cancer

Skin cancer is the most common cancer in the United States. Some people are at higher risk of skin cancer than others, but anyone can get it. The most preventable cause of skin cancer is overexposure to ultraviolet (UV) light, either from the sun or from artificial sources like tanning beds.

What Is Skin Cancer?

Skin cancer is the most common form of cancer in the United States. The two most common types of skin cancer—basal cell and squamous cell carcinomas (SCC)—are highly curable, but can be disfiguring and costly to treat. Melanoma, the third most common skin cancer, is more dangerous and causes the most deaths. The majority of these three types of skin cancer are caused by overexposure to ultraviolet (UV) light.

Ultraviolet (UV) Light

Ultraviolet (UV) rays are an invisible kind of radiation that comes from the sun, tanning beds, and sunlamps. UV rays can penetrate and change skin cells.

This chapter includes text excerpted from "Skin Cancer—Basic Information about Skin Cancer," Centers for Disease Control and Prevention (CDC), April 25, 2017.

The three types of UV rays are ultraviolet A (UVA), ultraviolet B (UVB), and ultraviolet C (UVC):

- More UVA rays reach the earth's surface than the other types of UV rays. UVA rays can reach deep into human skin, UVA rays can damaging connective tissue and the skin's deoxyribonucleic acid (DNA).
- Most UVB rays are absorbed by the ozone layer, so fewer of them reach the earth's surface compared to UVA rays. UVB rays, which help produce vitamin D in the skin, don't reach as far into the skin as UVA rays, but they can still cause sunburn and damage DNA.
- UVC rays are very dangerous, but they are absorbed completely by the ozone layer and do not reach the earth's surface.

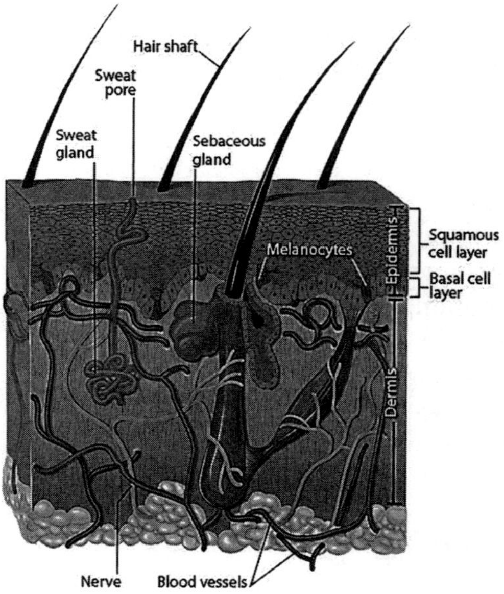

Figure 51.1. *Basal Cell Layer of the Skin*

Basal cell carcinoma begins in the basal cell layer of the skin. Squamous cell carcinoma begins in the squamous layer of the skin. Melanoma begins in the melanocytes, which are the cells that make melanin, the pigment that gives skin its color.

In addition to causing sunburn, too much exposure to UV rays can change skin texture, cause the skin to age prematurely, and can lead to skin cancer. UV rays also have been linked to eye conditions such as cataracts.

The National Weather Service (NWS) and the U.S. Environmental Protection Agency (EPA) developed the UV Index to forecast the risk of overexposure to UV rays. It lets you know how much caution you should take when spending time outdoors.

The UV Index predicts exposure levels on a 0–15 scale; higher levels indicate a higher risk of overexposure. Calculated on a next day basis for dozens of cities across the United States, the UV Index takes into account clouds and other local conditions that affect the amount of UV rays reaching the ground.

What Are the Risk Factors for Skin Cancer?

People with certain risk factors are more likely than others to develop skin cancer. Risk factors vary for different types of skin cancer, but some general risk factors are having:

- A lighter natural skin color
- Family history of skin cancer
- A personal history of skin cancer
- Exposure to the sun through work and play
- A history of sunburns, especially early in life
- A history of indoor tanning
- Skin that burns, freckles, reddens easily, or becomes painful in the sun
- Blue or green eyes
- Blond or red hair
- Certain types and a large number of moles

Tanning and Burning

Ultraviolet (UV) rays come from the sun or from indoor tanning (using a tanning bed, booth, or sunlamp to get tan). When UV rays reach the skin's inner layer, the skin makes more melanin.

Melanin is the pigment that colors the skin. It moves toward the outer layers of the skin and becomes visible as a tan.

A tan does not indicate good health. A tan is a response to injury, because skin cells signal that they have been hurt by UV rays by producing more pigment.

People burn or tan depending on their skin type, the time of year, and how long they are exposed to UV rays. The six types of skin, based on how likely it is to tan or burn, are:

- Always burns, never tans
- Burns easily, tans minimally
- Burns moderately, tans gradually to light brown
- Burns minimally, always tans well to moderately brown.
- Rarely burns, tans profusely to dark
- Never burns, deeply pigmented, least sensitive
- Although everyone's skin can be damaged by UV exposure, people with skin types I and II are at the highest risk

What Are the Symptoms of Skin Cancer?

A change in your skin is the most common sign of skin cancer. This could be a new growth, a sore that doesn't heal, or a change in a mole. Not all skin cancers look the same.

A simple way to remember the signs of melanoma is to remember the A-B-C-D-Es of melanoma:

- "A" stands for asymmetrical. Does the mole or spot have an irregular shape with two parts that look very different?
- "B" stands for border. Is the border irregular or jagged?
- "C" is for color. Is the color uneven?
- "D" is for diameter. Is the mole or spot larger than the size of a pea?
- "E" is for evolving. Has the mole or spot changed during the past few weeks or months?

Talk to your doctor if you notice changes in your skin such as a new growth, a sore that doesn't heal, a change in an old growth, or any of the A-B-C-D-Es of melanoma.

What Can I Do to Reduce My Risk of Skin Cancer?

Protection from ultraviolet (UV) radiation is important all year round, not just during the summer or at the beach. UV rays from the sun can reach you on cloudy and hazy days, as well as bright and sunny days. UV rays also reflect off of surfaces like water, cement, sand, and snow. Indoor tanning (using a tanning bed, booth, or sunlamp to get tan) exposes users to UV radiation.

The hours between 10 a.m. and 4 p.m. Daylight Saving Time (DST) (9 a.m. to 3 p.m. standard time) are the most hazardous for UV exposure outdoors in the continental United States. UV rays from sunlight are the greatest during the late spring and early summer in North America.

The Centers for Disease Control and Prevention (CDC) recommends easy options for protection from UV radiation:

- Stay in the shade, especially during midday hours
- Wear clothing that covers your arms and legs
- Wear a hat with a wide brim to shade your face, head, ears, and neck
- Wear sunglasses that wrap around and block both UVA and UVB rays
- Use sunscreen with a sun protection factor (SPF) of 15 or higher, and both UVA and UVB (broad spectrum) protection
- Avoid indoor tanning

What Screening Tests Are There?

The U.S. Preventive Services Task Force (USPSTF) has concluded there is not enough evidence to recommend for or against routine screening (total body examination by a doctor) to find skin cancers early. This recommendation is for people who do not have a history of skin cancer and who do not have any suspicious moles or other spots. Report any unusual moles or changes in your skin to your doctor. Also talk to your doctor if you are at increased risk of skin cancer.

Chapter 52

Melanoma

The skin is the body's largest organ. It protects against heat, sunlight, injury, and infection. Skin also helps control body temperature and stores water, fat, and vitamin D. The skin has several layers, but the two main layers are the epidermis (upper or outer layer) and the dermis (lower or inner layer). The epidermis is made up of three kinds of cells:

- **Squamous cells:** Thin, flat cells that form the top layer of the epidermis
- **Basal cells:** Round cells under the squamous cells
- **Melanocytes:** Cells that make melanin and are found in the lower part of the epidermis. Melanin is the pigment that gives skin its natural color. When skin is exposed to the sun or artificial light, melanocytes make more pigment and cause the skin to darken.

Skin cancer begins in the epidermis.

There are two forms of skin cancer: melanoma and nonmelanoma.

What Is Melanoma?

Melanoma is a disease in which malignant (cancer) cells form in melanocytes (cells that color the skin). It is a rare form of skin cancer. It is more likely to invade nearby tissues and spread to other parts of the body

---

This chapter includes text excerpted from "Melanoma Treatment (PDQ®)—Patient Version," National Cancer Institute (NCI), February 8, 2018.

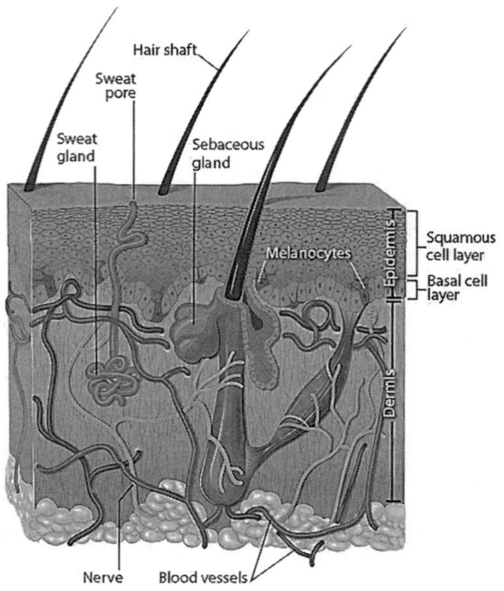

Figure 52.1. *Layer of Skin* (Source: "What Is Skin Cancer?" Centers for Disease Control and Prevention (CDC).)

than other types of skin cancer. When melanoma starts in the skin, it is called cutaneous melanoma. Melanoma may also occur in mucous membranes (thin, moist layers of tissue that cover surfaces such as the lips).

The most common types of skin cancer are basal cell carcinoma and squamous cell carcinoma. They are nonmelanoma skin cancers. Nonmelanoma skin cancers rarely spread to other parts of the body.

Where Do Melanoma Occur?

Melanoma can occur anywhere on the skin. In men, melanoma is often found on the trunk (the area from the shoulders to the hips) or the head and neck. In women, melanoma forms most often on the arms and legs.

When melanoma occurs in the eye, it is called intraocular or ocular melanoma.

What Are the Risk Factors for Melanoma?

Anything that increases your risk of getting a disease is called a risk factor. Having a risk factor does not mean that you will get cancer;

not having risk factors doesn't mean that you will not get cancer. Talk with your doctor if you think you may be at risk.

Unusual moles, exposure to sunlight, and health history can affect the risk of melanoma. Risk factors for melanoma include the following:

- Having a fair complexion, which includes the following:
    - Fair skin that freckles and burns easily, does not tan, or tans poorly
    - Blue or green or other light-colored eyes
    - Red or blond hair
- Being exposed to natural sunlight or artificial sunlight (such as from tanning beds) over long periods of time
- Being exposed to certain factors in the environment (in the air, your home or workplace, and your food and water). Some of the environmental risk factors for melanoma are radiation, solvents, vinyl chloride, and polychlorinated biphenyls (PCBs).
- Having a history of many blistering sunburns, especially as a child or teenager
- Having several large or many small moles
- Having a family history of unusual moles (atypical nevus syndrome)
- Having a family or personal history of melanoma
- Being white
- Having a weakened immune system
- Having certain changes in the genes that are linked to melanoma

Being white or having a fair complexion increases the risk of melanoma, but anyone can have melanoma, including people with dark skin.

What Are the Signs and Symptoms of Melanoma?

Signs of melanoma include a change in the way a mole or pigmented area looks. These and other signs and symptoms may be caused by melanoma or by other conditions. Check with your doctor if you have any of the following:

- A mole that:
    - changes in size, shape, or color

- has irregular edges or borders
- is more than one color
- is asymmetrical (if the mole is divided in half, the 2 halves are different in size or shape)
- itches
- oozes, bleeds, or is ulcerated (a hole forms in the skin when the top layer of cells breaks down and the tissue below shows through)

- A change in pigmented (colored) skin
- Satellite moles (new moles that grow near an existing mole)

How Is Melanoma Diagnosed?

Tests that examine the skin are used to detect (find) and diagnose melanoma. If a mole or pigmented area of the skin changes or looks abnormal, the following tests and procedures can help find and diagnose melanoma:

- **Skin exam:** A doctor or nurse checks the skin for moles, birthmarks, or other pigmented areas that look abnormal in color, size, shape, or texture.
- **Biopsy:** A procedure to remove the abnormal tissue and a small amount of normal tissue around it. A pathologist looks at the tissue under a microscope to check for cancer cells. It can be hard to tell the difference between a colored mole and an early melanoma lesion. Patients may want to have the sample of tissue checked by a second pathologist. If the abnormal mole or lesion is cancer, the sample of tissue may also be tested for certain gene changes.

It is important that abnormal areas of the skin not be shaved off or cauterized (destroyed with a hot instrument, an electric current, or a caustic substance) because cancer cells that remain may grow and spread.

Stages of Melanoma

After melanoma has been diagnosed, tests are done to find out if cancer cells have spread within the skin or to other parts of the body.

The process used to find out whether cancer has spread within the skin or to other parts of the body is called staging. The information gathered from the staging process determines the stage of the disease. It is important to know the stage in order to plan treatment.

The following tests and procedures may be used in the staging process:

- **Physical exam and history:** An exam of the body to check general signs of health, including checking for signs of disease, such as lumps or anything else that seems unusual. A history of the patient's health habits and past illnesses and treatments will also be taken.
- **Lymph node mapping and sentinel lymph node biopsy:** Procedures in which a radioactive substance and/or blue dye is injected near the tumor. The substance or dye flows through lymph ducts to the sentinel node or nodes (the first lymph node or nodes where cancer cells are likely to spread). The surgeon removes only the nodes with the radioactive substance or dye. A pathologist views a sample of tissue under a microscope to check for cancer cells. If no cancer cells are found, it may not be necessary to remove more nodes.
- **Computed tomography (CT)/computerized axial tomography (CAT) scan:** A procedure that makes a series of detailed pictures of areas inside the body taken from different angles. The pictures are made by a computer linked to an X-ray machine. A dye may be injected into a vein or swallowed to help the organs or tissues show up more clearly. For melanoma, pictures may be taken of the chest, abdomen, and pelvis.
- **Positron emission tomography (PET) scan:** A procedure to find malignant tumor cells in the body. A small amount of radioactive glucose (sugar) is injected into a vein. The PET scanner rotates around the body and makes a picture of where glucose is being used in the body. Malignant tumor cells show up brighter in the picture because they are more active and take up more glucose than normal cells do.
- **Magnetic resonance imaging (MRI) with gadolinium:** A procedure that uses a magnet, radio waves, and a computer to make a series of detailed pictures of areas inside the body, such as the brain. A substance called gadolinium is injected into a vein. The gadolinium collects around the cancer cells so they

show up brighter in the picture. This procedure is also called nuclear magnetic resonance imaging (NMRI).

- **Blood chemistry studies:** A procedure in which a blood sample is checked to measure the amounts of certain substances released into the blood by organs and tissues in the body. For melanoma, the blood is checked for an enzyme called lactate dehydrogenase (LDH). LDH levels that are higher than normal may be a sign of melanoma.

The results of these tests are viewed together with the results of the tumor biopsy to find out the stage of the melanoma.

What Is Method Used for Staging Melanoma Based Upon?

The method used to stage melanoma is based mainly on the thickness of the tumor and whether cancer has spread to lymph nodes or other parts of the body.

The staging of melanoma depends on the following:

- The thickness of the tumor. The thickness is described using the Breslow scale
- Whether the tumor is ulcerated (has broken through the skin)
- Whether the tumor has spread to the lymph nodes and if the lymph nodes are joined together (matted)
- Whether the tumor has spread to other parts of the body

The following stages are used for melanoma:

Stage 0 (melanoma in situ). In stage 0, abnormal melanocytes are found in the epidermis. These abnormal melanocytes may become cancer and spread into nearby normal tissue. Stage 0 is also called melanoma in situ.

Stage I. In stage I, cancer has formed. Stage I is divided into stages IA and IB.

- **Stage IA:** In stage IA, the tumor is not more than 1 millimeter thick, with no ulceration.
- **Stage IB:** In stage IB, the tumor is either:
    - not more than 1 millimeter thick and it has ulceration; or
    - more than 1 but not more than 2 millimeters thick, with no ulceration

Stage II. Stage II is divided into stages IIA, IIB, and IIC.

- **Stage IIA:** In stage IIA, the tumor is either:
    - more than 1 but not more than 2 millimeters thick, with ulceration; or
    - more than 2 but not more than 4 millimeters thick, with no ulceration
- **Stage IIB:** In stage IIB, the tumor is either:
    - more than 2 but not more than 4 millimeters thick, with ulceration; or
    - more than 4 millimeters thick, with no ulceration
- **Stage IIC:** In stage IIC, the tumor is more than 4 millimeters thick, with ulceration.

Stage III. In stage III, the tumor may be any thickness, with or without ulceration. One or more of the following is true:

- Cancer has spread to one or more lymph nodes.
- Lymph nodes are joined together (matted).
- Cancer is in a lymph vessel between the primary tumor and nearby lymph nodes. The cancer is more than 2 centimeters away from the primary tumor.
- Very small tumors are found on or under the skin, not more than 2 centimeters away from the primary tumor.

Stage IV. In stage IV, the cancer has spread to other places in the body, such as the lung, liver, brain, bone, soft tissue, or gastrointestinal (GI) tract. Cancer may have spread to places in the skin far away from where it first started.

Treatment Options

Five types of standard treatment are used:

Surgery

Surgery to remove the tumor is the primary treatment of all stages of melanoma. A wide local excision is used to remove the melanoma and some of the normal tissue around it. Skin grafting (taking skin from another part of the body to replace the skin that is removed) may be done to cover the wound caused by surgery.

It is important to know whether cancer has spread to the lymph nodes. Lymph node mapping and sentinel lymph node biopsy are done to check for cancer in the sentinel lymph node (the first lymph node the cancer is likely to spread to from the tumor) during surgery. A radioactive substance and/or blue dye is injected near the tumor. The substance or dye flows through the lymph ducts to the lymph nodes. The first lymph node to receive the substance or dye is removed. A pathologist views the tissue under a microscope to look for cancer cells. If cancer cells are found, more lymph nodes will be removed and tissue samples will be checked for signs of cancer. This is called a lymphadenectomy.

Even if the doctor removes all the melanoma that can be seen at the time of surgery, some patients may be given chemotherapy after surgery to kill any cancer cells that are left. Chemotherapy given after surgery, to lower the risk that the cancer will come back, is called adjuvant therapy.

Surgery to remove cancer that has spread to the lymph nodes, lung, gastrointestinal (GI) tract, bone, or brain may be done to improve the patient's quality of life by controlling symptoms.

Chemotherapy

Chemotherapy is a cancer treatment that uses drugs to stop the growth of cancer cells, either by killing the cells or by stopping them from dividing. When chemotherapy is taken by mouth or injected into a vein or muscle, the drugs enter the bloodstream and can reach cancer cells throughout the body (systemic chemotherapy). When chemotherapy is placed directly into the cerebrospinal fluid, an organ, or a body cavity such as the abdomen, the drugs mainly affect cancer cells in those areas (regional chemotherapy (RCT)).

One type of regional chemotherapy is hyperthermic isolated limb perfusion. With this method, anticancer drugs go directly to the arm or leg the cancer is in. The flow of blood to and from the limb is temporarily stopped with a tourniquet. A warm solution with the anticancer drug is put directly into the blood of the limb. This gives a high dose of drugs to the area where the cancer is.

The way the chemotherapy is given depends on the type and stage of the cancer being treated.

Radiation Therapy

Radiation therapy is a cancer treatment that uses high-energy X-rays or other types of radiation to kill cancer cells or keep them from growing. There are two types of radiation therapy:

- External radiation therapy uses a machine outside the body to send radiation toward the cancer.
- Internal radiation therapy uses a radioactive substance sealed in needles, seeds, wires, or catheters that are placed directly into or near the cancer.

The way the radiation therapy is given depends on the type and stage of the cancer being treated. External radiation therapy is used to treat melanoma, and may also be used as palliative therapy to relieve symptoms and improve quality of life.

Immunotherapy

Immunotherapy is a treatment that uses the patient's immune system to fight cancer. Substances made by the body or made in a laboratory are used to boost, direct, or restore the body's natural defenses against cancer. This type of cancer treatment is also called biotherapy or biologic therapy.

The following types of immunotherapy are being used in the treatment of melanoma:

- **Immune checkpoint inhibitor therapy:** Some types of immune cells, such as T cells, and some cancer cells have certain proteins, called checkpoint proteins, on their surface that keep immune responses in check. When cancer cells have large amounts of these proteins, they will not be attacked and killed by T cells. Immune checkpoint inhibitors block these proteins and the ability of T cells to kill cancer cells is increased. They are used to treat some patients with advanced melanoma or tumors that cannot be removed by surgery.

  There are two types of immune checkpoint inhibitor therapy:

  - **CTLA-4 inhibitor:** CTLA-4 is a protein on the surface of T cells that helps keep the body's immune responses in check. When CTLA-4 attaches to another protein called B7 on a cancer cell, it stops the T cell from killing the cancer cell.

CTLA-4 inhibitors attach to CTLA-4 and allow the T cells to kill cancer cells. Ipilimumab is a type of CTLA-4 inhibitor.

- **PD-1 inhibitor:** PD-1 is a protein on the surface of T cells that helps keep the body's immune responses in check. When PD-1 attaches to another protein called PDL-1 on a cancer cell, it stops the T cell from killing the cancer cell. PD-1 inhibitors attach to PDL-1 and allow the T cells to kill cancer cells. Pembrolizumab and nivolumab are types of PD-1 inhibitors.

- **Interferon:** Interferon affects the division of cancer cells and can slow tumor growth.
- **Interleukin-2 (IL-2):** IL-2 boosts the growth and activity of many immune cells, especially lymphocytes (a type of white blood cell). Lymphocytes can attack and kill cancer cells.
- **Tumor necrosis factor (TNF) therapy:** TNF is a protein made by white blood cells in response to an antigen or infection. TNF is made in the laboratory and used as a treatment to kill cancer cells. It is being studied in the treatment of melanoma.

Targeted Therapy

Targeted therapy is a type of treatment that uses drugs or other substances to attack cancer cells. Targeted therapies usually cause less harm to normal cells than chemotherapy or radiation therapy do. The following types of targeted therapy are used or being studied in the treatment of melanoma:

- **Signal transduction inhibitor (STI) therapy:** Signal transduction inhibitors block signals that are passed from one molecule to another inside a cell. Blocking these signals may kill cancer cells.
    - Vemurafenib, dabrafenib, trametinib, and cobimetinib are signal transduction inhibitors used to treat some patients with advanced melanoma or tumors that cannot be removed by surgery. Vemurafenib and dabrafenib block the activity of proteins made by mutant *BRAF* genes. Trametinib and cobimetinib affect the growth and survival of cancer cells.
- **Oncolytic virus therapy:** A type of targeted therapy that is used in the treatment of melanoma. Oncolytic virus therapy uses a virus that infects and breaks down cancer cells but not normal

cells. Radiation therapy or chemotherapy may be given after oncolytic virus therapy to kill more cancer cells.

- **Angiogenesis inhibitors:** A type of targeted therapy that is being studied in the treatment of melanoma. Angiogenesis inhibitors block the growth of new blood vessels. In cancer treatment, they may be given to prevent the growth of new blood vessels that tumors need to grow.

New targeted therapies and combinations of therapies are being studied in the treatment of melanoma.

What New Types of Treatment Are Being Tested in Clinical Trials?

Vaccine Therapy

Vaccine therapy uses a substance or group of substances meant to cause the immune system to respond to a tumor and kill it. Vaccine therapy is being studied in the treatment of stage III melanoma that can be removed by surgery.

Is There a Need for Follow-Up Tests?

Some of the tests that were done to diagnose the cancer or to find out the stage of the cancer may be repeated. Some tests will be repeated in order to see how well the treatment is working. Decisions about whether to continue, change, or stop treatment may be based on the results of these tests.

Some of the tests will continue to be done from time to time after treatment has ended. The results of these tests can show if your condition has changed or if the cancer has recurred (come back). These tests are sometimes called follow-up tests or check-ups.

What Is the Prognosis for Melanoma?

The prognosis (chance of recovery) and treatment options depend on the following:

- The thickness of the tumor and where it is in the body
- How quickly the cancer cells are dividing
- Whether there was bleeding or ulceration of the tumor
- How much cancer is in the lymph nodes

- The number of places cancer has spread to in the body
- The level of lactate dehydrogenase (LDH) in the blood
- Whether the cancer has certain mutations (changes) in a gene called *BRAF*
- The patient's age and general health

Chapter 53

Merkel Cell Carcinoma

What Is Merkel Cell Carcinoma?

Merkel cells are found in the top layer of the skin. These cells are very close to the nerve endings that receive the sensation of touch.

Merkel cell carcinoma, also called neuroendocrine carcinoma of the skin or trabecular cancer, is a very rare type of skin cancer that forms when Merkel cells grow out of control. It starts most often in areas of skin exposed to the sun, especially the head and neck, as well as the arms, legs, and trunk.

Merkel cell carcinoma tends to grow quickly and to metastasize (spread) at an early stage. It usually spreads first to nearby lymph nodes and then may spread to lymph nodes or skin in distant parts of the body, lungs, brain, bones, or other organs.

What Are the Risk Factors for Merkel Cell Carcinoma?

Anything that increases your risk of getting a disease is called a risk factor. Having a risk factor does not mean that you will get cancer; not having risk factors doesn't mean that you will not get cancer. Talk with your doctor if you think you may be at risk.

This chapter includes text excerpted from "Merkel Cell Carcinoma Treatment (PDQ®)—Patient Version," National Cancer Institute (NCI), January 19, 2018.

Sun exposure and having a weak immune system can affect the risk of Merkel cell carcinoma. Risk factors for Merkel cell carcinoma include the following:

- Being exposed to a lot of natural sunlight
- Being exposed to artificial sunlight, such as from tanning beds or psoralen and ultraviolet A (PUVA) therapy for psoriasis
- Having an immune system weakened by disease, such as chronic lymphocytic leukemia or human immunodeficiency virus (HIV) infection
- Taking drugs that make the immune system less active, such as after an organ transplant
- Having a history of other types of cancer
- Being older than 50 years, male, or white

What Are the Signs and Symptoms of Merkel Cell Carcinoma?

Merkel cell carcinoma usually appears as a single painless lump on sun-exposed skin. This and other changes in the skin may be caused by Merkel cell carcinoma or by other conditions. Check with your doctor if you see changes in your skin.

Merkel cell carcinoma usually appears on sun-exposed skin as a single lump that is:

- Fast growing
- Painless
- Firm and dome-shaped or raised
- Red or violet in color

How Is Merkel Cell Carcinoma Diagnosed?

Tests and procedures that examine the skin are used to detect (find) and diagnose Merkel cell carcinoma.

The following tests and procedures may be used:

- **Physical exam and history:** An exam of the body to check general signs of health, including checking for signs of disease, such as lumps or anything else that seems unusual. A history

of the patient's health habits and past illnesses and treatments will also be taken.

- **Full body skin exam:** A doctor or nurse checks the skin for bumps or spots that look abnormal in color, size, shape, or texture. The size, shape, and texture of the lymph nodes will also be checked.
- **Skin biopsy:** The removal of skin cells or tissues so they can be viewed under a microscope by a pathologist to check for signs of cancer.

Stages of Merkel Cell Carcinoma

After Merkel cell carcinoma has been diagnosed, tests are done to find out if cancer cells have spread to other parts of the body.

The process used to find out if cancer has spread to other parts of the body is called staging. The information gathered from the staging process determines the stage of the disease. It is important to know the stage in order to plan treatment.

The following tests and procedures may be used in the staging process:

- **Computed tomography (CT)/computerized axial tomography (CAT) scan:** A procedure that makes a series of detailed pictures of areas inside the body, taken from different angles. The pictures are made by a computer linked to an X-ray machine. A dye may be injected into a vein or swallowed to help the organs or tissues show up more clearly. A CT scan of the chest and abdomen may be used to check for primary small cell lung cancer, or to find Merkel cell carcinoma that has spread. A CT scan of the head and neck may also be used to find Merkel cell carcinoma that has spread to the lymph nodes.
- **Positron emission tomography (PET) scan:** A procedure to find malignant tumor cells in the body. A small amount of radioactive glucose (sugar) is injected into a vein. The PET scanner rotates around the body and makes a picture of where glucose is being used in the body. Malignant tumor cells show up brighter in the picture because they are more active and take up more glucose than normal cells do.
- **Lymph node biopsy:** There are two main types of lymph node biopsy used to stage Merkel cell carcinoma.

- **Sentinel lymph node biopsy:** The removal of the sentinel lymph node during surgery. The sentinel lymph node is the first lymph node to receive lymphatic drainage from a tumor. It is the first lymph node the cancer is likely to spread to from the tumor. A radioactive substance and/or blue dye is injected near the tumor. The substance or dye flows through the lymph ducts to the lymph nodes. The first lymph node to receive the substance or dye is removed. A pathologist views the tissue under a microscope to look for cancer cells. If cancer cells are not found, it may not be necessary to remove more lymph nodes.
- **Lymph node dissection:** A surgical procedure in which the lymph nodes are removed and a sample of tissue is checked under a microscope for signs of cancer. For a regional lymph node dissection, some of the lymph nodes in the tumor area are removed. For a radical lymph node dissection, most or all of the lymph nodes in the tumor area are removed. This procedure is also called lymphadenectomy.
- **Core needle biopsy:** A procedure to remove a sample of tissue using a wide needle. A pathologist views the tissue under a microscope to look for cancer cells.
- **Fine-needle aspiration biopsy:** A procedure to remove a sample of tissue using a thin needle. A pathologist views the tissue under a microscope to look for cancer cells.

- **Immunohistochemistry:** A test that uses antibodies to check for certain antigens in a sample of tissue. The antibody is usually linked to a radioactive substance or a dye that causes the tissue to light up under a microscope. This type of test may be used to tell the difference between different types of cancer.

The following stages are used for Merkel cell carcinoma:

Stage 0 (carcinoma in situ). In stage 0, abnormal Merkel cells are found in the top layer of skin. These abnormal cells may become cancer and spread into nearby normal tissue.

Stage I. In stage I, the tumor is 2 centimeters or smaller.

Stage II. Stage II Merkel cell carcinoma is divided into stages IIA and IIB.

- In stage IIA, the tumor is larger than 2 centimeters.

- In stage IIB, the tumor has spread to nearby connective tissue, muscle, cartilage, or bone.

Stage III. Stage III Merkel cell carcinoma is divided into stages IIIA and IIIB.

- In stage IIIA, either of the following is found:
    - the tumor may be any size and may have spread to nearby connective tissue, muscle, cartilage, or bone. A lymph node cannot be felt during a physical exam but cancer is found in the lymph node by sentinel lymph node biopsy or after the lymph node is removed and checked under a microscope for signs of cancer; or
    - a swollen lymph node is felt during a physical exam and/or seen on an imaging test. When the lymph node is removed and checked under a microscope for signs of cancer, cancer is found in the lymph node. The place where the cancer began is not known.
- In stage IIIB, the tumor may be any size and:
    - may have spread to nearby connective tissue, muscle, cartilage, or bone. A swollen lymph node is felt during a physical exam and/or seen on an imaging test. When the lymph node is removed and checked under a microscope for signs of cancer, cancer is found in the lymph node; or
    - cancer is in a lymph vessel between the primary tumor and lymph nodes that are near or far away. Cancer may have spread to lymph nodes.

Stage IV. In stage IV, the tumor has spread to skin that is not close to the primary tumor or to other parts of the body, such as the liver, lung, bone, or brain.

Treatment Options

Three types of standard treatment are used:

Surgery

One or more of the following surgical procedures may be used to treat Merkel cell carcinoma:

- **Wide local excision:** The cancer is cut from the skin along with some of the tissue around it. A sentinel lymph node biopsy may be done during the wide local excision procedure. If there is cancer in the lymph nodes, a lymph node dissection also may be done.

- **Lymph node dissection:** A surgical procedure in which the lymph nodes are removed and a sample of tissue is checked under a microscope for signs of cancer. For a regional lymph node dissection, some of the lymph nodes in the tumor area are removed; for a radical lymph node dissection, most or all of the lymph nodes in the tumor area are removed. This procedure is also called lymphadenectomy.

Even if the doctor removes all the cancer that can be seen at the time of the surgery, some patients may be given chemotherapy or radiation therapy after surgery to kill any cancer cells that are left. Treatment given after the surgery, to lower the risk that the cancer will come back, is called adjuvant therapy.

Radiation Therapy

Radiation therapy is a cancer treatment that uses high-energy X-rays or other types of radiation to kill cancer cells or keep them from growing. There are two types of radiation therapy:

- External radiation therapy uses a machine outside the body to send radiation toward the cancer.
- Internal radiation therapy uses a radioactive substance sealed in needles, seeds, wires, or catheters that are placed directly into or near the cancer.

The way the radiation therapy is given depends on the type and stage of the cancer being treated. External radiation therapy is used to treat Merkel cell carcinoma, and may also be used as palliative therapy to relieve symptoms and improve quality of life.

Chemotherapy

Chemotherapy is a cancer treatment that uses drugs to stop the growth of cancer cells, either by killing the cells or by stopping the cells from dividing. When chemotherapy is taken by mouth or injected into a vein or muscle, the drugs enter the bloodstream and can reach cancer cells throughout the body (systemic chemotherapy). When chemotherapy is placed directly into the cerebrospinal fluid, an organ, or a body cavity such as the abdomen, the drugs mainly affect cancer cells in those areas (regional chemotherapy). The way the chemotherapy is given depends on the type and stage of the cancer being treated.

Treatment for Merkel cell carcinoma may cause side effects.

Is There a Need for Follow-Up Tests?

Some of the tests that were done to diagnose the cancer or to find out the stage of the cancer may be repeated. Some tests will be repeated in order to see how well the treatment is working. Decisions about whether to continue, change, or stop treatment may be based on the results of these tests.

Some of the tests will continue to be done from time to time after treatment has ended. The results of these tests can show if your condition has changed or if the cancer has recurred (come back). These tests are sometimes called follow-up tests or check-ups.

What Is the Prognosis for Merkel Cell Carcinoma?

The prognosis (chance of recovery) and treatment options depend on the following:

- The stage of the cancer (the size of the tumor and whether it has spread to the lymph nodes or other parts of the body)
- Where the cancer is in the body
- Whether the cancer has just been diagnosed or has recurred (come back)
- The patient's age and general health

Prognosis also depends on how deeply the tumor has grown into the skin.

Chapter 54

Bone Cancers

Chapter Contents

Section 54.1

Overview of Bone Cancer

This section includes text excerpted from "Bone Cancer," National Cancer Institute (NCI), March 13, 2008. Reviewed March 2018.

What Is Bone Cancer?

Bone cancer is a malignant (cancerous) tumor of the bone that destroys normal bone tissue. Not all bone tumors are malignant. In fact, benign (noncancerous) bone tumors are more common than malignant ones. Both malignant and benign bone tumors may grow and compress healthy bone tissue, but benign tumors do not spread, do not destroy bone tissue, and are rarely a threat to life.

Malignant tumors that begin in bone tissue are called primary bone cancer. Cancer that metastasizes (spreads) to the bones from other parts of the body, such as the breast, lung, or prostate, is called metastatic cancer, and is named for the organ or tissue in which it began. Primary bone cancer is far less common than cancer that spreads to the bones.

Are There Different Types of Primary Bone Cancer?

Yes. Cancer can begin in any type of bone tissue. Bones are made up of osteoid (hard or compact), cartilaginous (tough, flexible), and fibrous (thread-like) tissue, as well as elements of bone marrow (soft, spongy tissue in the center of most bones).

Common types of primary bone cancer include the following:

- **Osteosarcoma,** which arises from osteoid tissue in the bone. This tumor occurs most often in the knee and upper arm.
- **Chondrosarcoma**, which begins in cartilaginous tissue. Cartilage pads the ends of bones and lines the joints. Chondrosarcoma occurs most often in the pelvis (located between the hip bones), upper leg, and shoulder. Sometimes a chondrosarcoma contains cancerous bone cells. In that case, doctors classify the tumor as an osteosarcoma.

- The **Ewing sarcoma family of tumors (ESFTs)**, which usually occur in bone but may also arise in soft tissue (muscle, fat, fibrous tissue, blood vessels, or other supporting tissue). Scientists think that ESFTs arise from elements of primitive nerve tissue in the bone or soft tissue. ESFTs occur most commonly along the backbone and pelvis and in the legs and arms.

Other types of cancer that arise in soft tissue are called soft tissue sarcomas. They are not bone cancer.

What Are the Possible Causes of Bone Cancer?

Although bone cancer does not have a clearly defined cause, researchers have identified several factors that increase the likelihood of developing these tumors. Osteosarcoma occurs more frequently in people who have had high dose external radiation therapy or treatment with certain anticancer drugs; children seem to be particularly susceptible. A small number of bone cancers are due to heredity. For example, children who have had hereditary retinoblastoma (an uncommon cancer of the eye) are at a higher risk of developing osteosarcoma, particularly if they are treated with radiation. Additionally, people who have hereditary defects of bones and people with metal implants, which doctors sometimes use to repair fractures, are more likely to develop osteosarcoma. Ewing sarcoma is not strongly associated with any hereditary cancer syndromes (HCS), congenital childhood diseases (CCD), or previous radiation exposure.

How Often Does Bone Cancer Occur?

Primary bone cancer is rare. It accounts for much less than 1 percent of all cancers. About 2,300 new cases of primary bone cancer are diagnosed in the United States each year. Different types of bone cancer are more likely to occur in certain populations:

- Osteosarcoma occurs most commonly between ages 10–19. However, people over age 40 who have other conditions, such as Paget disease (a benign condition characterized by abnormal development of new bone cells), are at increased risk of developing this cancer.
- Chondrosarcoma occurs mainly in older adults (over age 40). The risk increases with advancing age. This disease rarely occurs in children and adolescents.

- ESFTs occur most often in children and adolescents under 19 years of age. Boys are affected more often than girls. These tumors are extremely rare in African American children.

What Are the Symptoms of Bone Cancer?

Pain is the most common symptom of bone cancer, but not all bone cancers cause pain. Persistent or unusual pain or swelling in or near a bone can be caused by cancer or by other conditions. It is important to see a doctor to determine the cause.

How Is Bone Cancer Diagnosed?

To help diagnose bone cancer, the doctor asks about the patient's personal and family medical history. The doctor also performs a physical examination and may order laboratory and other diagnostic tests. These tests may include the following:

- **X-rays**, which can show the location, size, and shape of a bone tumor. If X-rays suggest that an abnormal area may be cancer, the doctor is likely to recommend special imaging tests. Even if X-rays suggest that an abnormal area is benign, the doctor may want to do further tests, especially if the patient is experiencing unusual or persistent pain.
    - A **bone scan**, which is a test in which a small amount of radioactive material is injected into a blood vessel and travels through the bloodstream; it then collects in the bones and is detected by a scanner.
    - A **computed tomography (CT)/computerized axial tomography (CAT) scan**, which is a series of detailed pictures of areas inside the body, taken from different angles, that are created by a computer linked to an X-ray machine.
    - A **magnetic resonance imaging (MRI) procedure**, which uses a powerful magnet linked to a computer to create detailed pictures of areas inside the body without using X-rays.
    - A **positron emission tomography (PET) scan**, in which a small amount of radioactive glucose (sugar) is injected into a vein, and a scanner is used to make detailed, computerized pictures of areas inside the body where the glucose is used. Because cancer cells often use more glucose than normal cells, the pictures can be used to find cancer cells in the body.

  - An **angiogram**, which is an X-ray of blood vessels.
- **Biopsy** (removal of a tissue sample from the bone tumor) to determine whether cancer is present. The surgeon may perform a needle biopsy or an incisional biopsy. During a needle biopsy, the surgeon makes a small hole in the bone and removes a sample of tissue from the tumor with a needle-like instrument. In an incisional biopsy, the surgeon cuts into the tumor and removes a sample of tissue. Biopsies are best done by an orthopedic oncologist (a doctor experienced in the treatment of bone cancer). A pathologist (a doctor who identifies disease by studying cells and tissues under a microscope) examines the tissue to determine whether it is cancerous.
- **Blood tests** to determine the level of an enzyme called alkaline phosphatase. A large amount of this enzyme is present in the blood when the cells that form bone tissue are very active—when children are growing, when a broken bone is mending, or when a disease or tumor causes production of abnormal bone tissue. Because high levels of alkaline phosphatase are normal in growing children and adolescents, this test is not a completely reliable indicator of bone cancer.

What Are the Treatment Options for Bone Cancer?

Treatment options depend on the type, size, location, and stage of the cancer, as well as the person's age and general health. Treatment options for bone cancer include surgery, chemotherapy, radiation therapy, and cryosurgery.

- **Surgery** is the usual treatment for bone cancer. The surgeon removes the entire tumor with negative margins (no cancer cells are found at the edge or border of the tissue removed during surgery). The surgeon may also use special surgical techniques to minimize the amount of healthy tissue removed with the tumor.

  Dramatic improvements in surgical techniques and preoperative tumor treatment have made it possible for most patients with bone cancer in an arm or leg to avoid radical surgical procedures (removal of the entire limb). However, most patients who undergo limb sparing surgery need reconstructive surgery to maximize limb function.
- **Chemotherapy** is the use of anticancer drugs to kill cancer cells. Patients who have bone cancer usually receive a

combination of anticancer drugs. However, chemotherapy is not currently used to treat chondrosarcoma.

- **Radiation therapy**, also called radiotherapy, involves the use of high energy X-rays to kill cancer cells. This treatment may be used in combination with surgery. It is often used to treat chondrosarcoma, which cannot be treated with chemotherapy, as well as ESFTs. It may also be used for patients who refuse surgery.
- **Cryosurgery** is the use of liquid nitrogen to freeze and kill cancer cells. This technique can sometimes be used instead of conventional surgery to destroy the tumor.

Is Follow-Up Treatment Necessary? What Does It Involve?

Yes. Bone cancer sometimes metastasizes, particularly to the lungs, or can recur (come back), either at the same location or in other bones in the body. People who have had bone cancer should see their doctor regularly and should report any unusual symptoms right away. Follow-up varies for different types and stages of bone cancer. Generally, patients are checked frequently by their doctor and have regular blood tests and X-rays. People who have had bone cancer, particularly children and adolescents, have an increased likelihood of developing another type of cancer, such as leukemia, later in life. Regular follow-up care ensures that changes in health are discussed and that problems are treated as soon as possible.

Section 54.2

Osteosarcoma and Malignant Fibrous Histiocytoma of Bone

This section includes text excerpted from "Osteosarcoma and Malignant Fibrous Histiocytoma of Bone Treatment (PDQ®)—Patient Version," National Cancer Institute (NCI), January 5, 2018.

What Is Osteosarcoma and Malignant Fibrous Histiocytoma (MFH) of the Bone

Osteosarcoma and malignant fibrous histiocytoma (MFH) of the bone are diseases in which malignant (cancer) cells form in bone.

Osteosarcoma usually starts in osteoblasts, which are a type of bone cell that becomes new bone tissue. Osteosarcoma is most common in adolescents. It commonly forms in the ends of the long bones of the body, which include bones of the arms and legs. In children and adolescents, it often forms in the long bones, near the knee. Rarely, osteosarcoma may be found in soft tissue or organs in the chest or abdomen.

Osteosarcoma is the most common type of bone cancer. MFH of bone is a rare tumor of the bone. It is treated like osteosarcoma.

What Are the Risk Factors for Osteosarcoma and MFH?

Having past treatment with radiation can increase the risk of osteosarcoma. Anything that increases your risk of getting a disease is called a risk factor. Having a risk factor does not mean that you will get cancer; not having risk factors doesn't mean that you will not get cancer. Talk with your child's doctor if you think your child may be at risk. Risk factors for osteosarcoma include the following:

- Past treatment with radiation therapy
- Past treatment with anticancer drugs called alkylating agents
- Having a certain change in the *RB1* gene
- Having certain conditions, such as the following:
    - Bloom syndrome

- Diamond-Blackfan anemia
- Li-Fraumeni syndrome
- Paget disease
- Hereditary retinoblastoma
- Rothmund-Thomson syndrome
- Werner syndrome

What Are the Signs and Symptoms of Osteosarcoma and MFH?

Signs and symptoms of osteosarcoma and MFH include swelling over a bone or a bony part of the body and joint pain. These and other signs and symptoms may be caused by osteosarcoma or MFH or by other conditions. Check with a doctor if your child has any of the following:

- Swelling over a bone or bony part of the body
- Pain in a bone or joint
- A bone that breaks for no known reason

How Is Osteosarcoma and MFH Diagnosed?

Imaging tests are used to detect (find) osteosarcoma and MFH. Imaging tests are done before a biopsy. The following tests and procedures may be used:

- **Physical exam and history:** An exam of the body to check general signs of health, including checking for signs of disease, such as lumps or anything else that seems unusual. A history of the patient's health habits and past illnesses and treatments will also be taken.
- **X-ray:** An X-ray of the organs and bones inside the body. An X-ray is a type of energy beam that can go through the body and onto film, making a picture of areas inside the body.
- **Computerized tomography (CT)/computerized axial tomography (CAT) scan:** A procedure that makes a series of detailed pictures of areas inside the body, taken from different

angles. The pictures are made by a computer linked to an X-ray machine. A dye may be injected into a vein or swallowed to help the organs or tissues show up more clearly.

- **Magnetic resonance imaging (MRI):** A procedure that uses a magnet, radio waves, and a computer to make a series of detailed pictures of areas inside the body. This procedure is also called nuclear magnetic resonance imaging (NMRI).

Biopsy

A biopsy is done to diagnose osteosarcoma. Cells and tissues are removed during a biopsy so they can be viewed under a microscope by a pathologist to check for signs of cancer. It is important that the biopsy be done by a surgeon who is an expert in treating cancer of the bone. It is best if that surgeon is also the one who removes the tumor. The biopsy and the surgery to remove the tumor are planned together. The way the biopsy is done affects which type of surgery can be done later.

The type of biopsy that is done will be based on the size of the tumor and where it is in the body. There are two types of biopsy that may be used:

- **Core biopsy:** The removal of tissue using a wide needle.
- **Incisional biopsy:** The removal of part of a lump or a sample of tissue that doesn't look normal.

The following test may be done on the tissue that is removed:

- **Electron microscopy:** A laboratory test in which cells in a sample of tissue are viewed under regular and high-powered microscopes to look for certain changes in the cells.

How Is Staging Done for Osteosarcoma and MFH of Bone?

After osteosarcoma or MFH has been diagnosed, tests are done to find out if cancer cells have spread to other parts of the body. The process used to find out if cancer has spread to other parts of the body is called staging. For osteosarcoma and MFH, most patients are grouped according to whether cancer is found in only one part of the body (localized) or has spread (metastatic).

The following tests and procedures may be used:

- **X-ray**: An X-ray of the organs, such as the chest, and bones inside the body. An X-ray is a type of energy beam that can go through the body and onto film, making a picture of areas inside the body. X-rays will be taken of the chest and the area where the tumor formed.
- **Computed tomography (CT/CAT) scan**: A procedure that makes a series of detailed pictures of areas inside the body, such as the chest, taken from different angles. The pictures are made by a computer linked to an X-ray machine. A dye may be injected into a vein or swallowed to help the organs or tissues show up more clearly. Pictures will be taken of the chest and the area where the tumor formed.
- **Positron emission tomography (PET)-CT scan**: A procedure that combines the pictures from a PET scan and a CT scan. The PET and CT scans are done at the same time on the same machine. The pictures from both scans are combined to make a more detailed picture than either test would make by itself. A PET scan is a procedure to find malignant tumor cells in the body. A small amount of radioactive glucose (sugar) is injected into a vein. The PET scanner rotates around the body and makes a picture of where glucose is being used in the body. Malignant tumor cells show up brighter in the picture because they are more active and take up more glucose than normal cells do.
- **Magnetic resonance imaging (MRI)**: A procedure that uses a magnet, radio waves, and a computer to make a series of detailed pictures of areas inside the body. This procedure is also called nuclear magnetic resonance imaging (NMRI).
- **Bone scan:** A procedure to check if there are rapidly dividing cells, such as cancer cells, in the bone. A very small amount of radioactive material is injected into a vein and travels through the bloodstream. The radioactive material collects in the bones with cancer and is detected by a scanner.

What Does the Healthcare Team for Children with Osteosarcoma or MFH Look Like?

Treatment will be overseen by a pediatric oncologist, a doctor who specializes in treating children with cancer. The pediatric oncologist works with other pediatric healthcare providers who are experts in treating osteosarcoma and MFH and who specialize in certain areas of medicine. These may include the following specialists:

- Pediatrician
- Orthopedic surgeon who has experience treating bone tumors
- Radiation oncologist
- Rehabilitation specialist
- Pediatric nurse specialist
- Social worker
- Child-life specialist
- Psychologist

Treatment for osteosarcoma or malignant fibrous histiocytoma may cause side effects.

Side effects from cancer treatment that begin after treatment and continue for months or years are called late effects. Late effects of cancer treatment may include the following:

- Physical problems
- Changes in mood, feelings, thinking, learning, or memory
- Second cancers (new types of cancer)

Some late effects may be treated or controlled. It is important to talk with your child's doctors about the effects cancer treatment can have on your child.

What Standard Treatment Options Are Available for People with Osteosarcoma and MFH?

Five types of standard treatment are used:

Surgery

Surgery to remove the entire tumor will be done when possible. Chemotherapy may be given before surgery to make the tumor smaller. This is called neoadjuvant chemotherapy. Chemotherapy is given so less bone tissue needs to be removed and there are fewer problems after surgery.

The following types of surgery may be done:

- **Wide local excision:** Surgery to remove the cancer and some healthy tissue around it.
- **Limb-sparing surgery:** Removal of the tumor in a limb (arm or leg) without amputation, so the use and appearance of the limb is saved. Most patients with osteosarcoma in a limb can be treated with limb-sparing surgery. The tumor is removed by wide local excision. Tissue and bone that are removed may be replaced with a graft using tissue and bone taken from another part of the patient's body, or with an implant such as artificial bone. If a fracture is found at the time of diagnosis or during chemotherapy before surgery, limb-sparing surgery may still be possible in some cases. If the surgeon is not able to remove all of the tumor and enough healthy tissue around it, an amputation may be done.
- **Amputation:** Surgery to remove part or all of an arm or leg. This may be done when it is not possible to remove all of the tumor in limb-sparing surgery. The patient may be fitted with a prosthesis (artificial limb) after amputation.
- **Rotationplasty:** Surgery to remove the tumor and the knee joint. The part of the leg that remains below the knee is then attached to the part of the leg that remains above the knee, with the foot facing backward and the ankle acting as a knee. A prosthesis may then be attached to the foot.

Studies have shown that survival is the same whether the first surgery done is a limb-sparing surgery or an amputation. Even if the doctor removes all the cancer that can be seen at the time of the surgery, patients are also given chemotherapy after surgery to kill any cancer cells that are left in the area where the tumor was removed or that have spread to other parts of the body. Treatment given after the surgery, to lower the risk that the cancer will come back, is called adjuvant therapy.

Chemotherapy

Chemotherapy is a cancer treatment that uses drugs to stop the growth of cancer cells, either by killing the cells or by stopping them from dividing. When chemotherapy is taken by mouth or injected into a vein or muscle, the drugs enter the bloodstream and can reach cancer cells throughout the body (systemic chemotherapy). When chemotherapy is placed directly into the cerebrospinal fluid, an organ, or a body cavity such as the abdomen, the drugs mainly affect cancer cells in those areas (regional chemotherapy).

Combination chemotherapy is the use of more than one anticancer drug.

Systemic chemotherapy is used to treat osteosarcoma and MFH of bone. Chemotherapy is usually given before and after surgery to remove the primary tumor.

Radiation Therapy

Radiation therapy is a cancer treatment that uses high-energy X-rays or other types of radiation to kill cancer cells or keep them from growing. There are two types of radiation therapy:

- External radiation therapy uses a machine outside the body to send radiation toward the cancer.
- Internal radiation therapy uses a radioactive substance sealed in needles, seeds, wires, or catheters that are placed directly into or near the cancer.

External radiation therapy is used to treat osteosarcoma and MFH of bone.

Osteosarcoma and MFH cells are not killed easily by external radiation therapy. It may be used when a small amount of cancer is left after surgery or used together with other treatments.

Samarium

Samarium is a radioactive drug that targets areas where bone cells are growing, such as tumor cells in bone. It helps relieve pain caused by cancer in the bone and it also kills blood cells in the bone marrow. It also is used to treat osteosarcoma that has come back after treatment in a different bone.

Treatment with samarium may be followed by stem cell transplant. Before treatment with samarium, stem cells (immature blood cells) are removed from the blood or bone marrow of the patient and are frozen and stored. After treatment with samarium is complete, the stored stem cells are thawed and given back to the patient through an infusion. These reinfused stem cells grow into (and restore) the body's blood cells.

Targeted Therapy

Targeted therapy is a treatment that uses drugs or other substances to find and attack specific cancer cells without harming normal cells. There are different types of targeted therapy being used to treat osteosarcoma or studied in clinical trials:

- **Kinase inhibitor therapy** blocks a protein needed for cancer cells to divide. Sorafenib is a type of kinase inhibitor therapy used to treat recurrent osteosarcoma.
- **Mammalian target of rapamycin (mTOR) inhibitors** block a protein called mTOR, which may keep cancer cells from growing and prevent the growth of new blood vessels that tumors need to grow. Everolimus is an mTOR inhibitor used to treat recurrent osteosarcoma.
- **Monoclonal antibody therapy** is a cancer treatment that uses antibodies made in the laboratory, from a single type of immune system cell. These antibodies can identify substances on cancer cells or normal substances that may help cancer cells grow. The antibodies attach to the substances and kill the cancer cells, block their growth, or keep them from spreading. Monoclonal antibodies are given by infusion. They may be used alone or to carry drugs, toxins, or radioactive material directly to cancer cells. Denosumab and dinutuximab are monoclonal antibodies being studied for the treatment of recurrent osteosarcoma.

What Is the Prognosis for Osteosarcoma and MFH?

Certain factors affect prognosis (chance of recovery) and treatment options.

The prognosis (chance of recovery) is affected by certain factors before and after treatment.

The prognosis of untreated osteosarcoma and MFH depends on the following:

- Where the tumor is in the body and whether tumors formed in more than one bone
- The size of the tumor
- Whether the cancer has spread to other parts of the body and where it has spread
- The type of tumor (based on how the cancer cells look under a microscope)

- The patient's age and weight at the time of diagnosis
- Whether the patient has had treatment for a different cancer
- Whether the tumor has caused a break in the bone
- Whether the patient has certain genetic diseases

After osteosarcoma or MFH is treated, prognosis also depends on the following:

- How much of the cancer was killed by chemotherapy
- How much of the tumor was taken out by surgery
- Whether the cancer has recurred (come back) within two years of diagnosis

Treatment options for osteosarcoma and MFH depend on the following:

- Where the tumor is in the body
- The size of the tumor
- The stage and grade of the cancer
- Whether the bones are still growing
- The patient's age and general health
- The desire of the patient and family for the patient to be able to take part in activities such as sports or to look a certain way
- Whether the cancer is newly diagnosed or has recurred after treatment

Section 54.3

Ewing Sarcoma Family of Tumors

This section includes text excerpted from "Ewing Sarcoma Treatment (PDQ®)—Patient Version," National Cancer Institute (NCI), December 6, 2017.

What Are the Signs and Symptoms of Ewing Sarcoma?

The signs and symptoms of Ewing sarcoma include swelling and pain near the tumor. These and other signs and symptoms may be caused by Ewing sarcoma or by other conditions.

Check with your child's doctor if your child has any of the following:

- Pain and/or swelling, usually in the arms, legs, chest, back, or pelvis
- A lump (which may feel soft and warm) in the arms, legs, chest, or pelvis
- Fever for no known reason
- A bone that breaks for no known reason

How Is Ewing Sarcoma Diagnosed?

Procedures that make pictures of the bones and soft tissues and nearby areas help diagnose Ewing sarcoma and show how far the cancer has spread. The process used to find out if cancer cells have spread within and around the bones and soft tissues is called staging.

In order to plan treatment, it is important to know if the cancer is in the area where it first formed or if it has spread to other parts of the body. Tests and procedures to detect, diagnose, and stage Ewing sarcoma are usually done at the same time.

The following tests and procedures may be used to diagnose or stage Ewing sarcoma:

- Physical exam and history
- Magnetic resonance imaging (MRI)

- Computerized tomography (CT) scan (CAT scan)
- Positron emission tomography (PET) scan
- Bone scan
- Bone marrow aspiration and biopsy
- X-ray
- Complete blood count (CBC)
- Blood chemistry studies

How Does Biopsy Help in Diagnosing Ewing Sarcoma?

A biopsy is done to diagnose Ewing sarcoma. Tissue samples are removed during a biopsy so they can be viewed under a microscope by a pathologist to check for signs of cancer. It is helpful if the biopsy is done at the same center where treatment will be given.

- **Needle biopsy**. For a needle biopsy, tissue is removed using a needle. This type of needle biopsy may be done if it's possible to remove tissue samples large enough to be used for testing.
- **Incisional biopsy**. For an incisional biopsy, a sample of tissue is removed through an incision in the skin.
- **Excisional biopsy**. The removal of an entire lump or area of tissue that doesn't look normal.

The specialists (pathologist, radiation oncologist, and surgeon) who will treat the patient usually work together to decide where the needle should be placed or the biopsy incision should be made. This is done so that the biopsy doesn't affect later treatment such as surgery to remove the tumor or radiation therapy.

If there is a chance that the cancer has spread to nearby lymph nodes, one or more lymph nodes may be removed and checked for signs of cancer. The following tests may be done on the tissue that is removed:

- **Cytogenetic analysis.** A laboratory test in which cells in a sample of tissue are viewed under a microscope to look for certain changes in the chromosomes.
- **Immunohistochemistry.** A test that uses antibodies to check for certain antigens in a sample of tissue. The antibody is usually linked to a radioactive substance or a dye that causes the

tissue to light up under a microscope. This type of test may be used to tell the difference between different types of cancer.

- **Flow cytometry.** A laboratory test that measures the number of cells in a sample, the percentage of live cells in a sample, and certain characteristics of cells, such as size, shape, and the presence of tumor markers on the cell surface. The cells are stained with a light-sensitive dye, placed in a fluid, and passed in a stream before a laser or other type of light. The measurements are based on how the light-sensitive dye reacts to the light.

What Treatment Is Available for Patients with Ewing Sarcoma?

Different types of treatments are available for children with Ewing sarcoma. Some treatments are standard (the currently used treatment), and some are being tested in clinical trials. A treatment clinical trial is a research study meant to help improve current treatments or obtain information on new treatments for patients with cancer. Because cancer in children is rare, taking part in a clinical trial should be considered. Some clinical trials are open only to patients who have not started treatment. Five types of standard treatment are used:

- **Chemotherapy.** Chemotherapy is a cancer treatment that uses drugs to stop the growth of cancer cells, either by killing the cells or by stopping them from dividing. When chemotherapy is taken by mouth or injected into a vein or muscle, the drugs enter the bloodstream and can reach cancer cells throughout the body (systemic chemotherapy). When chemotherapy is placed directly into the cerebrospinal fluid, an organ, or a body cavity such as the abdomen, the drugs mainly affect cancer cells in those areas (regional chemotherapy). Combination chemotherapy is treatment using more than one anticancer drug. Systemic chemotherapy is part of the treatment for all patients with Ewing tumors. It is often the first treatment given and lasts for about 6–12 months. Chemotherapy is often given to shrink the tumor before surgery or radiation therapy and to kill any tumor cells that may have spread to other parts of the body.
- **Radiation therapy.** Radiation therapy is a cancer treatment that uses high-energy X-rays or other types of radiation to kill cancer cells or keep them from growing. There are two types of radiation therapy:

- External radiation therapy uses a machine outside the body to send radiation toward the cancer.
- Internal radiation therapy uses a radioactive substance sealed in needles, seeds, wires, or catheters that are placed directly into or near the cancer.

External radiation therapy is used to treat Ewing sarcoma. Radiation therapy is used when the tumor cannot be removed by surgery or when surgery to remove the tumor will affect important body functions or the way the child will look. It may be used to make the tumor smaller and decrease the amount of tissue that needs to be removed during surgery. It may also be used to treat any tumor that remains after surgery and tumors that have spread to other parts of the body.

- **Surgery.** Surgery is usually done to remove cancer that is left after chemotherapy or radiation therapy. When possible, the whole tumor is removed by surgery. Tissue and bone that are removed may be replaced with a graft, which uses tissue and bone taken from another part of the patient's body or a donor. Sometimes an implant, such as artificial bone, is used. Even if the doctor removes all of the cancer that can be seen at the time of the operation, chemotherapy or radiation therapy may be given after surgery to kill any cancer cells that are left. Chemotherapy or radiation therapy given after surgery to lower the risk that the cancer will come back is called adjuvant therapy.
- **Targeted therapy.** Targeted therapy is a type of treatment that uses drugs or other substances to identify and attack specific cancer cells without harming normal cells. Monoclonal antibody therapy is a type of targeted therapy used in the treatment of recurrent Ewing sarcoma. It is being studied for the treatment of metastatic Ewing sarcoma. Monoclonal antibodies are made in the laboratory from a single type of immune system cell. These antibodies can identify substances on cancer cells or normal substances that may help cancer cells grow. The antibodies attach to the substances and kill the cancer cells, block their growth, or keep them from spreading. Monoclonal antibodies are given by infusion. They may be used alone or to carry drugs, toxins, or radioactive material directly to cancer cells.

New types of targeted therapy are being studied.

- **Kinase inhibitor therapy** is another type of targeted therapy. Kinase inhibitors are drugs that block a protein needed for cancer cells to divide. They are being studied in the treatment of recurrent Ewing sarcoma.

- **Poly (ADP-ribose) polymerase (PARP) inhibitor therapy** is another type of targeted therapy. PARP inhibitors are drugs that block deoxyribonucleic acid (DNA) repair and may cause cancer cells to die. They are being studied in the treatment of recurrent Ewing sarcoma.

- **High-dose chemotherapy with stem cell rescue**. High-dose chemotherapy with stem cell rescue is a way of giving high doses of chemotherapy to treat Ewing sarcoma and then replacing blood-forming cells destroyed by cancer treatment. Stem cells (immature blood cells) are removed from the blood or bone marrow of the patient and are frozen and stored. After chemotherapy is completed, the stored stem cells are thawed and given back to the patient through an infusion. These reinfused stem cells grow into (and restore) the body's blood cells. Chemotherapy with stem cell rescue is used to treat recurrent Ewing sarcoma.

Side Effects of Treatment for Ewing Sarcoma

Treatment for Ewing sarcoma may cause side effects. Side effects from cancer treatment that begin after treatment and continue for months or years are called late effects. Late effects of cancer treatment may include the following:

- Physical problems
- Changes in mood, feelings, thinking, learning, or memory
- Second cancers (new types of cancer). Patients treated for Ewing sarcoma have an increased risk of acute myeloid leukemia and myelodysplastic syndrome. There is also an increased risk of sarcoma in the area treated with radiation therapy.

Some late effects may be treated or controlled. It is important to talk with your child's doctors about the effects cancer treatment can have on your child.

What Is the Prognosis for Ewing Sarcoma?

The factors that affect prognosis (chance of recovery) are different before and after treatment. Before treatment, prognosis depends on:

- Whether the tumor has spread to lymph nodes or distant parts of the body
- Where in the body the tumor started
- Whether the tumor formed in the bone or in soft tissue
- How large the tumor is at when the tumor is diagnosed
- Whether the lactic acid dehydrogenase (LDH) in the blood is higher than normal
- How much radioactive glucose is taken up by the tumor during a PET scan
- Whether the tumor has certain gene changes
- Whether the child is younger than 15 years
- The patient's sex
- Whether the child has had treatment for a different cancer before Ewing sarcoma
- Whether the tumor has just been diagnosed or has recurred (come back)

After treatment, prognosis is affected by:

- Whether the tumor was completely removed by surgery
- Whether the tumor responds to chemotherapy or radiation therapy

If the cancer recurs after initial treatment, prognosis depends on:

- Whether the cancer came back more than two years after the initial treatment
- Where in the body the tumor came back
- The type of initial treatment given

Chapter 55

Soft Tissue Sarcomas

Chapter Contents

Section 55.1

Overview of Soft Tissue Sarcoma

This section contains text excerpted from the following sources: Text beginning with the heading "What Is Soft Tissue Sarcoma?" is excerpted from "Soft Tissue Sarcoma—Patient Version," National Cancer Institute (NCI), May 15, 2015; Text beginning with the heading "What Causes Soft Tissue Sarcoma?" is excerpted from "Soft Tissue Sarcoma," MedlinePlus, National Institutes of Health (NIH), July 27, 2016.

What Is Soft Tissue Sarcoma?

Soft tissue sarcoma is a cancer that starts in soft tissues of the body, including muscle, tendons, fat, lymph vessels, blood vessels, nerves, and tissue around joints. The tumors can be found anywhere in the body but often form in the arms, legs, chest, or abdomen.

What Are the Types of Soft Tissue Sarcoma?

There are many types of soft tissue sarcoma, based on the type of soft tissue cell in which the cancer formed. Different types may be treated differently.

Rhabdomyosarcoma is the most common type of soft tissue sarcoma in children. It begins in muscles that are attached to bones and help the body move. Most rhabdomyosarcomas are diagnosed in children younger than 10 years. Rhabdomyosarcomas usually form lumps near the surface of the body and are found early.

Gastrointestinal stromal tumors are soft tissue sarcomas that form in soft tissues of the gastrointestinal tract, usually in the stomach or small intestine. They are most common in adults, and may be benign (not cancer) or malignant (cancer). Gastrointestinal stromal tumors often do not cause early symptoms.

Ewing sarcoma, Kaposi sarcoma, and **uterine sarcoma** are other types of soft tissue sarcoma.

What Are the Signs and Symptoms of Soft Tissue Sarcoma?

Signs of soft tissue sarcoma include a lump or swelling in soft tissue. Sometimes there are no signs or symptoms until the tumor is big and presses on nearby nerves or other parts of the body.

Who Have the Risk of Getting Soft Tissue Sarcoma?

Both children and adults can develop soft tissue sarcoma. Treatment often works better in children and they may have a better chance of being cured than adults.

What Causes Soft Tissue Sarcoma?

No one knows exactly what causes these cancers. They are not common, but you have a higher risk if you have been exposed to certain chemicals, have had radiation therapy, or have certain genetic diseases.

How Is Soft Tissue Sarcoma Diagnosed?

Doctors diagnose soft tissue sarcomas with a biopsy.

What Is the Treatment for Soft Tissue Sarcoma?

Treatments include surgery to remove the tumor, radiation therapy, chemotherapy, or a combination.

Section 55.2

Childhood Soft Tissue Sarcoma

This section includes text excerpted from "Childhood Soft Tissue Sarcoma Treatment (PDQ®)—Patient Version," National Cancer Institute (NCI), August 18, 2017.

Soft tissues of the body connect, support, and surround other body parts and organs. The soft tissues include the following:

- Fat
- A mix of bone and cartilage
- Fibrous tissue
- Muscles
- Nerves
- Tendons (bands of tissue that connect muscles to bones)
- Synovial tissues (tissues around joints)
- Blood vessels
- Lymph vessels

Soft tissue sarcoma may be found anywhere in the body. In children, the tumors form most often in the arms, legs, or trunk (chest and abdomen). Childhood soft tissue sarcoma is a disease in which malignant (cancer) cells form in soft tissues of the body.

Types of Childhood Soft Tissue Sarcoma

There are many different types of soft tissue sarcomas. The soft tissue tumors are grouped based on the type of soft tissue cell where they first formed.

Fat Tissue Tumors

- **Liposarcoma.** This is a rare cancer of the fat cells. Liposarcoma usually forms in the fat layer just under the skin. In children and adolescents, liposarcoma is often low grade (likely to grow and spread slowly).

There are several different types of liposarcoma. Myxoid liposarcoma is usually low grade and responds well to treatment. The cells of myxoid liposarcoma have a certain genetic change called a translocation (part of one chromosome switches places with part of another chromosome). In order to diagnose myxoid liposarcoma, the tumor cells are checked for this genetic change. Pleomorphic liposarcoma is usually high grade (likely to grow and spread quickly) and is less likely to respond well to treatment.

Bone and Cartilage Tumors

Bone and cartilage tumors are a mix of bone cells and cartilage cells. Bone and cartilage tumors include the following types:

- **Extraskeletal mesenchymal chondrosarcoma.** This type of bone and cartilage tumor often affects young adults and occurs in the head and neck.
- **Extraskeletal osteosarcoma.** This type of bone and cartilage tumor is very rare in children and adolescents. It is likely to come back after treatment and may spread to the lungs.

Fibrous (Connective) Tissue Tumors

Fibrous (connective) tissue tumors include the following types:

- **Desmoid-type fibromatosis** (also called desmoid tumor or aggressive fibromatosis). This fibrous tissue tumor is low grade (likely to grow slowly). Desmoid tumors sometimes occur in children with changes in the *adenomatous polyposis coli* (APC) gene. Changes in this gene cause familial adenomatous polyposis (FAP). FAP is an inherited condition in which many polyps (growths on mucous membranes) form on the inside walls of the colon and rectum. Genetic counseling (a discussion with a trained professional about inherited diseases and a possible need for gene testing) may be needed.
- **Dermatofibrosarcoma protuberans.** This is a rare tumor of the deep layers of the skin found in children and adults. The cells of this tumor have a certain genetic change called a translocation (part of one chromosome switches places with part of

another chromosome). In order to diagnose dermatofibrosarcoma protuberans, the tumor cells are checked for this genetic change.

- **Fibrosarcoma.** There are two types of fibrosarcoma in children and adolescents:

- **Infantile fibrosarcoma (also called congenital fibrosarcoma).** This type of fibrosarcoma is found in children aged 4 years and younger.
- **Adult-type fibrosarcoma.** The cells of this tumor do not have the genetic change found in infantile fibrosarcoma. This is the same type of fibrosarcoma found in adults.
- **Inflammatory myofibroblastic tumor.** This is a fibrous tissue tumor that occurs in children and adolescents. It is likely to come back after treatment but rarely spreads to distant parts of the body. A certain genetic change has been found in about half of these tumors.
- **Low-grade fibromyxoid sarcoma.** This is a slow-growing tumor that affects young and middle-aged adults.
- **Myxofibrosarcoma.** This is a rare fibrous tissue tumor that is found less often in children than in adults.
- **Sclerosing epithelioid fibrosarcoma.** This is a rare fibrous tissue tumor that can come back and spread to other places years after treatment. Long-term follow-up is needed.

Skeletal Muscle Tumors

Skeletal muscle is attached to bones and helps the body move.

Rhabdomyosarcoma

Rhabdomyosarcoma is the most common childhood soft tissue sarcoma in children 14 years and younger.

Smooth Muscle Tumors

Smooth muscle lines the inside of blood vessels and hollow internal organs such as the stomach, intestines, bladder, and uterus.

- **Leiomyosarcoma**. This smooth muscle tumor has been linked with Epstein-Barr virus in children who also have human immunodeficiency virus (HIV) disease or acquired immune deficiency syndrome (AIDS). Leiomyosarcoma may also form as a second cancer in survivors of inherited retinoblastoma, sometimes many years after the initial treatment for retinoblastoma.

So-Called Fibrohistiocytic Tumors

- **Plexiform fibrohistiocytic tumor**. This is a rare tumor that usually affects children and young adults. The tumor usually starts as a painless growth on or just under the skin on the arm, hand, or wrist. It may rarely spread to nearby lymph nodes or to the lungs.

Peripheral Nervous System Tumors

Peripheral nervous system tumors include the following types:

- **Ectomesenchymoma.** This is a rare, fast-growing tumor of the nerve sheath (protective covering of nerves that are not part of the brain or spinal cord) that occurs mainly in children. Ectomesenchymomas may form in the head and neck, abdomen, perineum, scrotum, arms, or legs.
- **Malignant peripheral nerve sheath tumor.** This is a tumor that forms in the nerve sheath. Some children who have a malignant peripheral nerve sheath tumor have a rare genetic condition called neurofibromatosis type 1 (NF1). This tumor may be low grade or high grade.
- **Malignant triton tumor.** These are very rare, fast-growing tumors that occur most often in children with NF1.

Pericytic (Perivascular) Tumors

Pericytic tumors form in cells that wrap around blood vessels. Pericytic tumors include the following types:

- **Myopericytoma.** Infantile hemangiopericytoma is a type of myopericytoma. Children younger than 1 year at the time of diagnosis may have a better prognosis. In patients older than 1 year, infantile hemangiopericytoma is more likely to spread to other parts of the body, including the lymph nodes and lungs.
- **Infantile myofibromatosis.** Infantile myofibromatosis is another type of myopericytoma. It is a fibrous tumor that often

forms in the first 2 years of life. There may be one nodule under the skin, usually in the head and neck area (myofibroma), or nodules in several skin areas, muscle, and bone (myofibromatosis). These tumors may go away without treatment.

Tumors of Unknown Origin

Tumors of unknown origin (the place where the tumor first formed is not known) include the following types:

- **Alveolar soft part sarcoma.** This is a rare tumor of the soft supporting tissue that connects and surrounds the organs and other tissues. It is most commonly found in the limbs but can occur in the tissues of the mouth, jaws, and face. It may grow slowly and may have spread to other parts of the body at the time of diagnosis. Alveolar soft part sarcoma may have a better prognosis when the tumor is 5 centimeters or smaller or when the tumor is completely removed by surgery. The cells of this tumor usually have a certain genetic change called a translocation (part of one chromosome switches places with part of another chromosome). In order to diagnose alveolar soft part sarcoma, the tumor cells are checked for this genetic change.
- **Clear cell sarcoma of soft tissue.** This is a slow-growing soft tissue tumor that begins in a tendon (tough, fibrous, cord-like tissue that connects muscle to bone or to another part of the body). Clear cell sarcoma most commonly occurs in deep tissue of the foot, heel, and ankle. It may spread to nearby lymph nodes. The cells of this tumor usually have a certain genetic change called a translocation (part of one chromosome switches places with part of another chromosome). In order to diagnose clear cell sarcoma of soft tissue, the tumor cells are checked for this genetic change.
- **Desmoplastic small round cell tumor.** This tumor most often forms in the abdomen, pelvis or tissues around the testes, but it may form in the kidney. Desmoplastic small round cell tumor may also spread to the lungs and other parts of the body. The cells of this tumor usually have a certain genetic change called a translocation (part of one chromosome switches places with part of another chromosome). In order to diagnose desmoplastic small round cell tumor, the tumor cells are checked for this genetic change.

- **Epithelioid sarcoma.** This is a rare sarcoma that usually starts deep in soft tissue as a slow growing, firm lump and may spread to the lymph nodes.
- **Extrarenal (extracranial) rhabdoid tumor.** This is a rare, fast-growing tumor of soft tissues such as the liver and peritoneum. It usually occurs in young children, including newborns, but it can occur in older children and adults. Rhabdoid tumors may be linked to a change in a tumor suppressor gene called *SMARCB1*. This type of gene makes a protein that helps control cell growth. Changes in the *SMARCB1* gene may be inherited (passed on from parents to offspring). Genetic counseling (a discussion with a trained professional about inherited diseases and a possible need for gene testing) may be needed.
- **Extraskeletal myxoid chondrosarcoma.** This is a rare soft tissue sarcoma that may be found in children and adolescents. Over time, it tends to spread to other parts of the body, including the lymph nodes and lungs. The cells of this tumor usually have a genetic change, often a translocation (part of one chromosome switches places with part of another chromosome). In order to diagnose extraskeletal myxoid chondrosarcoma, the tumor cells are checked for this genetic change. The tumor may come back many years after treatment.
- **Perivascular epithelioid cell tumors (PEComas).** Benign (not cancer) PEComas may be found in children with an inherited condition called tuberous sclerosis. They occur in the stomach, intestines, lungs, female reproductive organs, and genitourinary organs.
- **Primitive neuroectodermal tumor (PNET)/extraskeletal Ewing tumor.**
- **Synovial sarcoma.** Synovial sarcoma is a common type of soft tissue sarcoma in children and adolescents. Synovial sarcoma usually forms in the tissues around the joints in the arms or legs, but may also form in the trunk, head, or neck. The cells of this tumor usually have a certain genetic change called a translocation (part of one chromosome switches places with part of another chromosome). Larger tumors have a greater risk of spreading to other parts of the body, including the lungs. Children younger than 10 years and those whose tumor is 5 centimeters or smaller have a better prognosis.

- **Undifferentiated /unclassified sarcoma**. These tumors usually occur in the muscles that are attached to bones and that help the body move.
    - **Undifferentiated pleomorphic sarcoma/malignant fibrous histiocytoma (high-grade).** This type of soft tissue tumor may form in parts of the body where patients have received radiation therapy in the past, or as a second cancer in children with retinoblastoma. The tumor is usually found on the arms or legs and may spread to other parts of the body.

Blood Vessel Tumors

Blood vessel tumors include the following types:

- **Angiosarcoma of the soft tissue.** Angiosarcoma of the soft tissue is a fast-growing tumor that forms in blood vessels or lymph vessels in any part of the body. Most angiosarcomas are in or just under the skin. Those in deeper soft tissue can form in the liver, spleen, and lung. They are very rare in children, who sometimes have more than one tumor in the skin or liver. Rarely, infantile hemangioma may become angiosarcoma of the soft tissue.
- **Epithelioid hemangioendothelioma.** Epithelioid hemangioendotheliomas can occur in children, but are most common in adults between 30 and 50 years of age. They usually occur in the liver, lung, or bone. They may be either fast growing or slow growing. In about a third of cases, the tumor spreads to other parts of the body very quickly.

Signs and Symptoms of Childhood Soft Tissue Sarcoma

The most common sign of childhood soft tissue sarcoma is a painless lump or swelling in soft tissues of the body. A sarcoma may appear as a painless lump under the skin, often on an arm, a leg, or the trunk. There may be no other signs or symptoms at first. As the sarcoma gets bigger and presses on nearby organs, nerves, muscles, or blood vessels, it may cause signs or symptoms, such as pain or weakness.

Other conditions may cause the same signs and symptoms.

Risk Factors for Childhood Soft Tissue Sarcoma

Having certain diseases and inherited disorders can increase the risk of childhood soft tissue sarcoma.

Risk factors for childhood soft tissue sarcoma include having the following inherited disorders:

- Li-Fraumeni syndrome
- Familial adenomatous polyposis (FAP)
- *Retinoblastoma 1* gene changes
- *SMARCB1 (INI1)* gene changes
- Neurofibromatosis type 1 (NF1)
- Werner syndrome

Other risk factors include the following:

- Past treatment with radiation therapy
- Having acquired immunodeficiency syndrome (AIDS) and Epstein-Barr virus infection at the same time

Diagnosis of Childhood Soft Tissue Sarcoma

The following tests and procedures may be used to detect (find) and diagnose childhood soft tissue sarcoma:

- Physical exam and history
- X-rays
- MRI
- CT scan
- Ultrasound exam

If tests show there may be a soft tissue sarcoma, a biopsy is done. One of the following types of biopsies is usually used:

- Core needle biopsy
- Incisional biopsy
- Excisional biopsy

Because soft tissue sarcoma can be hard to diagnose, the tissue sample should be checked by a pathologist who has experience in diagnosing soft tissue sarcoma.

One or more of the following laboratory tests may be done to study the tissue samples:

- Molecular test
- Reverse transcription–polymerase chain reaction (RT–PCR) test
- Cytogenetic analysis
- Immunocytochemistry

Treatment for Childhood Soft Tissue Sarcoma

Different types of treatments are available for patients with childhood soft tissue sarcoma. Treatment will be overseen by a pediatric oncologist, a doctor who specializes in treating children with cancer. The pediatric oncologist works with other healthcare providers who are experts in treating children with soft tissue sarcoma and who specialize in certain areas of medicine. These may include a pediatric surgeon with special training in the removal of soft tissue sarcomas. The following specialists may also be included:

- Pediatrician
- Radiation oncologist
- Pediatric hematologist
- Pediatric nurse specialist
- Rehabilitation specialist
- Psychologist
- Social worker
- Child-life specialist

Eight types of standard treatment are used:

Surgery. Surgery to completely remove the soft tissue sarcoma is done when possible. If the tumor is very large, radiation therapy or chemotherapy may be given first, to make the tumor smaller and decrease the amount of tissue that needs to be removed during surgery. The following types of surgery may be used:

- Wide local excision
- Amputation
- Lymphadenectomy

- Mohs surgery
- Hepatectomy

A second surgery may be needed to:

- Remove any remaining cancer cells
- Check the area around where the tumor was removed for cancer cells and then remove more tissue if needed

If cancer is in the liver, a hepatectomy and liver transplant may be done (the liver is removed and replaced with a healthy one from a donor).

Radiation therapy. Radiation therapy is a cancer treatment that uses high-energy X-rays or other types of radiation to kill cancer cells or keep them from growing. There are two types of radiation therapy:

- External radiation therapy
- Internal radiation therapy

The way the radiation therapy is given depends on the type and stage of the cancer being treated and whether the tumor was completely removed by surgery. External and internal radiation therapy are used to treat childhood soft tissue sarcoma.

Chemotherapy. Chemotherapy is a cancer treatment that uses drugs to stop the growth of cancer cells, either by killing the cells or by stopping them from dividing. The way the chemotherapy is given depends on the type of cancer being treated. Most types of soft tissue sarcoma do not respond to treatment with chemotherapy.

Observation. Observation is closely monitoring a patient's condition without giving any treatment until signs or symptoms appear or change. Observation may be done when:

- Complete removal of the tumor is not possible
- No other treatments are available
- The tumor is not likely to damage any vital organs

Hormone therapy. Hormone therapy is a cancer treatment that removes hormones or blocks their action and stops cancer cells from growing. Hormones are substances made by glands in the body and circulated in the bloodstream. Some hormones can cause certain cancers to grow. If tests show that the cancer cells have places where hormones can attach (receptors), drugs, surgery, or radiation therapy is used to reduce the production of hormones or block them from working. Antiestrogens (drugs that block estrogen), such as tamoxifen, may be used to treat desmoid-type fibromatosis.

Nonsteroidal anti-inflammatory drugs. Nonsteroidal anti-inflammatory drugs (NSAIDs) are drugs (such as aspirin, ibuprofen, and naproxen) that are commonly used to decrease fever, swelling, pain, and redness. In the treatment of desmoid-type fibromatosis, an NSAID called sulindac may be used to help block the growth of cancer cells.

Targeted therapy. Targeted therapy is a type of treatment that uses drugs or other substances to attack cancer cells. Targeted therapies usually cause less harm to normal cells than chemotherapy or radiation do.

Immunotherapy. Immunotherapy is a treatment that uses the patient's immune system to fight disease. Substances made by the body or made in a laboratory are used to boost, direct, or restore the body's natural defenses against disease. Interferon is a type of immunotherapy used to treat epithelioid hemangioendothelioma. It interferes with the division of tumor cells and can slow tumor growth.

Gene therapy. Gene therapy is being studied for childhood synovial sarcoma that has recurred, spread, or cannot be removed by surgery.

Prognosis for Childhood Soft Tissue Sarcoma

The prognosis (chance of recovery) and treatment options depend on the following:

- The part of the body where the tumor first formed
- The size and grade of the tumor
- The type of soft tissue sarcoma
- How deep the tumor is under the skin
- Whether the tumor has spread to other places in the body
- The amount of tumor remaining after surgery to remove it
- Whether radiation therapy was used to treat the tumor
- The age and sex of the patient
- Whether the cancer has just been diagnosed or has recurred (come back)

Section 55.3

Childhood Vascular Tumors

This section includes text excerpted from "Childhood Vascular Tumors Treatment (PDQ®)—Patient Version," National Cancer Institute (NCI), February 2, 2018.

- **Childhood vascular tumors form from cells that make blood vessels or lymph vessels.**
- Vascular tumors can form from abnormal blood vessel or lymph vessel cells anywhere in the body. They may be benign (not cancer) or malignant (cancer). There are many types of vascular tumors. The most common type of childhood vascular tumor is infantile hemangioma, which is a benign tumor that usually goes away on its own.
- Because malignant vascular tumors are rare in children, there is not a lot of information about what treatment works best.

Types of Childhood Vascular Tumors

Childhood vascular tumors may be classified into four groups.

- **Benign tumors.** Benign tumors are not cancer. This summary has information about the following benign vascular tumors:
  - Infantile hemangioma
  - Congenital hemangioma
  - Benign vascular tumors of the liver
  - Spindle cell hemangioma
  - Epithelioid hemangioma
  - Pyogenic granuloma (lobular capillary hemangioma)
  - Angiofibroma
  - Juvenile nasopharyngeal angiofibroma

- **Intermediate (locally aggressive) tumors.** Intermediate tumors that are locally aggressive often spread to the area around the tumor. This summary has information about the following locally aggressive vascular tumors:
    - Kaposiform hemangioendothelioma and tufted angioma.
- **Intermediate (rarely metastasizing) tumors.** Intermediate (rarely metastasizing) tumors sometimes spread to other parts of the body. This summary has information about the following vascular tumors that rarely metastasize:
    - Pseudomyogenic hemangioendothelioma
    - Retiform hemangioendothelioma
    - Papillary intralymphatic angioendothelioma
    - Composite hemangioendothelioma
    - Kaposi sarcoma
- **Malignant tumors.** Malignant tumors are cancer. This summary has information about the following malignant vascular tumors:
    - Epithelioid hemangioendothelioma
    - Angiosarcoma of soft tissue

Diagnosis of Childhood Vascular Tumors

Tests are used to detect (find) and diagnose childhood vascular tumors.

The following tests and procedures may be used:

- **Physical exam and history:** An exam of the body to check general signs of health, including checking for signs of disease, such as lumps, lesions, or anything else that seems unusual. A history of the patient's health habits and past illnesses and treatments will also be taken.
- **Ultrasound exam:** A procedure in which high-energy sound waves (ultrasound) are bounced off internal tissues or organs and make echoes. The echoes form a picture of body tissues called a sonogram. The picture can be printed to be looked at later.
- **CT scan (computed tomography scan):** A procedure that makes a series of detailed pictures of areas inside the body,

taken from different angles. The pictures are made by a computer linked to an X-ray machine. A dye may be injected into a vein or swallowed to help the organs or tissues show up more clearly. This procedure is also called computed tomography, computerized tomography, or computerized axial tomography.

- **Magnetic resonance imaging (MRI):** A procedure that uses a magnet, radio waves, and a computer to make a series of detailed pictures of areas inside the body. This procedure is also called nuclear magnetic resonance imaging (NMRI).
- **Biopsy:** The removal of cells or tissues so they can be viewed under a microscope by a pathologist to check for signs of cancer. A biopsy is not always needed to diagnose a vascular tumor.

Treatment of Childhood Vascular Tumors

Different types of treatment are available for children with vascular tumors. Some treatments are standard (the currently used treatment), and some are being tested in clinical trials. A treatment clinical trial is a research study meant to help improve current treatments or obtain information on new treatments. When clinical trials show that a new treatment is better than the standard treatment, the new treatment may become the standard treatment.

Because vascular tumors in children are rare, taking part in a clinical trial should be considered. Some clinical trials are open only to patients who have not started treatment.

Children with childhood vascular tumors should have their treatment planned by a team of healthcare providers who are experts in treating cancer in children.

Treatment will be overseen by a pediatric oncologist, a doctor who specializes in treating children with cancer. The pediatric oncologist works with other pediatric healthcare providers who are experts in treating children with cancer and who specialize in certain areas of medicine. These may include the following specialists:

- Pediatric vascular anomaly specialist (expert in treating children with vascular tumors)
- Pediatric surgeon
- Orthopedic surgeon
- Radiation oncologist
- Pediatric nurse specialist

- Rehabilitation specialist
- Psychologist
- Social worker

Some treatments cause side effects months or years after treatment has ended.

Some treatments, such as chemotherapy and radiation therapy, cause side effects that continue or appear months or years after treatment has ended. These are called late effects. Late effects of treatment may include:

- Physical problems
- Changes in mood, feelings, thinking, learning, or memory
- Second cancers (new types of cancer)

Some late effects may be treated or controlled. It is important to talk with your child's doctors about the possible late effects caused by some treatments.

Eleven types of standard treatment are used:

Beta Blocker Therapy

Beta blockers are drugs that decrease blood pressure and heart rate. When used in patients with vascular tumors, beta blockers may help shrink the tumors. Beta blocker therapy may be given by vein (IV), by mouth, or placed on the skin (topical). The way the beta blocker therapy is given depends on the type of vascular tumor and where the tumor first formed.

The beta blocker propranolol is usually the first treatment for hemangiomas. Infants treated with IV propranolol may need to have their treatment started in a hospital. Propranolol is also used to treat benign vascular tumor of liver and kaposiform hemangioendothelioma.

Other beta blockers used to treat vascular tumors include atenolol, nadolol, and timolol.

Infantile hemangioma may also be treated with propranolol and steroid therapy or propranolol and topical beta blocker therapy.

Surgery

The following types of surgery may be used to remove many types of vascular tumors:

- **Excision:** Surgery to remove the entire tumor and some of the healthy tissue around it.

- **Laser surgery:** A surgical procedure that uses a laser beam (a narrow beam of intense light) as a knife to make bloodless cuts in tissue or to remove a skin lesion such as a tumor. Surgery with a pulsed dye laser may be used for some hemangiomas. This type of laser uses a beam of light that targets blood vessels in the skin. The light is changed into heat and the blood vessels are destroyed without damaging nearby skin.
- **Curettage:** A procedure in which abnormal tissue is removed using a small, spoon-shaped instrument called a curette.
- **Total hepatectomy and liver transplant:** A surgical procedure to remove the entire liver followed by a transplant of a healthy liver from a donor.

The type of surgery used depends on the type of vascular tumor and where the tumor formed in the body.

For malignant tumors, even if the doctor removes all the cancer that can be seen at the time of the surgery, some patients may be given chemotherapy or radiation therapy after surgery to kill any cancer cells that are left. Treatment given after the surgery, to lower the risk that the tumor will come back, is called adjuvant therapy.

Photocoagulation

Photocoagulation is the use of an intense beam of light, such as a laser, to seal off blood vessels or destroy tissue. It is used to treat pyogenic granuloma.

Embolization

Embolization is a procedure that uses particles, such as tiny gelatin sponges or beads, to block blood vessels in the liver. It may be used to treat some benign vascular tumors of the liver and kaposiform hemangioendothelioma.

Chemotherapy

Chemotherapy is a treatment that uses drugs to stop the growth of tumor cells, either by killing the cells or by stopping them from dividing. There are different ways to give chemotherapy:

- **Systemic chemotherapy:** When chemotherapy is taken by mouth or injected into a vein or muscle, the drugs enter the bloodstream and can reach tumor cells throughout the body. Sometimes more than one anticancer drug is given. This is called combination chemotherapy.

- **Topical chemotherapy:** When chemotherapy is applied to the skin in a cream or lotion, the drugs mainly affect tumor cells in the treated area.
- **Regional chemotherapy:** When chemotherapy is placed directly into the cerebrospinal fluid, an organ, or a body cavity such as the abdomen, the drugs mainly affect tumor cells in those areas.

The way the chemotherapy is given depends on the type of the vascular tumor being treated. Systemic and topical chemotherapy are used to treat some vascular tumors.

Sclerotherapy

Sclerotherapy is a treatment used to destroy the blood vessel that leads to the tumor and the tumor. A liquid is injected into the blood vessel, causing it to scar and break down. Over time, the destroyed blood vessel is absorbed into normal tissue. The blood flows through nearby healthy veins instead. Sclerotherapy is used in the treatment of epithelioid hemangioma.

Radiation Therapy

Radiation therapy is a treatment that uses high-energy X-rays or other types of radiation to kill tumor cells or keep them from growing. There are two types of radiation therapy:

- External radiation therapy uses a machine outside the body to send radiation toward the tumor.
- Internal radiation therapy uses a radioactive substance sealed in needles, seeds, wires, or catheters that are placed directly into or near the tumor.

The way the radiation therapy is given depends on the type of the vascular tumor being treated. External radiation is used to treat some vascular tumors.

Targeted Therapy

Targeted therapy is a type of treatment that uses drugs or other substances to attack specific tumor cells. Targeted therapies usually cause less harm to normal cells than chemotherapy or radiation therapy do. Different types of targeted therapy are being used or studied to treat childhood vascular tumors:

- **Angiogenesis inhibitors:** Angiogenesis inhibitors are drugs that stop cells from dividing and prevent the growth of new blood vessels that tumors need to grow. The targeted therapy drugs thalidomide, sorafenib, pazopanib, and sirolimus are angiogenesis inhibitors used to treat childhood vascular tumors.
- **Mammalian target of rapamycin (mTOR) inhibitors:** mTOR inhibitors block a protein called mTOR, which may keep cancer cells from growing and prevent the growth of new blood vessels that tumors need to grow.
- **Kinase inhibitors:** Kinase inhibitors block signals needed for tumors to grow. Trametinib is being studied to treat epithelioid hemangioendothelioma.

Immunotherapy

Immunotherapy is a treatment that uses the patient's immune system to fight disease. Substances made by the body or made in a laboratory are used to boost, direct, or restore the body's natural defenses against disease.

Interferon is a type of immunotherapy used to treat childhood vascular tumors. It interferes with the division of tumor cells and can slow tumor growth. It is used in the treatment of juvenile nasopharyngeal angiofibroma, kaposiform hemangioendothelioma, and epithelioid hemangioendothelioma.

Other Drug Therapy

Other drugs used to treat childhood vascular tumors or manage their effects include the following:

- **Steroid therapy:** Steroids are hormones made naturally in the body. They can also be made in a laboratory and used as drugs. Steroid drugs help shrink some vascular tumors. Corticosteroids, such as prednisone and methylprednisolone, are used to treat infantile hemangioma.
- **Nonsteroidal anti-inflammatory drugs (NSAIDs):** NSAIDs are commonly used to decrease fever, swelling, pain, and redness. Examples of NSAIDs are aspirin, ibuprofen, and naproxen.

In the treatment of vascular tumors, NSAIDs can increase the flow of blood through the tumors and decrease the chance that an unwanted blood clot will form.

- **Antifibrinolytic therapy:** These drugs help the blood clot in patients who have Kasabach-Merritt syndrome. Fibrin is the main protein in a blood clot that helps stop bleeding and heal wounds. Some vascular tumors cause fibrin to break down and the patient's blood does not clot normally, causing uncontrolled bleeding. Antifibrinolytics help prevent the breakdown of fibrin.

Section 55.4

Adult Soft Tissue Sarcoma

This section includes text excerpted from "Adult Soft Tissue Sarcoma Treatment (PDQ®)—Patient Version," National Cancer Institute (NCI), May 15, 2017.

The soft tissues of the body include the muscles, tendons (bands of fiber that connect muscles to bones), fat, blood vessels, lymph vessels, nerves, and tissues around joints.

What Is Adult Soft Tissue Sarcoma?

Adult soft tissue sarcoma is a disease in which malignant (cancer) cells form in the soft tissues of the body. They can form almost anywhere in the body, but are most common in the head, neck, arms, legs, trunk, and abdomen.

There are many types of soft tissue sarcoma. The cells of each type of sarcoma look different under a microscope, based on the type of soft tissue in which the cancer began.

What Are the Signs and Symptoms of Adult Soft Tissue Sarcoma?

A sarcoma may appear as a painless lump under the skin, often on an arm or a leg. Sarcomas that begin in the abdomen may not cause signs or symptoms until they get very big. As the sarcoma grows bigger and presses on nearby organs, nerves, muscles, or blood vessels, signs and symptoms may include:

- Pain
- Trouble breathing

Other conditions may cause the same signs and symptoms. Check with your doctor if you have any of these problems.

What Are the Risk Factors for Adult Soft Tissue Sarcoma?

Anything that increases your risk of getting a disease is called a risk factor. Having a risk factor does not mean that you will get cancer; not having risk factors doesn't mean that you will not get cancer. Talk with your doctor if you think you may be at risk.

Having certain inherited disorders can increase the risk of adult soft tissue sarcoma. Risk factors for soft tissue sarcoma include the following inherited disorders:

- Retinoblastoma
- Neurofibromatosis type 1 (NF1; von Recklinghausen disease).
- Tuberous sclerosis (Bourneville disease)
- Familial adenomatous polyposis (FAP; Gardner syndrome).
- Li-Fraumeni syndrome
- Werner syndrome (adult progeria)
- Nevoid basal cell carcinoma syndrome (Gorlin syndrome)

Other risk factors for soft tissue sarcoma include the following:

- Past treatment with radiation therapy for certain cancers
- Being exposed to certain chemicals, such as Thorotrast (thorium dioxide), vinyl chloride, or arsenic
- Having swelling (lymphedema) in the arms or legs for a long time

How Is Adult Soft Tissue Sarcoma Diagnosed?

Adult soft tissue sarcoma is diagnosed with a biopsy. If your doctor thinks you may have a soft tissue sarcoma, a biopsy will be done. The type of biopsy will be based on the size of the tumor and where it is in the body. There are three types of biopsy that may be used:

- **Incisional biopsy:** The removal of part of a lump or a sample of tissue.
- **Core biopsy:** The removal of tissue using a wide needle.
- **Excisional biopsy:** The removal of an entire lump or area of tissue that doesn't look normal.

Samples will be taken from the primary tumor, lymph nodes, and other suspicious areas. A pathologist views the tissue under a microscope to look for cancer cells and to find out the grade of the tumor. The grade of a tumor depends on how abnormal the cancer cells look under a microscope and how quickly the cells are dividing. High-grade tumors usually grow and spread more quickly than low-grade tumors.

Because soft tissue sarcoma can be hard to diagnose, patients should ask to have tissue samples checked by a pathologist who has experience in diagnosing soft tissue sarcoma.

The following tests may be done on the tissue that was removed:

- **Immunohistochemistry:** A test that uses antibodies to check for certain antigens in a sample of tissue. The antibody is usually linked to a radioactive substance or a dye that causes the tissue to light up under a microscope. This type of test may be used to tell the difference between different types of cancer.
- **Light and electron microscopy:** A laboratory test in which cells in a sample of tissue are viewed under regular and high-powered microscopes to look for certain changes in the cells.
- **Cytogenetic analysis:** A laboratory test in which cells in a sample of tissue are viewed under a microscope to look for certain changes in the chromosomes.
- **Fluorescence in situ hybridization (FISH):** A laboratory test used to look at genes or chromosomes in cells and tissues. Pieces of deoxyribonucleic acid (DNA) that contain a fluorescent dye are made in the laboratory and added to cells or tissues on a glass slide. When these pieces of DNA attach to certain genes or areas of chromosomes on the slide, they light up when viewed under a microscope with a special light.

- **Flow cytometry:** A laboratory test that measures the number of cells in a sample, the percentage of live cells in a sample, and certain characteristics of cells, such as size, shape, and the presence of tumor markers on the cell surface. The cells are stained with a light-sensitive dye, placed in a fluid, and passed in a stream before a laser or other type of light. The measurements are based on how the light-sensitive dye reacts to the light.

How Is Staging Done for Adult Soft Tissue Sarcoma?

After adult soft tissue sarcoma has been diagnosed, tests are done to find out if cancer cells have spread within the soft tissue or to other parts of the body.

The process used to find out if cancer has spread within the soft tissue or to other parts of the body is called staging. Staging of soft tissue sarcoma is also based on the grade and size of the tumor, whether it is superficial (close to the skin's surface) or deep, and whether it has spread to the lymph nodes or other parts of the body. The information gathered from the staging process determines the stage of the disease. It is important to know the stage in order to plan treatment.

The following tests and procedures may be used in the staging process:

- **Physical exam and history:** An exam of the body to check general signs of health, including checking for signs of disease, such as lumps or anything else that seems unusual. A history of the patient's health habits and past illnesses and treatments will also be taken.
- **Chest X-ray:** An X-ray of the organs and bones inside the chest. An X-ray is a type of energy beam that can go through the body and onto film, making a picture of areas inside the body.
- **Blood chemistry studies:** A procedure in which a blood sample is checked to measure the amounts of certain substances released into the blood by organs and tissues in the body. An unusual (higher or lower than normal) amount of a substance can be a sign of disease.
- **Complete blood count (CBC):** A procedure in which a sample of blood is drawn and checked for the following:
    - The number of red blood cells, white blood cells, and platelets

- The amount of hemoglobin (the protein that carries oxygen) in the red blood cells
- The portion of the blood sample made up of red blood cells

- **Computerized tomography (CT)/computerized axial tomography (CAT) scan:** A procedure that makes a series of detailed pictures of areas inside of the body, such as the lung and abdomen, taken from different angles. The pictures are made by a computer linked to an X-ray machine. A dye may be injected into a vein or swallowed to help the organs or tissues show up more clearly.
- **Magnetic resonance imaging (MRI):** A procedure that uses a magnet, radio waves, and a computer to make a series of detailed pictures of areas inside the body. This procedure is also called nuclear magnetic resonance imaging (NMRI).
- **Positron emission tomography (PET) scan:** A procedure to find malignant tumor cells in the body. A small amount of radioactive glucose (sugar) is injected into a vein. The PET scanner rotates around the body and makes a picture of where glucose is being used in the body. Malignant tumor cells show up brighter in the picture because they are more active and take up more glucose than normal cells do.

The results of these tests are viewed together with the results of the tumor biopsy to find out the stage of the soft tissue sarcoma before treatment is given. Sometimes chemotherapy or radiation therapy is given as the initial treatment and afterward the soft tissue sarcoma is staged again.

Stages of Adult Soft Tissue Sarcoma

The following stages are used for adult soft tissue sarcoma:
Stage I. Stage I is divided into stages IA and IB:

- In stage IA, the tumor is low-grade (likely to grow and spread slowly) and 5 centimeters or smaller. It may be either superficial (in subcutaneous tissue with no spread into connective tissue or muscle below) or deep (in the muscle and may be in connective or subcutaneous tissue).
- In stage IB, the tumor is low-grade (likely to grow and spread slowly) and larger than 5 centimeters. It may be either superficial (in subcutaneous tissue with no spread into connective

tissue or muscle below) or deep (in the muscle and may be in connective or subcutaneous tissue).

Stage II. Stage II is divided into stages IIA and IIB:

- In stage IIA, the tumor is mid-grade (somewhat likely to grow and spread quickly) or high-grade (likely to grow and spread quickly) and 5 centimeters or smaller. It may be either superficial (in subcutaneous tissue with no spread into connective tissue or muscle below) or deep (in the muscle and may be in connective or subcutaneous tissue).
- In stage IIB, the tumor is mid-grade (somewhat likely to grow and spread quickly) and larger than 5 centimeters. It may be either superficial (in subcutaneous tissue with no spread into connective tissue or muscle below) or deep (in the muscle and may be in connective or subcutaneous tissue).

Stage III. In stage III, the tumor is either:

- high-grade (likely to grow and spread quickly), larger than 5 centimeters, and either superficial (in subcutaneous tissue with no spread into connective tissue or muscle below) or deep (in the muscle and may be in connective or subcutaneous tissue); or
- any grade, any size, and has spread to nearby lymph nodes.

Stage III cancer that has spread to the lymph nodes is advanced stage III.

Stage IV. In stage IV, the tumor is any grade, any size, and may have spread to nearby lymph nodes. Cancer has spread to distant parts of the body, such as the lungs.

What Standard Treatments Are Available for People with Adult Soft Tissue Sarcoma?

Surgery

Surgery is the most common treatment for adult soft tissue sarcoma. For some soft-tissue sarcomas, removal of the tumor in surgery may be the only treatment needed. The following surgical procedures may be used:

- **Mohs microsurgery:** A procedure in which the tumor is cut from the skin in thin layers. During surgery, the edges of the tumor and each layer of tumor removed are viewed through a microscope to check for cancer cells. Layers continue to be removed until no more cancer cells are seen. This type of surgery removes as little normal tissue as possible and is often used where appearance is important, such as on the skin.

- **Wide local excision:** Removal of the tumor along with some normal tissue around it. For tumors of the head, neck, abdomen, and trunk, as little normal tissue as possible is removed.
- **Limb-sparing surgery:** Removal of the tumor in an arm or leg without amputation, so the use and appearance of the limb is saved. Radiation therapy or chemotherapy may be given first to shrink the tumor. The tumor is then removed in a wide local excision. Tissue and bone that are removed may be replaced with a graft using tissue and bone taken from another part of the patient's body, or with an implant such as artificial bone.
- **Amputation:** Surgery to remove part or all of a limb or appendage, such as an arm or leg. Amputation is rarely used to treat soft tissue sarcoma of the arm or leg.
- **Lymphadenectomy:** A surgical procedure in which lymph nodes are removed and a sample of tissue is checked under a microscope for signs of cancer. This procedure is also called a lymph node dissection.

Radiation therapy or chemotherapy may be given before or after surgery to remove the tumor. When given before surgery, radiation therapy or chemotherapy will make the tumor smaller and reduce the amount of tissue that needs to be removed during surgery. Treatment given before surgery is called neoadjuvant therapy. When given after surgery, radiation therapy or chemotherapy will kill any remaining cancer cells. Treatment given after the surgery, to lower the risk that the cancer will come back, is called adjuvant therapy.

Radiation Therapy

Radiation therapy is a cancer treatment that uses high-energy X-rays or other types of radiation to kill cancer cells or keep them from growing. There are two types of radiation therapy:

- External radiation therapy uses a machine outside the body to send radiation toward the cancer.

- Internal radiation therapy uses a radioactive substance sealed in needles, seeds, wires, or catheters that are placed directly into or near the cancer.

Intensity-modulated radiation therapy (IMRT) is a type of 3-dimensional (3D) radiation therapy that uses a computer to make pictures of the size and shape of the tumor. Thin beams of radiation of different intensities (strengths) are aimed at the tumor from many angles. This type of external radiation therapy causes less damage to nearby healthy tissue and is less likely to cause dry mouth, trouble swallowing, and damage to the skin.

The way the radiation therapy is given depends on the type and stage of the cancer being treated. External radiation therapy and internal radiation therapy may be used to treat adult soft tissue sarcoma.

Chemotherapy

Chemotherapy is a cancer treatment that uses drugs to stop the growth of cancer cells, either by killing the cells or by stopping them from dividing. When chemotherapy is taken by mouth or injected into a vein or muscle, the drugs enter the bloodstream and can reach cancer cells throughout the body (systemic chemotherapy). The way the chemotherapy is given depends on the type and stage of the cancer being treated.

New types of treatment are being tested in clinical trials.

Regional chemotherapy. Clinical trials are studying ways to improve the effect of chemotherapy on tumor cells, including the following:

- **Regional hyperthermia therapy:** A treatment in which tissue around the tumor is exposed to high temperatures to damage and kill cancer cells or to make cancer cells more sensitive to chemotherapy.

- **Isolated limb perfusion:** A procedure that sends chemotherapy directly to an arm or leg in which the cancer has formed. The flow of blood to and from the limb is temporarily stopped with a tourniquet, and anticancer drugs are put directly into the blood of the limb. This sends a high dose of drugs to the tumor.

Treatment for adult soft tissue sarcoma may cause side effects.

Is There a Need for Follow-Up Tests?

Some of the tests that were done to diagnose the cancer or to find out the stage of the cancer may be repeated. Some tests will be repeated in order to see how well the treatment is working. Decisions about whether to continue, change, or stop treatment may be based on the results of these tests.

Some of the tests will continue to be done from time to time after treatment has ended. The results of these tests can show if your condition has changed or if the cancer has recurred (come back). These tests are sometimes called follow-up tests or check-ups.

What Is the Prognosis for Adult Soft Tissue Sarcoma?

The treatment options and prognosis (chance of recovery) depend on the following:

- The type of soft tissue sarcoma
- The size, grade, and stage of the tumor
- How fast the cancer cells are growing and dividing
- Where the tumor is in the body
- Whether all of the tumor is removed by surgery
- The patient's age and general health
- Whether the cancer has recurred (come back)

Section 55.5

Synovial Sarcoma

This section includes text excerpted from "Synovial Sarcoma," Genetic and Rare Diseases Information Center (GARD), National Center for Advancing Translational Sciences (NCATS), September 10, 2015.

What Is Synovial Sarcoma?

Synovial sarcoma is a rare and aggressive soft tissue sarcoma. In the early stages of the condition, it may cause no noticeable signs or symptoms. However, as the tumor grows larger, affected people may notice a lump or swelling. In some cases, the tumor can limit range of motion or cause numbness and/or pain if it presses on nearby nerves. Although synovial sarcoma does not have a clearly defined cause, genetic factors are believed to influence the development of this disease. Cells in these tumors are usually characterized by the presence of a translocation involving chromosomes X and 18. This translocation is specific to synovial sarcoma and is often used to diagnose the condition. Treatment generally includes a combination of surgery, radiation therapy and/or chemotherapy.

What Are the Signs and Symptoms of Synovial Sarcoma?

In the early stages of the condition, synovial sarcoma may cause no noticeable signs or symptoms. However, as the tumor grows larger, affected people may notice a lump or swelling. In some cases, the tumor can limit range of motion or cause numbness and/or pain if it presses on nearby nerves. The symptoms of synovial sarcoma can be mistaken for those of inflammation of the joints (arthritis) or other noncancerous conditions that cause inflammation such as bursitis and synovitis.

What Causes Synovial Sarcoma?

The exact underlying cause of synovial sarcoma is poorly understood. However, studies show that a certain genetic change is identified in more than 90 percent of cases. More specifically, a translocation between chromosome X and chromosome 18 appears to play a role in the development of synovial sarcoma. This alteration is known as a somatic mutation because it only develops in some cells of the body during a person's lifetime and is not inherited.

Certain inherited conditions such as Li Fraumeni syndrome or neurofibromatosis type 1 are associated with an increased risk of developing synovial sarcoma and other forms of soft tissue sarcoma. Some studies suggest that exposure to radiation therapy and/or certain chemical carcinogens may also be risk factors for soft tissue sarcoma.

How Is Synovial Sarcoma Diagnosed?

A diagnosis of synovial sarcoma may first be suspected based on the presence of characteristic signs and symptoms. Additional testing can then be ordered to confirm the diagnosis, determine the severity of the condition and inform treatment options. These tests may include:

- Imaging studies such as X-ray, computed tomography (CT), and/or magnetic resonance imaging (MRI) scan
- Genetic testing to detect the specific chromosomal translocation between chromosome 18 and chromosome X that is identified in most cases of synovial sarcoma
- A biopsy of the tumor

How Might Synovial Sarcoma Be Treated?

The treatment of synovial sarcoma depends on the age of the person; the size and location of the tumor and the severity of the disease. The most common treatment is surgery to remove the entire tumor. In some cases, radiation therapy and/or chemotherapy may also be necessary before and/or after the surgery. When given before surgery, radiation therapy and chemotherapy may reduce the size of the tumor, allowing less tissue to be removed. These therapies may be given after surgery to reduce the risk of recurrence.

What Is the Long-Term Outlook for People with Synovial Sarcoma?

The long-term outlook (prognosis) for people with synovial sarcoma depends on many factors, including the size, grade and stage of the tumor; where the tumor is located; and the affected person's age and overall health. In general, synovial sarcoma has a survival rate of 50–60 percent at 5 years and 40–50 percent at 10 years. Recurrence has been reported up to 69 months after treatment and suggests a worse prognosis with low survival rates.

Section 55.6

Gastrointestinal Stromal Tumors

This section includes text excerpted from "Gastrointestinal Stromal Tumors Treatment (PDQ®)—Patient Version," National Cancer Institute (NCI), May 15, 2017.

The gastrointestinal (GI) tract is part of the body's digestive system. It helps to digest food and takes nutrients (vitamins, minerals, carbohydrates, fats, proteins, and water) from food so they can be used by the body. The GI tract is made up of the following organs:

- Stomach
- Small intestine
- Large intestine (colon)

What Is Gastrointestinal Stromal Tumors (GISTs)?

Gastrointestinal stromal tumors (GISTs) is a disease in which abnormal cells form in the tissues of the gastrointestinal (GI) tract. It may be malignant (cancer) or benign (not cancer). They are most common in the stomach and small intestine but may be found anywhere in or near the GI tract. Some scientists believe that GISTs begin in cells called interstitial cells of Cajal (ICC), in the wall of the GI tract.

What Are the Risk Factors for GISTs?

Anything that increases your risk of getting a disease is called a risk factor. Having a risk factor does not mean that you will get cancer; not having risk factors doesn't mean that you will not get cancer. Talk with your doctor if you think you may be at risk.

The genes in cells carry the hereditary information received from a person's parents. Genetic factors can increase the risk of having a gastrointestinal stromal tumor. The risk of GIST is increased in people who have inherited a mutation (change) in a certain gene. In rare cases, GISTs can be found in several members of the same family.

GIST may be part of a genetic syndrome, but this is rare. A genetic syndrome is a set of symptoms or conditions that occur together and is usually caused by abnormal genes. The following genetic syndromes have been linked to GIST:

- Neurofibromatosis type 1 (NF1)
- Carney triad

What Are the Signs and Symptoms of GISTs?

Signs of GISTs include blood in the stool or vomit. These and other signs and symptoms may be caused by a GIST or by other conditions. Check with your doctor if you have any of the following:

- Blood (either bright red or very dark) in the stool or vomit
- Pain in the abdomen, which may be severe
- Feeling very tired
- Trouble or pain when swallowing
- Feeling full after only a little food is eaten

How Is GISTs Diagnosed?

Tests that examine the GI tract are used to detect (find) and diagnose gastrointestinal stromal tumors. The following tests and procedures may be used:

- **Physical exam and history:** An exam of the body to check general signs of health, including checking for signs of disease, such as lumps or anything else that seems unusual. A history of the patient's health habits and past illnesses and treatments will also be taken.
- **Computerized tomography (CT)/computerized axial tomography (CAT) scan:** A procedure that makes a series of detailed pictures of areas inside the body, taken from different angles. The pictures are made by a computer linked to an X-ray

machine. A dye may be injected into a vein or swallowed to help the organs or tissues show up more clearly.

- **Magnetic resonance imaging (MRI):** A procedure that uses a magnet, radio waves, and a computer to make a series of detailed pictures of areas inside the body. This procedure is also called nuclear magnetic resonance imaging (NMRI).
- **Endoscopic ultrasound and biopsy:** Endoscopy and ultrasound are used to make an image of the upper GI tract and a biopsy is done. An endoscope (a thin, tube-like instrument with a light and a lens for viewing) is inserted through the mouth and into the esophagus, stomach, and first part of the small intestine. A probe at the end of the endoscope is used to bounce high-energy sound waves (ultrasound) off internal tissues or organs and make echoes. The echoes form a picture of body tissues called a sonogram. This procedure is also called endosonography. Guided by the sonogram, the doctor removes tissue using a thin, hollow needle. A pathologist views the tissue under a microscope to look for cancer cells.

If cancer is found, the following tests may be done to study the cancer cells:

- **Immunohistochemistry:** A test that uses antibodies to check for certain antigens in a sample of tissue. The antibody is usually linked to a radioactive substance or a dye that causes the tissue to light up under a microscope. This type of test may be used to tell the difference between different types of cancer.
- **Mitotic rate:** A measure of how fast the cancer cells are dividing and growing. The mitotic rate is found by counting the number of cells dividing in a certain amount of cancer tissue.

Very Small GISTs Are Common

Sometimes GISTs are smaller than the eraser on top of a pencil. Tumors may be found during a procedure that is done for another reason, such as an X-ray or surgery. Some of these small tumors will not grow and cause signs or symptoms or spread to the abdomen or other parts of the body. Doctors do not agree on whether these small tumors should be removed or whether they should be watched to see if they begin to grow.

How Is Staging Done for GISTs?

After a GIST has been diagnosed, tests are done to find out if cancer cells have spread within the gastrointestinal tract or to other parts of the body.

The process used to find out if cancer has spread within the gastrointestinal (GI) tract or to other parts of the body is called staging. The information gathered from the staging process determines the stage of the disease. The following tests and procedures may be used in the staging process:

- **Positron emission tomography (PET) scan:** A procedure to find malignant tumor cells in the body. A small amount of radioactive glucose (sugar) is injected into a vein. The PET scanner rotates around the body and makes a picture of where glucose is being used in the body. Malignant tumor cells show up brighter in the picture because they are more active and take up more glucose than normal cells do.
- **CT/CAT scan:** A procedure that makes a series of detailed pictures of areas inside the body, taken from different angles. The pictures are made by a computer linked to an X-ray machine. A dye may be injected into a vein or swallowed to help the organs or tissues show up more clearly. This procedure is also called computed tomography, computerized tomography, or computerized axial tomography.
- **MRI:** A procedure that uses a magnet, radio waves, and a computer to make a series of detailed pictures of areas inside the body. This procedure is also called nuclear magnetic resonance imaging (NMRI).
- **Chest X-ray:** An X-ray of the organs and bones inside the chest. An X-ray is a type of energy beam that can go through the body and onto film, making a picture of areas inside the body.
- **Bone scan:** A procedure to check if there are rapidly dividing cells, such as cancer cells, in the bone. A very small amount of radioactive material is injected into a vein and travels through the bloodstream. The radioactive material collects in the bones with cancer and is detected by a scanner.

What Standard Treatments Are Available for People with GISTs?

Surgery

If the GIST has not spread and is in a place where surgery can be safely done, the tumor and some of the tissue around it may be removed. Sometimes surgery is done using a laparoscope (a thin, lighted tube) to see inside the body. Small incisions (cuts) are made in the wall of the abdomen and a laparoscope is inserted into one of the incisions. Instruments may be inserted through the same incision or through other incisions to remove organs or tissues.

Targeted Therapy

Targeted therapy is a type of treatment that uses drugs or other substances to identify and attack specific cancer cells without harming normal cells.

Tyrosine kinase inhibitors (TKIs) are targeted therapy drugs that block signals needed for tumors to grow. TKIs may be used to treat GISTs that cannot be removed by surgery or to shrink GISTs so they become small enough to be removed by surgery. Imatinib mesylate and sunitinib are two TKIs used to treat GISTs. TKIs are sometimes given for as long as the tumor does not grow and serious side effects do not occur.

Watchful Waiting

Watchful waiting is closely monitoring a patient's condition without giving any treatment until signs or symptoms appear or change.

Supportive Care

If a GIST gets worse during treatment or there are side effects, supportive care is usually given. The goal of supportive care is to prevent or treat the symptoms of a disease, side effects caused by treatment, and psychological, social, and spiritual problems related to a disease or its treatment. Supportive care helps improve the quality of life of patients who have a serious or life-threatening disease. Radiation therapy is sometimes given as supportive care to relieve pain in patients with large tumors that have spread.

Is There a Need for Follow-Up Tests?

Some of the tests that were done to diagnose the cancer or to find out the stage of the cancer may be repeated. Some tests will be repeated in order to see how well the treatment is working. Decisions about whether to continue, change, or stop treatment may be based on the results of these tests.

Some of the tests will continue to be done from time to time after treatment has ended. The results of these tests can show if your condition has changed or if the cancer has recurred (come back). These tests are sometimes called follow-up tests or check-ups.

Follow-up for GISTs that were removed by surgery may include CT scan of the liver and pelvis or watchful waiting. For GISTs that are treated with tyrosine kinase inhibitors, follow-up tests, such as CT, MRI, or PET scans, may be done to check how well the targeted therapy is working.

What Is the Prognosis for GISTs?

The prognosis (chance of recovery) and treatment options depend on the following:

- How quickly the cancer cells are growing and dividing
- The size of the tumor
- Where the tumor is in the body
- Whether the tumor can be completely removed by surgery
- Whether the tumor has spread to other parts of the body

Section 55.7

Kaposi Sarcoma

This section includes text excerpted from "Kaposi Sarcoma Treatment (PDQ®)—Patient Version," National Cancer Institute (NCI), February 14, 2018.

What Is Kaposi Sarcoma?

Kaposi sarcoma is a disease in which malignant tumors (cancer) can form in the skin, mucous membranes, lymph nodes, and other organs. It is a cancer that causes lesions (abnormal tissue) to grow in the skin; the mucous membranes lining the mouth, nose, and throat; lymph nodes; or other organs. The lesions are usually purple and are made of cancer cells, new blood vessels, red blood cells, and white blood cells. Kaposi sarcoma is different from other cancers in that lesions may begin in more than one place in the body at the same time.

How Many Types of Kaposi Sarcoma Are There?

There are several types of Kaposi sarcoma, including:

- Classic Kaposi sarcoma
- African Kaposi sarcoma
- Immunosuppressive therapy–related Kaposi sarcoma
- Epidemic Kaposi sarcoma
- Nonepidemic Kaposi sarcoma

What Causes Kaposi Sarcoma?

Human herpesvirus-8 (HHV-8) is found in the lesions of all patients with Kaposi sarcoma. This virus is also called Kaposi sarcoma herpesvirus (KSHV). Most people infected with HHV-8 do not get Kaposi sarcoma. Those infected with HHV-8 who are most likely to develop Kaposi sarcoma have immune systems weakened by disease or by drugs given after an organ transplant.

How Is Kaposi Sarcoma Diagnosed?

Tests that examine the skin, lungs, and gastrointestinal tract are used to detect (find) and diagnose Kaposi sarcoma. The following tests and procedures may be used:

- **Physical exam and history:** An exam of the body to check general signs of health, including checking skin and lymph nodes for signs of disease, such as lumps or anything else that seems unusual. A history of the patient's health habits and past illnesses and treatments will also be taken.
- **Chest X-ray:** An X-ray of the organs and bones inside the chest. An X-ray is a type of energy beam that can go through the body and onto film, making a picture of areas inside the body. This is used to find Kaposi sarcoma in the lungs.
- **Biopsy:** The removal of cells or tissues so they can be viewed under a microscope by a pathologist to check for signs of cancer.

One of the following types of biopsies may be done to check for Kaposi sarcoma lesions in the skin:

- **Excisional biopsy:** A scalpel is used to remove the entire skin growth.
- **Incisional biopsy:** A scalpel is used to remove part of a skin growth.
- **Core biopsy:** A wide needle is used to remove part of a skin growth.
- **Fine-needle aspiration (FNA) biopsy:** A thin needle is used to remove part of a skin growth.

An endoscopy or bronchoscopy may be done to check for Kaposi sarcoma lesions in the gastrointestinal tract or lungs.

- **Endoscopy for biopsy:** A procedure to look at organs and tissues inside the body to check for abnormal areas. An endoscope is inserted through an incision (cut) in the skin or opening in the body, such as the mouth. An endoscope is a thin, tube-like instrument with a light and a lens for viewing. It may also have a tool to remove tissue or lymph node samples, which are checked under a microscope for signs of disease. This is used to find Kaposi sarcoma lesions in the gastrointestinal tract.

- **Bronchoscopy for biopsy:** A procedure to look inside the trachea and large airways in the lung for abnormal areas. A bronchoscope is inserted through the nose or mouth into the trachea and lungs. A bronchoscope is a thin, tube-like instrument with a light and a lens for viewing. It may also have a tool to remove tissue samples, which are checked under a microscope for signs of disease. This is used to find Kaposi sarcoma lesions in the lungs.

After Kaposi sarcoma has been diagnosed, tests are done to find out if cancer cells have spread to other parts of the body.

The following tests and procedures may be used to find out if cancer has spread to other parts of the body:

- **Blood chemistry studies:** A procedure in which a blood sample is checked to measure the amounts of certain substances released into the blood by organs and tissues in the body. An unusual (higher or lower than normal) amount of a substance can be a sign of disease.
- **Computerized tomography (CT)/computerized axial tomography (CAT) scan:** A procedure that makes a series of detailed pictures of areas inside the body, such as the lung, liver, and spleen, taken from different angles. The pictures are made by a computer linked to an X-ray machine. A dye may be injected into a vein or swallowed to help the organs or tissues show up more clearly. This procedure is also called computed tomography, computerized tomography, or computerized axial tomography.
- **Positron emission tomography (PET) scan:** A procedure to find malignant tumor cells in the body. A small amount of radioactive glucose (sugar) is injected into a vein. The PET scanner rotates around the body and makes a picture of where glucose is being used in the body. Malignant tumor cells show up brighter in the picture because they are more active and take up more glucose than normal cells do. This imaging test checks for signs of cancer in the lung, liver, and spleen.
- **CD34 lymphocyte count:** A procedure in which a blood sample is checked to measure the amount of CD34 cells (a type of white blood cell). A lower than normal amount of CD34 cells can be a sign the immune system is not working well.

What Standard Treatments Are Available for Patients with Kaposi Sarcoma?

Four types of standard treatment are used to treat Kaposi sarcoma:

Radiation Therapy

Radiation therapy is a cancer treatment that uses high-energy X-rays or other types of radiation to kill cancer cells or keep them from growing. There are two types of radiation therapy:

- External radiation therapy uses a machine outside the body to send radiation toward the cancer.
- Internal radiation therapy uses a radioactive substance sealed in needles, seeds, wires, or catheters that are placed directly into or near the cancer.

The way the radiation therapy is given depends on the type of the cancer being treated. Certain types of external radiation therapy are used to treat Kaposi sarcoma lesions. Photon radiation therapy treats lesions with high-energy light. Electron beam radiation therapy uses tiny negatively charged particles called electrons.

Surgery

The following surgical procedures may be used for Kaposi sarcoma to treat small, surface lesions:

- **Local excision:** The cancer is cut from the skin along with a small amount of normal tissue around it.
- **Electrodesiccation and curettage:** The tumor is cut from the skin with a curette (a sharp, spoon-shaped tool). A needle-shaped electrode is then used to treat the area with an electric current that stops the bleeding and destroys cancer cells that remain around the edge of the wound. The process may be repeated one to three times during the surgery to remove all of the cancer.
- **Cryosurgery:** A treatment that uses an instrument to freeze and destroy abnormal tissue. This type of treatment is also called cryotherapy.

Chemotherapy

Chemotherapy is a cancer treatment that uses drugs to stop the growth of cancer cells, either by killing the cells or by stopping them

from dividing. When chemotherapy is taken by mouth or injected into a vein or muscle, the drugs enter the bloodstream and can reach cancer cells throughout the body (systemic chemotherapy). When chemotherapy is placed directly into the cerebrospinal fluid, an organ, tissue, or a body cavity such as the abdomen, the drugs mainly affect cancer cells in those areas (regional chemotherapy). In electrochemotherapy, intravenous chemotherapy is given and a probe is used to send electric pulses to the tumor. The pulses make an opening in the membrane around the tumor cell and allow the chemotherapy to get inside. Electrochemotherapy is being studied in the treatment of Kaposi sarcoma.

The way the chemotherapy is given depends on where the Kaposi sarcoma lesions occur in the body. In Kaposi sarcoma, chemotherapy may be given in the following ways:

- For local Kaposi sarcoma lesions, such as in the mouth, anticancer drugs may be injected directly into the lesion (intralesional chemotherapy).
- For local lesions on the skin, a topical agent may be applied to the skin as a gel. Electrochemotherapy may also be used.
- For widespread lesions on the skin, intravenous chemotherapy may be given.

Liposomal chemotherapy uses liposomes (very tiny fat particles) to carry anticancer drugs. Liposomal doxorubicin is used to treat Kaposi sarcoma. The liposomes build up in Kaposi sarcoma tissue more than in healthy tissue, and the doxorubicin is released slowly. This increases the effect of the doxorubicin and causes less damage to healthy tissue.

Biologic Therapy

Biologic therapy is a treatment that uses the patient's immune system to fight cancer. Substances made by the body or made in a laboratory are used to boost, direct, or restore the body's natural defenses against cancer. This type of cancer treatment is also called biotherapy or immunotherapy. Interferon alfa is a biologic agent used to treat Kaposi sarcoma.

Why Is Treatment of Epidemic Kaposi Sarcoma Combined with the Treatment for Acquired Immune Deficiency Syndrome (AIDS)?

Treatment of epidemic Kaposi sarcoma combines treatment for Kaposi sarcoma with treatment for AIDS. For the treatment of epidemic Kaposi sarcoma, combined antiretroviral therapy (cART) is used to slow the progression of AIDS. cART may be combined with anticancer drugs and medicines that prevent and treat infections.

What New Types of Treatment Are Being Tested in Clinical Trials?

Targeted Therapy

Targeted therapy is a type of treatment that uses drugs or other substances to identify and attack specific cancer cells without harming normal cells. Monoclonal antibody therapy and tyrosine kinase inhibitors (TKIs) are types of targeted therapy being studied in the treatment of Kaposi sarcoma.

Monoclonal antibody therapy is a cancer treatment that uses antibodies made in the laboratory from a single type of immune system cell. These antibodies can identify substances on cancer cells or normal substances that may help cancer cells grow. The antibodies attach to the substances and kill the cancer cells, block their growth, or keep them from spreading. Monoclonal antibodies are given by infusion. These may be used alone or to carry drugs, toxins, or radioactive material directly to cancer cells.

Bevacizumab is a monoclonal antibody that is being studied in the treatment of Kaposi sarcoma.

TKIs are targeted therapy drugs that block signals needed for tumors to grow. Imatinib mesylate is a TKI being studied in the treatment of Kaposi sarcoma.

Treatment for Kaposi sarcoma may cause side effects.

What Is the Prognosis for Kaposi Sarcoma?

The prognosis (chance of recovery) and treatment options depend on the following:

- The type of Kaposi sarcoma
- The general health of the patient, especially the patient's immune system
- Whether the cancer has just been diagnosed or has recurred (come back)

Is There a Need for Follow-Up Tests?

Some of the tests that were done to diagnose the cancer or to find out the stage of the cancer may be repeated. Some tests will be repeated in order to see how well the treatment is working. Decisions about whether to continue, change, or stop treatment may be based on the results of these tests.

Some of the tests will continue to be done from time to time after treatment has ended. The results of these tests can show if your condition has changed or if the cancer has recurred (come back). These tests are sometimes called follow-up tests or check-ups.

Chapter 56

Germ Cell Tumors

Chapter Contents

Section 56.1

Ovarian Germ Cell Tumors

This section includes text excerpted from "Ovarian Germ Cell Tumors Treatment (PDQ®)—Patient Version," National Cancer Institute (NCI), October 13, 2017.

The ovaries are a pair of organs in the female reproductive system. They are in the pelvis, one on each side of the uterus (the hollow, pear-shaped organ where a fetus grows). Each ovary is about the size and shape of an almond. The ovaries make eggs and female hormones.

What Is Ovarian Germ Cell Tumors?

Ovarian germ cell tumor is a disease in which malignant (cancer) cells form in the germ (egg) cells of the ovary. It is a general name that is used to describe several different types of cancer. The most common ovarian germ cell tumor is called dysgerminoma.

Germ cell tumors begin in the reproductive cells (egg or sperm) of the body. Ovarian germ cell tumors usually occur in teenage girls or young women and most often affect just one ovary.

What Are the Signs and Symptoms of Ovarian Germ Cell Tumors?

Signs of ovarian germ cell tumor are swelling of the abdomen or vaginal bleeding after menopause.

Ovarian germ cell tumors can be hard to diagnose (find) early. Often there are no symptoms in the early stages, but tumors may be found during regular gynecologic exams (checkups). Check with your doctor if you have either of the following:

- Swollen abdomen without weight gain in other parts of the body
- Bleeding from the vagina after menopause (when you are no longer having menstrual periods)

How Is Ovarian Germ Cell Tumors Diagnosed?

Tests that examine the ovaries, pelvic area, blood, and ovarian tissue are used to detect (find) and diagnose ovarian germ cell tumor. The following tests and procedures may be used:

- **Physical exam and history:** An exam of the body to check general signs of health, including checking for signs of disease, such as lumps or anything else that seems unusual. A history of the patient's health habits and past illnesses and treatments will also be taken.
- **Pelvic exam:** An exam of the vagina, cervix, uterus, fallopian tubes, ovaries, and rectum. A speculum is inserted into the vagina and the doctor or nurse looks at the vagina and cervix for signs of disease. A pap test of the cervix is usually done. The doctor or nurse also inserts one or two lubricated, gloved fingers of one hand into the vagina and places the other hand over the lower abdomen to feel the size, shape, and position of the uterus and ovaries. The doctor or nurse also inserts a lubricated, gloved finger into the rectum to feel for lumps or abnormal areas.
- **Laparotomy:** A surgical procedure in which an incision (cut) is made in the wall of the abdomen to check the inside of the abdomen for signs of disease. The size of the incision depends on the reason the laparotomy is being done. Sometimes organs are removed or tissue samples are taken and checked under a microscope for signs of disease.
- **Computed tomography (CT)/computerized axial tomography (CAT) scan:** A procedure that makes a series of detailed pictures of areas inside the body, taken from different angles. The pictures are made by a computer linked to an X-ray machine. A dye may be injected into a vein or swallowed to help the organs or tissues show up more clearly. This procedure is also called computed tomography, computerized tomography, or computerized axial tomography.
- **Serum tumor marker test:** A procedure in which a sample of blood is checked to measure the amounts of certain substances released into the blood by organs, tissues, or tumor cells in the body. Certain substances are linked to specific types of cancer when found in increased levels in the blood. These are called

tumor markers. An increased level of alpha-fetoprotein (AFP) or human chorionic gonadotropin (HCG) in the blood may be a sign of ovarian germ cell tumor.

How Is Staging Done for Ovarian Germ Cell Tumors?

After ovarian germ cell tumor has been diagnosed, tests are done to find out if cancer cells have spread within the ovary or to other parts of the body.

The process used to find out whether cancer has spread within the ovary or to other parts of the body is called staging. The information gathered from the staging process determines the stage of the disease. Unless a doctor is sure the cancer has spread from the ovaries to other parts of the body, an operation called a laparotomy is done to see if the cancer has spread. The doctor must cut into the abdomen and carefully look at all the organs to see if they have cancer in them. The doctor will cut out small pieces of tissue so they can be checked under a microscope for signs of cancer. The doctor may also wash the abdominal cavity with fluid, which is also checked under a microscope to see if it has cancer cells in it. Usually the doctor will remove the cancer and other organs that have cancer in them during the laparotomy. It is important to know the stage in order to plan treatment.

Many of the tests used to diagnose ovarian germ cell tumor are also used for staging. The following tests and procedures may also be used for staging:

- **Positron emission tomography (PET) scan:** A procedure to find malignant tumor cells in the body. A small amount of radioactive glucose (sugar) is injected into a vein. The PET scanner rotates around the body and makes a picture of where glucose is being used in the body. Malignant tumor cells show up brighter in the picture because they are more active and take up more glucose than normal cells do.
- **Magnetic resonance imaging (MRI):** A procedure that uses a magnet, radio waves, and a computer to make a series of detailed pictures of areas inside the body. This procedure is also called nuclear magnetic resonance imaging (NMRI).
- **Transvaginal ultrasound exam:** A procedure used to examine the vagina, uterus, fallopian tubes, and bladder. An ultrasound transducer (probe) is inserted into the vagina and used to bounce high-energy sound waves (ultrasound) off internal tissues or organs and make echoes. The echoes form a picture of

body tissues called a sonogram. The doctor can identify tumors by looking at the sonogram.

Stages of Ovarian Germ Cell Tumors

The following stages are used for ovarian germ cell tumors:

Stage I. In stage I, cancer is found in one or both ovaries. Stage I is divided into stage IA, stage IB, and stage IC.

- **Stage IA:** Cancer is found inside a single ovary.
- **Stage IB:** Cancer is found inside both ovaries.
- **Stage IC:** Cancer is found inside one or both ovaries and one of the following is true:

cancer is also found on the outside surface of one or both ovaries; or

the capsule (outer covering) of the ovary has ruptured (broken open); or

cancer cells are found in the fluid of the peritoneal cavity (the body cavity that contains most of the organs in the abdomen) or in washings of the peritoneum (tissue lining the peritoneal cavity).

Stage II. In stage II, cancer is found in one or both ovaries and has spread into other areas of the pelvis. Stage II is divided into stage IIA, stage IIB, and stage IIC.

- **Stage IIA:** Cancer has spread to the uterus and/or fallopian tubes (the long slender tubes through which eggs pass from the ovaries to the uterus).
- **Stage IIB:** Cancer has spread to other tissue within the pelvis.
- **Stage IIC:** Cancer is found inside one or both ovaries and has spread to the uterus and/or fallopian tubes, or to other tissue within the pelvis. Also, one of the following is true:
    - cancer is found on the outside surface of one or both ovaries; or
    - the capsule (outer covering) of the ovary has ruptured (broken open); or
    - cancer cells are found in the fluid of the peritoneal cavity (the body cavity that contains most of the organs in the abdomen) or in washings of the peritoneum (tissue lining the peritoneal cavity).

Stage III. In stage III, cancer is found in one or both ovaries and has spread outside the pelvis to other parts of the abdomen and/or nearby lymph nodes. Stage III is divided into stage IIIA, stage IIIB, and stage IIIC.

- **Stage IIIA:** The tumor is found in the pelvis only, but cancer cells that can be seen only with a microscope have spread to the surface of the peritoneum (tissue that lines the abdominal wall and covers most of the organs in the abdomen), the small intestines, or the tissue that connects the small intestines to the wall of the abdomen.
- **Stage IIIB:** Cancer has spread to the peritoneum and the cancer in the peritoneum is 2 centimeters or smaller.
- **Stage IIIC:** Cancer has spread to the peritoneum and the cancer in the peritoneum is larger than 2 centimeters and/or cancer has spread to lymph nodes in the abdomen.

Cancer that has spread to the surface of the liver is also considered stage III ovarian cancer.

Stage IV. In stage IV, cancer has spread beyond the abdomen to other parts of the body, such as the lungs or tissue inside the liver.

Cancer cells in the fluid around the lungs is also considered stage IV ovarian cancer.

What Standard Treatments Are Available for People with Ovarian Germ Cell Tumors?

Four types of standard treatment are used:

Surgery

Surgery is the most common treatment of ovarian germ cell tumor. A doctor may take out the cancer using one of the following types of surgery.

- **Unilateral salpingo-oophorectomy:** A surgical procedure to remove one ovary and one fallopian tube.
- **Total hysterectomy:** A surgical procedure to remove the uterus, including the cervix. If the uterus and cervix are taken out through the vagina, the operation is called a vaginal hysterectomy. If the uterus and cervix are taken out through a

large incision (cut) in the abdomen, the operation is called a total abdominal hysterectomy. If the uterus and cervix are taken out through a small incision (cut) in the abdomen using a laparoscope, the operation is called a total laparoscopic hysterectomy.

- **Bilateral salpingo-oophorectomy:** A surgical procedure to remove both ovaries and both fallopian tubes.
- **Tumor debulking:** A surgical procedure in which as much of the tumor as possible is removed. Some tumors cannot be completely removed.

Even if the doctor removes all the cancer that can be seen at the time of the operation, some patients may be offered chemotherapy or radiation therapy after surgery to kill any cancer cells that are left. Treatment given after the surgery, to lower the risk that the cancer will come back, is called adjuvant therapy.

After chemotherapy for an ovarian germ cell tumor, a second-look laparotomy may be done. This is similar to the laparotomy that is done to find out the stage of the cancer. Second-look laparotomy is a surgical procedure to find out if tumor cells are left after primary treatment. During this procedure, the doctor will take samples of lymph nodes and other tissues in the abdomen to see if any cancer is left. This procedure is not done for dysgerminomas.

Observation

Observation is closely watching a patient's condition without giving any treatment unless signs or symptoms appear or change.

Chemotherapy

Chemotherapy is a cancer treatment that uses drugs to stop the growth of cancer cells, either by killing the cells or by stopping them from dividing. When chemotherapy is taken by mouth or injected into a vein or muscle, the drugs enter the bloodstream and can reach cancer cells throughout the body (systemic chemotherapy). When chemotherapy is placed directly into the cerebrospinal fluid, an organ, or a body cavity such as the abdomen, the drugs mainly affect cancer cells in those areas (regional chemotherapy). Combination chemotherapy is treatment using more than one anticancer drug. The way the chemotherapy is given depends on the type and stage of the cancer being treated.

Radiation Therapy

Radiation therapy is a cancer treatment that uses high-energy X-rays or other types of radiation to kill cancer cells or keep them from growing. There are two types of radiation therapy:

- External radiation therapy uses a machine outside the body to send radiation toward the cancer.
- Internal radiation therapy uses a radioactive substance sealed in needles, seeds, wires, or catheters that are placed directly into or near the cancer.

The way the radiation therapy is given depends on the type and stage of the cancer being treated. External radiation therapy is used to treat ovarian germ cell tumors.

Treatment for ovarian germ cell tumors may cause side effects.

Is There a Need for Follow-Up Tests?

Some of the tests that were done to diagnose the cancer or to find out the stage of the cancer may be repeated. Some tests will be repeated in order to see how well the treatment is working. Decisions about whether to continue, change, or stop treatment may be based on the results of these tests.

Some of the tests will continue to be done from time to time after treatment has ended. The results of these tests can show if your condition has changed or if the cancer has recurred (come back). These tests are sometimes called follow-up tests or check-ups.

What Is the Prognosis for Ovarian Germ Cell Tumors?

The prognosis (chance of recovery) and treatment options depend on the following:

- The type of cancer
- The size of the tumor
- The stage of cancer (whether it affects part of the ovary, involves the whole ovary, or has spread to other places in the body)
- The way the cancer cells look under a microscope
- The patient's general health

Ovarian germ cell tumors are usually cured if found and treated early.

Section 56.2

Extragonadal Germ Cell Tumors

This section includes text excerpted from "Extragonadal Germ Cell Tumors Treatment (PDQ®)—Patient Version," National Cancer Institute (NCI), May 24, 2016.

What Is Extragonadal Germ Cell Tumors?

"Extragonadal" means outside of the gonads (sex organs). When cells that are meant to form sperm in the testicles or eggs in the ovaries travel to other parts of the body, they may grow into extragonadal germ cell tumors. These tumors may begin to grow anywhere in the body but usually begin in organs such as the pineal gland in the brain, in the mediastinum (area between the lungs), or in the retroperitoneum (the back wall of the abdomen).

Extragonadal germ cell tumors can be benign (noncancer) or malignant (cancer). Benign extragonadal germ cell tumors are called benign teratomas. These are more common than malignant extragonadal germ cell tumors and often are very large.

Malignant extragonadal germ cell tumors are divided into two types, nonseminoma and seminoma. Nonseminomas tend to grow and spread more quickly than seminomas. They usually are large and cause signs and symptoms. If untreated, malignant extragonadal germ cell tumors may spread to the lungs, lymph nodes, bones, liver, or other parts of the body.

What Are the Risk Factors of Extragonadal Germ Cell Tumors?

Anything that increases your chance of getting a disease is called a risk factor. Having a risk factor does not mean that you will get cancer; not having risk factors doesn't mean that you will not get cancer. Talk with your doctor if you think you may be at risk.

Age and gender can affect the risk of extragonadal germ cell tumors. Risk factors for malignant extragonadal germ cell tumors include the following:

- Being male
- Being age 20 or older
- Having Klinefelter syndrome (KS)

What Are the Signs and Symptoms of Extragonadal Germ Cell Tumors?

Signs and symptoms of extragonadal germ cell tumors include breathing problems and chest pain.

Malignant extragonadal germ cell tumors may cause signs and symptoms as they grow into nearby areas. Other conditions may cause the same signs and symptoms. Check with your doctor if you have any of the following:

- Chest pain
- Breathing problems
- Cough
- Fever
- Headache
- Change in bowel habits
- Feeling very tired
- Trouble walking
- Trouble in seeing or moving the eyes

How Is Extragonadal Germ Cell Tumors Diagnosed?

Imaging and blood tests are used to detect (find) and diagnose extragonadal germ cell tumors. The following tests and procedures may be used:

- **Physical exam and history:** An exam of the body to check general signs of health, including checking for signs of disease, such as lumps or anything else that seems unusual. The testicles may be checked for lumps, swelling, or pain. A history of the patient's health habits and past illnesses and treatments will also be taken.

- **Chest X-ray:** An X-ray of the organs and bones inside the chest. An X-ray is a type of energy beam that can go through the body and onto film, making a picture of areas inside the body.
- **Serum tumor marker test:** A procedure in which a sample of blood is examined to measure the amounts of certain substances released into the blood by organs, tissues, or tumor cells in the body. Certain substances are linked to specific types of cancer when found in increased levels in the blood. These are called tumor markers. The following three tumor markers are used to detect extragonadal germ cell tumor:
  - Alpha-fetoprotein (AFP)
  - Beta-human chorionic gonadotropin (β-hCG)
  - Lactate dehydrogenase (LDH)

Blood levels of the tumor markers help determine if the tumor is a seminoma or nonseminoma.

- **Computed tomography (CT)/computerized axial tomography (CAT) scan:** A procedure that makes a series of detailed pictures of areas inside the body, taken from different angles. The pictures are made by a computer linked to an X-ray machine. A dye may be injected into a vein or swallowed to help the organs or tissues show up more clearly.

Sometimes a CT scan and a positron emission tomography (PET) scan are done at the same time. A PET scan is a procedure to find malignant tumor cells in the body. A small amount of radioactive glucose (sugar) is injected into a vein. The PET scanner rotates around the body and makes a picture of where glucose is being used in the body. Malignant tumor cells show up brighter in the picture because they are more active and take up more glucose than normal cells do. When a PET scan and CT scan are done at the same time, it is called a PET-CT.

- **Biopsy:** The removal of cells or tissues so they can be viewed under a microscope by a pathologist to check for signs of cancer. The type of biopsy used depends on where the extragonadal germ cell tumor is found.
  - **Excisional biopsy:** The removal of an entire lump of tissue.
  - **Incisional biopsy:** The removal of part of a lump or sample of tissue.
  - **Core biopsy:** The removal of tissue using a wide needle.

- **Fine-needle aspiration (FNA) biopsy:** The removal of tissue or fluid using a thin needle.

How Is Staging Done for Extragonadal Germ Cell Tumors?

After an extragonadal germ cell tumor has been diagnosed, tests are done to find out if cancer cells have spread to other parts of the body.

The extent or spread of cancer is usually described as stages. For extragonadal germ cell tumors, prognostic groups are used instead of stages. The tumors are grouped according to how well the cancer is expected to respond to treatment. It is important to know the prognostic group in order to plan treatment.

What Standard Treatments Are Available for People with Extragonadal Germ Cell Tumors?

Three types of standard treatment are used:

Radiation Therapy

Radiation therapy is a cancer treatment that uses high-energy X-rays or other types of radiation to kill cancer cells or keep them from growing. There are two types of radiation therapy:

- External radiation therapy uses a machine outside the body to send radiation toward the cancer.
- Internal radiation therapy uses a radioactive substance sealed in needles, seeds, wires, or catheters that are placed directly into or near the cancer.

The way the radiation therapy is given depends on the type and stage of the cancer being treated. External radiation therapy is used to treat seminoma.

Chemotherapy

Chemotherapy is a cancer treatment that uses drugs to stop the growth of cancer cells, either by killing the cells or by stopping them from dividing. When chemotherapy is taken by mouth or injected into a vein or muscle, the drugs enter the bloodstream and can reach cancer cells throughout the body (systemic chemotherapy). When chemotherapy is placed directly in the cerebrospinal fluid, an organ, or a body cavity such as the abdomen, the drugs mainly affect cancer cells in those areas (regional chemotherapy). The way the chemotherapy is given depends on the type and stage of the cancer being treated.

Surgery

Patients who have benign tumors or tumor remaining after chemotherapy or radiation therapy may need to have surgery.

High-Dose Chemotherapy with Stem Cell Transplant

High-dose chemotherapy with stem cell transplant is a method of giving high doses of chemotherapy and replacing blood-forming cells destroyed by the cancer treatment. Stem cells (immature blood cells) are removed from the blood or bone marrow of the patient or a donor and are frozen and stored. After the chemotherapy is completed, the stored stem cells are thawed and given back to the patient through an infusion. These reinfused stem cells grow into (and restore) the body's blood cells.

What Is the Prognosis for Extragonadal Germ Cell Tumors Diagnosed?

The prognosis (chance of recovery) and treatment options depend on the following:

- Whether the tumor is nonseminoma or seminoma
- The size of the tumor and where it is in the body
- The blood levels of AFP, β-hCG, and LDH
- Whether the tumor has spread to other parts of the body
- The way the tumor responds to initial treatment
- Whether the tumor has just been diagnosed or has recurred (come back)

The following prognostic groups are used for extragonadal germ cell tumors:

Good Prognosis

A nonseminoma extragonadal germ cell tumor is in the good prognosis group if:

- the tumor is in the back of the abdomen; and

- the tumor has not spread to organs other than the lungs; and
- the levels of tumor markers AFP and β-hCG are normal and LDH is slightly above normal

A seminoma extragonadal germ cell tumor is in the good prognosis group if:

- the tumor has not spread to organs other than the lungs; and
- the level of AFP is normal; β-hCG and LDH may be at any level

Intermediate Prognosis

A nonseminoma extragonadal germ cell tumor is in the intermediate prognosis group if:

- the tumor is in the back of the abdomen; and
- the tumor has not spread to organs other than the lungs; and
- the level of any one of the tumor markers (AFP, β-hCG, or LDH) is more than slightly above normal

A seminoma extragonadal germ cell tumor is in the intermediate prognosis group if:

- the tumor has spread to organs other than the lungs; and
- the level of AFP is normal; β-hCG and LDH may be at any level

Poor Prognosis

A nonseminoma extragonadal germ cell tumor is in the poor prognosis group if:

- the tumor is in the chest; or
- the tumor has spread to organs other than the lungs; or
- the level of any one of the tumor markers (AFP, β-hCG, or LDH) is high

Seminoma extragonadal germ cell tumor does not have a poor prognosis group.

Is There a Need for Follow-Up Tests?

Some of the tests that were done to diagnose the cancer or to find out the stage of the cancer may be repeated. Some tests will be repeated

in order to see how well the treatment is working. Decisions about whether to continue, change, or stop treatment may be based on the results of these tests.

Some of the tests will continue to be done from time to time after treatment has ended. The results of these tests can show if your condition has changed or if the cancer has recurred (come back). These tests are sometimes called follow-up tests or check-ups.

After initial treatment for extragonadal germ cell tumors, blood levels of AFP and other tumor markers continue to be checked to find out how well the treatment is working.

Section 56.3

Childhood Extracranial Germ Cell Tumors

This section includes text excerpted from "Childhood Extracranial Germ Cell Tumors Treatment (PDQ®)—Patient Version," National Cancer Institute (NCI), August 12, 2016.

What Are Childhood Extracranial Germ Cell Tumors?

Childhood extracranial germ cell tumors form from germ cells in parts of the body other than the brain.

A germ cell is a type of cell that forms as a fetus (unborn baby) develops. These cells later become sperm in the testicles or eggs in the ovaries. Sometimes while the fetus is forming, germ cells travel to parts of the body where they should not be and grow into a germ cell tumor. The tumor may form before or after birth.

Extracranial germ cell tumors usually form in the following areas of the body:

- Testicles
- Ovaries
- Sacrum or coccyx (bottom part of the spine)
- Retroperitoneum (the back wall of the abdomen)
- Mediastinum (area between the lungs)

Extracranial germ cell tumors are most common in adolescents 15–19 years of age. It may be benign (noncancer) or malignant (cancer).

What Are the Types of Childhood Extracranial Germ Cell Tumors?

There are three types of extracranial germ cell tumors. Extracranial germ cell tumors are grouped into mature teratomas, immature teratomas, and malignant germ cell tumors:

1. **Mature teratomas.** Mature teratomas are the most common type of extracranial germ cell tumor. Mature teratomas are benign tumors and not likely to become cancer. They usually occur in the sacrum or coccyx (bottom part of the spine) in newborns or in the ovaries of girls at the start of puberty. The cells of mature teratomas look almost like normal cells under a microscope. Some mature teratomas release enzymes or hormones that cause signs and symptoms of disease.
2. **Immature teratomas.** Immature teratomas also usually occur in the sacrum or coccyx (bottom part of the spine) in newborns or the ovaries of girls at the start of puberty. Immature teratomas have cells that look very different from normal cells under a microscope. Immature teratomas may be cancer. They often have several different types of tissue in them, such as hair, muscle, and bone. Some immature teratomas release enzymes or hormones that cause signs and symptoms of disease.
3. **Malignant germ cell tumors.** Malignant germ cell tumors are cancer. There are two main types of malignant germ cell tumors:
   - Germinomas. Tumors that make a hormone called beta-human chorionic gonadotropin (β-hCG). There are three types of germinomas:
     - Dysgerminomas form in the ovary in girls
     - Seminomas form in the testicle in boys
     - Germinomas form in areas of the body that are not the ovary or testicle
   - Nongerminomas. There are four types of nongerminomas:

- Yolk sac tumors make a hormone called alpha-fetoprotein (AFP). They can form in the ovary, testicle, or other areas of the body.
- Choriocarcinomas make a hormone called beta-human chorionic gonadotropin (β-hCG). They can form in the ovary, testicle, or other areas of the body.
- Embryonal carcinomas may make a hormone called β-hCG and/or a hormone called AFP. They can form in the testicle or other parts of the body, but not in the ovary.
- Mixed germ cell tumors are made up of both malignant germ cell tumor and teratoma. They can form in the ovary, testicle, or other areas of the body.

Childhood extracranial germ cell tumors are grouped as gonadal or extragonadal. Malignant extracranial germ cell tumors are gonadal or extragonadal.

- Gonadal germ cell tumors. Gonadal germ cell tumors form in the testicles in boys or ovaries in girls.
    - Testicular germ cell tumors. Testicular germ cell tumors are divided into two main types, seminoma, and nonseminoma
        - Seminomas make a hormone called beta-human chorionic gonadotropin (β-hCG)
        - Nonseminomas are usually large and cause signs or symptoms. They tend to grow and spread more quickly than seminomas

Testicular germ cell tumors usually occur before the age of 4 years or in adolescents and young adults. Testicular germ cell tumors in adolescents and young adults are different from those that form in early childhood. Boys older than 14 years with testicular germ cell tumors are treated in pediatric cancer centers, but the treatment is much like the treatment used in adults.

- Ovarian germ cell tumors. Ovarian germ cell tumors are more common in adolescent girls and young women. Most ovarian germ cell tumors are benign teratomas. Sometimes immature teratomas, dysgerminomas, yolk sac tumors, and mixed germ cell tumors (cancer) occur.

- Extragonadal extracranial germ cell tumors. Extragonadal extracranial germ cell tumors form in areas other than the brain, testicles, or ovaries. Most extragonadal extracranial germ cell tumors form along the midline of the body. This includes the following:
  - Sacrum (the large, triangle shaped bone in the lower spine that forms part of the pelvis)
  - Coccyx (the small bone at the bottom of the spine, also called the tailbone)
  - Mediastinum (the area between the lungs)
  - Back of the abdomen
  - Neck

In younger children, extragonadal extracranial germ cell tumors usually occur at birth or in early childhood. Most of these tumors are teratomas in the sacrum or coccyx. In older children, adolescents, and young adults, extragonadal extracranial germ cell tumors are often in the mediastinum.

The cause of most childhood extracranial germ cell tumors is unknown.

What Are the Risks of Childhood Extracranial Germ Cell Tumors?

Having certain inherited disorders can increase the risk of an extracranial germ cell tumor. Anything that increases your risk of getting a disease is called a risk factor. Having a risk factor does not mean that you will get cancer; not having risk factors doesn't mean that you will not get cancer. Talk with your child's doctor if you think your child may be at risk.

Possible risk factors for extracranial germ cell tumors include the following:

Having certain genetic syndromes:

- Klinefelter syndrome (KS) may increase the risk of germ cell tumors in the mediastinum.
  - Swyer syndrome may increase the risk of germ cell tumors in the testicles or ovaries.
  - Turner syndrome (TS) may increase the risk of germ cell tumors in the ovaries.

- Having an undescended testicle may increase the risk of developing a testicular germ cell tumor.

What Are the Signs of Childhood Extracranial Germ Cell Tumors?

The signs of childhood extracranial germ cell tumors depend on the type of tumor and where it is in the body. Different tumors may cause the following signs and symptoms. Other conditions may cause these same signs and symptoms. Check with a doctor if your child has any of the following:

- A lump in the abdomen or lower back
- A painless lump in the testicle
- Pain in the abdomen
- Fever
- Constipation
- In females, no menstrual periods
- In females, unusual vaginal bleeding

How Are Childhood Extracranial Germ Cell Tumors Diagnosed?

Imaging studies and blood tests are used to detect (find) and diagnose childhood extracranial germ cell tumors. The following tests and procedures may be used:

- **Physical exam and history.** An exam of the body to check general signs of health, including checking for signs of disease, such as lumps or anything else that seems unusual. The testicles may be checked for lumps, swelling, or pain. A history of the patient's health habits and past illnesses and treatments will also be taken.
- **Serum tumor marker test.** A procedure in which a sample of blood is checked to measure the amounts of certain substances released into the blood by organs, tissues, or tumor cells in the body. Certain substances are linked to specific types of cancer when found in increased levels in the blood. These are called tumor markers. Most malignant germ cell tumors release tumor

markers. The following tumor markers are used to detect extracranial germ cell tumors:

- Alpha-fetoprotein (AFP)
- Beta-human chorionic gonadotropin (β-hCG)

For testicular germ cell tumors, blood levels of the tumor markers help show if the tumor is a seminoma or nonseminoma.

- **Blood chemistry studies.** A procedure in which a blood sample is checked to measure the amounts of certain substances released into the blood by organs and tissues in the body. An unusual (higher or lower than normal) amount of a substance can be a sign of disease.
- **Chest X-ray.** An X-ray of the organs and bones inside the chest. An X-ray is a type of energy beam that can go through the body and onto film, making a picture of areas inside the body.
- **Computed tomography (CT) scan (Computerized axial tomography (CAT) scan).** A procedure that makes a series of detailed pictures of areas inside the body, taken from different angles. The pictures are made by a computer linked to an X-ray machine. A dye may be injected into a vein or swallowed to help the organs or tissues show up more clearly. This procedure is also called computed tomography, computerized tomography, or computerized axial tomography.
- **Magnetic resonance imaging (MRI).** A procedure that uses a magnet, radio waves, and a computer to make a series of detailed pictures of areas inside the body. This procedure is also called nuclear magnetic resonance imaging (NMRI).
- **Ultrasound exam.** A procedure in which high-energy sound waves (ultrasound) are bounced off internal tissues or organs and make echoes. The echoes form a picture of body tissues called a sonogram. The picture can be printed to be looked at later.
- **Biopsy.** The removal of cells or tissues so they can be viewed under a microscope by a pathologist to check for signs of cancer. In some cases, the tumor is removed during surgery and then a biopsy is done.

The following tests may be done on the sample of tissue that is removed:

- **Cytogenetic analysis.** A laboratory test in which cells in a sample of tissue are viewed under a microscope to look for certain changes in the chromosomes.
- **Immunohistochemistry.** A test that uses antibodies to check for certain antigens in a sample of tissue. The antibody is usually linked to a radioactive substance or a dye that causes the tissue to light up under a microscope. This type of test may be used to tell the difference between different types of cancer.

What Are the Treatment Options for Childhood Extracranial Germ Cell Tumors?

Three types of standard treatment are used:

Surgery

Surgery to completely remove the tumor is done whenever possible. If the tumor is very large, chemotherapy may be given first, to make the tumor smaller and decrease the amount of tissue that needs to be removed during surgery. A goal of surgery is to keep reproductive function. The following types of surgery may be used:

- **Resection.** Surgery to remove tissue or part or all of an organ.
- **Radical inguinal orchiectomy.** Surgery to remove one or both testicles through an incision (cut) in the groin.
- **Unilateral salpingo-oophorectomy.** Surgery to remove one ovary and one fallopian tube on the same side.

Even if the doctor removes all the cancer that can be seen at the time of the surgery, some patients may be given chemotherapy after surgery to kill any cancer cells that are left. Treatment given after the surgery, to lower the risk that the cancer will come back, is called adjuvant therapy.

Observation

Observation is closely monitoring a patient's condition without giving any treatment until signs or symptoms appear or change. For childhood extracranial germ cell tumors, this includes:

- physical exams
- imaging tests and
- tumor marker tests

Chemotherapy

Chemotherapy is a cancer treatment that uses drugs to stop the growth of cancer cells, either by killing the cells or by stopping them from dividing. When chemotherapy is taken by mouth or injected into a vein or muscle, the drugs enter the bloodstream and can reach cancer cells throughout the body (systemic chemotherapy). When chemotherapy is placed directly into the cerebrospinal fluid, an organ, or a body cavity such as the abdomen, the drugs mainly affect cancer cells in those areas (regional chemotherapy). Combination chemotherapy is treatment using more than one anticancer drug.

The way the chemotherapy is given depends on the type and stage of the cancer being treated.

High Dose Chemotherapy with Stem Cell Transplant

High dose chemotherapy with stem cell transplant is a way of giving high doses of chemotherapy and replacing blood-forming cells destroyed by the cancer treatment. Stem cells (immature blood cells) are removed from the blood or bone marrow of the patient or a donor and are frozen and stored. After the chemotherapy is completed, the stored stem cells are thawed and given back to the patient through an infusion. These reinfused stem cells grow into (and restore) the body's blood cells.

Radiation Therapy

Radiation therapy is a cancer treatment that uses high-energy X-rays or other types of radiation to kill cancer cells or keep them from growing. There are two types of radiation therapy:

- External radiation therapy uses a machine outside the body to send radiation toward the cancer.
- Internal radiation therapy uses a radioactive substance sealed in needles, seeds, wires, or catheters that are placed directly into or near the cancer.

The way the radiation therapy is given depends on the type of cancer and whether it has come back. External radiation therapy is being studied for the treatment of childhood extracranial germ cell tumors that have come back.

What Are the Side Effects of Treatment?

Some cancer treatments cause side effects months or years after treatment has ended. Side effects from cancer treatment that begin during or after treatment and continue for months or years are called late effects. Late effects of cancer treatment may include the following:

- Physical problems
- Changes in mood, feelings, thinking, learning, or memory
- Second cancers (new types of cancer)

For example, late effects of surgery to remove tumors in the sacrum or coccyx include:

- Constipation
- Loss of bowel and bladder control
- Scars

Some late effects may be treated or controlled. It is important to talk with your child's doctors about the effects cancer treatment can have on your child.

What Is the Prognosis for Childhood Extracranial Germ Cell Tumors?

Certain factors affect prognosis (chance of recovery) and treatment options.

- The type of germ cell tumor
- Where the tumor first began to grow
- The stage of the cancer (whether it has spread to nearby areas or to other places in the body)
- How well the tumor responds to treatment (lower AFP and β-hCG levels)
- Whether the tumor can be completely removed by surgery.
- The patient's age and general health
- Whether the cancer has just been diagnosed or has recurred (come back)

The prognosis for childhood extracranial germ cell tumors, especially ovarian germ cell tumors, is good.

Chapter 57

Carcinoma of Unknown Primary Origin

What Is Carcinoma of Unknown Primary (CUP)?

Cancer can form in any tissue of the body. The primary cancer (the cancer that first formed) can spread to other parts of the body. This process is called metastasis. Cancer cells usually look like the cells in the type of tissue in which the cancer began. For example, breast cancer cells may spread to the lung. Because the cancer began in the breast, the cancer cells in the lung look like breast cancer cells.

Sometimes doctors find where the cancer has spread but cannot find where in the body the cancer first began to grow. This type of cancer is called a cancer of unknown primary (CUP) or occult primary tumor.

Tests are done to find where the primary cancer began and to get information about where the cancer has spread. When tests are able to find the primary cancer, the cancer is no longer a CUP and treatment is based on the type of primary cancer.

This chapter includes text excerpted from "Carcinoma of Unknown Primary Treatment (PDQ®)–Patient Version," National Cancer Institute (NCI), January 12, 2018.

Why Is the Primary Cancer Occasionally Not Traceable?

The primary cancer (the cancer that first formed) may not be found for one of the following reasons:

- The primary cancer is very small and grows slowly
- The body's immune system killed the primary cancer
- The primary cancer was removed during surgery for another condition and doctors didn't know cancer had formed. For example, a uterus with cancer may be removed during a hysterectomy to treat a serious infection.

What Are the Signs and Symptoms of CUP?

The signs and symptoms of CUP are different, depending on where the cancer has spread in the body. Sometimes CUP does not cause any signs or symptoms. Signs and symptoms may be caused by CUP or by other conditions. Check with your doctor if you have any of the following:

- Lump or thickening in any part of the body
- Pain that is in one part of the body and does not go away
- A cough that does not go away or hoarseness in the voice
- Change in bowel or bladder habits, such as constipation, diarrhea, or frequent urination
- Unusual bleeding or discharge
- Fever for no known reason that does not go away
- Night sweats
- Weight loss for no known reason or loss of appetite

How Is CUP Diagnosed?

Different tests are used to detect (find) cancer. The following tests and procedures may be used:

Physical exam and history: An exam of the body to check general signs of health, including checking for signs of disease, such as lumps or anything else that seems unusual. A history of the patient's health habits and past illnesses and treatments will also be taken.

Urinalysis: A test to check the color of urine and its contents, such as sugar, protein, blood, and bacteria.

- **Blood chemistry studies:** A procedure in which a blood sample is checked to measure the amounts of certain substances released into the blood by organs and tissues in the body. An unusual (higher or lower than normal) amount of a substance can be a sign of disease.
- **Complete blood count (CBC):** A procedure in which a sample of blood is drawn and checked for the following:
  - The number of red blood cells, white blood cells, and platelets
  - The amount of hemoglobin (the protein that carries oxygen) in the red blood cells
  - The portion of the sample made up of red blood cells
- **Fecal occult blood test:** A test to check stool (solid waste) for blood that can only be seen with a microscope. Small samples of stool are placed on special cards and returned to the doctor or laboratory for testing. Because some cancers bleed, blood in the stool may be a sign of cancer in the colon or rectum.

If tests show there may be cancer, a biopsy is done.

Biopsy: A biopsy is the removal of cells or tissues so they can be viewed under a microscope by a pathologist. The pathologist views the tissue under a microscope to look for cancer cells and to find out the type of cancer. The type of biopsy that is done depends on the part of the body being tested for cancer. One of the following types of biopsies may be used:

- **Excisional biopsy:** The removal of an entire lump of tissue.
- **Incisional biopsy:** The removal of part of a lump or a sample of tissue.
- **Core biopsy:** The removal of tissue using a wide needle.
- **Fine-needle aspiration (FNA) biopsy:** The removal tissue or fluid using a thin needle.

If cancer is found, one or more of the following laboratory tests may be used to study the tissue samples and find out the type of cancer:

- **Histologic study:** A laboratory test in which stains are added to a sample of cancer cells or tissue and viewed under a microscope to look for certain changes in the cells. Certain changes in the cells are linked to certain types of cancer.

- **Immunohistochemistry:** A test that uses antibodies to check for certain antigens in a sample of tissue. The antibody is usually linked to a radioactive substance or a dye that causes the tissue to light up under a microscope. This type of test may be used to tell the difference between different types of cancer.
- **Reverse transcription–polymerase chain reaction (RT-PCR) test:** A laboratory test in which cells in a sample of tissue are studied using chemicals to look for certain changes in the genes.
- **Cytogenetic analysis:** A laboratory test in which cells in a sample of tissue are viewed under a microscope to look for certain changes in the chromosomes. Changes in certain chromosomes are linked to certain types of cancer.
- **Light and electron microscopy:** A laboratory test in which cells in a sample of tissue are viewed under regular and high-powered microscopes to look for certain changes in the cells.

When Is Diagnosis of CUP Possible?

When the type of cancer cells or tissue removed is different from the type of cancer cells expected to be found, a diagnosis of CUP may be made.

The cells in the body have a certain look that depends on the type of tissue they come from. For example, a sample of cancer tissue taken from the breast is expected to be made up of breast cells. However, if the sample of tissue is a different type of cell (not made up of breast cells), it is likely that the cells have spread to the breast from another part of the body. In order to plan treatment, doctors first try to find the primary cancer (the cancer that first formed).

What Tests and Procedures Are Used to Find the Primary Cancer?

Tests and procedures used to find the primary cancer depend on where the cancer has spread.

- **Computerized tomography (CT)/computerized axial tomography (CAT) scan:** A procedure that makes a series of detailed pictures of areas inside the body, such as the chest or abdomen, taken from different angles. The pictures are made by a computer linked to an X-ray machine. A dye may be injected into a vein or swallowed to help the organs or tissues show up more clearly.

- **Magnetic resonance imaging (MRI):** A procedure that uses a magnet, radio waves, and a computer to make a series of detailed pictures of areas inside the body. This procedure is also called nuclear magnetic resonance imaging (NMRI).
- **Positron emission tomography (PET) scan:** A procedure to find malignant tumor cells in the body. A small amount of radioactive glucose (sugar) is injected into a vein. The PET scanner rotates around the body and makes a picture of where glucose is being used in the body. Malignant tumor cells show up brighter in the picture because they are more active and take up more glucose than normal cells do.
- **Mammogram:** An X-ray of the breast.
- **Endoscopy:** A procedure to look at organs and tissues inside the body to check for abnormal areas. An endoscope is inserted through an incision (cut) in the skin or opening in the body, such as the mouth. An endoscope is a thin, tube-like instrument with a light and a lens for viewing. It may also have a tool to remove tissue or lymph node samples, which are checked under a microscope for signs of disease. For example, a colonoscopy may be done.
- **Tumor marker test:** A procedure in which a sample of blood, urine, or tissue is checked to measure the amounts of certain substances made by organs, tissues, or tumor cells in the body. Certain substances are linked to specific types of cancer when found in increased levels in the body. These are called tumor markers. The blood may be checked for the levels of CA-125, CgA, alpha-fetoprotein (AFP), beta-human chorionic gonadotropin (β-hCG), or prostate-specific antigen (PSA).

Sometimes, none of the tests can find the primary cancer site. In these cases, treatment may be based on what the doctor thinks is the most likely type of cancer.

Stages of CUP

There is no staging system for CUP. The extent or spread of cancer is usually described as stages. The stage of the cancer is usually used to plan treatment. However, CUP has already spread to other parts of the body when it is found.

The information that is known about the cancer is used to plan treatment.

Doctors use the following types of information to plan treatment:

- The place in the body where the cancer is found, such as the peritoneum or the cervical (neck), axillary (armpit), or inguinal (groin) lymph nodes
- The type of cancer cell, such as melanoma
- Whether the cancer cell is poorly differentiated (looks very different from normal cells when viewed under a microscope)
- The signs and symptoms caused by the cancer
- The results of tests and procedures
- Whether the cancer is newly diagnosed or has recurred (come back)

Treatment Option Overview

Four types of standard treatment are used:

Surgery

Surgery is a common treatment for CUP. A doctor may remove the cancer and some of the healthy tissue around it.

Even if the doctor removes all the cancer that can be seen at the time of the surgery, some patients may be given chemotherapy or radiation therapy after surgery to kill any cancer cells that are left. Treatment given after the surgery, to increase the chances of a cure, is called adjuvant therapy.

Radiation Therapy

Radiation therapy is a cancer treatment that uses high-energy X-rays or other types of radiation to kill cancer cells or keep them from growing. There are two types of radiation therapy:

- External radiation therapy uses a machine outside the body to send radiation toward the cancer. Certain ways of giving radiation therapy can help keep radiation from damaging nearby healthy tissue. This type of radiation therapy may include the following:

- **Intensity-modulated radiation therapy (IMRT):** IMRT is a type of 3-dimensional (3D) radiation therapy that uses a computer to make pictures of the size and shape of the tumor. Thin beams of radiation of different intensities (strengths) are aimed at the tumor from many angles. This type of external radiation therapy causes less damage to nearby healthy tissue and is less likely to cause dry mouth, trouble swallowing, and damage to the skin.

- Internal radiation therapy uses a radioactive substance sealed in needles, seeds, wires, or catheters that are placed directly into or near the cancer.

The way the radiation therapy is given depends on the type and stage of the cancer being treated. External and internal radiation therapy are used to treat CUP.

Chemotherapy

Chemotherapy is a cancer treatment that uses drugs to stop the growth of cancer cells, either by killing the cells or by stopping them from dividing. When chemotherapy is taken by mouth or injected into a vein or muscle, the drugs enter the bloodstream and can reach cancer cells throughout the body (systemic chemotherapy). When chemotherapy is placed directly into the cerebrospinal fluid, an organ, or a body cavity such as the abdomen, the drugs mainly affect cancer cells in those areas (regional chemotherapy). Combination chemotherapy is the use of two or more anticancer drugs.

Hormone Therapy

Hormone therapy is a cancer treatment that removes hormones or blocks their action and stops cancer cells from growing. Hormones are substances made by glands in the body and circulated in the bloodstream. Some hormones can cause certain cancers to grow. If tests show that the cancer cells have places where hormones can attach (receptors), drugs, surgery, or radiation therapy are used to reduce the production of hormones or block them from working.

What Is the Prognosis for CUP?

The prognosis (chance of recovery) depends on the following:

- Where the cancer began in the body and where it has spread
- The number of organs with cancer in them
- The way the tumor cells look when viewed under a microscope
- Whether the patient is male or female
- Whether the cancer has just been diagnosed or has recurred

For most patients with CUP, current treatments do not cure the cancer. Patients may want to take part in one of the many clinical trials being done to improve treatment. Clinical trials for CUP are taking place in many parts of the country.

Part Three

Cancer-Related Tests and Treatments

Chapter 58

Cancer Diagnosis, Staging, and Prognosis

Cancer can cause many different symptoms. Most often these symptoms are not caused by cancer, but by benign tumors or other problems. If you have symptoms that last for a couple of weeks, your doctor will do a physical exam and order tests or other procedures to find out what is causing your symptoms. If you do find out you have cancer, your doctor will order another set of tests or procedures to figure out its stage. Stage refers to the extent of your cancer and is based on factors such as how large the tumor is and if it has spread. Once your doctor knows the stage of your cancer, he will be able to suggest treatment and discuss your prognosis with you. Understanding your cancer and knowing what to expect can help you and your loved ones feel more in control and cope with your diagnosis.

Symptoms of Cancer

Cancer can cause many different symptoms. These are some of them:

- Skin changes, such as:
    - A new mole or a change in an existing mole
    - A sore that does not heal

This chapter includes text excerpted from "Diagnosis and Staging," National Cancer Institute (NCI), March 5, 2015.

- Breast changes, such as:
  - Change in size or shape of the breast or nipple
  - Change in texture of breast skin
- A thickening or lump on or under the skin
- Hoarseness or cough that does not go away
- Changes in bowel habits
- Difficult or painful urination
- Problems with eating, such as:
  - Discomfort after eating
  - A hard time swallowing
  - Changes in appetite
- Weight gain or loss with no known reason
- Abdominal pain
- Unexplained night sweats
- Unusual bleeding or discharge, including:
  - Blood in the urine
  - Vaginal bleeding
  - Blood in the stool
- Feeling weak or very tired

Most often, these symptoms are not due to cancer. They may also be caused by benign tumors or other problems. If you have symptoms that last for a couple of weeks, it is important to see a doctor so that problems can be diagnosed and treated as early as possible. Usually, early cancer does not cause pain. If you have symptoms, do not wait to feel pain before seeing a doctor.

How Cancer Is Diagnosed

If you have a symptom or your screening test result suggests cancer, the doctor must find out whether it is due to cancer or some other cause. The doctor may ask about your personal and family medical history and do a physical exam. The doctor also may order lab tests, scans, or other tests or procedures.

Lab Tests

High or low levels of certain substances in your body can be a sign of cancer. So, lab tests of the blood, urine, or other body fluids that measure these substances can help doctors make a diagnosis. However, abnormal lab results are not a sure sign of cancer. Lab tests are an important tool, but doctors cannot rely on them alone to diagnose cancer.

Imaging Procedures

Imaging procedures create pictures of areas inside your body that help the doctor see whether a tumor is present. These pictures can be made in the following ways:

- **Computed tomography (CT) scan:** An X-ray machine linked to a computer takes a series of detailed pictures of your organs. You may receive a dye or other contrast material to highlight areas inside the body. Contrast material helps make these pictures easier to read.
- **Nuclear scan:** For this scan, you receive an injection of a small amount of radioactive material, which is sometimes called a tracer. It flows through your bloodstream and collects in certain bones or organs. A machine called a scanner detects and measures the radioactivity. The scanner creates pictures of bones or organs on a computer screen or on film. Your body gets rid of the radioactive substance quickly. This type of scan may also be called radionuclide scan.
- **Ultrasound:** An ultrasound device sends out sound waves that people cannot hear. The waves bounce off tissues inside your body like an echo. A computer uses these echoes to create a picture of areas inside your body. This picture is called a sonogram.
- **Magnetic resonance imaging (MRI):** A strong magnet linked to a computer is used to make detailed pictures of areas in your body. Your doctor can view these pictures on a monitor and print them on film.
- **Positron emission tomography (PET) scan:** For this scan, you receive an injection of a tracer. Then, a machine makes 3D pictures that show where the tracer collects in the body. These scans show how organs and tissues are working.
- **X-rays:** X-rays use low doses of radiation to create pictures of the inside of your body.

Biopsy

In most cases, doctors need to do a biopsy to make a diagnosis of cancer. A biopsy is a procedure in which the doctor removes a sample of tissue. A pathologist then looks at the tissue under a microscope to see if it is cancer. The sample may be removed in the following ways:

- **With a needle:** The doctor uses a needle to withdraw tissue or fluid.
- **With an endoscope:** The doctor looks at areas inside the body using a thin, lighted tube called an endoscope. The scope is inserted through a natural opening, such as the mouth. Then, the doctor uses a special tool to remove tissue or cells through the tube.
- **With surgery:** Surgery may be excisional or incisional.
- In an excisional biopsy, the surgeon removes the entire tumor. Often some of the normal tissue around the tumor also is removed.
- In an incisional biopsy, the surgeon removes just part of the tumor.

Cancer Staging

Stage refers to the extent of your cancer, such as how large the tumor is, and if it has spread. Knowing the stage of your cancer helps your doctor:

- Understand how serious your cancer is and your chances of survival.
- Plan the best treatment for you.
- Identify clinical trials that may be treatment options for you.

A cancer is always referred to by the stage it was given at diagnosis, even if it gets worse or spreads. New information about how a cancer has changed over time gets added to the original stage. So, the stage doesn't change, even though the cancer might.

Systems That Describe Stage

There are many staging systems. Some, such as the tumor, node, and metastasis (TNM) staging system, are used for many types of cancer. Others are specific to a particular type of cancer. Most staging systems include the following information:

- Where the tumor is located in the body
- The cell type (such as, adenocarcinoma or squamous cell carcinoma)
- The size of the tumor
- Whether the cancer has spread to nearby lymph nodes
- Whether the cancer has spread to a different part of the body
- Tumor grade, which refers to how abnormal the cancer cells look and how likely the tumor is to grow and spread

The TNM Staging System

The TNM system is the most widely used cancer staging system. Most hospitals and medical centers use the TNM system as their main method for cancer reporting. You are likely to see your cancer described by this staging system in your pathology report, unless you have a cancer for which a different staging system is used. Examples of cancers with different staging systems include brain and spinal cord tumors and blood cancers.

In the TNM system:

- The T refers to the size and extent of the main tumor. The main tumor is usually called the primary tumor.
- The N refers to the number of nearby lymph nodes that have cancer.
- The M refers to whether the cancer has metastasized. This means that the cancer has spread from the primary tumor to other parts of the body.

When your cancer is described by the TNM system, there will be numbers after each letter that give more details about the cancer—for example, T1N0MX or T3N1M0. The following explains what the letters and numbers mean:

Primary tumor (T)

- **TX:** Main tumor cannot be measured.
- **T0:** Main tumor cannot be found.

- **T1, T2, T3, T4:** Refers to the size and/or extent of the main tumor. The higher the number after the T, the larger the tumor or the more it has grown into nearby tissues. T's may be further divided to provide more detail, such as T3a and T3b.

Regional lymph nodes (N)

- **NX:** Cancer in nearby lymph nodes cannot be measured.
- **N0:** There is no cancer in nearby lymph nodes.
- **N1, N2, N3:** Refers to the number and location of lymph nodes that contain cancer. The higher the number after the N, the more lymph nodes that contain cancer.

Distant metastasis (M)

- **MX:** Metastasis cannot be measured.
- **M0:** Cancer has not spread to other parts of the body.
- **M1:** Cancer has spread to other parts of the body.

Other Ways to Describe Stage

The TNM system helps describe cancer in great detail. But, for many cancers, the TNM combinations are grouped into five less-detailed stages. When talking about your cancer, your doctor or nurse may describe it as one of these following stages:

Table 58.1. Cancer Stages

Stage	What It Means
Stage 0	Abnormal cells are present but have not spread to nearby tissue. Also called carcinoma in situ, or CIS. CIS is not cancer, but it may become cancer.
Stage I, Stage II, and Stage III	Cancer is present. The higher the number, the larger the cancer tumor and the more it has spread into nearby tissues.
Stage IV	The cancer has spread to distant parts of the body.

Another staging system that is used for all types of cancer groups the cancer into one of five main categories. This staging system is more often used by cancer registries than by doctors. But, you may still hear your doctor or nurse describe your cancer in one of the following ways:

- **In situ**—Abnormal cells are present but have not spread to nearby tissue.
- **Localized**—Cancer is limited to the place where it started, with no sign that it has spread.
- **Regional**—Cancer has spread to nearby lymph nodes, tissues, or organs.
- **Distant**—Cancer has spread to distant parts of the body.
- **Unknown**—There is not enough information to figure out the stage.

Understanding Cancer Prognosis

If you have cancer, you may have questions about how serious your cancer is and your chances of survival. The estimate of how the disease will go for you is called prognosis. It can be hard to understand what prognosis means and also hard to talk about, even for doctors.

Many Factors Can Affect Your Prognosis

Some of the factors that affect prognosis include the following:

- The type of cancer and where it is in your body
- The stage of the cancer, which refers to the size of the cancer and if it has spread to other parts of your body
- The cancer's grade, which refers to how abnormal the cancer cells look under a microscope. Grade provides clues about how quickly the cancer is likely to grow and spread.
- Certain traits of the cancer cells
- Your age and how healthy you were before cancer
- How you respond to treatment

Seeking Information about Your Prognosis Is a Personal Decision

When you have cancer, you and your loved ones face many unknowns. Understanding your cancer and knowing what to expect can help you and your loved ones make decisions. Some of the decisions you may face include the following:

- Which treatment is best for you
- If you want treatment
- How to best take care of yourself and manage treatment side effects
- How to deal with financial and legal matters

Many people want to know their prognosis. They find it easier to cope when they know more about their cancer. You may ask your doctor about survival statistics or search for this information on your own. Or, you may find statistics confusing and frightening, and think they are too impersonal to be of value to you. It is up to you to decide how much information you want. If you do decide you want to know more, the doctor who knows the most about your situation is in the best position to discuss your prognosis and explain what the statistics may mean.

Understanding Statistics about Survival

Doctors estimate prognosis by using statistics that researchers have collected over many years about people with the same type of cancer. Several types of statistics may be used to estimate prognosis. The most commonly used statistics include the following:

- **Cancer-specific survival:** This is the percentage of patients with a specific type and stage of cancer who have not died from their cancer during a certain period of time after diagnosis. The period of time may be 1 year, 2 years, 5 years, etc., with 5 years being the time period most often used. Cancer-specific survival is also called disease-specific survival. In most cases, cancer-specific survival is based on causes of death listed in medical records.
- **Relative survival:** This statistic is another method used to estimate cancer-specific survival that does not use information about the cause of death. It is the percentage of cancer patients who have survived for a certain period of time after diagnosis compared to people who do not have cancer.
- **Overall survival:** This is the percentage of people with a specific type and stage of cancer who have not died from any cause during a certain period of time after diagnosis.

- **Disease-free survival:** This statistic is the percentage of patients who have no signs of cancer during a certain period of time after treatment. Other names for this statistic are recurrence-free or progression-free survival.

Because statistics are based on large groups of people, they cannot be used to predict exactly what will happen to you. Everyone is different. Treatments and how people respond to treatment can differ greatly. Also, it takes years to see the benefit of new treatments and ways of finding cancer. So, the statistics your doctor uses to make a prognosis may not be based on treatments being used today. Still, your doctor may tell you that you have a good prognosis if statistics suggest that your cancer is likely to respond well to treatment. Or, he may tell you that you have a poor prognosis if the cancer is harder to control. Whatever your doctor tells you, keep in mind that a prognosis is an educated guess. Your doctor cannot be certain how it will go for you.

If You Decide Not to Have Treatment

If you decide not to have treatment, the doctor who knows your situation best is in the best position to discuss your prognosis. Survival statistics most often come from studies that compare treatments with each other, rather than treatment with no treatment. So, it may not be easy for your doctor to give you an accurate prognosis.

Understanding the Difference between Cure and Remission

Cure means that there are no traces of your cancer after treatment and the cancer will never come back. Remission means that the signs and symptoms of your cancer are reduced. Remission can be partial or complete. In a complete remission, all signs and symptoms of cancer have disappeared. If you remain in complete remission for 5 years or more, some doctors may say that you are cured. Still, some cancer cells can remain in your body for many years after treatment. These cells may cause the cancer to come back one day. For cancers that return, most do so within the first 5 years after treatment. But, there is a chance that cancer will come back later. For this reason, doctors cannot say for sure that you are cured. The most they can say is that there are no signs of cancer at this time. Because of the chance that cancer can come back, your doctor will monitor you for many years and do tests to look for signs of cancer's return. They will also look for signs of late side effects from the cancer treatments you received.

Chapter 59

Finding Healthcare Services

If you have been diagnosed with cancer, finding a doctor and a treatment facility for your cancer care is an important step to getting the best treatment possible. You will have many things to consider when choosing a doctor. It's important for you to feel comfortable with the specialist that you choose because you will be working closely with that person to make decisions about your cancer treatment.

Choosing a Doctor

When choosing a doctor for your cancer care, it may be helpful to know some of the terms used to describe a doctor's training and credentials. Most physicians who treat people with cancer are medical doctors (they have an M.D. degree) or osteopathic doctors (they have a D.O. degree). Standard training includes 4 years of study at a college or university, 4 years of medical school, and 3–7 years of postgraduate medical education through internships and residencies. Doctors must pass an exam to become licensed to practice medicine in their state.

Specialists are doctors who have done their residency training in a specific field such as internal medicine. Independent specialty boards certify physicians after they have met needed requirements, including meeting certain education and training standards, being licensed to practice medicine, and passing an examination given by their specialty board. Once they have met these requirements, physicians are said to be "board certified."

This chapter includes text excerpted from "Finding Health Care Services," National Cancer Institute (NCI), August 25, 2017.

Some specialists who treat cancer are:

- **Medical oncologist:** Specializes in treating cancer
- **Hematologist:** Focuses on diseases of the blood and related tissues, including the bone marrow, spleen, and lymph nodes
- **Radiation oncologist:** Uses X-rays and other forms of radiation to diagnose and treat disease
- **Surgeon:** Performs operations on almost any area of the body and may specialize in a certain type of surgery

Finding a Doctor Who Specializes in Cancer Care

To find a doctor who specializes in cancer care, ask your primary care doctor to suggest someone. Or you may know of a specialist through the experience of a friend of family member. Also, your local hospital should be able to provide you with a list of specialists who practice there. Another option for finding a doctor is your nearest National Cancer Institute (NCI)-designated cancer center. The Find a Cancer Center page (www.cancer.gov/research/nci-role/cancer-centers/find) provides contact information to help healthcare providers and cancer patients with referrals to all NCI-designated cancer centers in the United States.

The online directories listed below may also help you find a cancer care specialist:

- The American Board of Medical Specialists (ABMS), which creates and implements the standards for certifying and evaluating doctors, has a list of doctors that have met specific requirements and passed specialty exams.
- The American Medical Association's (AMA) DoctorFinder (apps.ama-assn.org/doctorfinder/recaptcha.jsp) provides information on licensed doctors in the United States.
- The American Society of Clinical Oncology (ASCO) member database (www.cancer.net/find-cancer-doctor) has the names and affiliations of nearly 30,000 oncologists worldwide.
- The American College of Surgeons (ACS) lists member surgeons by region and specialty in their Find a Surgeon database (www.facs.org/search/find-a-surgeon). The ACS can also be reached at 800-621-4111.
- The American Osteopathic Association's (AOA) Find a Doctor database (doctorsthatdo.org) provides an online list of practicing

osteopathic physicians who are AOA members. The AOA can also be reached at 800-621-1773.

Local medical societies may also maintain lists of doctors in each specialty for you to check. Public and medical libraries may have print directories of doctors' names listed geographically by specialty. Depending on your health insurance plan, your choice may be limited to doctors who participate in your plan. Your insurance company can give you a list of doctors who take part in your plan. It's important to contact the office of the doctor you're considering to be sure that he or she is accepting new patients through your plan. It's also important to do this if you're using a federal or state health insurance program such as Medicare or Medicaid.

If you can change health insurance plans, you may want to decide which doctor you would like to use first and then choose the plan that includes your chosen physician. You also have the option of seeing a doctor outside your plan and paying more of the costs yourself.

To help make your decision when you're considering what doctor to choose, think about if the doctor:

- Has the education and training needed to meet your needs
- Has someone who covers for them if they are unavailable and who would have access to your medical records
- Has a helpful support staff
- Explains things clearly, listens to you, and treats you with respect
- Encourages you to ask questions
- Has office hours that meet your needs
- Is easy to get an appointment with

If you are choosing a surgeon, you will want to ask:

- Are they board certified?
- How often do they perform the type of surgery you need?
- How many of these procedures have they performed?
- At what hospital(s) do they practice?

It's important for you to feel good about the doctor you choose. You will be working with this person closely as you make decisions about your cancer treatment.

Getting a Second Opinion

After you talk to a doctor about the diagnosis and treatment plan for your cancer, you may want to get another doctor's opinion before you begin treatment. This is known as getting a second opinion. You can do this by asking another specialist to review all the materials related to your case. The doctor who gives the second opinion may agree with the treatment plan proposed by your first doctor, or they may suggest changes or another approach. Either way, getting a second opinion may:

- Give you more information
- Answer any questions you may have
- Give you a greater sense of control
- Help you feel more confident, knowing you have explored all your options

Getting a second opinion is very common. Yet some patients worry that their doctor will be offended if they ask for a second opinion. Usually the opposite is true. Most doctors welcome a second opinion. And many health insurance companies pay for a second opinion or even require them, particularly if a doctor recommends surgery.

When talking with your doctor about getting a second opinion, it may be helpful to express that you're satisfied with your care but want to be certain you're as informed as possible about your treatment options. It's best to involve your doctor in the process of getting a second opinion, because he or she will need to make your medical records (such as your test results and X-rays) available to the doctor giving the second opinion. You may wish to bring a family member along for support when asking for a second opinion. If your doctor can't suggest another specialist for a second opinion, many of the resources listed above for finding a doctor can help you find a specialist for a second opinion. You can also call National Cancer Institute's (NCI) Contact Center at 800-4-CANCER (800-422-6237) for guidance.

Choosing a Treatment Facility

As with choosing a doctor, your choice of facilities may be limited to those that take part in your health insurance plan. If you have already found a doctor for your cancer treatment, you may need to choose a treatment facility based on where your doctor practices. Or your doctor may be able to recommend a facility that provides quality care to meet your needs.

Some questions to ask when considering a treatment facility are as follows:

- Does it have experience and success in treating my condition?
- Has it been rated by state, consumer, or other groups for its quality of care?
- How does it check on and work to improve its quality of care?
- Has it been approved by a nationally recognized accrediting body, such as the American Cancer Society's (ACS) Commission on Cancer (CoC) and/or The Joint Commission?
- Does it explain patients' rights and responsibilities? Are copies of this information available to patients?
- Does it offer support services, such as social workers and resources, to help me find financial assistance if I need it?
- Is it conveniently located?

If you belong to a health insurance plan, ask your insurance company if the facility you are choosing is approved by your plan. If you decide to pay for treatment yourself because you choose to go outside of your network or don't have insurance, discuss the possible costs with your doctor beforehand. You will want to talk to the hospital billing department as well. Nurses and social workers may also be able to give you more information about coverage, eligibility, and insurance issues.

The following resources may help you find a hospital or treatment facility for your care:

- NCI's Find a Cancer Center page (www.cancer.gov/research/nci-role/cancer-centers/find) provides contact information for NCI-designated cancer centers located throughout the country.
- The American College of Surgeon's (ACS) Commission on Cancer (CoC). The ACS website has a searchable database (www.facs.org/search/cancer-programs) of cancer care programs they have accredited. They can also be reached at 312-202-5085 or by e-mail at CoC@facs.org.
- The Joint Commission (www.jointcommission.org) evaluates and accredits healthcare organizations and programs in the United States. It also provides guidance about choosing a treatment facility, and offers an online Quality Check® service (www.

qualitycheck.org) that patients can use to check whether a specific facility has been accredited by the Joint Commission and to view its performance reports. They also can be reached at 630-792-5000.

For more information or assistance about finding a treatment facility, call NCI's Contact Center at 800-4-CANCER (800-422-6237).

Getting Treatment in the United States If You Are Not a U.S. Citizen

Some people who live outside the United States may wish to obtain a second opinion or have their cancer treatment in this country. Many facilities in the United States offer these services to international cancer patients. They may also provide support services, such as language interpretation or help with travel and finding lodging near the treatment facility.

If you live outside the United States and would like to get cancer treatment in this country, you should contact cancer treatment facilities directly to find out whether they have an international patient office. The NCI-Designated Cancer Centers Find a Cancer Center page offers contact information for NCI-designated cancer centers throughout the United States.

Citizens of other countries who are planning to travel to the United States for cancer treatment must first obtain a nonimmigrant visa for medical treatment from the U.S. Embassy or Consulate in their home country. Visa applicants must show that they:

- Want to come to the United States for medical treatment
- Plan to stay for a specific, limited period
- Have funds to cover expenses in the United States
- Have a residence and social and economic ties outside the United States
- Intend to return to their home country

To find out the fees and documents needed for the nonimmigrant visa and to learn more about the application process, contact the U.S. Embassy and Consulate in your home country. A list of links to the websites of U.S. Embassies and Consulates worldwide can be found on the U.S. Department of State's (DOS) website.

Finding a Treatment Facility outside the United States

Cancer information services are available in many countries to provide information and answer questions about cancer. They may also be able to help you find a cancer treatment facility close to where you live. The International Cancer Information Service Group (ICISG), a worldwide network of more than 70 organizations that deliver cancer information, has a list of cancer information services on their website. Or you can email ICISG for questions or comments.

The Union for International Cancer Control (UICC) is another resource for people living outside the United States who want to find a cancer treatment facility. The UICC consists of international cancer-related organizations devoted to the worldwide fight against cancer. These organizations serve as resources for the public and may have helpful information about cancer and treatment facilities. To find a resource in or near your country, you may send the UICC an email or contact them at:

Union for International Cancer Control (UICC)
62 route de Frontenex
1207 Geneva
Switzerland
+41 22 809 1811

Finding Health Insurance

The Affordable Care Act (ACA) changes how health insurance works in the United States, with implications for the prevention, screening, and treatment of cancer. Under this healthcare law, most Americans are required to have health insurance. If you do not have health insurance or want to look at new options, the online Health Insurance Marketplace lets you compare plans in your state based on price, benefits, quality, and other needs you may have. To learn about the Health Insurance Marketplace and your new coverage options, please go to Healthcare.gov or CuidadoDeSalud.gov or call toll-free at 800-318-2596 (TTY: 855-889-4325).

Home Care Services

Sometimes patients want to be cared for at home so they can be in familiar surroundings with family and friends. Home care services can help patients stay at home by using a team approach with doctors, nurses, social workers, physical therapists, and others.

If the patient qualifies for home care services, such services may include the following:

- Managing symptoms and monitoring care
- Delivery of medications
- Physical therapy
- Emotional and spiritual care
- Help with preparing meals and personal hygiene
- Providing medical equipment

For many patients and families, home care can be both rewarding and demanding. It can change relationships and require families to cope with all aspects of patient care. New issues may also arise that families need to address such as the logistics of having home care providers coming into the home at regular intervals. To prepare for these changes, patients and caregivers should ask questions and get as much information as possible from the home care team or organization. A doctor, nurse, or social worker can provide information about a patient's specific needs, the availability of services, and the local home care agencies.

Getting Financial Assistance for Home Care

Help with paying for home care services may be available from public or private sources. Private health insurance may cover some home care services, but benefits vary from plan to plan.

Some public resources to help pay for home care are:

- Centers for Medicare and Medicaid Services (CMS): A government agency responsible for the administration of several key federal healthcare programs.
    - Medicare: A government health insurance program for the elderly or disabled. For information, visit their website or call 800-MEDICARE (800-633-4227).
    - Medicaid: A joint federal and state health insurance program for those who need help with medical expenses. Coverage varies by state.

Both Medicare and Medicaid may cover home care services for patients who qualify, but some rules apply. Talk to a social worker and other members of the healthcare team to find out more about home care providers and agencies. For more information contact the CMS online or call 877-267-2323.

- Eldercare Locator: Run by the U.S. Administration on Aging (AOA), it provides information about local Area Agencies on Aging and other assistance for older people. These agencies may provide funds for home care. Eldercare Locator can be reached at 800-677-1116 for more information.
- U.S. Department of Veterans Affairs (VA) Veterans who are disabled as a result of military service can receive home care services from the U.S. Department of Veterans Affairs (VA). However, only home care services provided by VA hospitals may be used. More information about these benefits can be found on their website or by calling 877-222-VETS (877-222-8387).

Chapter 60

Common Medical Procedures and Tests for Cancer

Chapter Contents

Section 60.1

Cancer Imaging

This section includes text excerpted from "Cancer Imaging Program (CIP)—Cancer Imaging Basics," National Cancer Institute (NCI), December 22, 2016.

Cancer may be difficult to detect, but for some types of cancer, the earlier it is detected, the better are the chances of treating it effectively. Imaging techniques—methods of producing pictures of the body—have become an important element of early detection for many cancers. But imaging is not simply used for detection. Imaging is also important for determining the stage (telling how advanced the cancer is) and the precise locations of cancer to aid in directing surgery and other cancer treatments, or to check if a cancer has returned.

Uses of Imaging

Imaging, by itself, is not a treatment but is a tool that can help in making better decisions about treatments. The same imaging technique can help doctors find cancer, tell how far a cancer has spread, guide delivery of specific treatments, or find out if a treatment is working.

Here is some information about the uses of imaging:

- **Screening for cancer:** Imaging can be used to determine if a person has any suspicious areas or abnormalities that might be cancerous. Mammograms are an example of a familiar imaging tool used to screen for breast cancer. Screening for cancer is usually recommended for people who are at increased risk (due to their family history, lifestyle, or age) for developing a particular type of cancer.
- **Diagnosis and staging:** Imaging can be used to find out where a cancer is located in the body, if it has spread, and how much is present. Used in this way, imaging can help determine what stage (how advanced) the cancer is, and if the cancer is in, around, or near important organs and blood vessels. If a biopsy

(taking a small amount of the tumor for laboratory examination) is necessary, imaging may be used to help guide doctors to the tumor and take a sample of it.

- **Guiding cancer treatments:** Imaging can help guide delivery of cancer treatments in numerous ways. Imaging can help make cancer treatments less invasive by narrowly focusing treatments on the tumors. For instance, ultrasound (US), magnetic resonance imaging (MRI), or computed tomography (CT) scans may be used to determine exact tumor locations so that therapy procedures can be focused on the tumor, minimizing damage to surrounding tissue.
- **Determining if a treatment is working:** Imaging can be used to see if a tumor is shrinking or if the tumor has changed and is using less of the body's resources than before treatment. For example, in some current cancer treatment trials, X-rays, MRIs, and CT scans are done at intervals to see if a treatment is working and the tumor is shrinking. Positron emission tomography (PET) and other molecular imaging and nuclear medicine techniques are used to monitor the ways the tumor uses the body's resources. Magnetic resonance spectroscopy is used to study chemical changes in the tumor.
- **Monitoring for cancer recurrence:** Imaging can be used to see if a previously treated cancer has returned or if the cancer is spreading to other locations.

X-Ray Imaging

X-ray imaging is perhaps the most familiar type of imaging. Most adults have had a chest X-ray to look for an infection or maybe just as part of an employment health check. Some people have had X-rays obtained of a hand or a foot looking for a fracture or metallic splinter. Images produced by X-rays are due to the different absorption rates of different tissues. Calcium in bones absorbs X-rays the most, so bones look white on a film recording of the X-ray image, called a radiograph. Fat and other soft tissues absorb less, and look gray. Air absorbs least, so lungs look black on a radiograph. The most familiar use of X-rays is checking for broken bones. We can also use X-rays to look for cancer. X-rays are also used in cancer diagnosis. For example, chest radiographs and mammograms are often used for early cancer detection or to see if cancer has spread to the lungs or other areas in the chest. Mammograms use X-rays to look for tumors or suspicious areas in the breasts.

Computed Tomography (CT) Scans

A computed tomography scan (CT scan, also called a CAT scan) uses computer-controlled X-rays to create images of the body. However, a radiograph and a CT scan show different types of information. Although an experienced radiologist can get a sense for the approximate three-dimensional location of a tumor from a radiograph, in general, a plain radiograph is two-dimensional.

An arm or chest radiograph looks all the way through a body without being able to tell how deep anything is. A CT scan is three-dimensional. By imaging and looking at several three-dimensional slices of a body (like slices of bread) a doctor could not only tell if a tumor is present, but roughly how deep it is in the body. A CT scan can be three dimensional because the information about how much of the X-rays are passing through a body is collected not just on a flat piece of film, but on a computer.

The data from a CT scan can be enhanced to be more vivid than a plain radiograph. For both plain radiographs and CT scans, the patient may be given a contrast agent to drink and/or by injection to more clearly show the boundaries between organs or between organs and tumors.

Technical advances in CT scanning dramatically increased its speed and effectiveness by a process called multi-slice or helical (spiral) scanning.

Conventional CT scans take pictures of slices of the body (like slices of bread). These slices are a few millimeters apart. The newer spiral (also called helical) CT scan takes continuous pictures of the body in a rapid spiral motion, so that there are no gaps in the pictures collected. CT scanning is very common. Doctors will order a CT scan or MRI exam on every patient with a suspect cancer.

Molecular and Nuclear Imaging (PET and SPECT)

Molecular and nuclear imaging use low doses of radioactive substances linked to compounds used by the body's cells or compounds that attach to tumor cells. Using special detection equipment, the radioactive substances can be traced in the body to see where and when they concentrate.

PET Scan

The positron emission tomography (PET) scan creates computerized images of chemical changes, such as sugar metabolism, that take place in tissue. Typically, the patient is given an injection of a substance that consists of a combination of a sugar and a small amount of radioactively labeled sugar. The radioactive sugar can help in locating a tumor, because cancer cells take up or absorb sugar more avidly than other tissues in the body.

After receiving the radioactive sugar, the patient lies still for about 60 minutes while the radioactively labeled sugar circulates throughout the body. If a tumor is present, the radioactive sugar will accumulate in the tumor. The patient then lies on a table, which gradually moves through the PET scanner incrementally several times during a 15- to 60-minute period. The PET scanner is used to detect the distribution of the sugar in the tumor and in the body. By the combined matching of a CT scan with PET images, there is an improved capacity to discriminate normal from abnormal tissues. A computer translates this information into the images that are interpreted by a radiologist.

PET scans may play a role in determining whether a mass is cancerous. However, PET scans are more accurate in detecting larger and more aggressive tumors than they are in locating tumors that are smaller than 8 mm a pinky nail (or half of a thumbnail) and/or less aggressive cancers. The size of smallest tumor mass that can be found at PET is constantly improving. They may also detect cancer when other imaging techniques show normal results. PET scans may be helpful in evaluating and staging recurrent disease (cancer that has come back). PET scans are beginning to be also commonly used to check if a treatment is working—if tumor cells are dying and thus using less sugar.

SPECT Scan

Similar to PET, single photon emission computed tomography (SPECT) uses radioactive tracers and a scanner to record data that a computer constructs into two- or three-dimensional images. A small amount of a radioactive drug is injected into a vein and a scanner is used to make detailed images of areas inside the body where the radioactive material is taken up by the cells. SPECT can give information about blood flow to tissues and chemical reactions (metabolism) in the body.

In this procedure, antibodies (proteins that recognize and stick to tumor cells) can be linked to a radioactive substance. If a tumor is present, the antibodies will stick to it. Then a SPECT scan can be done to detect the radioactive substance and reveal where the tumor is located.

Ultrasound

Ultrasound (US) uses sound waves with frequencies above those humans can hear. A transducer sends sound waves traveling into the body which are reflected back from organs and tissues, allowing a picture to be made of the internal organs. Ultrasound can show tumors, and can also guide doctors doing biopsies or treating tumors. Most people know about US images when a woman is pregnant, for example—boy or girl. As with diagnostic MRI, there is no harmful radiation from diagnostic ultrasound. (Keep in mind, both MRI and US can be used for treatment under certain conditions—but this is very uncommon currently.) Unfortunately, while US is very useful for imaging certain body parts, it is not as useful as other imaging techniques for looking at the brain, lungs, or an entire abdomen or pelvis. Because masses can sometimes be tiny and far from the skin surface, we usually need CT, MRI, and/or PET to find these places of suspect tumor spread.

Magnetic Resonance Imaging (MRI)

MRI uses radio waves in the presence of a strong magnetic field that surrounds the opening of the MRI machine where the patient lies to get tissues to emit radio waves of their own.

Different tissues (including tumors) emit a more or less intense signal based on their chemical makeup, so a picture of the body organs can be displayed on a computer screen. Much like CT scans, MRI can produce three-dimensional images of sections of the body, but MRI is sometimes more sensitive than CT scans for distinguishing soft tissues.

Many people know that MR scanners are noisy. Most every MRI technologist has a big supply of earplugs or an over-the-ear headphone for the patient to use. Some people get claustrophobic in the MR units. The doctors and technologists are accustomed to helping patients deal with this.

MR is safe—so long as there is no metal in your body. MR is safe for pregnant women and kids—there is no harmful radiation from MRI.

Digital Mammography

Conventional mammography uses X-rays to look for tumors or suspicious areas in the breasts. Digital mammography also uses X-rays, but the data is collected on computer instead of on a piece of film. This means that the image can be computer-enhanced, or areas can be magnified. Eventually, a computer could in certain appropriate situations, screen digital mammograms, theoretically detecting suspicious areas that human error might miss. There are both 2D and 3D forms of mammography available now.

In addition to "regular" mammograms, additional or spot views might be needed if a suspicious finding is noted on a screening mammogram (meaning no tumor was suspected by history nor by physical exam when the test was ordered).

Ultrasound and MRI (magnetic resonance imaging) are other types of diagnostic tests that might be obtained to assess the breast.

Sometimes a biopsy is recommended in order to get a piece of tissue for the Pathologist to examine. This will determine if a tumor might be present.

In every part of the body except for the breast, most biopsies find cancer or something else bad. In the breast, 80–90 percent of biopsies do not show any tumor. However, because imaging findings for cancer and noncancerous abnormalities are similar, a way to improve on this low yield has not yet been found. Breast cancer also occurs in men. So a man with a new chest mass should also see his doctor.

Virtual Colonoscopy

Virtual colonoscopy (VC) (or computerized tomographic colonography (CTC)) uses X-rays and computers to produce two- and three-dimensional images of the colon (large intestine) from the lowest part, the rectum, all the way to the lower end of the small intestine and display them on a screen. The procedure is used to diagnose colon and bowel disease, including polyps, diverticulosis, and cancer. VC can be performed with computed tomography (CT), sometimes called a computerized axial tomography (CAT) scan, or with magnetic resonance imaging (MRI).

Virtual Colonoscopy Procedure

While preparations for VC vary, you will usually be asked to take laxatives or other oral agents at home the day before the procedure to clear stool from your colon. You may also be asked to use a suppository to cleanse your rectum of any remaining fecal matter.

VC takes place in the radiology department of a hospital or medical center. The examination takes about 10 minutes and does not require sedatives. During the procedure:

- The doctor will ask you to lie on your back on a table.

- A thin tube will be inserted into your rectum, and air will be pumped through the tube to inflate the colon for better viewing.
- The table moves through the scanner to produce a series of two-dimensional cross-sections along the length of the colon. A computer program puts these images together to create a three-dimensional picture that can be viewed on the video screen.
- You will be asked to hold your breath during the scan to avoid distortion on the images.
- The scanning procedure is then repeated with you lying on your stomach.

After the examination, the information from the scanner must be processed to create the computer picture or image of your colon. A radiologist evaluates the results to identify any abnormalities.

You may resume normal activity after the procedure, although your doctor may ask you to wait while the test results are analyzed. If abnormalities are found and you need conventional colonoscopy, it may be performed the same day.

Conventional Colonoscopy

In a conventional colonoscopy, the doctor inserts a colonoscope—a long, flexible, lighted tube—into the patient's rectum and slowly guides it up through the colon. Pain medication and a mild sedative help the patient stay relaxed and comfortable during the 30- to 60-minute procedure. A tiny camera in the scope transmits an image of the lining of the colon, so the doctor can examine it on a video monitor. If an abnormality is detected, the doctor can remove it or take tissue samples using tiny instruments passed through the scope.

Advantages of Virtual Colonoscopy

VC is more comfortable than conventional colonoscopy for some people because it does not use a colonoscope. As a result, no sedation is needed, and you can return to your usual activities or go home after the procedure without the aid of another person. VC provides clearer, more detailed images than a conventional X-ray using a barium enema, sometimes called a lower gastrointestinal (GI) series. It also takes less time than either a conventional colonoscopy or a lower GI series.

Disadvantages of Virtual Colonoscopy

The doctor cannot take tissue samples or remove polyps during VC, so a conventional colonoscopy must be performed if abnormalities are found. Also, VC does not show as much detail as a conventional colonoscopy, so polyps smaller than 10 millimeters in diameter may not show up on the images.

Sentinel Node Mapping

This technique illustrates how imaging may be able to reduce the need for extensive diagnostic surgery. When patients are being diagnosed with breast cancer it has been standard practice to surgically remove all of the lymph nodes under the arm to determine if the cancer has spread beyond the breast and what treatment is appropriate. Removing all the lymph nodes can result in long-term complications and discomfort for the patient from bad arm swelling called lymphedema (a condition where excess lymph fluid collects in tissues and causes swelling). Trials are underway now; however, to test an alternative, less damaging procedure in which imaging plays an important role.

In this alternative procedure, called sentinel node mapping, only the sentinel node (the first lymph node to which breast cancer is likely to spread) is removed rather than all the lymph nodes. In order to identify the sentinel node, the doctors inject either a blue dye or a relatively nontoxic radioactive substance and see which lymph node it reaches first. This lymph node is the sentinel node, and is surgically removed.

This has been done since the 1990s at many centers. It is becoming more common outside of assessment of breast tumor spread.

Image-Guided Surgery (IGS)

IGS is most commonly used by brain surgeons. When you hear about a brain surgery patient having a big metal or plastic frame around their head, this is part of the localization system.

Various techniques for this have been around since the 1990s. These systems fuse imaging data from a presurgical CT or MRI to location information which can be used by the surgeon during the neurosurgical procedure. This can make the procedure both faster and safer.

There are multiple techniques for using imaging to guide surgery in the body, for example in the liver. This is an area where technique changes occur often.

Section 60.2

Computed Tomography (CT)

This section includes text excerpted from "Computed Tomography (CT) Scans and Cancer," National Cancer Institute (NCI), July 16, 2013. Reviewed March 2018.

What Is Computed Tomography?

Computed tomography (CT) is an imaging procedure that uses special X-ray equipment to create detailed pictures, or scans, of areas inside the body. It is also called computerized tomography and computerized axial tomography (CAT).

The term tomography comes from the Greek words tomos (a cut, a slice, or a section) and graphein (to write or record). Each picture created during a CT procedure shows the organs, bones, and other tissues in a thin "slice" of the body. The entire series of pictures produced in CT is like a loaf of sliced bread—you can look at each slice individually (2-dimensional pictures), or you can look at the whole loaf (a 3-dimensional picture). Computer programs are used to create both types of pictures.

Most modern CT machines take continuous pictures in a helical (or spiral) fashion rather than taking a series of pictures of individual slices of the body, as the original CT machines did. Helical CT has several advantages over older CT techniques: it is faster, produces better 3D pictures of areas inside the body, and may detect small abnormalities better. The newest CT scanners, called multislice CT or multidetector CT scanners, allow more slices to be imaged in a shorter period of time.

In addition to its use in cancer, CT is widely used to help diagnose circulatory (blood) system diseases and conditions, such as coronary artery disease (atherosclerosis), blood vessel aneurysms, and blood clots; spinal conditions; kidney and bladder stones; abscesses; inflammatory diseases, such as ulcerative colitis and sinusitis; and injuries to the head, skeletal system, and internal organs. CT can be a life-saving tool for diagnosing illness and injury in both children and adults.

What Can a Person Expect during a CT Procedure?

During a CT procedure, the person lies very still on a table, and the table passes slowly through the center of a large X-ray machine. With some types of CT scanners, the table stays still and the machine moves around the person. The person might hear whirring sounds during the procedure. At times during a CT procedure, the person may be asked to hold their breath to prevent blurring of the images.

Sometimes, CT involves the use of a contrast (imaging) agent, or "dye." The dye may be given by mouth, injected into a vein, given by enema, or given in all three ways before the procedure. The contrast dye highlights specific areas inside the body, resulting in clearer pictures. Iodine and barium are two dyes commonly used in CT.

In very rare cases, the contrast agents used in CT can cause allergic reactions. Some people experience mild itching or hives (small bumps on the skin). Symptoms of a more serious allergic reaction include shortness of breath and swelling of the throat or other parts of the body. People should tell the technologist immediately if they experience any of these symptoms, so they can be treated promptly. Very rarely, the contrast agents used in CT can also cause kidney problems in certain patients. These kidney problems usually do not have any symptoms, but they can be detected by running a simple test on a blood sample.

CT does not cause any pain. However, lying in one position during the procedure may be slightly uncomfortable. The length of a CT procedure depends on the size of the area being scanned, but it usually lasts only a few minutes to half an hour. For most people, the CT is performed on an outpatient basis at a hospital or a radiology center, without an overnight hospital stay.

Some people are concerned about experiencing claustrophobia during a CT procedure. However, most CT scanners surround only portions of the body, not the whole body. Therefore, people are not enclosed in a machine and are unlikely to feel claustrophobic.

Women should let their healthcare provider and the technologist know if there is any possibility that they are pregnant, because radiation from CT can harm a growing fetus.

How Is CT Used in Cancer?

CT is used in cancer in the following ways:

- To detect abnormal growths
- To help diagnose the presence of a tumor

- To provide information about the stage of a cancer
- To determine exactly where to perform (i.e., guide) a biopsy procedure
- To guide certain local treatments, such as cryotherapy, radiofrequency ablation, and the implantation of radioactive seeds
- To help plan external-beam radiation therapy or surgery
- To determine whether a cancer is responding to treatment
- To detect recurrence of a tumor

How Is CT Used in Cancer Screening?

Studies have shown that CT can be effective in both colorectal cancer screening (including screening for large polyps) and lung cancer screening.

Colorectal Cancer

CT colonography (also known as virtual colonoscopy) can be used to screen for both large colorectal polyps and colorectal tumors. CT colonography uses the same dose of radiation that is used in standard CT of the abdomen and pelvis, which is about 10 millisieverts (mSv). (By comparison, the estimated average annual dose received from natural sources of radiation is about 3 mSv.) As with standard (optical) colonoscopy, a thorough cleansing of the colon is performed before this test. During the examination, air or carbon dioxide gas is pumped into the colon to expand it for better viewing.

The National CT Colonography Trial, a National Cancer Institute (NCI)-sponsored clinical trial, found that the accuracy of CT colonography is similar to that of standard colonoscopy. CT colonography is less invasive than standard colonoscopy and has a lower risk of complications. However, if polyps or other abnormal growths are found on CT colonography, a standard colonoscopy is usually performed to remove them.

Whether CT colonography can help reduce the death rate from colorectal cancer is not yet known, and most insurance companies (and Medicare) do not currently reimburse the costs of this procedure. Also, because CT colonography can produce images of organs and tissues outside the colon, it is possible that noncolorectal abnormalities may be found. Some of these "extra-colonic" findings will be serious, but many will not be, leading to unnecessary additional tests and surgeries.

Lung Cancer

The NCI-sponsored National Lung Screening Trial (NLST) showed that people aged 55–74 years with a history of heavy smoking are 20 percent less likely to die from lung cancer if they are screened with low-dose helical CT than if they are screened with standard chest X-rays. (Previous studies had shown that screening with standard chest X-rays does not reduce the death rate from lung cancer.) The estimated amount of radiation in a low-dose helical CT procedure is 1.5 mSv.

Despite the effectiveness of low-dose helical CT for lung cancer screening in heavy smokers, the NLST identified risks as well as benefits. For example, people screened with low-dose helical CT had a higher overall rate of false-positive results (that is, findings that appeared to be abnormal even though no cancer was present), a higher rate of false-positive results that led to an invasive procedure (such as bronchoscopy or biopsy), and a higher rate of serious complications from an invasive procedure than those screened with standard X-rays.

The benefits of helical CT in screening for lung cancer may vary, depending on how similar someone is to the people who participated in the NLST. The benefits may also be greater for those with a higher lung cancer risk, and the harms may be more pronounced for those who have more medical problems (like heart or other lung disease), which could increase problems arising from biopsies and other surgery.

People who think that they have an increased risk of lung cancer and are interested in screening with low-dose helical CT should discuss the appropriateness and the benefits and risks of lung cancer screening with their doctors. They should also be aware that, because the technique is fairly new, some insurance plans do not currently cover it.

What Is Total, or Whole-Body, CT?

Total, or whole-body, CT creates pictures of nearly every area of the body—from the chin to below the hips. This procedure, which is used routinely in patients who already have cancer, can also be used in people who do not have any symptoms of disease. However, whole-body CT has not been shown to be an effective screening method for healthy people. Most abnormal findings from this procedure do not indicate a serious health problem, but the tests that must be done to follow up and rule out a problem can be expensive, inconvenient, and uncomfortable. In addition, whole-body CT can expose people to relatively large amounts of ionizing radiation—about 12 mSv, or four times the estimated average annual dose received from natural sources of radiation. Most doctors recommend against whole-body CT for people without any signs or symptoms of disease.

What Is Combined PET/CT?

Combined PET/CT uses two imaging methods, CT and positron emission tomography (PET), in one procedure. CT is done first to create anatomic pictures of the organs and structures in the body, and then PET is done to create colored pictures that show chemical or other functional changes in tissues.

Different types of positron-emitting (radioactive) substances can be used in PET. Depending on the substance used, different kinds of chemical or functional changes can be imaged. The most common type of PET procedure uses an imaging agent called fluorodeoxyglucose (FDG) (a radioactive form of the sugar glucose), which shows the metabolic activity of tissues. Because cancerous tumors are usually more metabolically active than normal tissues, they appear different from other tissues on a PET scan. Other PET imaging agents can provide information about the level of oxygen in a particular tissue, the formation of new blood vessels, the presence of bone growth, or whether tumor cells are actively dividing and growing.

Combining CT and PET may provide a more complete picture of a tumor's location and growth or spread than either test alone. The combined procedure may improve the ability to diagnose cancer, to determine how far a tumor has spread, to plan treatment, and to monitor response to treatment. Combined PET/CT may also reduce the number of additional imaging tests and other procedures a patient needs.

Is the Radiation from CT Harmful?

Some people may be concerned about the amount of radiation they receive during CT. CT imaging involves the use of X-rays, which are a form of ionizing radiation. Exposure to ionizing radiation is known to increase the risk of cancer. Standard X-ray procedures, such as routine chest X-rays and mammography, use relatively low levels of ionizing radiation. The radiation exposure from CT is higher than that from standard X-ray procedures, but the increase in cancer risk from one CT scan is still small. Not having the procedure can be much more risky than having it, especially if CT is being used to diagnose cancer or another serious condition in someone who has signs or symptoms of disease.

It is commonly thought that the extra risk of any one person developing a fatal cancer from a typical CT procedure is about 1 in 2,000. In contrast, the lifetime risk of dying from cancer in the United States population is about 1 in 5.

It is also important to note that everyone is exposed to some background level of naturally occurring ionizing radiation every day. The average person in the United States receives an estimated effective dose of about 3 millisieverts (mSv) per year from naturally occurring radioactive materials, such as radon and radiation from outer space. By comparison, the radiation exposure from one low-dose CT scan of the chest (1.5 mSv) is comparable to 6 months of natural background radiation, and a regular-dose CT scan of the chest (7 mSv) is comparable to 2 years of natural background radiation.

The widespread use of CT and other procedures that use ionizing radiation to create images of the body has raised concerns that even small increases in cancer risk could lead to large numbers of future cancers. People who have CT procedures as children may be at higher risk because children are more sensitive to radiation and have a longer life expectancy than adults. Women are at a somewhat higher risk than men of developing cancer after receiving the same radiation exposures at the same ages.

People considering CT should talk with their doctors about whether the procedure is necessary for them and about its risks and benefits. Some organizations recommend that people keep a record of the imaging examinations they have received in case their doctors don't have access to all of their health records.

What Are the Risks of CT Scans for Children?

Radiation exposure from CT scans affects adults and children differently. Children are considerably more sensitive to radiation than adults because of their growing bodies and the rapid pace at which the cells in their bodies divide. In addition, children have a longer life expectancy than adults, providing a larger window of opportunity for radiation-related cancers to develop.

Individuals who have had multiple CT scans before the age of 15 were found to have an increased risk of developing leukemia, brain tumors, and other cancers in the decade following their first scan. However, the lifetime risk of cancer from a single CT scan was small—about one case of cancer for every 10,000 scans performed on children.

In talking with healthcare providers, three key questions that the parents can ask are: why is the test needed? Will the results change the treatment decisions? Is there an alternative test that doesn't involve radiation? If the test is clinically justified, then the parents can be reassured that the benefits will outweigh the small long-term risks.

What Is Being Done to Reduce the Level of Radiation Exposure from CT?

In response to concerns about the increased risk of cancer associated with CT and other imaging procedures that use ionizing radiation, several organizations and government agencies have developed guidelines and recommendations regarding the appropriate use of these procedures.

- In 2010, the U.S. Food and Drug Administration (FDA) launched the Initiative to Reduce Unnecessary Radiation Exposure from Medical Imaging. This initiative focuses on the safe use of medical imaging devices, informed decision-making about when to use specific imaging procedures, and increasing patients' awareness of their radiation exposure. Key components of the initiative include avoiding repeat procedures, keeping doses as low as possible while maximizing image quality, and using imaging only when appropriate. The FDA also produced Reducing Radiation from Medical X-rays, a guide for consumers that includes information about the risks of medical X-rays, steps consumers can take to reduce radiation risks, and a table that shows the radiation dose of some common medical X-ray exams.
- The National Institutes of Health (NIH) Clinical Center (CC) requires that radiation dose exposures from CT and other imaging procedures be included in the electronic medical records of patients treated at the center. In addition, all imaging equipment purchased by NIH must provide data on exposure in a form that can be tracked and reported electronically. This patient protection policy is being adopted by other hospitals and imaging facilities.
- National Cancer Institute (NCI) website includes a guide for healthcare providers, Radiation Risks and Pediatric Computed Tomography (CT): A Guide for Healthcare Providers. The guide addresses the value of CT as a diagnostic tool in children, unique considerations for radiation exposure in children, risks to children from radiation exposure, and measures to minimize exposure.

- The American College of Radiology (ACR) has developed the *ACR Appropriateness Criteria*®, evidence-based guidelines to help providers make appropriate imaging and treatment decisions for a number of clinical conditions. These guidelines and supporting documents are available on ACR's website.
- ACR has also established the Dose Index Registry, which collects anonymized information related to dose indices for all CT exams at participating facilities. Data from the registry can be used to compare radiology facilities and to establish national benchmarks.
- CT scanner manufacturers are developing newer cameras and detector systems that can provide higher quality images at much lower radiation doses.

Where Can People Get More Information about CT?

Additional information about CT imaging is available from the U.S. Food and Drug Administration (FDA), the federal agency that regulates food, drugs, medical devices, cosmetics, biologics, and radiation-emitting products. The FDA can be contacted at:

U.S. Food and Drug Administration (FDA)
10903 New Hampshire Avenue
Silver Spring, MD 20993
Toll-Free: 888-INFO-FDA (888-463-6332)
Website: www.fda.gov

Section 60.3

Tumor Markers

This section includes text excerpted from "Tumor Markers," National Cancer Institute (NCI), November 4, 2015.

What Are Tumor Markers?

Tumor markers are substances that are produced by cancer or by other cells of the body in response to cancer or certain benign (noncancerous) conditions. Most tumor markers are made by normal cells as well as by cancer cells; however, they are produced at much higher levels in cancerous conditions. These substances can be found in the blood, urine, stool, tumor tissue, or other tissues or bodily fluids of some patients with cancer. Most tumor markers are proteins. However, more recently, patterns of gene expression and changes to deoxyribonucleic acid (DNA) have also begun to be used as tumor markers.

Many different tumor markers have been characterized and are in clinical use. Some are associated with only one type of cancer, whereas others are associated with two or more cancer types. No "universal" tumor marker that can detect any type of cancer has been found.

There are some limitations to the use of tumor markers. Sometimes, noncancerous conditions can cause the levels of certain tumor markers to increase. In addition, not everyone with a particular type of cancer will have a higher level of a tumor marker associated with that cancer. Moreover, tumor markers have not been identified for every type of cancer.

How Are Tumor Markers Used in Cancer Care?

Tumor markers are used to help detect, diagnose, and manage some types of cancer. Although an elevated level of a tumor marker may suggest the presence of cancer, this alone is not enough to diagnose cancer. Therefore, measurements of tumor markers are usually combined with other tests, such as biopsies, to diagnose cancer.

Tumor marker levels may be measured before treatment to help doctors plan the appropriate therapy. In some types of cancer, the level of a tumor marker reflects the stage (extent) of the disease and/or the patient's prognosis (likely outcome or course of disease).

Tumor markers may also be measured periodically during cancer therapy. A decrease in the level of a tumor marker or a return to the marker's normal level may indicate that the cancer is responding to treatment, whereas no change or an increase may indicate that the cancer is not responding.

Tumor markers may also be measured after treatment has ended to check for recurrence (the return of cancer).

How Are Tumor Markers Measured?

A doctor takes a sample of tumor tissue or bodily fluid and sends it to a laboratory, where various methods are used to measure the level of the tumor marker.

If the tumor marker is being used to determine whether treatment is working or whether there is a recurrence, the marker's level will be measured in multiple samples taken over time. Usually, these "serial measurements," which show whether the level of a marker is increasing, staying the same, or decreasing, are more meaningful than a single measurement.

What Tumor Markers Are Currently Being Used, and for Which Cancer Types?

A number of tumor markers are currently being used for a wide range of cancer types. Although most of these can be tested in laboratories that meet standards set by the Clinical Laboratory Improvement Amendments, some cannot be and may, therefore, be considered experimental. Tumor markers that are currently in common use are listed below.

ALK gene rearrangements and overexpression

- Cancer types: Nonsmall cell lung cancer and anaplastic large cell lymphoma
- Tissue analyzed: Tumor
- How used: To help determine treatment and prognosis

Alpha-fetoprotein (AFP)

- Cancer types: Liver cancer and germ cell tumors
- Tissue analyzed: Blood

- How used: To help diagnose liver cancer and follow response to treatment; to assess stage, prognosis, and response to treatment of germ cell tumors

Beta-2-microglobulin (B2M)

- Cancer types: Multiple myeloma, chronic lymphocytic leukemia, and some lymphomas
- Tissue analyzed: Blood, urine, or cerebrospinal fluid
- How used: To determine prognosis and follow response to treatment

Beta-human chorionic gonadotropin (Beta-hCG)

- Cancer types: Choriocarcinoma and germ cell tumors
- Tissue analyzed: Urine or blood
- How used: To assess stage, prognosis, and response to treatment

BRCA1 and *BRCA2* gene mutations

- Cancer type: Ovarian cancer
- Tissue analyzed: Blood
- How used: To determine whether treatment with a particular type of targeted therapy is appropriate

BCR-ABL fusion gene (Philadelphia chromosome)

- Cancer type: Chronic myeloid leukemia, acute lymphoblastic leukemia, and acute myelogenous leukemia
- Tissue analyzed: Blood and/or bone marrow
- How used: To confirm diagnosis, predict response to targeted therapy, and monitor disease status

BRAF V600 mutations

- Cancer types: Cutaneous melanoma and colorectal cancer
- Tissue analyzed: Tumor
- How used: To select patients who are most likely to benefit from treatment with certain targeted therapies

C-kit/CD117

- Cancer types: Gastrointestinal stromal tumor and mucosal melanoma
- Tissue analyzed: Tumor
- How used: To help in diagnosing and determining treatment

CA15-3/CA27.29

- Cancer type: Breast cancer
- Tissue analyzed: Blood
- How used: To assess whether treatment is working or disease has recurred

CA19-9

- Cancer types: Pancreatic cancer, gallbladder cancer, bile duct cancer, and gastric cancer
- Tissue analyzed: Blood
- How used: To assess whether treatment is working

CA-125

- Cancer type: Ovarian cancer
- Tissue analyzed: Blood
- How used: To help in diagnosis, assessment of response to treatment, and evaluation of recurrence

Calcitonin

- Cancer type: Medullary thyroid cancer
- Tissue analyzed: Blood
- How used: To aid in diagnosis, check whether treatment is working, and assess recurrence

Carcinoembryonic antigen (CEA)

- Cancer types: Colorectal cancer and some other cancers
- Tissue analyzed: Blood
- How used: To keep track of how well cancer treatments are working or check if cancer has come back

CD20

- Cancer type: Non-Hodgkin lymphoma
- Tissue analyzed: Blood
- How used: To determine whether treatment with a targeted therapy is appropriate

Chromogranin A (CgA)

- Cancer type: Neuroendocrine tumors
- Tissue analyzed: Blood
- How used: To help in diagnosis, assessment of treatment response, and evaluation of recurrence

Chromosomes 3, 7, 17, and 9p21

- Cancer type: Bladder cancer
- Tissue analyzed: Urine
- How used: To help in monitoring for tumor recurrence

Circulating tumor cells of epithelial origin (CELLSEARCH®)

- Cancer types: Metastatic breast, prostate, and colorectal cancers
- Tissue analyzed: Blood
- How used: To inform clinical decision making, and to assess prognosis

Cytokeratin fragment 21-1

- Cancer type: Lung cancer
- Tissue analyzed: Blood
- How used: To help in monitoring for recurrence

EGFR gene mutation analysis

- Cancer type: Nonsmall cell lung cancer
- Tissue analyzed: Tumor
- How used: To help determine treatment and prognosis

Estrogen receptor (ER)/progesterone receptor (PR)

- Cancer type: Breast cancer

- Tissue analyzed: Tumor
- How used: To determine whether treatment with hormone therapy and some targeted therapies is appropriate

Fibrin/fibrinogen

- Cancer type: Bladder cancer
- Tissue analyzed: Urine
- How used: To monitor progression and response to treatment

HE4

- Cancer type: Ovarian cancer
- Tissue analyzed: Blood
- How used: To plan cancer treatment, assess disease progression, and monitor for recurrence

HER2/neu gene amplification or protein overexpression

- Cancer types: Breast cancer, gastric cancer, and gastroesophageal junction adenocarcinoma
- Tissue analyzed: Tumor
- How used: To determine whether treatment with certain targeted therapies is appropriate

Immunoglobulins (Ig)

- Cancer types: Multiple myeloma and Waldenström macroglobulinemia
- Tissue analyzed: Blood and urine
- How used: To help diagnose disease, assess response to treatment, and look for recurrence

KRAS gene mutation analysis

- Cancer types: Colorectal cancer and nonsmall cell lung cancer
- Tissue analyzed: Tumor
- How used: To determine whether treatment with a particular type of targeted therapy is appropriate

Lactate dehydrogenase (LDH)

- Cancer types: Germ cell tumors, lymphoma, leukemia, melanoma, and neuroblastoma

- Tissue analyzed: Blood
- How used: To assess stage, prognosis, and response to treatment

Neuron-specific enolase (NSE)

- Cancer types: Small cell lung cancer and neuroblastoma
- Tissue analyzed: Blood
- How used: To help in diagnosis and to assess response to treatment

Nuclear matrix protein 22

- Cancer type: Bladder cancer
- Tissue analyzed: Urine
- How used: To monitor response to treatment

Programmed death ligand 1 (PD-L1)

- Cancer type: Nonsmall cell lung cancer
- Tissue analyzed: Tumor
- How used: To determine whether treatment with a particular type of targeted therapy is appropriate

Prostate-specific antigen (PSA)

- Cancer type: Prostate cancer
- Tissue analyzed: Blood
- How used: To help in diagnosis, assess response to treatment, and look for recurrence

Thyroglobulin (Tg)

- Cancer type: Thyroid cancer
- Tissue analyzed: Blood
- How used: To evaluate response to treatment and look for recurrence

Urokinase plasminogen activator (uPA) and plasminogen activator inhibitor (PAI-1)

- Cancer type: Breast cancer

- Tissue analyzed: Tumor
- How used: To determine aggressiveness of cancer and guide treatment

5-Protein signature (OVA1®)

- Cancer type: Ovarian cancer
- Tissue analyzed: Blood
- How used: To preoperatively assess pelvic mass for suspected ovarian cancer

21-Gene signature (Oncotype DX®)

- Cancer type: Breast cancer
- Tissue analyzed: Tumor
- How used: To evaluate risk of recurrence

70-Gene signature (Mammaprint®)

- Cancer type: Breast cancer
- Tissue analyzed: Tumor
- How used: To evaluate risk of recurrence

Can Tumor Markers Be Used in Cancer Screening?

Because tumor markers can be used to assess the response of a tumor to treatment and for prognosis, researchers have hoped that they might also be useful in screening tests that aim to detect cancer early, before there are any symptoms. For a screening test to be useful, it should have very high sensitivity (ability to correctly identify people who have the disease) and specificity (ability to correctly identify people who do not have the disease). If a test is highly sensitive, it will identify most people with the disease—that is, it will result in very few false-negative results. If a test is highly specific, only a small number of people will test positive for the disease who do not have it—in other words, it will result in very few false-positive results.

Although tumor markers are extremely useful in determining whether a tumor is responding to treatment or assessing whether it has recurred, no tumor marker identified to date is sufficiently sensitive or specific to be used on its own to screen for cancer.

For example, the prostate-specific antigen (PSA) test, which measures the level of PSA in the blood, is often used to screen men for prostate cancer. However, an increased PSA level can be caused by benign prostate conditions as well as by prostate cancer, and most men with an elevated PSA level do not have prostate cancer. Initial results from two large randomized controlled trials, the NCI-sponsored Prostate, Lung, Colorectal, and Ovarian Cancer Screening Trial (PLCO), and the European Randomized Study of Screening for Prostate Cancer (ERSPC) showed that PSA testing at best leads to only a small reduction in the number of prostate cancer deaths. Moreover, it is not clear whether the benefits of PSA screening outweigh the harms of follow-up diagnostic tests and treatments for cancers that in many cases would never have threatened a man's life.

Similarly, results from the PLCO trial showed that CA-125, a tumor marker that is sometimes elevated in the blood of women with ovarian cancer but can also be elevated in women with benign conditions, is not sufficiently sensitive or specific to be used together with transvaginal ultrasound to screen for ovarian cancer in women at average risk of the disease. An analysis of 28 potential markers for ovarian cancer in blood from women who later went on to develop ovarian cancer found that none of these markers performed even as well as CA-125 at detecting the disease in women at average risk.

What Kind of Research Is Underway to Develop More Accurate Tumor Markers?

Cancer researchers are turning to proteomics (the study of protein structure, function, and patterns of expression) in hopes of developing new biomarkers that can be used to identify disease in its early stages, to predict the effectiveness of treatment, or to predict the chance of cancer recurrence after treatment has ended.

Scientists are also evaluating patterns of gene expression for their ability to help determine a patient's prognosis or response to therapy. For example, results of the National Cancer Institute (NCI)-sponsored Trial Assigning IndividuaLized Options for Treatment (Rx), or TAILORx, showed that for women recently diagnosed with lymph node–negative, hormone receptor–positive, HER2-negative breast cancer who had undergone surgery, those with the lowest 21-gene (Oncotype Dx®) recurrence scores had very low recurrence rates when given hormone therapy alone and thus can be spared chemotherapy. The trial is ongoing to see whether women at intermediate risk of recurrence, based on the 21-gene test, do better with chemotherapy in addition to hormone therapy than with hormone therapy alone.

Chapter 61

Surgical Procedures and Cancer

Chapter Contents

Section 61.1

What You Need to Know about Surgery

This section includes text excerpted from "Surgery to Treat Cancer," National Cancer Institute (NCI), April 29, 2015.

Surgery, when used to treat cancer, is a procedure in which a surgeon removes cancer from your body. Surgeons are medical doctors with special training in surgery.

How Surgery Is Performed

Surgeons often use small, thin knives, called scalpels, and other sharp tools to cut your body during surgery. Surgery often requires cuts through skin, muscles, and sometimes bone. After surgery, these cuts can be painful and take some time to recover from.

Anesthesia keeps you from feeling pain during surgery. Anesthesia refers to drugs or other substances that cause you to lose feeling or awareness. The following are the three types of anesthesia:

- Local anesthesia causes loss of feeling in one small area of the body.
- Regional anesthesia causes loss of feeling in a part of the body, such as an arm or leg.
- General anesthesia causes loss of feeling and a complete loss of awareness that seems like a very deep sleep.

There are other ways of performing surgery that do not involve cuts with scalpels. Some of these include:

- **Cryosurgery.** Cryosurgery is a type of treatment in which extreme cold produced by liquid nitrogen or argon gas is used to destroy abnormal tissue. Cryosurgery may be used to treat early-stage skin cancer, retinoblastoma, and precancerous growths on the skin and cervix. Cryosurgery is also called cryotherapy.

- **Lasers.** This is a type of treatment in which powerful beams of light are used to cut through tissue. Lasers can focus very accurately on tiny areas, so they can be used for precise surgeries. Lasers can also be used to shrink or destroy tumors or growths that might turn into cancer.

  Lasers are most often used to treat tumors on the surface of the body or on the inside lining of internal organs. Examples include basal cell carcinoma, cervical changes that might turn into cancer, and cervical, vaginal, esophageal, and nonsmall cell lung cancer.

- **Hyperthermia.** Hyperthermia is a type of treatment in which small areas of body tissue are exposed to high temperatures. The high heat can damage and kill cancer cells or make them more sensitive to radiation and certain chemotherapy drugs. Radiofrequency ablation is one type of hyperthermia that uses high-energy radio waves to generate heat. Hyperthermia is not widely available and is being studied in clinical trials.

- **Photodynamic therapy (PDT).** Photodynamic therapy is a type of treatment that uses drugs which react to a certain type of light. When the tumor is exposed to this light, these drugs become active and kill nearby cancer cells. Photodynamic therapy is used most often to treat or relieve symptoms caused by skin cancer, mycosis fungoides, and nonsmall cell lung cancer.

Types of Surgery

There are many types of surgery. The types differ based on the purpose of the surgery, the part of the body that requires surgery, the amount of tissue to be removed, and, in some cases, what the patient prefers.

Surgery may be open or minimally invasive.

- In open surgery, the surgeon makes one large cut to remove the tumor, some healthy tissue, and maybe some nearby lymph nodes.

- In minimally invasive surgery, the surgeon makes a few small cuts instead of one large one. She inserts a long, thin tube with a tiny camera into one of the small cuts. This tube is called a laparoscope. The camera projects images from the inside of the body onto a monitor, which allows the surgeon to see what she is doing. She uses special surgery tools that are inserted through the other small cuts to remove the tumor and some healthy tissue.

Because minimally invasive surgery requires smaller cuts, it takes less time to recover from than open surgery.

Who Has Surgery

Many people with cancer are treated with surgery. Surgery works best for solid tumors that are contained in one area. It is a local treatment, meaning that it treats only the part of your body with the cancer. It is not used for leukemia (a type of blood cancer) or for cancers that have spread.

Sometimes surgery will be the only treatment you need. But most often, you will also have other cancer treatments.

How Surgery Works against Cancer

Depending on your type of cancer and how advanced it is, surgery can be used to:

- **Remove the entire tumor.** Surgery removes cancer that is contained in one area.
- **Debulk a tumor.** Surgery removes some, but not all, of a cancer tumor. Debulking is used when removing an entire tumor might damage an organ or the body. Removing part of a tumor can help other treatments work better.
- **Ease cancer symptoms.** Surgery is used to remove tumors that are causing pain or pressure.

Risks of Surgery

Surgeons are highly trained and will do everything they can to prevent problems during surgery. Even so, sometimes problems do occur.

Common problems are as follows:

- **Pain.** After surgery, most people will have pain in the part of the body that was operated on. How much pain you feel will depend on the extent of the surgery, the part of your body where you had surgery, and how you feel pain.

Your doctor or nurse can help you manage pain after surgery. Talk with your doctor or nurse before surgery about ways to control pain. After surgery, tell them if your pain is not controlled.

- **Infection.** Infection is another problem that can happen after surgery. To help prevent infection, follow your nurse's instructions about caring for the area where you had surgery. If you do develop an infection, your doctor can prescribe a medicine (called an antibiotic) to treat it.

Other risks of surgery include bleeding, damage to nearby tissues, and reactions to the anesthesia. Talk to your doctor about possible risks for the type of surgery you will have.

How Much Surgery Costs

The cost of surgery depends on the following factors:

- The type of surgery you have
- How many specialists are involved in your surgery
- If you need local, regional, or general anesthesia
- Where you have surgery—at an outpatient clinic, a doctor's office, or the hospital
- If you need to stay in the hospital, and for how long
- The part of the country where you live

Talk with your health insurance company about what services it will pay for. Most insurance plans pay for surgery to treat cancer. To learn more, talk with the business office of the clinic or hospital where you go for treatment. If you need financial assistance, there are organizations that may be able to help. To find such organizations, go to the National Cancer Institute (NCI) database, Organizations that Offer Support Services (supportorgs.cancer.gov/home.aspx?js=1) and search for "financial assistance." Or call toll-free 800-4-CANCER (800-422-6237) to ask for information on organizations that may help.

Where You Have Surgery

Where you have surgery depends on the following:

- The type of surgery
- How extensive it is
- Where the surgeon practices
- The type of facility your insurance will cover

You can have outpatient surgery in a doctor's office, surgery center, or hospital. Outpatient means that you do not spend the night. Or, you may have surgery in the hospital and stay the night. How many nights you stay will depend on the type of surgery you have and how quickly you recover.

What to Expect before, during, and after Surgery

Before Surgery

Before surgery, a nurse may call you to tell you how to prepare. He or she may tell you about tests and exams you need to have before the surgery. Common tests that you may need, if you have not had them lately, are:

- Blood tests
- Chest X-ray
- Electrocardiogram (ECG)

You may not be able to eat or drink for a certain period of time before the surgery. It is important to follow the instructions about eating and drinking. If you don't, your surgery may need to be rescheduled.

You may also be asked to have supplies on hand for taking care of your wounds after surgery. Supplies might include antiseptic ointment and bandages.

During Surgery

Once you are under anesthesia, the surgeon removes the cancer, usually along with some healthy tissue around it. Removing this healthy tissue helps improve the chances that all the cancer has been removed.

Sometimes, the surgeon might also remove lymph nodes or other tissues near the tumor. These tissues will be checked under a microscope to see if the cancer has spread. Knowing if the nearby tissue contains cancer will help your doctors suggest the best treatment plan for you after surgery.

After Surgery

Once you are ready to go home after surgery, the nurse will tell you how to take care of yourself. He or she will explain the following:

- How to control pain
- Activities you should and should not do
- How to take care of your wound
- How to spot signs of infection and steps to take if you do
- When you can return to work

You will have at least one more visit with the surgeon a week or two after you go home. For more complex surgeries, you may need to see the surgeon more often. You may have stitches removed, and the surgeon will check to make sure you are healing as you should.

Special Diet Needs before and after Surgery

Surgery increases your need for good nutrition. If you are weak or underweight, you may need to eat a high-protein, high-calorie diet before surgery.

Some types of surgery may change how your body uses food. Surgery can also affect eating if you have surgery of the mouth, stomach, intestines, or throat. If you have trouble eating after surgery, you may be given nutrients through a feeding tube or intravenous (IV)—through a needle directly into a vein.

Talk with a dietitian for help with eating problems caused by surgery.

Working after Surgery

You will need to take time off from work to have and recover from surgery. You may need only 1 day or many weeks.

How long you need to recover depends on many factors, such as:

- The type of anesthesia you have. If you have local or regional anesthesia, you will probably return to work more quickly than if you have general anesthesia.
- The type of surgery you have, and how extensive it is
- The type of work you do. If you have an active job, you may need to take off more time than if you sit at a desk. If your job allows, you may want to see if you can work at home, or start back part-time, to help you ease back into a full workday.

Ask your doctor how long you will need to recover from your surgery. If you expect a longer recovery time, talk with your employer to find out if you can take medical leave. Check to make sure your health insurance will cover costs if you are on medical leave and not working for a time.

Section 61.2

Lasers in Cancer Treatment

This section includes text excerpted from "Lasers in Cancer Treatment," National Cancer Institute (NCI), September 13, 2011. Reviewed March 2018.

What Is Laser Light?

The term "laser" stands for light amplification by stimulated emission of radiation. Ordinary light, such as that from a light bulb, has many wavelengths and spreads in all directions. Laser light, on the other hand, has a specific wavelength. It is focused in a narrow beam and creates a very high-intensity light. This powerful beam of light may be used to cut through steel or to shape diamonds. Because lasers can focus very accurately on tiny areas, they can also be used for very precise surgical work or for cutting through tissue (in place of a scalpel).

What Is Laser Therapy, and How Is It Used in Cancer Treatment?

Laser therapy uses high-intensity light to treat cancer and other illnesses. Lasers can be used to shrink or destroy tumors or precancerous growths. Lasers are most commonly used to treat superficial cancers (cancers on the surface of the body or the lining of internal organs) such as basal cell skin cancer and the very early stages of some cancers, such as cervical, penile, vaginal, vulvar, and nonsmall cell lung cancer.

Lasers also may be used to relieve certain symptoms of cancer, such as bleeding or obstruction. For example, lasers can be used to shrink or destroy a tumor that is blocking a patient's trachea (windpipe) or esophagus. Lasers also can be used to remove colon polyps or tumors that are blocking the colon or stomach.

Laser therapy can be used alone, but most often it is combined with other treatments, such as surgery, chemotherapy, or radiation therapy. In addition, lasers can seal nerve endings to reduce pain after surgery and seal lymph vessels to reduce swelling and limit the spread of tumor cells.

How Is Laser Therapy Given to the Patient?

Laser therapy is often given through a flexible endoscope (a thin, lighted tube used to look at tissues inside the body). The endoscope is fitted with optical fibers (thin fibers that transmit light). It is inserted through an opening in the body, such as the mouth, nose, anus, or vagina. Laser light is then precisely aimed to cut or destroy a tumor.

Laser-induced interstitial thermotherapy (LITT), or interstitial laser photocoagulation, also uses lasers to treat some cancers. LITT is similar to a cancer treatment called hyperthermia, which uses heat to shrink tumors by damaging or killing cancer cells. During LITT, an optical fiber is inserted into a tumor. Laser light at the tip of the fiber raises the temperature of the tumor cells and damages or destroys them. LITT is sometimes used to shrink tumors in the liver.

Photodynamic therapy (PDT) is another type of cancer treatment that uses lasers. In PDT, a certain drug, called a photosensitizer or photosensitizing agent, is injected into a patient and absorbed by cells all over the patient's body. After a couple of days, the agent is found mostly in cancer cells. Laser light is then used to activate the agent and destroy cancer cells. Because the photosensitizer makes the skin and eyes sensitive to light afterward patients are advised to avoid direct sunlight and bright indoor light during that time.

What Types of Lasers Are Used in Cancer Treatment?

Three types of lasers are used to treat cancer: carbon dioxide (CO_2) lasers, argon lasers, and neodymium: yttrium-aluminum-garnet (Nd:YAG) lasers. Each of these can shrink or destroy tumors and can be used with endoscopes.

CO_2 and argon lasers can cut the skin's surface without going into deeper layers. Thus, they can be used to remove superficial cancers, such as skin cancer. In contrast, the Nd:YAG laser is more commonly applied through an endoscope to treat internal organs, such as the uterus, esophagus, and colon.

Nd:YAG laser light can also travel through optical fibers into specific areas of the body during LITT. Argon lasers are often used to activate the drugs used in PDT.

What Are the Advantages of Laser Therapy?

Lasers are more precise than standard surgical tools (scalpels), so they do less damage to normal tissues. As a result, patients usually have less pain, bleeding, swelling, and scarring. With laser therapy, operations are usually shorter. In fact, laser therapy can often be done on an outpatient basis. It takes less time for patients to heal after laser surgery, and they are less likely to get infections. Patients should consult with their healthcare provider about whether laser therapy is appropriate for them.

What Are the Disadvantages of Laser Therapy?

Laser therapy also has several limitations. Surgeons must have specialized training before they can do laser therapy, and strict safety precautions must be followed. Laser therapy is expensive and requires bulky equipment. In addition, the effects of laser therapy may not last long, so doctors may have to repeat the treatment for a patient to get the full benefit.

Chapter 62

Chemotherapy

Chemotherapy (also called chemo) is a type of cancer treatment that uses drugs to kill cancer cells.

How Chemotherapy Works against Cancer

Chemotherapy works by stopping or slowing the growth of cancer cells, which grow and divide quickly. Chemotherapy is used to:

- **Treat cancer.** Chemotherapy can be used to cure cancer, lessen the chance it will return, or stop or slow its growth.
- **Ease cancer symptoms.** Chemotherapy can be used to shrink tumors that are causing pain and other problems.

Who Receives Chemotherapy

Chemotherapy is used to treat many types of cancer. For some people, chemotherapy may be the only treatment you receive. But most often, you will have chemotherapy and other cancer treatments. The types of treatment that you need depends on the type of cancer you have, if it has spread and where, and if you have other health problems.

This chapter includes text excerpted from "Chemotherapy to Treat Cancer," National Cancer Institute (NCI), April 29, 2015.

How Chemotherapy Is Used with Other Cancer Treatments

When used with other treatments, chemotherapy can:

- Make a tumor smaller before surgery or radiation therapy. This is called neoadjuvant chemotherapy (NAC)
- Destroy cancer cells that may remain after treatment with surgery or radiation therapy. This is called adjuvant chemotherapy
- Help other treatments work better
- Kill cancer cells that have returned or spread to other parts of your body

Chemotherapy Can Cause Side Effects

Chemotherapy not only kills fast growing cancer cells, but also kills or slows the growth of healthy cells that grow and divide quickly. Examples are cells that line your mouth and intestines and those that cause your hair to grow. Damage to healthy cells may cause side effects, such as mouth sores, nausea, and hair loss. Side effects often get better or go away after you have finished chemotherapy.

The most common side effect is fatigue, which is feeling exhausted and worn out. You can prepare for fatigue in the following ways:

- Asking someone to drive you to and from chemotherapy
- Planning time to rest on the day of and day after chemotherapy
- Asking for help with meals and child care on the day of and at least one day after chemotherapy

There are many ways you can help manage chemotherapy side effects.

How Much Chemotherapy Costs

The cost of chemotherapy depends on the following:

- The types and doses of chemotherapy used
- How long and how often chemotherapy is given
- Whether you get chemotherapy at home, in a clinic or office, or during a hospital stay
- The part of the country where you live

Talk with your health insurance company about what services it will pay for. Most insurance plans pay for chemotherapy. To learn more, talk with the business office where you go for treatment.

If you need financial assistance, there are organizations that may be able to help.

What to Expect When Receiving Chemotherapy

Chemotherapy may be given in many ways. Some common ways include the following:

- **Oral.** The chemotherapy comes in pills, capsules, or liquids that you swallow.
- **Intravenous (IV).** The chemotherapy goes directly into a vein.
- **Injection.** The chemotherapy is given by a shot in a muscle in your arm, thigh, or hip, or right under the skin in the fatty part of your arm, leg, or belly.
- **Intrathecal.** The chemotherapy is injected into the space between the layers of tissue that cover the brain and spinal cord.
- **Intraperitoneal (IP).** The chemotherapy goes directly into the peritoneal cavity, which is the area in your body that contains organs such as your intestines, stomach, and liver.
- **Intraarterial (IA).** The chemotherapy is injected directly into the artery that leads to the cancer.
- **Topical.** The chemotherapy comes in a cream that you rub onto your skin.

Chemotherapy is often given through a thin needle that is placed in a vein on your hand or lower arm. Your nurse will put the needle in at the start of each treatment and remove it when treatment is over. Intravenous (IV) chemotherapy may also be given through catheters or ports, sometimes with the help of a pump.

- **Catheter.** A catheter is a thin, soft tube. A doctor or nurse places one end of the catheter in a large vein, often in your chest area. The other end of the catheter stays outside your body. Most catheters stay in place until you have finished your chemotherapy treatments. Catheters can also be used to give you other drugs and to draw blood. Be sure to watch for signs of infection around your catheter.

- **Port.** A port is a small, round disc that is placed under your skin during minor surgery. A surgeon puts it in place before you begin your course of treatment, and it remains there until you have finished. A catheter connects the port to a large vein, most often in your chest. Your nurse can insert a needle into your port to give you chemotherapy or draw blood. This needle can be left in place for chemotherapy treatments that are given for longer than one day. Be sure to watch for signs of infection around your port.
- **Pump.** Pumps are often attached to catheters or ports. They control how much and how fast chemotherapy goes into a catheter or port, allowing you to receive your chemotherapy outside of the hospital. Pumps can be internal or external. External pumps remain outside your body. Internal pumps are placed under your skin during surgery.

How Your Doctor Decides Which Chemotherapy Drugs to Give You

There are many different chemotherapy drugs. Which ones are included in your treatment plan depends mostly on the following factors:

- The type of cancer you have and how advanced it is
- Whether you have had chemotherapy before
- Whether you have other health problems, such as diabetes or heart disease

Where You Go for Chemotherapy

You may receive chemotherapy during a hospital stay, at home, or as an outpatient at a doctor's office, clinic, or hospital. Outpatient (OP) means you do not stay overnight. No matter where you go for chemotherapy, your doctor and nurse will watch for side effects and help you manage them.

How Often You Receive Chemotherapy

Treatment schedules for chemotherapy vary widely. How often and how long you get chemotherapy depends on the following factors:

- Your type of cancer and how advanced it is

- Whether chemotherapy is used to:
    - Cure your cancer
    - Control its growth
    - Ease symptoms
- The type of chemotherapy you are getting
- How your body responds to the chemotherapy

You may receive chemotherapy in cycles. A cycle is a period of chemotherapy treatment followed by a period of rest. For instance, you might receive chemotherapy every day for one week followed by three weeks with no chemotherapy. These four weeks make up one cycle. The rest period gives your body a chance to recover and build new healthy cells.

Missing a Chemotherapy Treatment

It is best not to skip a chemotherapy treatment. But, sometimes your doctor may change your chemotherapy schedule if you are having certain side effects. If this happens, your doctor or nurse will explain what to do and when to start treatment again.

How Chemotherapy May Affect You

Chemotherapy affects people in different ways. How you feel depends on the following factors:

- The type of chemotherapy you are getting
- The dose of chemotherapy you are getting
- Your type of cancer
- How advanced your cancer is
- How healthy you are before treatment

Since everyone is different and people respond to chemotherapy in different ways, your doctor and nurses cannot know for sure how you will feel during chemotherapy.

How You'll Know If Chemotherapy Is Working

You will see your doctor often. During these visits, she will ask you how you feel, do a physical exam, and order medical tests and scans.

Tests might include blood tests. Scans might include magnetic resonance imaging (MRI), computed tomography (CT), or positron emission tomography (PET) scans.

You cannot tell if chemotherapy is working based on its side effects. Some people think that severe side effects mean that chemotherapy is working well, or that no side effects mean that chemotherapy is not working. The truth is that side effects have nothing to do with how well chemotherapy is fighting your cancer.

Special Diet Needs

Chemotherapy can damage the healthy cells that line your mouth and intestines and cause eating problems. Tell your doctor or nurse if you have trouble eating while you are receiving chemotherapy. You might also find it helpful to speak with a dietitian.

Working during Chemotherapy

Many people can work during chemotherapy, as long as they match their work schedule to how they feel. Whether or not you can work may depend on what kind of job you have. If your job allows, you may want to see if you can work part-time or from home on days you do not feel well.

Many employers are required by law to change your work schedule to meet your needs during cancer treatment. Talk with your employer about ways to adjust your work during chemotherapy. You can learn more about these laws by talking with a social worker.

Chapter 63

Radiation Therapy

Radiation therapy (also called radiotherapy) is a cancer treatment that uses high doses of radiation to kill cancer cells and shrink tumors. At low doses, radiation is used in X-rays to see inside your body, as with X-rays of your teeth or broken bones.

How Radiation Therapy Works against Cancer

At high doses, radiation therapy kills cancer cells or slows their growth by damaging their deoxyribonucleic acid (DNA). Cancer cells whose DNA is damaged beyond repair stop dividing or die. When the damaged cells die, they are broken down and removed by the body. Radiation therapy does not kill cancer cells right away. It takes days or weeks of treatment before DNA is damaged enough for cancer cells to die. Then, cancer cells keep dying for weeks or months after radiation therapy ends.

Types of Radiation Therapy

There are two main types of radiation therapy, external beam and internal.

External Beam Radiation Therapy

External beam radiation therapy comes from a machine that aims radiation at your cancer. The machine is large and may be noisy. It

---

This chapter includes text excerpted from "Cancer Treatment—Radiation Therapy to Treat Cancer," National Cancer Institute (NCI), July 19, 2017.

does not touch you, but can move around you, sending radiation to a part of your body from many directions. External beam radiation therapy is a local treatment, which means it treats a specific part of your body. For example, if you have cancer in your lung, you will have radiation only to your chest, not to your whole body.

Internal Radiation Therapy

Internal radiation therapy is a treatment in which a source of radiation is put inside your body. The radiation source can be solid or liquid. Internal radiation therapy with a solid source is called brachytherapy. In this type of treatment, seeds, ribbons, or capsules that contain a radiation source are placed in your body in or near the tumor. Like external beam radiation therapy, brachytherapy is a local treatment and treats only a specific part of your body.

Internal radiation therapy with a liquid source is called systemic therapy. Systemic means that the treatment travels in the blood to tissues throughout your body, seeking out and killing cancer cells. You receive systemic radiation therapy by swallowing or through a vein, via an intravenous (IV) line.

The type of radiation therapy that you may have depends on the following factors:

- The type of cancer
- The size of the tumor
- The tumor's location in the body
- How close the tumor is to normal tissues that are sensitive to radiation
- Your general health and medical history
- Whether you will have other types of cancer treatment
- Other factors, such as your age and other medical conditions

Why People with Cancer Receive Radiation Therapy

Radiation therapy is used to treat cancer and ease cancer symptoms. When treatments are used to ease symptoms, they are known as palliative treatments. External beam radiation may shrink tumors to treat pain and other problems caused by the tumor, such as trouble breathing or loss of bowel and bladder control. Pain from cancer that has spread to the bone can be treated with systemic radiation therapy drugs called radiopharmaceuticals. When used to treat cancer, radiation therapy can cure cancer, prevent it from returning, or stop or slow its growth.

Types of Cancer That Are Treated with Radiation Therapy

External beam radiation therapy is used to treat many types of cancer. Brachytherapy is often used to treat cancers of the head and neck, breast, cervix, prostate, and eye. Systemic radiation therapy is most often used to treat certain types of thyroid cancer. This treatment uses radioactive iodine, which is also known as I-131.

How Radiation Is Used with Other Cancer Treatments

For some people, radiation may be the only treatment you need. But, most often, you will have radiation therapy with other cancer treatments, such as surgery, chemotherapy, and immunotherapy. Radiation therapy may be given before, during, or after these other treatments to improve the chances that treatment will work. The timing of when radiation therapy is given depends on the type of cancer being treated and whether the goal of radiation therapy is to treat the cancer or ease symptoms.

When radiation is combined with surgery, it can be given in the following ways:

- Before surgery, to shrink the size of the cancer so it can be removed by surgery and be less likely to return.
- During surgery, so that it goes straight to the cancer without passing through the skin. Radiation therapy used this way is called intraoperative radiation. With this technique, doctors can more easily protect nearby normal tissues from radiation.
- After surgery to kill any cancer cells that remain.

Radiation Therapy Can Cause Side Effects

Radiation not only kills or slows the growth of cancer cells, it can also affect nearby healthy cells. Damage to healthy cells can cause side effects. Many people who get radiation therapy have fatigue. Fatigue is feeling exhausted and worn out. It can happen all at once or come on slowly. People feel fatigue in different ways and you may feel more or less fatigue than someone else who is getting the same amount of radiation therapy to the same part of the body.

Other radiation therapy side effects you may have depend on the part of the body that is treated. To see which side effects you might expect, find the part of your body being treated in the following (Table 63.1). Discuss this with your doctor or nurse. Ask them about your chances of getting each side effect.

Table 63.1. Treatment Areas and Possible Side Effects

Part of the Body Being Treated	Possible Side Effects
Brain	• Fatigue • Hair loss • Nausea and vomiting • Skin changes • Headache • Blurry vision
Breast	• Fatigue • Hair loss • Skin changes • Swelling (Edema) • Tenderness
Chest	• Fatigue • Hair loss • Skin changes • Throat changes, such as trouble swallowing • Cough • Shortness of breath
Head and neck	• Fatigue • Hair loss • Mouth changes • Skin changes • Taste changes • Throat changes, such as trouble swallowing • Less active thyroid gland
Pelvis	• Diarrhea • Fatigue • Hair loss • Nausea and vomiting • Sexual problems (men) • Fertility problems (men) • Sexual problems (women) • Fertility problems (women) • Skin changes • Urinary and bladder changes

Table 63.1. Continued

Part of the Body Being Treated	Possible Side Effects
Rectum	• Diarrhea • Fatigue • Hair loss • Sexual problems (men) • Fertility problems (men) • Sexual problems (women) • Fertility problems (women) • Skin changes • Urinary and bladder changes
Stomach and abdomen	• Diarrhea • Fatigue • Hair loss • Nausea and vomiting • Skin changes • Urinary and bladder change

Healthy cells that are damaged during radiation treatment usually recover within a few months after treatment is over. But sometimes people may have side effects that do not improve. Other side effects may show up months or years after radiation therapy is over. These are called late effects. Whether you might have late effects, and what they might be, depends on the part of your body that was treated, other cancer treatments you've had, genetics, and other factors, such as smoking. Ask your doctor or nurse which late effects you should watch for.

How Much Radiation Therapy Costs

Radiation therapy can be expensive. It uses complex machines and involves the services of many healthcare providers. The exact cost of your radiation therapy depends on the cost of healthcare where you live, what type of radiation therapy you get, and how many treatments you need.

Talk with your health insurance company about what services it will pay for. Most insurance plans pay for radiation therapy. To learn more, talk with the business office at the clinic or hospital where you go for treatment.

What to Expect When Having External Beam Radiation Therapy

How Often You Will Have External Beam Radiation Therapy

Most people have external beam radiation therapy once a day, five days a week, Monday through Friday. Radiation is given in a series of treatments to allow healthy cells to recover and to make radiation more effective. How many weeks you have treatment depends on the type of cancer you have, the goal of your treatment, the radiation dose, and the radiation schedule.

The span of time from your first radiation treatment to the last is called a course of treatment.

Researchers are looking at different ways to adjust the radiation dose or schedule in order to reach the total dose of radiation more quickly or to limit damage to healthy cells. Different ways of delivering the total radiation dose include the following:

- Accelerated fractionation, which is treatment given in larger daily or weekly doses to reduce the number of weeks of treatment
- Hyperfractionation, which is a smaller dose than the usual daily dose of radiation given more than once a day
- Hypofractionation, which is larger doses given once a day or less often to reduce the number of treatments

Researchers hope these different schedules for delivering radiation may be more effective and cause fewer side effects than the usual way of doing it or be as effective but more convenient.

Where You Go for External Beam Radiation Therapy

Most of the time, you will get external beam radiation therapy as an outpatient. This means that you will have treatment at a clinic or radiation therapy center and will not stay the night in the hospital.

What Happens before Your First External Beam Radiation Therapy Treatment

You will have a 1- to 2-hour meeting with your doctor or nurse before you begin radiation therapy. At this time, you will have a physical exam, talk about your medical history, and maybe have imaging tests. Your doctor or nurse will discuss external beam radiation therapy, its benefits and side effects, and ways you can care for yourself during and after treatment. You can then choose whether to have external beam radiation therapy.

If you decide to have external beam radiation therapy, you will be scheduled for a treatment planning session called a simulation. At this time:

- A radiation oncologist (a doctor who specializes in using radiation to treat cancer) and radiation therapist will figure out your treatment area. You may also hear the treatment area referred to as the treatment port or treatment field. These terms refer to the places in your body that will get radiation. You will be asked to lie very still while X-rays or scans are taken.
- The radiation therapist will tattoo or draw small dots of colored ink on your skin to mark the treatment area. These dots will be needed throughout your course of radiation therapy. The radiation therapist will use them to make sure you are in exactly the same position for every treatment. The dots are about the size of a freckle. If the dots are tattooed, they will remain on your skin for the rest of your life. Ink markings will fade over time. Be careful not to remove them and tell the radiation therapist if they have faded or lost color.
- A body mold may be made of the part of the body that is being treated. This is a plastic or plaster form that keeps you from moving during treatment. It also helps make sure that you are in exactly the same position for each treatment
- If you are getting radiation to the head and neck area you may be fitted for a mask. The mask has many air holes. It attaches to the table where you will lie for your treatments. The mask helps keep your head from moving so that you are in exactly the same position for each treatment.

What to Wear for Your Treatments

Wear clothes that are comfortable and made of soft fabric, such as fleece or cotton. Choose clothes that are easy to take off, since you may need to expose the treatment area or change into a hospital gown. Do not wear clothes that are tight, such as close-fitting collars or waistbands, near your treatment area. Also, do not wear jewelry, adhesive bandages, or powder in the treatment area.

What Happens during a Treatment Session

- You may be asked to change into a hospital gown or robe.
- You will go to the treatment room where you will receive radiation. The temperature in this room will be very cool.

- Depending on where your cancer is, you will either lie down on a treatment table or sit in a special chair. The radiation therapist will use the dots on your skin and body mold or face mask, if you have one, to help you get into the right position.
- You may see colored lights pointed at your skin marks. These lights are harmless and help the therapist position you for treatment.
- You will need to stay very still so the radiation goes to the exact same place each time. You will get radiation for 1–5 minutes. During this time, you can breathe normally.

The radiation therapist will leave the room just before your treatment begins. He or she will go to a nearby room to control the radiation machine. The therapist watches you on a TV screen or through a window and talks with you through a speaker in the treatment room. Make sure to tell the therapist if you feel sick or are uncomfortable. He or she can stop the radiation machine at any time. You will hear the radiation machine and see it moving around, but you won't be able to feel, hear, see, or smell the radiation. Most visits last from 30 minutes to an hour, with most of that time spent helping you get into the correct position.

How to Relax for Treatment Sessions

Keep yourself busy while you wait:

- Read a book or magazine.
- Work on crossword puzzles or needlework.
- Use headphones to listen to music or recorded books.
- Meditate, breathe deeply, pray, use imagery, or find other ways to relax.

External Beam Radiation Therapy Will Not Make You Radioactive

People often wonder if they will be radioactive when they are having treatment with radiation. External beam radiation therapy will not make you radioactive. You may safely be around other people, even pregnant women, babies, and young children.

What to Expect When Having Internal Radiation Therapy

What Happens before Your First Internal Radiation Therapy Treatment

You will have a 1- to 2-hour meeting with your doctor or nurse to plan your treatment before you begin internal radiation therapy. At this time, you will have a physical exam, talk about your medical history, and maybe have imaging tests. Your doctor will discuss the type of internal radiation therapy that is best for you, its benefits and side effects, and ways you can care for yourself during and after treatment. You can then decide whether to have internal radiation therapy.

How Brachytherapy Is Put in Place

Most brachytherapy is put in place through a catheter, which is a small, stretchy tube. Sometimes, brachytherapy is put in place through a larger device called an applicator. The way the brachytherapy is put in place depends on your type of cancer. Your doctor will place the catheter or applicator into your body before you begin treatment.

Techniques for placing brachytherapy include the following:

- Interstitial brachytherapy, in which the radiation source is placed within the tumor. This technique is used for prostate cancer, for instance.
- Intracavity brachytherapy, in which the radiation source is placed within a body cavity or a cavity created by surgery. For example, radiation can be placed in the vagina to treat cervical or endometrial cancer.
- Episcleral brachytherapy, in which the radiation source is attached to the eye. This technique is used to treat melanoma of the eye.

Once the catheter or applicator is in place, the radiation source is placed inside it. The radiation source may be kept in place for a few minutes, for many days, or for the rest of your life. How long it remains in place depends on the type of radiation source, your type of cancer, where the cancer is in your body, your health, and other cancer treatments you have had.

Types of Brachytherapy

There are three types of brachytherapy:

1. **Low-dose rate (LDR) implants.** In this type of brachytherapy, the radiation source stays in place for 1–7 days. You are likely to be in the hospital during this time. Once your treatment is finished, your doctor will remove the radiation source and the catheter or applicator.
2. **High-dose rate (HDR) implants.** In this type of brachytherapy, the radiation source is left in place for just 10–20 minutes at a time and then taken out. You may have treatment twice a day for 2–5 days or once a week for 2–5 weeks. The schedule depends on your type of cancer. During the course of treatment, your catheter or applicator may stay in place, or it may be put in place before each treatment. You may be in the hospital during this time, or you may make daily trips to the hospital to have the radiation source put in place. As with LDR implants, your doctor will remove the catheter or applicator once you have finished treatment.
3. **Permanent implants.** After the radiation source is put in place, the catheter is removed. The implants remain in your body for the rest of your life, but the radiation gets weaker each day. As time goes on, almost all the radiation will go away. When the radiation is first put in place, you may need to limit your time around other people and take other safety measures. Be extra careful not to spend time with children or pregnant women.

Internal Radiation Therapy Makes You Give off Radiation

With systemic radiation, your body fluids (urine, sweat, and saliva) will give off radiation for a while. With brachytherapy, your body fluids will not give off radiation, but the radiation source in your body will. If the radiation you receive is a very high dose, you may need to follow some safety measures. These measures may include the following:

- Staying in a private hospital room to protect others from radiation coming from your body.
- Being treated quickly by nurses and other hospital staff. They will provide all the care you need, but may stand at a distance, talk with you from the doorway of your room, and wear protective clothing.

Your visitors will also need to follow safety measures, which may include the following:

- Not being allowed to visit when the radiation is first put in
- Needing to check with the hospital staff before they go to your room
- Standing by the doorway rather than going into your hospital room
- Keeping visits short (30 minutes or less each day). The length of visits depends on the type of radiation being used and the part of your body being treated
- Not having visits from pregnant women and children younger than a year old

You may also need to follow safety measures once you leave the hospital, such as not spending much time with other people. Your doctor or nurse will talk with you about any safety measures you should follow when you go home.

What to Expect When the Catheter Is Removed

Once you finish treatment with light dependent resistor (LDR) or HDR implants, the catheter will be removed. Here are some things to expect:

- You will get medicine for pain before the catheter or applicator is removed.
- The area where the catheter or applicator was might be tender for a few months.
- There is no radiation in your body after the catheter or applicator is removed. It is safe for people to be near you—even young children and pregnant women.

For a week or two, you may need to limit activities that take a lot of effort. Ask your doctor what kinds of activities are safe for you and which ones you should avoid.

Special Diet Needs

Radiation can cause side effects that make it hard to eat, such as nausea, mouth sores, and throat problems called esophagitis. Since your body uses a lot of energy to heal during radiation therapy, it is important that you eat enough calories and protein to maintain your weight during treatment. If you are having trouble eating and maintaining your weight, talk to your doctor or nurse. You might also find it helpful to speak with a dietitian.

Working during Radiation Therapy

Some people are able to work full-time during radiation therapy. Others can work only part-time or not at all. How much you are able to work depends on how you feel. Ask your doctor or nurse what you may expect from the treatment you will have.

You are likely to feel well enough to work when you first start your radiation treatments. As time goes on, do not be surprised if you are more tired, have less energy, or feel weak. Once you have finished treatment, it may take just a few weeks for you to feel better—or it could take months.

You may get to a point during your radiation therapy when you feel too sick to work. Talk with your employer to find out if you can go on medical leave. Check that your health insurance will pay for treatment while you are on medical leave.

Chapter 64

Immunotherapy

Immunotherapy is a type of biological therapy. Biological therapy is a type of treatment that uses substances made from living organisms to treat cancer.

Types of Immunotherapy

Many different types of immunotherapy are used to treat cancer. They include the following:

- **Monoclonal antibodies**, which are drugs that are designed to bind to specific targets in the body. They can cause an immune response that destroys cancer cells.

Other types of monoclonal antibodies can "mark" cancer cells so it is easier for the immune system to find and destroy them. These types of monoclonal antibodies may also be referred to as targeted therapy.

- **Adoptive cell transfer**, which is a treatment that attempts to boost the natural ability of your T cells to fight cancer. T cells are a type of white blood cell and part of the immune system. Researchers take T cells from the tumor. They then isolate the T cells that are most active against your cancer or modify the genes in them to make them better able to find and destroy your cancer cells. Researchers then grow large batches of these T cells in the lab.

This chapter includes text excerpted from "Cancer Treatment—Immunotherapy to Treat Cancer," National Cancer Institute (NCI), May 4, 2017.

You may have treatments to reduce your immune cells. After these treatments, the T cells that were grown in the lab will be given back to you via a needle in your vein. The process of growing your T cells in the lab can take 2–8 weeks, depending on how fast they grow.

- **Cytokines**, which are proteins that are made by your body's cells. They play important roles in the body's normal immune responses and also in the immune system's ability to respond to cancer. The two main types of cytokines used to treat cancer are called interferons and interleukins.
- **Treatment vaccines**, which work against cancer by boosting your immune system's response to cancer cells. Treatment vaccines are different from the ones that help prevent disease.
- **BCG**, which stands for Bacillus Calmette-Guérin, is an immunotherapy that is used to treat bladder cancer. It is a weakened form of the bacteria that causes tuberculosis. When inserted directly into the bladder with a catheter, BCG causes an immune response against cancer cells. It is also being studied in other types of cancer.

Who Receives Immunotherapy

Immunotherapy is not yet as widely used as surgery, chemotherapy, and radiation therapy. However, immunotherapies have been approved to treat people with many types of cancer.

Many other immunotherapies are being studied in clinical trials, which are research studies involving people.

How Immunotherapy Works against Cancer

One reason that cancer cells thrive is because they are able to hide from your immune system. Certain immunotherapies can mark cancer cells so it is easier for the immune system to find and destroy them. Other immunotherapies boost your immune system to work better against cancer.

Immunotherapy Can Cause Side Effects

Immunotherapy can cause side effects, which affect people in different ways. The side effects you may have and how they make you feel will depend on how healthy you are before treatment, your type of cancer, how advanced it is, the type of therapy you are getting, and the dose. Doctors and nurses cannot know for certain how you will feel during treatment.

The most common side effects are skin reactions at the needle site. These side effects include the following:

- Pain
- Swelling
- Soreness
- Redness
- Itchiness
- Rash

You may have flu-like symptoms, which include the following:

- Fever
- Chills
- Weakness
- Dizziness
- Nausea or vomiting
- Muscle or joint aches
- Fatigue
- Headache
- Trouble breathing
- Low or high blood pressure

Other side effects might include the following:

- Swelling and weight gain from retaining fluid
- Heart palpitations
- Sinus congestion
- Diarrhea
- Risk of infection

Immunotherapies may also cause severe or even fatal allergic reactions. However, these reactions are rare.

How Immunotherapy Is Given

Different forms of immunotherapy may be given in different ways. These include the following:

- **Intravenous (IV).** The immunotherapy goes directly into a vein.
- **Oral.** The immunotherapy comes in pills or capsules that you swallow.
- **Topical.** The immunotherapy comes in a cream that you rub onto your skin. This type of immunotherapy can be used for very early skin cancer.

- **Intravesical.** The immunotherapy goes directly into the bladder.

Where You Go for Your Immunotherapy Treatment

You may receive immunotherapy in a doctor's office, clinic, or outpatient unit in a hospital. Outpatient means you do not spend the night in the hospital.

How Often You Will Receive Immunotherapy Treatment

How often and how long you receive immunotherapy depends on the following factors:

- Your type of cancer and how advanced it is
- The type of immunotherapy you get
- How your body reacts to treatment

You may have treatment every day, week, or month. Some immunotherapies are given in cycles. A cycle is a period of treatment followed by a period of rest. The rest period gives your body a chance to recover, respond to the immunotherapy, and build new healthy cells.

How to Tell Whether Immunotherapy Is Working

You will see your doctor often. He or she will give you physical exams and ask you how you feel. You will have medical tests, such as blood tests and different types of scans. These tests will measure the size of your tumor and look for changes in your blood work.

Chapter 65

Stem Cell Transplant

Stem cell transplants are procedures that restore blood-forming stem cells in people who have had theirs destroyed by the very high doses of chemotherapy or radiation therapy that are used to treat certain cancers.

Blood-forming stem cells are important because they grow into different types of blood cells. The following are the main types of blood cells:

1. White blood cells, which are part of your immune system and help your body fight infection.
2. Red blood cells, which carry oxygen throughout your body.
3. Platelets, which help the blood clot.

You need all three types of blood cells to be healthy.

Types of Stem Cell Transplants

In a stem cell transplant, you receive healthy blood-forming stem cells through a needle in your vein. Once they enter your bloodstream, the stem cells travel to the bone marrow, where they take the place of the cells that were destroyed by treatment. The blood-forming stem cells that are used in transplants can come from the bone marrow, bloodstream, or umbilical cord. Transplants can be done in the following ways:

This chapter includes text excerpted from "Cancer Treatment—Stem Cell Transplants in Cancer Treatment," National Cancer Institute (NCI), April 29, 2015.

- Autologous, which means the stem cells come from you, the patient
- Allogeneic, which means the stem cells come from someone else. The donor may be a blood relative but can also be someone who is not related.
- Syngeneic, which means the stem cells come from your identical twin, if you have one

To reduce possible side effects and improve the chances that an allogeneic transplant will work, the donor's blood-forming stem cells must match yours in certain ways.

How Stem Cell Transplants Work against Cancer

Stem cell transplants do not usually work against cancer directly. Instead, they help you recover your ability to produce stem cells after treatment with very high doses of radiation therapy, chemotherapy, or both.

However, in multiple myeloma and some types of leukemia, the stem cell transplant may work against cancer directly. This happens because of an effect called graft-versus-tumor that can occur after allogeneic transplants. Graft-versus-tumor occurs when white blood cells from your donor (the graft) attack any cancer cells that remain in your body (the tumor) after high-dose treatments. This effect improves the success of the treatments.

Who Receives Stem Cell Transplants

Stem cell transplants are most often used to help people with leukemia and lymphoma. They may also be used for neuroblastoma and multiple myeloma. Stem cell transplants for other types of cancer are being studied in clinical trials, which are research studies involving people.

Stem Cell Transplants Can Cause Side Effects

The high doses of cancer treatment that you have before a stem cell transplant can cause problems such as bleeding and an increased risk of infection. Talk with your doctor or nurse about other side effects that you might have and how serious they might be.

If you have an allogeneic transplant, you might develop a serious problem called graft-versus-host disease. Graft-versus-host disease (GvHD) can occur when white blood cells from your donor (the graft) recognize cells in your body (the host) as foreign and attack them. This problem can cause damage to your skin, liver, intestines, and many other organs. It can occur a few weeks after the transplant or much later. Graft-versus-host disease can be treated with steroids or other drugs that suppress your immune system.

The closer your donor's blood-forming stem cells match yours, the less likely you are to have graft-versus-host disease. Your doctor may also try to prevent it by giving you drugs to suppress your immune system.

How Much Stem Cell Transplants Cost

Stem cells transplants are complicated procedures that are very expensive. Most insurance plans cover some of the costs of transplants for certain types of cancer. Talk with your health plan about which services it will pay for. Talking with the business office where you go for treatment may help you understand all the costs involved.

What To Expect When Receiving A Stem Cell Transplant

Where You Go for a Stem Cell Transplant

When you need an allogeneic stem cell transplant, you will need to go to a hospital that has a specialized transplant center. The National Marrow Donor Program® maintains a list of transplant centers in the United States that can help you find a transplant center.

Unless you live near a transplant center, you may need to travel from home for your treatment. You might need to stay in the hospital during your transplant, you may be able to have it as an outpatient, or you may need to be in the hospital only part of the time. When you are not in the hospital, you will need to stay in a hotel or apartment nearby. Many transplant centers can assist with finding nearby housing.

How Long It Takes to Have a Stem Cell Transplant

A stem cell transplant can take a few months to complete. The process begins with treatment of high doses of chemotherapy, radiation therapy, or a combination of the two. This treatment goes on for a week or two. Once you have finished, you will have a few days to rest.

Next, you will receive the blood-forming stem cells. The stem cells will be given to you through an intravenous (IV) catheter. This process is like receiving a blood transfusion. It takes 1–5 hours to receive all the stem cells.

After receiving the stem cells, you begin the recovery phase. During this time, you wait for the blood cells you received to start making new blood cells.

Even after your blood counts return to normal, it takes much longer for your immune system to fully recover—several months for autologous transplants and 1–2 years for allogeneic or syngeneic transplants.

How Stem Cell Transplants May Affect You

Stem cell transplants affect people in different ways. How you feel depends on the following factors:

- The type of transplant that you have
- The doses of treatment you had before the transplant
- How you respond to the high-dose treatments
- Your type of cancer
- How advanced your cancer is
- How healthy you were before the transplant

Since people respond to stem cell transplants in different ways, your doctor or nurses cannot know for sure how the procedure will make you feel.

How to Tell If Your Stem Cell Transplant Worked

Doctors will follow the progress of the new blood cells by checking your blood counts often. As the newly transplanted stem cells produce blood cells, your blood counts will go up.

Special Diet Needs

The high-dose treatments that you have before a stem cell transplant can cause side effects that make it hard to eat, such as mouth sores and nausea. Tell your doctor or nurse if you have trouble eating while you are receiving treatment. You might also find it helpful to speak with a dietitian.

Working during Your Stem Cell Transplant

Whether or not you can work during a stem cell transplant may depend on the type of job you have. The process of a stem cell transplant, with the high-dose treatments, the transplant, and recovery, can take weeks or months. You will be in and out of the hospital during this time. Even when you are not in the hospital, sometimes you will need to stay near it, rather than staying in your own home. So, if your job allows, you may want to arrange to work remotely part-time.

Many employers are required by law to change your work schedule to meet your needs during cancer treatment. Talk with your employer about ways to adjust your work during treatment. You can learn more about these laws by talking with a social worker.

Chapter 66

Hormone Therapy

Hormone therapy is a cancer treatment that slows or stops the growth of cancer that uses hormones to grow. Hormone therapy is also called hormonal therapy, hormone treatment, or endocrine therapy.

How Hormone Therapy Works against Cancer

Hormone therapy is used to:

- **Treat cancer.** Hormone therapy can lessen the chance that cancer will return or stop or slow its growth.
- **Ease cancer symptoms.** Hormone therapy may be used to reduce or prevent symptoms in men with prostate cancer who are not able to have surgery or radiation therapy.

Types of Hormone Therapy

Hormone therapy falls into two broad groups, those that block the body's ability to produce hormones and those that interfere with how hormones behave in the body.

Who Receives Hormone Therapy

Hormone therapy is used to treat prostate and breast cancers that use hormones to grow. Hormone therapy is most often used along with

---

This chapter includes text excerpted from "Cancer Treatment—Hormone Therapy to Treat Cancer," National Cancer Institute (NCI), April 29, 2015.

other cancer treatments. The types of treatment that you need depend on the type of cancer, if it has spread and how far, if it uses hormones to grow, and if you have other health problems.

How Hormone Therapy Is Used with Other Cancer Treatments

When used with other treatments, hormone therapy can:

- Make a tumor smaller before surgery or radiation therapy. This is called neoadjuvant therapy.
- Lower the risk that cancer will come back after the main treatment. This is called adjuvant therapy.
- Destroy cancer cells that have returned or spread to other parts of your body.

Hormone Therapy Can Cause Side Effects

Because hormone therapy blocks your body's ability to produce hormones or interferes with how hormones behave, it can cause unwanted side effects. The side effects you have will depend on the type of hormone therapy you receive and how your body responds to it. People respond differently to the same treatment, so not everyone gets the same side effects. Some side effects also differ if you are a man or a woman.

Some common side effects for men who receive hormone therapy for prostate cancer include the following:

- Hot flashes
- Loss of interest in or ability to have sex
- Weakened bones
- Diarrhea
- Nausea
- Enlarged and tender breasts
- Fatigue

Some common side effects for women who receive hormone therapy for breast cancer include the following:

- Hot flashes

- Vaginal dryness
- Changes in your periods if you have not yet reached menopause
- Loss of interest in sex
- Nausea
- Mood changes
- Fatigue

How Much Hormone Therapy Costs

The cost of hormone therapy depends on:

- The types of hormone therapy you receive
- How long and how often you receive hormone therapy
- The part of the country where you live

Talk with your health insurance company about what services it will pay for. Most insurance plans pay for hormone therapy for their members.

What to Expect When Receiving Hormone Therapy

How Hormone Therapy Is Given

Hormone therapy may be given in the following ways:

- **Oral.** Hormone therapy comes in pills that you swallow.
- **Injection.** The hormone therapy is given by a shot in a muscle in your arm, thigh, or hip, or right under the skin in the fatty part of your arm, leg, or belly.
- **Surgery.** You may have surgery to remove organs that produce hormones. In women, the ovaries are removed. In men, the testicles are removed.

Where You Receive Hormone Therapy

Where you receive treatment depends on which hormone therapy you are getting and how it is given. You may take hormone therapy at home. Or, you may receive hormone therapy in a doctor's office, clinic, or hospital.

How Hormone Therapy May Affect You

Hormone therapy affects people in different ways. How you feel depends on the type of cancer you have, how advanced it is, the type of hormone therapy you are getting, and the dose. Your doctors and nurses cannot know for certain how you will feel during hormone therapy.

How to Tell If Hormone Therapy Is Working

If you are taking hormone therapy for prostate cancer, you will have regular prostate-specific antigen (PSA) tests. If hormone therapy is working, your PSA levels will stay the same or may even go down. But, if your PSA levels go up, this may be a sign that the treatment is no longer working. If this happens, your doctor will discuss treatment options with you.

Special Diet Needs

Hormone therapy for prostate cancer may cause weight gain. Talk with your doctor, nurse, or dietitian if weight gain becomes a problem for you.

Working during Hormone Therapy

Hormone therapy should not interfere with your ability to work.

Chapter 67

Targeted Therapies

What Are Targeted Cancer Therapies?

Targeted cancer therapies are drugs or other substances that block the growth and spread of cancer by interfering with specific molecules ("molecular targets") that are involved in the growth, progression, and spread of cancer. Targeted cancer therapies are sometimes called "molecularly targeted drugs," "molecularly targeted therapies," "precision medicines," or similar names.

Targeted therapies differ from standard chemotherapy in the following ways:

- Targeted therapies act on specific molecular targets that are associated with cancer, whereas most standard chemotherapies act on all rapidly dividing normal and cancerous cells.
- Targeted therapies are deliberately chosen or designed to interact with their target, whereas many standard chemotherapies were identified because they kill cells.
- Targeted therapies are often cytostatic (that is, they block tumor cell proliferation), whereas standard chemotherapy agents are cytotoxic (that is, they kill tumor cells).

Targeted therapies are currently the focus of much anticancer drug development. They are a cornerstone of precision medicine, a form of

---

This chapter includes text excerpted from "Cancer Treatment—Targeted Cancer Therapies," National Cancer Institute (NCI), February 9, 2018.

medicine that uses information about a person's genes and proteins to prevent, diagnose, and treat disease.

Many targeted cancer therapies have been approved by the U.S. Food and Drug Administration (FDA) to treat specific types of cancer. Others are being studied in clinical trials (research studies with people), and many more are in preclinical testing (research studies with animals).

How Are Targets for Targeted Cancer Therapies Identified?

The development of targeted therapies requires the identification of good targets—that is, targets that play a key role in cancer cell growth and survival. (It is for this reason that targeted therapies are sometimes referred to as the product of "rational" drug design.)

One approach to identify potential targets is to compare the amounts of individual proteins in cancer cells with those in normal cells. Proteins that are present in cancer cells but not normal cells or that are more abundant in cancer cells would be potential targets, especially if they are known to be involved in cell growth or survival. An example of such a differentially expressed target is the human epidermal growth factor receptor 2 protein (HER-2). HER-2 is expressed at high levels on the surface of some cancer cells. Several targeted therapies are directed against HER-2, including trastuzumab (Herceptin®), which is approved to treat certain breast and stomach cancers that overexpress HER-2.

Another approach to identify potential targets is to determine whether cancer cells produce mutant (altered) proteins that drive cancer progression. For example, the cell growth signaling protein BRAF is present in an altered form (known as BRAF V600E) in many melanomas. Vemurafenib (Zelboraf®) targets this mutant form of the BRAF protein and is approved to treat patients with inoperable or metastatic melanoma that contains this altered BRAF protein.

Researchers also look for abnormalities in chromosomes that are present in cancer cells but not in normal cells. Sometimes these chromosome abnormalities result in the creation of a fusion gene (a gene that incorporates parts of two different genes) whose product, called a fusion protein, may drive cancer development. Such fusion proteins are potential targets for targeted cancer therapies. For example, imatinib mesylate (Gleevec®) targets the BCR-ABL fusion protein, which is made from pieces of two genes that get joined together in some leukemia cells and promotes the growth of leukemic cells.

How Are Targeted Therapies Developed?

Once a candidate target has been identified, the next step is to develop a therapy that affects the target in a way that interferes with its ability to promote cancer cell growth or survival. For example, a targeted therapy could reduce the activity of the target or prevent it from binding to a receptor that it normally activates, among other possible mechanisms.

Most targeted therapies are either small molecules or monoclonal antibodies. Small-molecule compounds are typically developed for targets that are located inside the cell because such agents are able to enter cells relatively easily. Monoclonal antibodies are relatively large and generally cannot enter cells, so they are used only for targets that are outside cells or on the cell surface.

Candidate small molecules are usually identified in what are known as "high-throughput screens," in which the effects of thousands of test compounds on a specific target protein are examined. Compounds that affect the target (sometimes called "lead compounds") are then chemically modified to produce numerous closely related versions of the lead compound. These related compounds are then tested to determine which are most effective and have the fewest effects on nontarget molecules.

Monoclonal antibodies are developed by injecting animals (usually mice) with purified target proteins, causing the animals to make many different types of antibodies against the target. These antibodies are then tested to find the ones that bind best to the target without binding to nontarget proteins.

Before monoclonal antibodies are used in humans, they are "humanized" by replacing as much of the mouse antibody molecule as possible with corresponding portions of human antibodies. Humanizing is necessary to prevent the human immune system from recognizing the monoclonal antibody as "foreign" and destroying it before it has a chance to bind to its target protein. Humanization is not an issue for small-molecule compounds because they are not typically recognized by the body as foreign.

What Types of Targeted Therapies Are Available?

Many different targeted therapies have been approved for use in cancer treatment. These therapies include hormone therapies, signal transduction inhibitors, gene expression modulators, apoptosis inducers, angiogenesis inhibitors, immunotherapies, and toxin delivery molecules.

- **Hormone therapies** slow or stop the growth of hormone-sensitive tumors, which require certain hormones to grow. Hormone therapies act by preventing the body from producing the hormones or by interfering with the action of the hormones. Hormone therapies have been approved for both breast cancer and prostate cancer.
- **Signal transduction inhibitors** block the activities of molecules that participate in signal transduction, the process by which a cell responds to signals from its environment. During this process, once a cell has received a specific signal, the signal is relayed within the cell through a series of biochemical reactions that ultimately produce the appropriate response(s). In some cancers, the malignant cells are stimulated to divide continuously without being prompted to do so by external growth factors. Signal transduction inhibitors interfere with this inappropriate signaling.
- **Gene expression modulators** modify the function of proteins that play a role in controlling gene expression.
- **Apoptosis inducers** cause cancer cells to undergo a process of controlled cell death called apoptosis. Apoptosis is one method the body uses to get rid of unneeded or abnormal cells, but cancer cells have strategies to avoid apoptosis. Apoptosis inducers can get around these strategies to cause the death of cancer cells.
- **Angiogenesis inhibitors** block the growth of new blood vessels to tumors (a process called tumor angiogenesis). A blood supply is necessary for tumors to grow beyond a certain size because blood provides the oxygen and nutrients that tumors need for continued growth. Treatments that interfere with angiogenesis may block tumor growth. Some targeted therapies that inhibit angiogenesis interfere with the action of vascular endothelial growth factor (VEGF), a substance that stimulates new blood vessel formation. Other angiogenesis inhibitors target other molecules that stimulate new blood vessel growth.
- **Immunotherapies** trigger the immune system to destroy cancer cells. Some immunotherapies are monoclonal antibodies that recognize specific molecules on the surface of cancer cells. Binding of the monoclonal antibody to the target molecule results in the immune destruction of cells that express that target

molecule. Other monoclonal antibodies bind to certain immune cells to help these cells better kill cancer cells.

- **Monoclonal antibodies that deliver toxic molecules** can cause the death of cancer cells specifically. Once the antibody has bound to its target cell, the toxic molecule that is linked to the antibody—such as a radioactive substance or a poisonous chemical—is taken up by the cell, ultimately killing that cell. The toxin will not affect cells that lack the target for the antibody—i.e., the vast majority of cells in the body.

Cancer vaccines and **gene therapy** are sometimes considered targeted therapies because they interfere with the growth of specific cancer cells.

How Is It Determined Whether a Patient Is a Candidate for Targeted Therapy?

For some types of cancer, most patients with that cancer will have an appropriate target for a particular targeted therapy and, thus, will be candidates to be treated with that therapy. CML is an example: most patients have the *BCR-ABL* fusion gene. For other cancer types, however, a patient's tumor tissue must be tested to determine whether or not an appropriate target is present. The use of a targeted therapy may be restricted to patients whose tumor has a specific gene mutation that codes for the target; patients who do not have the mutation would not be candidates because the therapy would have nothing to target.

Sometimes, a patient is a candidate for a targeted therapy only if he or she meets specific criteria (for example, their cancer did not respond to other therapies, has spread, or is inoperable). These criteria are set by the FDA when it approves a specific targeted therapy.

What Are the Limitations of Targeted Cancer Therapies?

Targeted therapies do have some limitations. One is that cancer cells can become resistant to them. Resistance can occur in two ways: the target itself changes through mutation so that the targeted therapy no longer interacts well with it, and/or the tumor finds a new pathway to achieve tumor growth that does not depend on the target.

For this reason, targeted therapies may work best in combination. For example, a recent study found that using two therapies that target different parts of the cell signaling pathway that is altered in melanoma by the BRAF V600E mutation slowed the development of resistance and disease progression to a greater extent than using just one targeted therapy.

Another approach is to use a targeted therapy in combination with one or more traditional chemotherapy drugs. For example, the targeted therapy trastuzumab (Herceptin®) has been used in combination with docetaxel, a traditional chemotherapy drug, to treat women with metastatic breast cancer that overexpresses the protein HER2/neu.

Another limitation of targeted therapy at present is that drugs for some identified targets are difficult to develop because of the target's structure and/or the way its function is regulated in the cell. One example is Ras, a signaling protein that is mutated in as many as one-quarter of all cancers (and in the majority of certain cancer types, such as pancreatic cancer). To date, it has not been possible to develop inhibitors of Ras signaling with existing drug development technologies. However, promising new approaches are offering hope that this limitation can soon be overcome.

What Are the Side Effects of Targeted Cancer Therapies?

Scientists had expected that targeted cancer therapies would be less toxic than traditional chemotherapy drugs because cancer cells are more dependent on the targets than are normal cells. However, targeted cancer therapies can have substantial side effects.

The most common side effects seen with targeted therapies are diarrhea and liver problems, such as hepatitis and elevated liver enzymes. Other side effects seen with targeted therapies include the following:

- Skin problems (acneiform rash, dry skin, nail changes, hair depigmentation)
- Problems with blood clotting and wound healing
- High blood pressure
- Gastrointestinal perforation (a rare side effect of some targeted therapies)

Certain side effects of some targeted therapies have been linked to better patient outcomes. For example, patients who develop acneiform rash (skin eruptions that resemble acne) while being treated with the signal transduction inhibitors erlotinib (Tarceva®) or gefitinib (Iressa®), both of which target the epidermal growth factor receptor, have tended to respond better to these drugs than patients who do not develop the rash. Similarly, patients who develop high blood pressure while being treated with the angiogenesis inhibitor bevacizumab generally have had better outcomes. The few targeted therapies that are approved for use in children can have different side effects in children than in adults, including immunosuppression and impaired sperm production.

What Targeted Therapies Have Been Approved for Specific Types of Cancer?

The FDA has approved targeted therapies for the treatment of some patients with the following types of cancer (some targeted therapies have been approved to treat more than one type of cancer):

Table 67.1. Targeted Therapies for Different Type of Cancers

Types of Cancers	Targeted Therapies
Adenocarcinoma of the stomach or gastroesophageal junction	• Trastuzumab (Herceptin®) • Ramucirumab (Cyramza®)
Bladder cancer	• Atezolizumab (Tecentriq™) • Nivolumab (Opdivo®) • Durvalumab (Imfinzi™) • Avelumab (Bavencio®) • Pembrolizumab (Keytruda®)
Brain cancer	• Bevacizumab (Avastin®) • Everolimus (Afinitor®)
Breast cancer	• Everolimus (Afinitor®) • Tamoxifen (Nolvadex) • Toremifene (Fareston®) • Trastuzumab (Herceptin®) • Fulvestrant (Faslodex®) • Anastrozole (Arimidex®) • Exemestane (Aromasin®) • Lapatinib (Tykerb®) • Letrozole (Femara®) • Pertuzumab (Perjeta®) • Ado-Trastuzumab Emtansine (Kadcyla®) • Palbociclib (Ibrance®) • Ribociclib (Kisqali®) • Neratinib Maleate (Nerlynx™) • Abemaciclib (Verzenio™) • Olaparib (Lynparza™)

Table 67.1. Continued

Types of Cancers	Targeted Therapies
Cervical cancer	• Bevacizumab (Avastin®)
Colorectal cancer	• Cetuximab (Erbitux®) • Panitumumab (Vectibix®) • Bevacizumab (Avastin®) • Ziv-Aflibercept (Zaltrap®) • Regorafenib (Stivarga®) • Ramucirumab (Cyramza®) • Nivolumab (Opdivo®)
Dermatofibrosarcoma protuberans	• Imatinib Mesylate (Gleevec®)
Endocrine/neuroendocrine tumors	• Lanreotide Acetate (Somatuline® Depot) • Avelumab (Bavencio®) • Lutetium Lu 177-Dotatate (Lutathera®)
Head and neck cancer	• Cetuximab (Erbitux®) • Pembrolizumab (Keytruda®) • Nivolumab (Opdivo®)
Gastrointestinal stromal tumor	• Imatinib mesylate (Gleevec®) • Sunitinib (Sutent®) • Regorafenib (Stivarga®)
Giant cell tumor of the bone	• Denosumab (Xgeva®)
Kidney cancer	• Bevacizumab (Avastin®) • Sorafenib (Nexavar®) • Sunitinib (Sutent®) • Pazopanib (Votrient®) • Temsirolimus (Torisel®) • Everolimus (Afinitor®) • Axitinib (Inlyta®) • Nivolumab (Opdivo®) • Cabozantinib (Cabometyx™) • Lenvatinib Mesylate (Lenvima®)

Table 67.1. Continued

Types of Cancers	Targeted Therapies
Leukemia	• Tretinoin (Vesanoid®) • Imatinib Mesylate (Gleevec®) • Dasatinib (Sprycel®) • Nilotinib (Tasigna®) • Bosutinib (Bosulif®) • Rituximab (Rituxan®) • Alemtuzumab (Campath®) • Ofatumumab (Arzerra®) • Obinutuzumab (Gazyva®) • Ibrutinib (Imbruvica®) • Idelalisib (Zydelig®) • Blinatumomab (Blincyto®) • Venetoclax (Venclexta™) • Ponatinib Hydrochloride (Iclusig®) • Midostaurin (Rydapt®) • Enasidenib Mesylate (Idhifa®) • Inotuzumab Ozogamicin (Besponsa®) • Tisagenlecleucel (Kymriah®) • Gemtuzumab Ozogamicin (Mylotarg™) • Rituximab And Hyaluronidase Human (Rituxan Hycela™)
Liver cancer	• Sorafenib (Nexavar®) • Regorafenib (Stivarga®) • Nivolumab (Opdivo®)
Lung cancer	• Bevacizumab (Avastin®) • Crizotinib (Xalkori®) • Erlotinib (Tarceva®) • Gefitinib (Iressa®) • Afatinib Dimaleate (Gilotrif®) • Ceritinib (Ldk378/Zykadia™) • Ramucirumab (Cyramza®) • Nivolumab (Opdivo®) • Pembrolizumab (Keytruda®) • Osimertinib (Tagrisso™) • Necitumumab (Portrazza™) • Alectinib (Alecensa®) • Atezolizumab (Tecentriq™) • Brigatinib (Alunbrig™) • Trametinib (Mekinist®) • Dabrafenib (Tafinlar®)

Table 67.1. Continued

Types of Cancers	Targeted Therapies
Lymphoma	• Ibritumomab Tiuxetan (Zevalin®) • Denileukin Diftitox (Ontak®) • Brentuximab Vedotin (Adcetris®) • Rituximab (Rituxan®) • Vorinostat (Zolinza®) • Romidepsin (Istodax®) • Bexarotene (Targretin®) • Bortezomib (Velcade®) • Pralatrexate (Folotyn®) • Ibrutinib (Imbruvica®) • Siltuximab (Sylvant®) • Idelalisib (Zydelig®) • Belinostat (Beleodaq®) • Obinutuzumab (Gazyva®) • Nivolumab (Opdivo®) • Pembrolizumab (Keytruda®) • Rituximab and Hyaluronidase Human (Rituxan Hycela™) • Copanlisib Hydrochloride (Aliqopa™) • Axicabtagene Ciloleucel (Yescarta™) • Acalabrutinib (Calquence®)
Microsatellite instability-high or mismatch repair-deficient solid tumors	• Pembrolizumab (Keytruda®)
Multiple myeloma	• Bortezomib (Velcade®) • Carfilzomib (Kyprolis®) • Panobinostat (Farydak®) • Daratumumab (Darzalex™) • Ixazomib Citrate (Ninlaro®) • Elotuzumab (Empliciti™)
Myelodysplastic/myeloproliferative disorders	• Imatinib Mesylate (Gleevec®) • Ruxolitinib Phosphate (Jakafi®)
Neuroblastoma	• Dinutuximab (Unituxin™)
Ovarian epithelial/fallopian tube/primary peritoneal cancers	• Bevacizumab (Avastin®) • Olaparib (Lynparza™) • Rucaparib Camsylate (Rubraca™) • Niraparib Tosylate Monohydrate (Zejula™)
Pancreatic cancer	• Erlotinib (Tarceva®) • Everolimus (Afinitor®) • Sunitinib (Sutent®)

Table 67.1. Continued

Types of Cancers	**Targeted Therapies**
Prostate cancer	• Cabazitaxel (Jevtana®) • Enzalutamide (Xtandi®) • Abiraterone Acetate (Zytiga®) • Radium 223 Dichloride (Xofigo®)
Skin cancer	• Vismodegib (Erivedge®) • Sonidegib (Odomzo®) • Ipilimumab (Yervoy®) • Vemurafenib (Zelboraf®) • Trametinib (Mekinist®) • Dabrafenib (Tafinlar®) • Pembrolizumab (Keytruda®) • Nivolumab (Opdivo®) • Cobimetinib (Cotellic™) • Alitretinoin (Panretin®) • Avelumab (Bavencio®)
Soft tissue sarcoma	• Pazopanib (Votrient®) • Olaratumab (Lartruvo™) • Alitretinoin (Panretin®)
Stomach cancer	• Pembrolizumab (Keytruda®)
Systemic mastocytosis	• Imatinib Mesylate (Gleevec®) • Midostaurin (Rydapt®)
Thyroid cancer	• Cabozantinib (Cometriq®) • Vandetanib (Caprelsa®) • Sorafenib (Nexavar®) • Lenvatinib Mesylate (Lenvima®)

Chapter 68

Precision Medicine

Precision medicine is an approach to patient care that allows doctors to select treatments that are most likely to help patients based on a genetic understanding of their disease. This may also be called personalized medicine. The idea of precision medicine is not new, but recent advances in science and technology have helped speed up the pace of this area of research.

When you are diagnosed with cancer, you usually receive the same treatment as others who have same type and stage of cancer. Even so, different people may respond differently, and doctors didn't know why. After decades of research, scientists now understand that patients' tumors have genetic changes that cause cancer to grow and spread. They have also learned that the changes that occur in one person's cancer may not occur in others who have the same type of cancer. And, the same cancer-causing changes may be found in different types of cancer.

The Promise of Precision Medicine

The hope of precision medicine is that treatments will one day be tailored to the genetic changes in each person's cancer. Scientists see a future when genetic tests will help decide which treatments a patient's tumor is most likely to respond to, sparing the patient from receiving treatments that are not likely to help. Research studies are going on now to test whether treating patients with treatments that target the cancer-causing genetic changes in their tumors, no matter

---

This chapter includes text excerpted from "Cancer Treatment—Precision Medicine in Cancer Treatment," National Cancer Institute (NCI), October 3, 2017.

where the cancer develops in the body, will help them. Many of these treatments are drugs known as targeted therapies.

If you need treatment for cancer, you may receive a combination of treatments, including surgery, chemotherapy, radiation therapy, and immunotherapy. Which treatments you receive usually will depend on the type of cancer, its size, and whether it has spread. With precision medicine, information about genetic changes in your tumor can help decide which treatment will work best for you.

There are drugs that have been proven effective against cancers with specific genetic changes and are approved by the U.S. Food and Drug Administration (FDA). Approved treatments should be available wherever you have cancer treatment.

Precision Medicine as a Treatment Approach

Even though researchers are making progress every day, the precision medicine approach to cancer treatment is not yet part of routine care for most patients. Many new treatments designed to target a specific change are being tested right now in precision medicine clinical trials. Some clinical trials are accepting patients with specific types and stages of cancer. Others accept patients with a variety of cancer types and stages. To be eligible for precision medicine trials, your tumor must have a genetic change that can be targeted by a treatment being tested.

Precision Medicine Does Not Yet Apply to Everyone

If there is a targeted drug or other treatment approved for your type of cancer, you will likely be tested to see if the genetic change targeted by the treatment is present in your cancer. For instance, people with melanoma, some leukemias, and breast, lung, colon, and rectal cancers usually have their cancers tested for certain genetic changes when they are diagnosed. Since additional genetic changes that can drive cancer may occur over time, you might also have your cancer tested if it comes back or gets worse.

If there is not an approved targeted treatment for your type of cancer, you still may be tested for genetic changes. For instance, your cancer may be tested to see if you can join a precision medicine clinical trial.

How Genetic Changes in Your Cancer Are Identified

To figure out which genetic changes are in your cancer, you may need to have a biopsy. A biopsy is a procedure in which your doctor removes a sample of the cancer. This sample will be sent to a special lab, where a machine called a deoxyribonucleic acid (DNA) sequencer looks for genetic changes that may be causing the cancer to grow. The process of looking for genetic changes in cancer may be called DNA sequencing, genomic testing, molecular profiling, or tumor profiling.

Paying for Precision Medicine

Testing for genetic changes in your cancer may be covered by your insurance.

If you join a precision medicine clinical trial, the cost of testing for genetic changes may be covered by the organization sponsoring the trial. To be sure, check with the trial staff and make sure that you understand your consent form.

Treatment using precision medicine can be expensive. It takes many years, sometimes decades, of research to develop treatments that target the changes that cause cancer to develop, grow, and spread. So, by the time these treatments are available on the market, they are often very expensive.

Chapter 69

Cancer and Complementary and Alternative Medicine (CAM)

Chapter Contents

Section 69.1

Thinking about CAM

This section includes text excerpted from "Complementary and Alternative Medicine," National Cancer Institute (NCI), April 10, 2015.

Complementary and alternative medicine (CAM) is the term for medical products and practices that are not part of standard medical care.

- **Standard medical care** is medicine that is practiced by health professionals who hold an M.D. (medical doctor) or D.O. (doctor of osteopathy) degree. It is also practiced by other health professionals, such as physical therapists, physician assistants, psychologists, and registered nurses. Standard medicine may also be called biomedicine or allopathic, Western, mainstream, orthodox, or regular medicine. Some standard medical care practitioners are also practitioners of CAM.
- **Complementary medicine** is treatments that are used along with standard medical treatments but are not considered to be standard treatments. One example is using acupuncture to help lessen some side effects of cancer treatment.
- **Alternative medicine** is treatments that are used instead of standard medical treatments. One example is using a special diet to treat cancer instead of anticancer drugs that are prescribed by an oncologist.
- **Integrative medicine** is a total approach to medical care that combines standard medicine with the CAM practices that have been shown to be safe and effective. They treat the patient's mind, body, and spirit.

Are CAM Approaches Safe?

Some CAM therapies have undergone careful evaluation and have been found to be safe and effective. However, there are others that have been found to be ineffective or possibly harmful. Less is known about many CAM therapies, and research has been slower for a number of reasons including the following:

- Time and funding issues
- Problems finding institutions and cancer researchers to work with on the studies
- Regulatory issues

CAM therapies need to be evaluated with the same long and careful research process used to evaluate standard treatments. Standard cancer treatments have generally been studied for safety and effectiveness through an intense scientific process that includes clinical trials with large numbers of patients.

Natural Does Not Mean Safe

CAM therapies include a wide variety of botanicals and nutritional products, such as dietary supplements, herbal supplements, and vitamins. Many of these "natural" products are considered to be safe because they are present in, or produced by, nature. However, that is not true in all cases. In addition, some may affect how well other medicines work in your body. For example, the herb St. John's wort, which some people use for depression, may cause certain anticancer drugs not to work as well as they should.

Herbal supplements may be harmful when taken by themselves, with other substances, or in large doses. For example, some studies have shown that kava-kava, an herb that has been used to help with stress and anxiety, may cause liver damage.

Vitamins can also have unwanted effects in your body. For example, some studies show that high doses of vitamins, even vitamin C, may affect how chemotherapy and radiation work. Too much of any vitamin is not safe, even in a healthy person.

Tell your doctor if you're taking any dietary supplements, no matter how safe you think they are. This is very important. Even though there may be ads or claims that something has been used for years, they do not prove that it's safe or effective.

Supplements do not have to be approved by the federal government before being sold to the public. Also, a prescription is not needed to buy them. Therefore, it's up to consumers to decide what is best for them.

National Cancer Institute (NCI) and the National Center for Complementary and Integrative Health (NCCIH) are currently sponsoring or cosponsoring various clinical trials that test CAM treatments and therapies in people. Some study the effects of complementary approaches used in addition to conventional treatments, and some compare alternative therapies with conventional treatments.

What Should Patients Do When Using or Considering CAM Therapies?

Cancer patients who are using or considering using complementary or alternative therapy should talk with their doctor or nurse. Some therapies may interfere with standard treatment or even be harmful. It is also a good idea to learn whether the therapy has been proven to do what it claims to do.

To find a CAM practitioner, ask your doctor or nurse to suggest someone. Or ask if someone at your cancer center, such as a social worker or physical therapist can help you. Choosing a CAM practitioner should be done with as much care as choosing a primary care provider.

Patients, their families, and their healthcare providers can learn about CAM therapies and practitioners from the following government agencies:

- National Center for Complementary and Integrative Health (NCCIH)
- NCI Office of Cancer Complementary and Alternative Medicine (OCCAM)
- Office of Dietary Supplements (ODS)

Section 69.2

Acupuncture

This section includes text excerpted from "Acupuncture (PDQ®)—Patient Version—Questions and Answers about Acupuncture," National Cancer Institute (NCI), October 27, 2017.

Frequently Asked Questions (FAQs)

What Is Acupuncture?

Acupuncture applies needles, heat, pressure, and other treatments to certain places on the skin, called acupuncture points (or acupoints), to cause a change in the physical functions of the body. The use of acupuncture is part of traditional Chinese medicine (TCM). TCM is a medical system that has been used for thousands of years to prevent, diagnose, and treat disease.

Acupuncture is based on the belief that qi (vital energy) flows through the body along a network of paths, called meridians. Qi is said to affect a person's spiritual, emotional, mental, and physical condition. According to TCM, qi has two forces, yin and yang. Yin and yang are opposite forces that work together to form a whole. The forces of yin and yang depend on each other and are made from each other in an unending cycle, such as hot and cold, day and night, and health and disease. Nothing is ever all yin or all yang, both exist in all things, including people. Many of the major organs of the body are believed to be yin-yang pairs that must be in balance to be healthy. When a person's yin and yang are not in balance, qi can become blocked. Blocked qi causes pain, illness, or other health problems. TCM uses acupuncture, diet, herbal therapy, meditation, physical exercise, and massage to restore health by unblocking qi and correcting the balance of yin and yang within the person. Most acupuncturists in the United States practice acupuncture according to the traditions of Chinese medicine. However, there are other types of acupuncture, including some used for medical treatment, that have different theories about meridians and acupoint locations.

What Is the History of the Discovery and Use of Acupuncture as a Complementary Treatment for Cancer?

The oldest known medical book in China (second century BC) describes the use of needles to treat medical problems. The use of the treatment spread to other Asian countries and to other regions of the world, including to Europe by the 1700s. In the United States, acupuncture has been used for about 200 years.

Research on acupuncture began in the United States in 1976. Twenty years later, the U.S. Food and Drug Administration (FDA) approved the acupuncture needle as a medical device. Many illnesses are treated with acupuncture. In cancer treatment, its main use is to control symptoms, including the following:

- Pain
- Fatigue
- Nausea and vomiting caused by chemotherapy
- Weight loss
- Anxiety
- Depression
- Insomnia
- Poor appetite
- Dry mouth
- Hot flashes
- Nerve problems
- Constipation and diarrhea
- Failure of gastrointestinal (GI) muscles to move food through the GI tract following surgery

For cancer patients, acupuncture is used as complementary therapy, which is treatment given in addition to conventional (standard) therapy.

What Is the Theory behind the Claim That Acupuncture Is Useful in Treating Cancer?

According to TCM, qi can be unblocked by using acupuncture at certain places on the skin, called acupoints. Acupoints are places where the meridians come to the surface of the body. There are more than 360 acupoints on the human body, with specific acupoints for each condition being treated.

What Physical Effects May Acupuncture Have When Used in Cancer Patients?

Acupuncture may cause physical responses in nerve cells, the pituitary gland, and parts of the brain. These responses can cause the body to release proteins, hormones, and brain chemicals that control a number of body functions. It is proposed that, in this way, acupuncture affects blood pressure and body temperature, boosts immune system activity, and causes the body's natural painkillers, such as endorphins, to be released.

How Is Acupuncture Administered?

The acupuncture method most well-known uses needles. Disposable, stainless steel needles that are slightly thicker than a human hair are inserted into the skin at acupoints. The acupuncture practitioner determines the correct acupoints to use for the problem being treated. The inserted needles may be twirled, moved up and down at different speeds and depths, heated, or charged with a weak electric current. There are other acupuncture methods that do not use needles.

Some acupuncture techniques include the following:

- **Auricular acupuncture:** The placing of acupuncture needles at acupoints on the outer ear that match up with certain parts of the body.
- **Electroacupuncture:** A procedure in which pulses of weak electrical current are sent through acupuncture needles into acupoints in the skin.
- **Trigger point acupuncture:** The placing of acupuncture needles in a place on the skin that is away from the painful part of the body. Trigger points have to do with referred pain, pain that is not felt at the site of injury, but is sent along nerves and felt elsewhere in the body.
- **Laser acupuncture:** The use of a weak laser beam instead of an acupuncture needle to stimulate an acupoint.
- **Acupuncture point injection:** The use of a syringe and needle to inject drugs, vitamins, herbal extracts, or other fluids into the body at an acupoint.

- **Microwave acupuncture:** The use of a microwave device attached to an acupuncture needle to deliver microwave radiation to an acupoint.
- **Acupressure:** A type of massage therapy in which the fingers are used to press on an acupoint. In cancer patients, acupressure has been used to control symptoms such as pain or nausea and vomiting.
- **Moxibustion:** A type of heat therapy in which an herb is burned above the body to warm a meridian at an acupoint and increase the flow of blood and qi. The herb may be placed directly on the skin, held close to the skin for several minutes, or placed on the tip of an acupuncture needle. Heat lamps may also be used to warm the acupoints.
- **Cupping:** A procedure in which a rounded glass cup is warmed and placed upside down over an area of the body, making a vacuum that holds the cup to the skin. Cupping is used to increase the flow of blood and qi. It is believed to open up the skin's pores and allow toxins to leave the body.

What Do Patients Feel during Acupuncture?

Patients may have a needling feeling during acupuncture, known as de qi sensation, making them feel heaviness, numbness, or tingling.

Have Any Preclinical (Laboratory or Animal) Studies Been Conducted Using Acupuncture?

Scientific studies on the use of acupuncture to treat cancer and side effects of cancer have begun. Laboratory and animal studies suggest that acupuncture can reduce vomiting caused by chemotherapy and may help the immune system be stronger during chemotherapy. Animal studies support the use of electroacupuncture to relieve cancer pain. Laboratory and animal studies have also looked at how acupuncture works for cancer treatment, such as the role of acupuncture in stimulating nerve cells that trigger the release of hormones into the blood and immune functions, including increasing blood cell count and enhancing lymphocyte and natural killer cell activity.

Have Any Clinical Trials (Research Studies with People) of Acupuncture Been Conducted?

In 1997, the National Institutes of Health (NIH) began evaluating the safety and effectiveness of acupuncture as a complementary therapy for relieving cancer-related symptoms and side effects of cancer treatments.

Studies of acupuncture in cancer care also have been done in China and other countries, including England, France, Australia, Japan, and Sweden.

- **Studies of the effect of acupuncture on the immune system**

  Human studies on the effect of acupuncture on the immune system have been done and suggest that acupuncture may improve immune response.

- **Studies of the effect of acupuncture on pain**

  In clinical studies, acupuncture reduced the amount of cancer pain in some patients. In one study, most of the patients treated with acupuncture were able to stop taking drugs for pain relief or to take smaller doses. The findings from these studies are not considered strong, however, because of weaknesses in study design and size. Studies using strict scientific methods are needed to prove how acupuncture affects pain.

In four of five randomized clinical trials on pain after surgery, acupuncture reduced the pain. The studies included small numbers of patients and unknown additional treatments, and there was no placebo treatment in some of them. More trials are needed to answer all questions.

- **Studies of the effect of acupuncture on muscle and joint pain from aromatase inhibitors**

Aromatase inhibitors, a type of hormone therapy for postmenopausal women who have hormone-dependent breast cancer, may cause muscle and joint pain.

Studies of acupuncture for pain caused by aromatase inhibitors include the following:

- Four randomized controlled trials compared the effects of real and sham acupuncture in reducing these symptoms. In sham acupuncture, needles do not go as deep and are not used at the same points on the body. All four trials showed no side effects from either real acupuncture or sham acupuncture. One trial showed real acupuncture was much better than sham acupuncture in relieving joint and muscle pain, but the other three trials did not show that. In one of the studies, patients receiving real acupuncture had more pain relief than a control group of patients who were waiting to receive treatment later.

- An observational study showed that acupuncture is safe, patients are helped by both real and sham acupuncture, and both real acupuncture and sham acupuncture may relieve pain more than standard care.
- A review of 17,922 patients reported that real acupuncture relieved pain much better than sham acupuncture.

An ongoing randomized clinical trial of 228 patients is comparing real acupuncture, sham acupuncture, and standard care in breast cancer survivors with muscle and joint pain from aromatase inhibitors.

- **Studies of the effect of acupuncture on nausea and vomiting caused by cancer therapies**

The strongest evidence of the effect of acupuncture has come from clinical trials on the use of acupuncture to relieve nausea and vomiting.

Nausea and vomiting caused by chemotherapy, surgery, and morning sickness:

- A 2013 review that included 41 randomized controlled trials found that acupuncture was helpful as a complementary treatment for nausea and vomiting caused by chemotherapy.
- Another review, of 11 randomized clinical trials published between 1987 and 2003, found that fewer chemotherapy patients in the acupuncture groups had vomiting. Not all of the studies had a sham acupuncture group as a control. The review also found that acupressure may relieve nausea caused by chemotherapy, even though the studies did not have a placebo-controlled group.
- A comparison of studies suggests that the specific acupuncture point used may make a difference in how well acupuncture works to relieve nausea caused by chemotherapy.

Nausea and vomiting caused by radiation therapy:

- Patients who received either true acupuncture or sham acupuncture were compared to patients who received only standard care to prevent nausea and vomiting. The study found that patients in both the true and sham acupuncture groups had less nausea and vomiting than those in the standard care group.

- **Studies of the effect of acupuncture on hot flashes in patients treated for cancer**

Hormone therapy may cause hot flashes in women with breast cancer and men with prostate cancer. Studies of the use of acupuncture to relieve hot flashes have shown mixed results:

- Six randomized clinical trials studied the use of acupuncture to prevent hot flashes in breast cancer survivors. These trials found that acupuncture was safe and decreased hot flashes significantly. It was not clear in these trials whether real acupuncture works better than sham acupuncture.
- A 2015 randomized trial of electroacupuncture in breast cancer survivors with hot flashes had four groups for treatment: electroacupuncture, sham acupuncture, medicine, and a placebo. The trial looked at how well sham acupuncture worked compared to the placebo and also compared hot flash relief in all groups. The study found that sham acupuncture worked much better than the medicine or the placebo, and both electroacupuncture and sham acupuncture gave longer-lasting relief than the medicine did.
- A 2016 randomized trial compared acupuncture plus self-care to self-care alone in breast cancer survivors. The study found that adding acupuncture reduced hot flashes after 12 weeks of treatment and at the 3- and 6-month follow-up visits. The study also found that acupuncture markedly improved the patients' quality of life.
- A 2016 review of 12 randomized trials in breast cancer survivors with hot flashes included 6 studies that compared real acupuncture with sham acupuncture. Of these, only 2 studies found that real acupuncture had a benefit compared with the sham treatment. The other studies found that acupuncture was no better than hormone therapy, venlafaxine, or relaxation therapy in relieving hot flashes.
- Some studies have reported that acupuncture may relieve hot flashes in prostate cancer patients on androgen-deprivation therapy.

- **Studies of the effect of acupuncture on fatigue in patients treated for cancer**

Fatigue is a common symptom in patients with cancer and a frequent side effect of chemotherapy and radiation therapy.

- Several randomized clinical trials have studied the use of acupuncture in reducing cancer-related fatigue. These trials found that acupuncture significantly improved fatigue when compared to standard care alone. It is not clear whether real acupuncture works better than sham acupuncture.

- **Studies of the effect of acupuncture on xerostomia (dry mouth) in patients treated for cancer**

Several clinical trials have been done to study the effect of acupuncture in the treatment and prevention of xerostomia (dry mouth) caused by radiation therapy given to patients with nasopharyngeal carcinoma and head and neck cancer.

- Two studies compared acupuncture with standard care for preventing xerostomia in patients being treated with radiation therapy. The studies found that patients treated with acupuncture during radiation therapy had fewer symptoms and increased saliva flow.
- In studies that compared acupuncture to standard care for treating xerostomia caused by radiation therapy, acupuncture improved xerostomia symptoms better than standard care.
- Two randomized controlled trials compared real and sham acupuncture for the prevention and treatment of xerostomia. These trials found that both real and sham acupuncture increased the flow of saliva.
- A prevention study compared acupuncture to standard care for xerostomia and found that patients treated with acupuncture reported fewer symptoms and had better saliva flow than the standard care group.
- A study on the long-term effects of acupuncture on xerostomia found that patients had better salivary flow at 6 months compared to before treatment. Patients who received additional acupuncture had increased saliva flow at 3 years compared to patients who did not continue acupuncture treatment.

Other trials are ongoing.

- **Studies of the effect of acupuncture on peripheral neuropathy caused by anticancer drugs**

Peripheral neuropathy is a nerve problem that causes pain, numbness, tingling, swelling, or muscle weakness in different parts of the body. It usually begins in the hands or feet and gets worse over time.

Peripheral neuropathy may be caused by chemotherapy or other treatments or conditions. It can become serious enough that cancer treatment has to be reduced or stopped. If left untreated, it can disable the patient and lower the quality of life.

Several small studies have been done on the use of acupuncture in treating peripheral neuropathy caused by chemotherapy or other anticancer drugs. Most of these studies found acupuncture decreased pain and improved nerve function. A randomized controlled trial, however, found that acupuncture did not work better than a placebo. Larger randomized controlled trials are needed.

- **Studies of the effect of acupuncture on lymphedema in breast cancer patients**

Lymphedema is a condition in which lymph fluid builds up in tissues and causes swelling. It may occur in an arm or leg if lymph vessels are blocked, damaged, or removed by surgery. Lymphedema is a lifelong concern for many breast cancer patients.

There have been a number of case reports and studies that show acupuncture is safe and may decrease swelling and relieve symptoms in patients with lymphedema in the arms and legs. In one randomized clinical trial, acupuncture was found to keep lymphedema from getting worse but did not decrease swelling or symptoms. More studies are needed.

- **Studies of the effect of acupuncture on ileus caused by cancer surgery**

After cancer surgery, some patients develop ileus, the failure of gastrointestinal (GI) muscles to move food through the GI tract. Three randomized clinical trials studied acupuncture for this condition and had different findings:

- A trial that compared acupuncture to standard care reported that acupuncture was not effective.
- A trial that compared real and sham acupuncture found no difference between the two.
- A trial that compared real acupuncture, sham acupuncture, and no acupuncture found that real acupuncture shortened the length of time ileus lasted.

- **Studies of the effect of acupuncture on sleeping problems**

A study that compared acupuncture with the drug fluoxetine (used to treat depression) found that acupuncture worked better in relieving depression and improving sleep. Another study found that acupuncture improved sleep slightly better than standard care. More studies are needed.

- **Studies of the effect of acupuncture on other symptoms of cancer and side effects of cancer treatment**

The aim of most acupuncture clinical observation and clinical trials in cancer patients has been to study the effects of acupuncture on cancer symptoms and side effects caused by cancer treatment, including weight loss, cough, coughing up blood, fever, anxiety, depression, proctitis, speech problems, blocked esophagus, and hiccups. Studies have shown that, for many patients, treatment with acupuncture either relieves symptoms or keeps them from getting worse.

Have Any Side Effects or Risks Been Reported from Acupuncture?

There have been few complications reported. Problems are caused by using needles that are not sterile (free of germs) and from placing the needle in the wrong place, movement of the patient, or a defect in the needle. Problems include soreness and pain during treatment; feeling tired, lightheaded, or sleepy; and infections. Because chemotherapy and radiation therapy weaken the body's immune system, a strict clean needle method must be used when acupuncture treatment is given to cancer patients. It is important to seek treatment from a qualified acupuncture practitioner who uses a new set of disposable (single-use) needles for each patient.

Is Acupuncture Approved by the U.S. Food and Drug Administration (FDA) for Use as a Cancer Treatment in the United States?

The U.S. Food and Drug Administration (FDA) approved acupuncture needles for use by licensed practitioners in 1996. The FDA requires that sterile, nontoxic needles be used and that they be labeled for single use by qualified practitioners only. More than 40 states and the District of Columbia (DC) have laws regulating acupuncture practice. The National Certification Commission for Acupuncture and Oriental Medicine (NCCAOM) certifies practitioners of acupuncture and traditional Chinese medicine (TCM). Most states require this certification.

Section 69.3

Aromatherapy

This section includes text excerpted from "Aromatherapy and Essential Oils (PDQ®)—Patient Version—Questions and Answers about Aromatherapy," National Cancer Institute (NCI), February 23, 2018.

Frequently Asked Questions (FAQs)

What Is Aromatherapy?

Aromatherapy is the use of essential oils from plants to support and balance the mind, body, and spirit. It is used by patients with cancer mainly as a form of supportive care that may improve quality of life and reduce stress, anxiety, and nausea and vomiting caused by chemotherapy. Aromatherapy may be combined with other complementary treatments like massage therapy and acupuncture, as well as with standard treatments, for symptom management.

Essential oils (also known as volatile oils) are the basic materials of aromatherapy. They represent the fragrant essences found in many plants. These essences are made in special plant cells, often under the surface of leaves, bark, or peel, using energy from the sun and elements from the air, soil, and water. If the plant is crushed, the essence and its unique fragrance are released.

When essences are extracted from plants, they become essential oils. They may be distilled with steam and/or water, or mechanically pressed. Essential oils that are made by processes that modify their chemistry are not considered true essential oils.

There are many essential oils used in aromatherapy, including those from Roman chamomile, geranium, lavender, tea tree, lemon, ginger, cedarwood, and bergamot. Each plant's essential oil has a different chemical composition that affects how it smells, how it is absorbed, and how it is used by the body. Even the essential oils from varieties of the same plant species may have chemical compositions different from each other. The same applies to plants that are grown or harvested in different ways or locations. Essential oils are very concentrated. For example, it takes about 220 lbs of lavender flowers to make about 1 pound of essential oil. Essential oils are volatile, evaporating quickly when they are exposed to open air.

What Is the History of the Discovery and Use of Aromatherapy as a Complementary and Alternative Treatment for Cancer?

Fragrant plants have been used in healing practices for thousands of years across many cultures, including ancient China, India, and Egypt. Ways to extract essential oils from plants were first discovered during the Middle Ages. The history of modern aromatherapy began in the early 20th century, when French chemist Rene Gattefosse coined the term aromatherapy and studied the effects of essential oils on many kinds of diseases. In the 1980s and 1990s, aromatherapy was rediscovered in Western countries as interest in complementary and alternative medicine (CAM) began to grow.

What Is the Theory behind the Claim That Aromatherapy Is Useful in Treating Cancer?

Aromatherapy is rarely suggested as a treatment for cancer, but rather as a form of supportive care to manage symptoms of cancer or side effects of cancer treatment. There are different theories about how aromatherapy and essential oils work. A leading theory is that smell receptors in the nose may respond to the smells of essential oils by sending chemical messages along nerve pathways to the brain's limbic system, which affects moods and emotions. Imaging studies in humans help show the effects of smells on the limbic system and its emotional pathways.

How Is Aromatherapy Administered?

Aromatherapy is used in various ways. Following are examples:

- Indirect inhalation (patient breathes in an essential oil by using a room diffuser or placing drops nearby)
- Direct inhalation (patient breathes in an essential oil by using an individual inhaler with drops floated on top of hot water) to treat a sinus headache
- Aromatherapy massage (massaging of one or more essential oils, diluted in a carrier oil, into the skin)
- Applying essential oils to the skin by combining them with bath salts, lotions, or dressings

Aromatherapy is rarely taken by mouth.

There are some essential oils commonly chosen to treat specific conditions. However, the types of oils used and the ways they are combined may vary, depending on the experience and training of the aromatherapist. This lack of standard methods has led to some conflicting research on the effects of aromatherapy.

Have Any Preclinical (Laboratory or Animal) Studies Been Conducted Using Aromatherapy?

Many studies of essential oils have found that they have antibacterial effects when applied to the skin. Some essential oils have antiviral activity against the herpes simplex virus. Others have antifungal activity against certain vaginal and oropharyngeal fungal infections. In addition, studies in rats have shown that different essential oils can be calming or energizing. When rats were exposed to certain fragrances under stressful conditions, their behavior and immune responses were improved.

One study showed that after essential oils were inhaled, markers of the fragrance compounds were found in the bloodstream, suggesting that aromatherapy affects the body directly like a drug, in addition to indirectly through the central nervous system.

Have Any Clinical Trials (Research Studies with People) of Aromatherapy Been Conducted?

Clinical trials of aromatherapy have mainly studied its use in the treatment of nausea and vomiting caused by chemotherapy, stress, anxiety, and other health-related conditions in seriously ill patients. Several clinical trials of aromatherapy in patients with cancer have been published with mixed results.

A few early studies have shown that aromatherapy may improve quality of life in patients with cancer. Some patients receiving aromatherapy have reported improvement in symptoms such as nausea or pain, and have lower blood pressure, pulse, and respiratory rates. Studies of aromatherapy massage have had mixed results, with some studies reporting improvement in mood, anxiety, pain, and constipation and other studies reporting no effect.

A study of inhaled ginger essential oil in women receiving chemotherapy for breast cancer showed improvements in acute nausea, but no improvement in vomiting or chronic nausea.

A study of inhaled bergamot essential oil in children and adolescents receiving stem cell transplants reported an increase in anxiety and nausea and no effect on pain. Parents receiving the aromatherapy and parents receiving the placebo both showed less anxiety after their children's transplants. In a study of adult patients receiving stem cell transplants, tasting or sniffing sliced oranges was more effective at reducing nausea, retching, and coughing than inhaling an orange essential oil.

A small study of tea tree essential oil as a topical treatment to clear antibiotic-resistant methicillin-resistant *Staphylococcus aureus* (MRSA) bacteria from the skin of hospital patients found that it was as effective as the standard treatment. Antibacterial essential oils have been studied to lessen odor in necrotic ulcers.

No studies in scientific or medical literature discuss aromatherapy as a treatment for cancer specifically.

Have Any Side Effects or Risks Been Reported from Aromatherapy?

Safety testing on essential oils shows very few side effects or risks when they are used as directed. Some essential oils have been approved as ingredients in food and are classified as GRAS (generally recognized as safe) by the U.S. Food and Drug Administration (FDA), within specific limits. Swallowing large amounts of essential oils is not recommended.

Allergic reactions and skin irritation may occur in aromatherapists or in patients, especially when essential oils are in contact with the skin for long periods of time. Sun sensitivity may develop when citrus or other essential oils are applied to the skin before sun exposure.

Lavender and tea tree essential oils have been found to have some hormone-like effects. They have effects similar to estrogen (female sex hormone) and also block or decrease the effect of androgens (male sex hormones). Applying lavender and tea tree essential oils to the skin over a long period of time has been linked in one study to breast enlargement in boys who have not yet reached puberty. It is recommended that patients with tumors that need estrogen to grow avoid using lavender and tea tree essential oils.

Is Aromatherapy Approved by the U.S. Food and Drug Administration (FDA) for Use as a Cancer Treatment in the United States?

Aromatherapy products do not need approval by the U.S. Food and Drug Administration (FDA) because no specific claims are made for the treatment of cancer or other diseases. Aromatherapy is not regulated by state law, and there is no licensing required to practice aromatherapy in the United States. Professionals often combine aromatherapy training with another field in which they are licensed, for example, massage therapy, registered nursing, acupuncture, or naturopathy. Some aromatherapy courses for healthcare providers offer medical credit hours and include conducting research and measuring results.

The National Association for Holistic Aromatherapy (NAHA) and the Alliance of International Aromatherapists (AIA) are two organizations that have national educational standards for aromatherapists. The NAHA plans to have a standard aromatherapy certification in the United States. There are many schools that offer certificate programs approved by NAHA. The Canadian Federation of Aromatherapists (CFA) certifies aromatherapists in Canada.

Section 69.4

Cannabis *and Cannabinoids*

This section includes text excerpted from "*Cannabis* and Cannabinoids (PDQ®)—Patient Version—Questions and Answers about *Cannabis*," National Cancer Institute (NCI), December 20, 2017.

Frequently Asked Questions (FAQs)

What Is Cannabis?

Cannabis, also known as marijuana, is a plant from Central Asia that is grown in many parts of the world today. The *Cannabis* plant produces a resin containing compounds called cannabinoids. Some cannabinoids are psychoactive (acting on the brain and changing mood or consciousness). In the United States, *Cannabis* is a controlled substance and has been classified as a Schedule I agent (a drug with a high potential for abuse and no currently accepted medical use).

Clinical trials that study medicinal *Cannabis* in cancer are limited. To do research with *Cannabis* in the United States, researchers must file an Investigational New Drug (IND) application with the U.S. Food and Drug Administration (FDA), receive a Schedule I license from the Drug Enforcement Administration (DEA), and gain approval from the National Institute on Drug Abuse (NIDA).

By federal law, the possession of *Cannabis* (marijuana) is illegal in the United States outside of approved research settings. However, a growing number of states, territories, and the District of Columbia have enacted laws to legalize medical marijuana.

What Are Cannabinoids?

Cannabinoids are active chemicals in *Cannabis* that cause drug-like effects throughout the body, including the central nervous system and the immune system. They are also known as phytocannabinoids. The main active cannabinoid in *Cannabis* is delta-9-tetrahydrocannabinol (delta-9-THC). Another active cannabinoid is cannabidiol (CBD), which may relieve pain and lower inflammation without causing the "high" of delta-9-THC.

Cannabinoids may be useful in treating the side effects of cancer and cancer treatment.

Other possible effects of cannabinoids include the following:

- Anti-inflammatory activity
- Blocking cell growth
- Preventing the growth of blood vessels that supply tumors
- Antiviral activity
- Relieving muscle spasms caused by multiple sclerosis

What Is the History of the Medical Use of Cannabis?

The use of *Cannabis* for medicinal purposes dates back at least 3,000 years. It came into use in Western medicine in the 19th century and was said to relieve pain, inflammation, spasms, and convulsions.

In 1937, the U.S. Treasury began taxing *Cannabis* under the Marijuana Tax Act at one dollar per ounce for medicinal use and one hundred dollars per ounce for nonmedical use. The American Medical Association (AMA) opposed this regulation of *Cannabis* and did not want studies of its potential medicinal benefits to be limited. In 1942, *Cannabis* was removed from the U.S. Pharmacopoeia (USP) because of continuing concerns about its safety. In 1951, Congress passed the

Boggs Act, which included *Cannabis* with narcotic drugs for the first time.

Under the Controlled Substances Act (CSA) passed by Congress in 1970, marijuana was classified as a Schedule I drug. Other Schedule I drugs include heroin, LSD, mescaline, methaqualone, and gamma-hydroxybutyrate (GHB).

Although *Cannabis* was not believed to have any medicinal use, the U.S. government distributed it to patients on a case-by-case basis under the Compassionate Use Investigational New Drug (IND) program started in 1978. This program was closed to new patients in 1992.

Researchers have studied how cannabinoids act on the brain and other parts of the body. Cannabinoid receptors (molecules that bind cannabinoids) have been discovered in brain cells and nerve cells in other parts of the body. The presence of cannabinoid receptors on immune system cells suggests that cannabinoids may have a role in immunity.

Nabiximols (Sativex) is a *Cannabis* extract that contains delta-9-THC and cannabidiol (CBD). Nabiximols is approved in Canada (under the Notice of Compliance with Conditions) for relief of pain in patients with advanced cancer or multiple sclerosis.

How Is **Cannabis** *Administered?*

Cannabis may be taken by mouth or may be inhaled. When taken by mouth (in baked products or as an herbal tea), the main psychoactive ingredient in *Cannabis* (delta-9-THC) is processed by the liver, making an additional psychoactive chemical.

When *Cannabis* is smoked and inhaled, cannabinoids quickly enter the bloodstream. The additional psychoactive chemical is produced in smaller amounts than when taken by mouth.

A growing number of clinical trials are studying a medicine made from an extract of *Cannabis* that contains specific amounts of cannabinoids. This medicine is sprayed under the tongue.

Have Any Preclinical (Laboratory or Animal) Studies Been Conducted Using **Cannabis** *or Cannabinoids?*

Preclinical studies of cannabinoids have investigated the following:

Antitumor Activity

- Studies in mice and rats have shown that cannabinoids may inhibit tumor growth by causing cell death, blocking cell growth, and blocking the development of blood vessels needed by tumors to grow. Laboratory and animal studies have shown that cannabinoids may be able to kill cancer cells while protecting normal cells.

- A study in mice showed that cannabinoids may protect against inflammation of the colon and may have potential in reducing the risk of colon cancer, and possibly in its treatment.
- A laboratory study of delta-9-THC in hepatocellular carcinoma (liver cancer) cells showed that it damaged or killed the cancer cells. The same study of delta-9-THC in mouse models of liver cancer showed that it had antitumor effects. Delta-9-THC has been shown to cause these effects by acting on molecules that may also be found in nonsmall cell lung cancer cells and breast cancer cells.
- A laboratory study of cannabidiol (CBD) in estrogen receptor positive and estrogen receptor negative breast cancer cells showed that it caused cancer cell death while having little effect on normal breast cells. Studies in mouse models of metastatic breast cancer showed that cannabinoids may lessen the growth, number, and spread of tumors.
- A review of 34 studies of cannabinoids in glioma tumor models found that all but one study showed that cannabinoids can kill cancer cells without harming normal cells.
- A laboratory study of cannabidiol (CBD) in human glioma cells showed that when given along with chemotherapy, CBD may make chemotherapy more effective and increase cancer cell death without harming normal cells. Studies in mouse models of cancer showed that CBD together with delta-9-THC may make chemotherapy such as temozolomide more effective.

Stimulating Appetite

- Many animal studies have shown that delta-9-THC and other cannabinoids stimulate appetite and can increase food intake.

Pain Relief

- Cannabinoid receptors (molecules that bind cannabinoids) have been studied in the brain, spinal cord, and nerve endings throughout the body of animals to understand their roles in pain relief.

- Cannabinoids have been studied for anti-inflammatory effects that may play a role in pain relief.
- Animal studies have shown that cannabinoids may prevent nerve problems (pain, numbness, tingling, swelling, and muscle weakness) caused by some types of chemotherapy.

Nausea and Vomiting

- Cannabinoid receptors found in brain cells may have a role in controlling nausea and vomiting. Animal studies have shown that delta-9-THC and other cannabinoids may act on cannabinoid receptors to prevent vomiting caused by certain types of chemotherapy.

Anxiety and Sleep

- Cannabinoid receptors found in the brain and other parts of the nervous system may be involved in controlling mood and anxiety.
- Antianxiety effects of cannabidiol (CBD) have been shown in several animal models.

Have Any Clinical Trials (Research Studies with People) of Cannabis or Cannabinoid Use by Cancer Patients Been Conducted?

No ongoing clinical trials of *Cannabis* as a treatment for cancer in humans have been found in the CAM on PubMed database maintained by the National Institutes of Health (NIH).

Cannabis and cannabinoids have been studied in clinical trials for ways to manage side effects of cancer and cancer therapies, including the following:

Cancer

- Cannabidiol (CBD) by mouth to treat solid tumors that have recurred (come back)
- An oral spray combining 2 cannabinoids (delta-9-THC and CBD) given with temozolomide to treat recurrent glioblastoma multiforme
- Cannabidiol (CBD) to treat acute graft-versus-host disease in patients who have undergone allogeneic hematopoietic stem cell transplantation

Nausea and Vomiting

- **Delta-9-THC taken by mouth:** Two cannabinoid drugs approved in the United States are available under the names dronabinol and nabilone. Both dronabinol and nabilone are approved by the U.S. Food and Drug Administration (FDA) for the treatment of chemotherapy-related nausea and vomiting in patients who have not responded to standard therapy. Many clinical trials have shown that both dronabinol and nabilone worked as well as or better than some of the weaker FDA-approved drugs to relieve nausea and vomiting. Newer drugs given for chemotherapy-related nausea have not been directly compared with *Cannabis* or cannabinoids in cancer patients.
- **Inhaled *Cannabis*:** Ten small trials have studied inhaled *Cannabis* for the treatment of chemotherapy-related nausea and vomiting. Various study methods and chemotherapy agents were used with mixed results. There is not enough information to interpret these findings.
- **Oral spray with delta-9-THC and cannabidiol (CBD):** Nabiximols, a *Cannabis* extract given as a mouth spray, was shown in a small randomized, placebo-controlled, double-blinded clinical trial in Spain to treat chemotherapy-related nausea and vomiting.
- There is growing interest in treating children for symptoms such as nausea with *Cannabis* and cannabinoids, although studies are limited. The American Academy of Pediatrics (AAP) has not endorsed *Cannabis* and cannabinoid use because of concerns about brain development.

Stimulating Appetite

- **Delta-9-THC taken by mouth:** A clinical trial compared delta-9-THC (dronabinol) and a standard drug (megestrol) in patients with advanced cancer and loss of appetite. Results showed that delta-9-THC was not as effective in increasing appetite or weight gain in advanced cancer patients compared with standard therapy. However, a clinical trial of patients with human immunodeficiency virus (HIV)/acquired immunodeficiency syndrome (AIDS) and weight loss found that those who took delta-9-THC had increased appetite and stopped losing weight compared with patients who took a placebo.

- **Inhaled *Cannabis*:** There are no published studies of the effect of inhaled *Cannabis* on cancer patients with loss of appetite. Studies of healthy people who inhaled *Cannabis* showed that they consumed more calories, especially high-fat and sweet snacks.

Pain Relief

- **Combining cannabinoids with opioids:** In a small study of 21 patients with chronic pain, combining vaporized *Cannabis* with morphine relieved pain better than morphine alone, while combining vaporized *Cannabis* with oxycodone did not produce significantly greater pain relief. These findings should be tested in further studies.
- **Delta-9-THC taken by mouth:** Two small clinical trials of oral delta-9-THC showed that it relieved cancer pain. In the first study, patients had good pain relief as well as relief of nausea and vomiting and better appetite. A second study showed that delta-9-THC could be given in doses that gave pain relief comparable to codeine. An observational study of nabilone also showed that it relieved cancer pain along with nausea, anxiety, and distress when compared with no treatment. Neither dronabinol nor nabilone is approved by the U.S. Food and Drug Administration (FDA) for pain management.
- ***Cannabis* plant extract medicine:** A study of an extract of *Cannabis* that contained specific amounts of cannabinoids, which was sprayed under the tongue, found it was effective in patients with advanced cancer whose pain was not relieved by strong opioids alone. Patients who received the lower doses of cannabinoid spray showed markedly better pain control and less sleep loss compared with patients who received a placebo. Results showed that, for some patients, control of their cancer-related pain continued without needing higher doses of spray or higher doses of their other pain medicines.

Anxiety and Sleep

- **Inhaled *Cannabis*:** A small case series found that patients who inhaled *Cannabis* had improved mood, improved sense of well-being, and less anxiety.

Have Any Side Effects or Risks Been Reported from Cannabis *and Cannabinoids?*

Adverse side effects of cannabinoids may include the following:

- Rapid beating of the heart
- Low blood pressure
- Muscle relaxation
- Bloodshot eyes
- Slowed digestion and movement of food by the stomach and intestines
- Dizziness
- Depression
- Hallucinations
- Paranoia

Because *Cannabis* smoke contains many of the same substances as tobacco smoke, there are concerns about how inhaled *Cannabis* affects the lungs. A study of over 5,000 men and women without cancer over a period of 20 years found that smoking tobacco was linked with some loss of lung function but that occasional and low use of *Cannabis* was not linked with loss of lung function.

Because use of *Cannabis* over a long time may have harmful effects on the endocrine and reproductive systems, rates of testicular germ cell tumors (TGCTs) in *Cannabis* users have been studied. Larger studies that follow patients over time and laboratory studies of cannabinoid receptors in TGCTs are needed to find if there is a link between *Cannabis* use and a higher risk of TGCTs.

A review of bladder cancer rates in *Cannabis* users and nonusers was done in over 84,000 men who took part in the California Men's Health Study (CMHS). Over 16 years of follow-up and adjusting for age, race/ethnic group and body mass index (BMI), rates of bladder cancer were found to be 45 percent lower in *Cannabis* users than in men who did not report *Cannabis* use.

Both *Cannabis* and cannabinoids may be addictive.

Symptoms of withdrawal from cannabinoids may include the following:

- Irritability
- Trouble sleeping

- Restlessness
- Hot flashes
- Nausea and cramping (rarely occur)

These symptoms are mild compared to withdrawal from opiates and usually lessen after a few days.

Are Cannabis *or Cannabinoids Approved by the U.S. Food and Drug Administration (FDA) for Use as a Cancer Treatment in the United States?*

The U.S. Food and Drug Administration (FDA) has not approved *Cannabis* or cannabinoids for use as a cancer treatment.

Are Cannabis *or Cannabinoids Approved by the FDA for Use as a Treatment for Cancer-Related Symptoms or Side Effects of Cancer Therapy?*

Cannabis is not approved by the FDA for the treatment of any cancer-related symptom or side effect of cancer therapy. Two cannabinoids (dronabinol and nabilone) are approved by the FDA for the treatment of chemotherapy-related nausea and vomiting in patients who have not responded to standard therapy.

Section 69.5

Cartilage (Bovine and Shark)

This section includes text excerpted from "Cartilage (Bovine and Shark) (PDQ®)—Patient Version—Questions and Answers about Cartilage (Bovine and Shark)," National Cancer Institute (NCI), September 7, 2017.

Frequently Asked Questions (FAQs)

What Is Cartilage?

Cartilage is a type of tough, flexible connective tissue that forms parts of the skeleton in many animals. Cartilage contains cells called chondrocytes, which are surrounded by collagen (a fibrous protein) and proteoglycans, which are made of protein and carbohydrate.

Products containing cartilage are sold in the United States as dietary supplements. Companies that make cartilage products may not have a process in place to check that all batches they make are exactly the same. This means different batches of a cartilage product may contain different amounts or strengths of ingredients. Different binding agents (substances that make loose mixtures stick together) and fillers may be used in different batches. Therefore, the results of a particular clinical trial may be true only for the batch that was used in the study.

What Is the History of the Discovery and Use of Cartilage as a Complementary or Alternative Treatment for Cancer?

Cartilage from cows (bovine cartilage) and sharks has been studied as a treatment for cancer and other medical conditions for more than 30 years. It was once believed that sharks, whose skeletons are made mostly from cartilage, do not develop cancer. This caused interest in cartilage as a possible treatment for cancer. Although malignant tumors are rare in sharks, cancers have been found in these animals.

Early studies used extracts of bovine cartilage.

- In the 1960s, it was first reported that bovine cartilage decreased inflammation (redness, swelling, pain, and feeling of heat).
- In the 1970s, it was first reported that bovine cartilage contains a substance that blocks angiogenesis (the forming of new blood vessels). If blood vessel growth into a tumor can be blocked, the tumor will stop growing or shrink.
- In the 1980s, researchers first described laboratory and animal studies and clinical trials (research studies in people) testing bovine cartilage as a treatment for cancer.

Interest in using shark cartilage grew because it was believed that shark cartilage may be more active than bovine cartilage in preventing new blood vessels from being formed. Since a shark's skeleton is made mostly of cartilage, shark cartilage is more plentiful than bovine cartilage.

- In the 1980s, it was first published that shark cartilage contains a substance that blocks blood vessel growth.
- In 1998 and 2005, there were published reports of clinical trials of shark cartilage as a treatment for cancer.

What Is the Theory behind the Claim That Cartilage Is Useful in Treating Cancer?

Three theories have been suggested to explain how cartilage acts against cancer:

- As cartilage is broken down by the body, it releases products that kill cancer cells.
- Cartilage increases the action of the body's immune system to kill cancer cells.
- Cartilage makes substances that block tumor angiogenesis (the growth of new blood vessels that feed a tumor and help it grow).

Based on laboratory and animal studies, the third theory may be most likely. Cartilage does not contain blood vessels, so cancer cannot easily grow in it. It is suggested that a cancer treatment using cartilage may keep blood vessels from forming in a tumor, causing the tumor to stop growing or shrink.

How Is Cartilage Administered?

In animal studies, cartilage products have been given by mouth; injected into a vein or the abdomen; applied to the skin; or placed in slow-release plastic pellets that were surgically implanted (put into the body).

In studies with people, cartilage products have been given by mouth; applied to the skin; injected under the skin; or given by enema (injected as a liquid into the rectum). The dose and length of time the cartilage treatment was given was different for each study, in part because different types of products were used.

Have Any Preclinical (Laboratory or Animal) Studies Been Conducted Using Cartilage?

A number of preclinical studies have been done with cartilage. Preclinical studies in a laboratory or using animals are done to find out if a drug, procedure, or treatment is likely to be safe and useful in humans. These preclinical studies are done before testing in humans is begun. Some research studies are published in scientific journals. Most scientific journals have experts who review research reports before they are published, to make sure that the evidence and conclusions are sound. Preclinical studies of cartilage looked at whether bovine and shark cartilage products can kill cancer cells in the laboratory, make the immune system more active against cancer, and prevent blood vessels from forming.

Powdered Cartilage

The following have been reported from preclinical studies of the effect of powdered cartilage on cancer cells *in vitro* (outside of the body):

- In a published laboratory study, a powdered form of bovine cartilage called Catrix slowed the growth of human cancer cells by half or more. It is not clear if Catrix had this effect only on cancer cells, because its effect the growth of normal cells was not tested. It is also not known if the dose used in the laboratory study could safely be used in people.
- In a published laboratory study of powdered shark cartilage, there was no effect on the growth of human astrocytoma cells (cancer cells that begin in the brain or spinal cord).

The following have been reported from preclinical studies of the effect of powdered cartilage on the immune system:

- One published study reported that Catrix injected into mice caused their immune systems to be more active. This effect did not happen when Catrix was given by mouth.
- A laboratory study on the effect of shark cartilage on a tumor model reported an increase in tumor-fighting immune cells in the tumor but not in the blood.
- A study on the effect of shark cartilage on immune system response in mice reported a number of different effects, both helpful and harmful. It increased antibody response but decreased the activity of natural killer cells (tumor-fighting white blood cells). The study also reported a decrease in blood vessel growth.

A large number of laboratory and animal studies on the effect of powdered cartilage on angiogenesis have been published. The following have been reported from these studies:

- Powdered shark cartilage given by mouth to rats decreased the growth of abdominal tissue cells.
- Powdered shark cartilage given by mouth to rats decreased the growth of gliosarcomas, a type of brain cancer.
- Two powdered shark cartilage products (Sharkilage and MIA Shark Powder) given by mouth to mice did not stop the growth or spread of squamous cell skin cancer.
- Three substances that prevent blood vessel growth were found in bovine cartilage. These substances have not shown an effect on the growth of normal cells or tumor cells.
- Two substances that prevent blood vessel growth were found in shark cartilage. These substances have not shown an effect on the growth of normal cells or tumor cells.

Liquid Cartilage

The following have been reported from preclinical studies of liquid cartilage products:

- In a laboratory study, a liquid form of shark cartilage called AE-941/Neovastat was reported to stop the growth of a number of cancer cell types. The results have not been published in a scientific journal.

- Several studies have shown that AE-941/Neovastat blocks the growth of new blood vessels.
- AE-941/Neovastat given by mouth to mice slowed the growth of breast cancer cells and the spread of lung cancer. In the lung cancer study, AE-941/Neovastat increased the effect of the anticancer drug cisplatin.
- A substance made from human cartilage slowed the spread of pancreatic cancer cells in an animal study and prevented blood vessel growth in both animal and laboratory studies.

Have Any Clinical Trials (Research Studies with People) Been Conducted Using Cartilage?

Clinical trials are a type of research study that tests how well new drugs or other treatments work in people. Since the 1970s, there have been at least a dozen clinical studies of cartilage as a treatment for cancer.

There has been one randomized clinical trial of cartilage as cancer treatment published in a peer-reviewed scientific journal. This trial compared treatment using a form of shark cartilage to treatment using a placebo (an inactive substance that looks the same as, and is given the same way as, the substance being tested). Patients also received standard care. In 83 patients having either advanced breast or advanced colon cancer, there was no difference in the quality of life or survival rate between the group that received the shark cartilage product and the group that received the placebo.

Powdered Cartilage

The following have been reported from clinical trials of powdered cartilage products:

- Case series (a collection of detailed information about individual patients) of 31 patients who were treated with Catrix by injection and/or by mouth:

The cancer went into remission (signs and symptoms of cancer went away) in 19 patients and then recurred (came back) in about half of them. Some of these patients also received standard cancer treatment and there was no control group (a group of patients who do not receive the treatment being studied, to show if the treatment being studied makes a difference). For these reasons, the effectiveness of cartilage as a cancer treatment is not proven by this case series.

- A clinical trial of Cartilade by mouth in 60 patients with advanced cancer:

  All but 1 patient had been treated with standard therapy before the trial. The cancer stopped growing in 10 of the patients for 12 weeks or more and then began to grow again. The cancer did not shrink or go into remission in any of the patients.

Liquid Cartilage

The following have been reported from clinical trials of liquid cartilage products:

- A clinical trial of Catrix in 9 patients whose cancers did not respond to radiation therapy and/or chemotherapy:

  Catrix was given by injection. One patient's cancer went into remission for more than 39 weeks and the other 8 patients did not respond to treatment with Catrix.

- Clinical studies on the safety of the liquid shark cartilage product AE-941/Neovastat have reported that it has little harmful effect.
- A randomized clinical trial studied the effect of AE-941/Neovastat on blood vessel growth related to wound healing after surgery. This study reported that one of the ingredients that prevents blood vessel growth can be absorbed and used by the body when taken by mouth.
- A clinical trial of oral AE-941/Neovastat in 379 patients with advanced nonsmall cell lung cancer reported that there was no difference in how long patients lived between the group receiving the shark cartilage product and chemoradiotherapy compared to the group receiving the placebo and chemoradiotherapy. Both kinds of treatment were well tolerated.

Have Any Side Effects or Risks Been Reported from Cartilage?

The side effects of cartilage treatment are usually mild or moderate.

The most common side effects of treatment with the bovine cartilage product Catrix include the following:

- Inflammation at the injection location
- A bad taste in the mouth
- Feeling very tired
- Nausea
- Upset stomach
- Fever
- Feeling dizzy
- Swelling of the scrotum (the sac that contains the testicles)

The most common side effects of treatment with the shark cartilage include the following:

- Nausea
- Vomiting
- Abdominal cramps and/or bloating
- Constipation
- Lower than normal blood pressure
- Higher than normal blood sugar
- General weakness
- A higher than normal level of calcium in the blood

Nausea, vomiting, and upset stomach are the side effects reported most often from treatment with the shark cartilage product AE–941/Neovastat. There has been one report of hepatitis occurring in a person who used shark cartilage.

Is Cartilage Approved by the U.S. Food and Drug Administration (FDA) for Use as a Cancer Treatment in the United States?

The U.S. Food and Drug Administration (FDA) has not approved cartilage as a treatment for cancer. A number of cartilage products are sold in the United States as dietary supplements. Dietary supplements are products meant to be added to the diet. They are not drugs and are not meant to treat, prevent, or cure diseases. The manufacturer is responsible for ensuring that the product is safe and that the label claims are truthful and not misleading. The FDA does not approve dietary supplements as safe or effective before they are sold.

Section 69.6

Laetrile/Amygdalin

This section includes text excerpted from "Laetrile/Amygdalin (PDQ®)—Patient Version—Questions and Answers about Laetrile/Amygdalin," National Cancer Institute (NCI), April 13, 2017.

Frequently Asked Questions (FAQs)

What Is Laetrile?

Laetrile is a compound that has been used as a treatment for people with cancer worldwide. It is not approved by the U.S. Food and Drug Administration (FDA) as a treatment for cancer or any other medical condition. The term laetrile comes from 2 words (laevorotatory and mandelonitrile) and is used to describe a purified form of the chemical amygdalin. Amygdalin is a plant compound that contains sugar and produces hydrogen cyanide. Hydrogen cyanide is thought to be the main anticancer compound formed from laetrile when broken down in the body. Amygdalin is found in the pits of many fruits and in raw nuts. It is also found in other plants such as lima beans, clover, and sorghum.

The names laetrile, Laetrile, vitamin B-17, and amygdalin are often used in place of one another, but they are not the same product. The chemical makeup of Laetrile patented in the United States is different from the laetrile/amygdalin produced in Mexico. The patented Laetrile is a partly synthetic (man-made) form of amygdalin, while the laetrile/amygdalin made in Mexico comes from crushed apricot pits. The studies discussed in this section either Mexican laetrile/amygdalin or Laetrile. The generic term laetrile will be used throughout this section except in cases when the patented version of Laetrile is known to have been used in a study.

What Is the History of the Discovery and Use of Laetrile as a Complementary or Alternative Treatment for Cancer?

Amygdalin was first isolated in 1830 and was used as an anticancer agent in Russia as early as 1845. Its first recorded use in the United States as a treatment for cancer was in the 1920s. The early pill form of amygdalin was found to be too toxic, and work with the compound was stopped. In the 1950s, a reportedly nontoxic, partly synthetic form of amygdalin was made and patented in the United States as Laetrile. Laetrile gained popularity in the 1970s as a single anticancer agent and as part of a metabolic therapy program that included a special diet, high-dose vitamin supplements, and pancreatic enzymes (a group of proteins that aid in the digestion of food). By 1978, more than 70,000 people in the United States had reportedly been treated with Laetrile. In 1980, the U.S. Supreme Court upheld a ban on the shipment of laetrile between states in the United States. It is still used in Mexico and at some clinics in the United States.

What Is the Theory behind the Claim That Laetrile Is Useful in Treating Cancer?

Hydrogen cyanide is thought to be the main anticancer ingredient in laetrile. Two other breakdown products of amygdalin, prunasin (which is similar in structure to laetrile) and benzaldehyde, may also be cancer cell blockers. The following theories have been proposed to support the use of laetrile for cancer:

- Two of the theories state that the balance of certain enzymes in cancer cells allows laetrile to be toxic to the cancer cells. There is some evidence that normal tissues and malignant tissues do have different amounts of these enzymes.
- Another theory states that cancer is the result of a vitamin deficiency and that laetrile, or amygdalin/vitamin B-17, is the missing vitamin needed by the body to restore health. There is currently no evidence that laetrile is needed by the body or that laetrile can act as a vitamin in animals or humans.
- The fourth theory states that the cyanide released by laetrile has a toxic effect that results in killing the cancer cells and stopping them from growing. The theory also states that the damage to the cells causes a boost to the immune system.

How Is Laetrile Administered?

Laetrile is given by mouth (orally) as a pill. It can also be given by injection into a vein (intravenously) or muscle. Laetrile is commonly given intravenously over a period of time and then orally as maintenance therapy (treatment given to help extend the benefit of previous therapy).

Have Any Preclinical (Laboratory or Animal) Studies Been Conducted Using Laetrile?

Preclinical studies have been done with laetrile either alone or combined with other substances. These studies tested the benefits of laetrile against cancer, the side effects of laetrile treatment, where and how laetrile breaks down in the body, and how laetrile and its breakdown products leave the body. Laboratory and animal studies have shown mixed results on the anticancer effects of laetrile (amygdalin).

Two animal studies of amygdalin by the National Cancer Institute (NCI) reported no response when it was given alone or with an enzyme that activates the release of cyanide from amygdalin in the body. The animals had more side effects when the enzyme was given at the same time as the amygdalin. Similar results were reported when human breast and colon tumors were implanted into mice.

Other studies have reported the following responses to amygdalin:

- A laboratory study of amygdalin reported that it somewhat slowed the growth of colon cancer cells.
- A laboratory study of amygdalin reported the higher the dose of amygdalin, the more likely the prostate cancer cells were to respond.
- A laboratory study of amygdalin given with beta-D-glucosidase reported a time and dose-dependent response in hepatoma cells. The longer amount of time that amygdalin and beta-D-glucoside were given and the higher the dose, the more likely the hepatoma cells were to respond.
- A laboratory study of amygdalin reported the higher the dose of amygdalin, the more likely the cervical cancer cells were to respond.
- One study in rats reported that amygdalin was not effective at treating, preventing, or delaying development of tumors.
- One study reported tumor response in mice with mammary tumors when amygdalin was given with enzymes and vitamin A, but not when given alone.

Have Any Clinical Trials (Research Studies with People) of Laetrile Been Conducted?

No controlled clinical trials (trials that compare groups of patients who receive the new treatment to groups who do not) of laetrile have been reported. Although many anecdotal reports (incomplete descriptions of the medical/treatment history of one or more patients) and case reports (detailed reports of the diagnosis, treatment, and follow-up of individual patients) are available, they provide little evidence to support laetrile as a treatment for cancer.

The following has been reported from case series about the use of laetrile in patients with cancer:

- A case series (a group or series of case reports involving patients who were given similar treatment) of 44 patients treated with laetrile was published in 1953. Most of the patients who showed some improvement also received radiation therapy or anticancer drugs, so it is not known which treatment produced the benefit.
- In another series of case reports published in 1962, 10 patients with metastatic cancer (cancer that has spread from one part of the body to another) were treated with a wide range of doses of intravenous Laetrile. Pain relief was the main reported benefit. Reduced swelling of lymph nodes and decreased tumor size were also reported. Long-term follow-up with these patients was not done, however, so it is not known how long the benefits lasted after treatment.
- Benzaldehyde, which is made when laetrile is broken down by the body, has also been tested for anticancer activity in humans. In two clinical series (case reports of a number of patients who are treated consecutively in a clinic), patients with advanced cancer who had not responded to standard therapy were treated with benzaldehyde. Some patients had a complete response (the disappearance of all signs and symptoms of cancer), while some had a decrease in tumor size. The responses to benzaldehyde lasted as long as the treatment continued. Almost all of the patients had been treated previously with chemotherapy or radiation therapy, but it is not known how soon treatment with benzaldehyde began after the other treatment ended.
- In 1978, the National Cancer Institute (NCI) requested case reports from practitioners who believed their patients were helped by treatment with laetrile. Ninety-three cases were

submitted; 67 of these were complete enough to be evaluated. An expert panel concluded that 2 of the 67 patients had complete responses and 4 others had a decrease in tumor size. Based on these 6 cases, NCI sponsored clinical studies with laetrile.

Findings from only 2 clinical trials with laetrile have been published. These trials, sponsored by NCI, were done in the late 1970s and early 1980s, and did not include a control group for comparison.

The following has been reported from these 2 clinical trials about the use of laetrile in patients with cancer:

- The first trial, a phase I study, tested doses, schedules, and ways to give amygdalin in 6 cancer patients. Researchers found that amygdalin caused very few side effects when given by mouth or intravenously. Two patients who ate raw almonds while taking amygdalin, however, developed symptoms of cyanide poisoning.
- In 1982, a phase II study with 175 patients looked at which types of cancer might benefit from treatment with amygdalin. Most of the patients in this study had breast, colon, or lung cancer. Amygdalin was given by injection for 21 days, followed by oral maintenance therapy using doses and procedures similar to those in the phase I study. Vitamins and pancreatic enzymes were also given as part of a metabolic therapy program that also included dietary changes. One stomach cancer patient showed a decrease in tumor size, which was maintained for 10 weeks while the patient was on amygdalin therapy. In about half of the patients, cancer had grown at the end of the treatment. Cancer had grown in all patients 7 months after completing treatment. Some patients reported an improvement in their ability to work or do other activities, and other patients said their symptoms improved. These improvements, however, did not last after treatment ended.

Have Any Side Effects or Risks Been Reported from Laetrile?

The following are the side effects of laetrile treatment are like the signs and symptoms of cyanide poisoning.

- Nausea and vomiting
- Headache
- Dizziness
- Blue color of the skin due to a lack of oxygen in the blood

- Liver damage
- Abnormally low blood pressure
- Droopy upper eyelid
- Trouble walking due to damaged nerves
- Fever
- Mental confusion
- Coma
- Death

The side effects of laetrile appear to depend on the way it is given. Side effects are more severe when laetrile is given by mouth than when it is given by injection. These side effects may be increased by the following factors:

- Eating raw almonds or crushed fruit pits
- Eating certain types of fruits and vegetables, including celery, peaches, bean sprouts, and carrots
- Taking high doses of vitamin C

Is Laetrile Approved by the FDA for Use as a Cancer Treatment in the United States?

The FDA has not approved laetrile as a treatment for cancer in the United States. The drug is made and used as a cancer treatment in Mexico. Laetrile compounds from Mexico, which is the primary supplier of laetrile, may vary in purity and contents. Products containing bacteria and other substances and products labeled incorrectly have been found.

Section 69.7

Milk Thistle

This section includes text excerpted from "Milk Thistle (PDQ®)—Patient Version—Questions and Answers about Milk Thistle," National Cancer Institute (NCI), June 26, 2017.

Frequently Asked Questions (FAQs)

What Is Milk Thistle?

Milk thistle is a plant whose fruit and seeds have been used for more than 2,000 years as a treatment for disorders of the liver, bile ducts, and gallbladder. Milk thistle is native to Europe but can also be found in the United States and South America.

The medicinal ingredient found in milk thistle is silymarin, an extract of milk thistle seeds. Silymarin is a mixture that contains several closely related compounds, including silybin (consisting of the silybins A and B), isosilybin (consisting of the isosilybins A and B), silychristin and isosilychristin, silydianin, and taxifolin. Most research has studied silymarin or its major component silybin, instead of the plant in its whole form.

The botanical name for milk thistle is Silybum marianum. Milk thistle is also called holy thistle, Marian thistle, Mary thistle, St. Mary thistle, Our Lady's thistle, wild artichoke, Mariendistel (German), and Chardon-Marie (French).

What Is the History of the Discovery and Use of Milk Thistle as a Complementary and Alternative Therapy?

The ancient Greeks and Romans used milk thistle as a treatment for liver ailments and snake bites. During the Middle Ages, milk thistle was recommended to treat liver toxins. Modern homeopathic practitioners have used compounds from milk thistle seeds to treat a range of disorders including jaundice, gallstones, and peritonitis. The German Commission E, which studies the safety and efficacy of herbs for the German government, recommends milk thistle for liver damage due to toxins, cirrhosis of the liver, and as a supportive therapy for chronic inflammation of the liver.

Despite milk thistle's long history of use for liver complaints, it was not until 1968 that researchers extracted silymarin from milk thistle seeds and suggested that it might be the plant's active ingredient. Silymarin was later discovered to be a mixture of flavonolignans, a family of plant-based substances.

What Is the Theory behind the Claim That Milk Thistle Is Useful in Treating Cancer?

The active substance in milk thistle is silymarin, containing silybin as its major compound. To research the claim that milk thistle is useful in treating cancer, silymarin and silybin have been the most widely studied ingredients.

Silymarin and silybin may protect the liver against damage from toxic chemicals by blocking toxins from entering the cell or by moving toxins out of the cell before damage begins.

Silymarin and silybin have been studied in the laboratory in cancer cells as well as in animal tumors of the tongue, skin, bladder, colon, and small intestine. They have been tested for their potential to:

- Make chemotherapy less toxic
- Make chemotherapy more effective
- Stop or slow the growth of cancer cells and block tumors from starting or continuing to grow
- Help to repair liver tissue

Can Milk Thistle Make Anticancer Medications or Other Drugs More Effective?

It is not known if milk thistle may make anticancer medications or other drugs more effective, less effective, or have no effect when taken with them. Specifically, it has not yet been determined whether milk thistle will increase or decrease how well chemotherapy works, or have no effect on it.

How Is Milk Thistle Administered?

Milk thistle is usually taken by mouth in capsules or tablets. Since it does not dissolve well in water, it is not commonly taken as an herbal tea. In Europe, the active compound silybin is given by intravenous infusion as the only effective antidote for Amanita phalloides, a mushroom toxin that causes deadly liver failure.

Most milk thistle supplements are measured by how much silybin they contain. Special forms of silybin made to be easily absorbed and used by the body are sold under the names Legalon, silipide, and Siliphos.

Have Any Preclinical (Laboratory or Animal) Studies Been Conducted Using Milk Thistle?

Research in a laboratory or using animals is done to find out if a drug, procedure, or treatment is likely to be useful in humans. Preclinical studies are done before clinical trials (in humans) are begun. Silymarin, the active substance found in milk thistle seeds, has been studied in laboratory research. These studies have shown that it:

- Strengthens cell walls to prevent toxins from crossing into the cell
- Stimulates enzymes that make toxins less harmful to the body
- Blocks damaging substances called free radicals from attacking cells

Silybin A and B, the major components of silymarin, have been studied in laboratory experiments using cancer cell lines (cells adapted to grow in the laboratory). These studies suggest that these silybins:

- May help cisplatin and doxorubicin (chemotherapy drugs) work better against ovarian and breast cancer cells
- May have direct anticancer effects against prostate, breast, and cervical cancer cells, and may also prevent the development of cancer
- May slow down cell growth, as shown in prostate cancer cell lines
- In laboratory tests using rat livers, silymarin and silybin have also been found to boost the regrowth of liver tissue

In laboratory tests using rats and mice whose ovaries have been removed, milk thistle has been found to help stop bone loss.

Tests on colorectal cancer cells transplanted into mice found that silybin given twice a day decreased tumor growth.

Have Any Clinical Trials (Research Studies with People) of Milk Thistle Been Conducted?

Several small studies have looked at whether milk thistle can be used to treat cancer and to decrease harmful effects of cancer treatment. A randomized clinical trial in children with acute lymphoblastic leukemia found that silymarin decreased the harmful effects of chemotherapy on the liver without working against the cancer treatment. The children taking silymarin needed fewer chemotherapy dose reductions because of side effects than the children who did not take milk thistle.

A randomized clinical trial in men who had surgery to remove their prostate found that a combination of silymarin and selenium improved quality of life, decreased cholesterol, and increased the amount of selenium in the blood.

A randomized clinical trial studied 30 patients with head and neck cancer who received radiation therapy. The study found that those who took silymarin for 6 weeks had markedly lower rates of radiation-related mucositis compared to those who did not.

A nonrandomized observational study in women with breast cancer who had surgery and radiation therapy found that a silymarin-based cream helped prevent patients from having skin reactions to radiation therapy.

A phase I clinical trial in 3 patients with advanced liver cancer and poor liver function aimed to find out the maximum dose of silybin-phosphatidylcholine that patients can safely handle. One patient showed some improvement in liver function and signs of inflammation.

A number of clinical trials have studied milk thistle or silymarin in the treatment of patients with hepatitis, cirrhosis, or disorders of the bile ducts. These trials have used a wide range of doses with mixed results. In a trial of biologic therapy for patients with chronic hepatitis, patients taking silymarin had fewer symptoms and a better quality of life compared to patients not taking silymarin. The beneficial effects of silymarin shown in some studies suggest it might play a role in preventing hepatitis and/or liver cancer, but no clinical trials have studied the use of silymarin for prevention. Silymarin has been found to increase the effectiveness of iron chelation therapy, which removes extra iron in the blood of patients who have had many blood transfusions.

Have Any Side Effects or Risks Been Reported from Milk Thistle?

Very few side effects from the use of milk thistle or silymarin have been reported when taken as recommended. Several large, carefully designed studies in patients with liver disorders have found that taking silymarin may rarely have a laxative effect or cause nausea, heartburn, or stomach upset. At high doses, mild allergic reactions have been seen (more than 1,500 milligrams a day).

Is Milk Thistle Approved by the U.S. Food and Drug Administration (FDA) for Use as a Cancer Treatment in the United States?

The U.S. Food and Drug Administration (FDA) has not approved the use of milk thistle as a treatment for cancer or any other medical condition. Milk thistle is available in the United States as a dietary supplement. Dietary supplements are products meant to be added to the diet. They are not drugs and are not meant to treat, prevent, or cure diseases. The manufacturer is responsible for ensuring that the product is safe and that the label claims are truthful and not misleading. The FDA does not approve dietary supplements as safe or effective before they are sold. Given the limited research done with milk thistle in patients with cancer, using it as a cancer treatment cannot be recommended except in carefully designed clinical trials.

Section 69.8

Mistletoe Extracts

This section includes text excerpted from "Mistletoe Extracts (PDQ®)—Patient Version—Questions and Answers about Mistletoe," National Cancer Institute (NCI), February 15, 2017.

Frequently Asked Questions (FAQs)

What Is Mistletoe?

Mistletoe is a semiparasitic plant that grows on several types of trees, including apple, oak, maple, elm, pine, and birch. It has been used for centuries to treat medical conditions such as epilepsy, hypertension, headaches, menopausal symptoms, infertility, arthritis, and rheumatism.

Mistletoe is one of the most widely studied complementary and alternative medicine therapies for cancer. In certain European countries, extracts made from European mistletoe are among the most prescribed therapies for cancer patients. These products are made and sold under the following brand names:

- Iscador (also called Iscar)
- Helixor
- Iscucin
- Lektinol (also called Plenosol)
- abnobaVISCUM

Brand names including Eurixor, Isorel, and Vysorel are no longer sold.

The chemical makeup of mistletoe products varies, depending on the following factors:

- The type of host tree on which the mistletoe plant grows
- The time of year the plant is harvested
- The exact species of mistletoe
- Whether the extract is fermented or unfermented
- Whether the extract is prepared with homeopathic methods
- The company that makes the product

Mistletoe extracts are prepared as water-based solutions or solutions of water and alcohol. Mistletoe products may be named according to the type of host tree on which the plant grows. For example, IscadorM is from apple trees, IscadorP comes from pine trees, IscadorQu is from oak trees, and IscadorU comes from elm trees. Some users believe that the type of mistletoe extract chosen should depend on the type of tumor and the sex of the patient.

What Is the History of the Discovery and Use of Mistletoe as a Complementary or Alternative Treatment for Cancer?

Mistletoe was used by the Druids and the ancient Greeks, and appears in legend and folklore as a panacea or "cure-all." Modern interest in mistletoe as a possible treatment for cancer began in the 1920s.

Extracts of mistletoe have been shown to kill cancer cells in the laboratory and to boost the immune system (the complex group of organs and cells that defends the body against infection or disease). For this reason, mistletoe has been classified as a type of biological response modifier (a substance that stimulates the body's response to infection and disease). Extracts of mistletoe have also been shown in the laboratory to prevent the growth of new blood vessels needed for tumors to grow.

Ingredients in mistletoe that have been studied for their usefulness in treating cancer include the following:

- Alkaloids
- Viscotoxins
- Polysaccharides
- Lectins

What Is the Theory behind the Claim That Mistletoe Is Useful in Treating Cancer?

Mistletoe extract is studied as a possible anticancer agent because it has been shown to:

- Have effects on the immune system
- Kill mouse, rat, and human cancer cells in the laboratory
- Protect the DNA in white blood cells in the laboratory, including cells that have been exposed to DNA-damaging chemotherapy drugs

How Is Mistletoe Administered?

Mistletoe extracts are usually given by injection under the skin (subcutaneous). Less common ways to give mistletoe include by mouth, into a vein (intravenous or IV), into the pleural cavity, or into the tumor. In most reported studies, injections under the skin were given 2 to 3 times a week for various lengths of time.

What Preclinical (Laboratory or Animal) Studies Have Been Conducted Using Mistletoe?

Many laboratory and animal studies have been done with mistletoe, either alone or combined with other agents. Laboratory studies have suggested that mistletoe may support the immune system by increasing the number and activity of various types of white blood cells.

Studies testing mistletoe's ability to stop cancer cell growth in animals have yielded mixed and inconsistent results, depending on the extract used, the dose tested, the way it was given (injected under the skin or into the peritoneal cavity), and the type of cancer studied.

Have Any Clinical Trials (Research Studies with People) Been Conducted Using Mistletoe?

Most clinical trials using mistletoe to treat cancer have been done in Europe. Most study results have been published in German. Although many of these trials have reported mistletoe to be effective, there are major weaknesses in almost all that raise doubts about their findings. Weaknesses have included small numbers of patients, incomplete patient data, lack of information about mistletoe dose, and problems with study design.

Many studies involve using mistletoe as adjuvant therapy in patients with cancer. One retrospective cohort study done in Europe between 1993 and 2000 looked at the use of a mistletoe extract (Iscador) as long-term adjuvant therapy in 800 patients treated with chemotherapy and/or radiation therapy for colorectal cancer that had not spread. The study found that patients treated with Iscador had fewer adverse events, better symptom relief, and improved disease-free survival compared to patients who did not receive Iscador as adjuvant therapy.

A European study published in 2013 looked at the use of Iscador QU in advanced or metastatic pancreatic cancer. Patients received best supportive care and were randomly assigned to receive either Iscador QU or no anticancer therapy. Results in 220 patients showed that those treated with Iscador had improved survival and less severe disease-related symptoms (including pain, weight loss, fatigue, nausea, diarrhea, and anxiety) compared with those who did not receive Iscador QU.

A European study done between 1978 and 1987 looked at the use of Iscador U and Iscador QU in nonsmall cell lung cancer that could not be treated with surgery. Patients were randomly assigned to receive one of 3 treatments: Iscador injections; Polyerga Neu injections (a sheep spleen preparation said to stimulate the immune system and have antitumor effects); or placebo injections of a vitamin B mixture. Results in 312 patients showed no differences among the 3 groups in survival or tumor response. It was noted that more patients in the Iscador group reported an improved sense of well-being compared with patients in the other groups.

Before researchers can conduct clinical drug research in the United States, they must file an Investigational New Drug (IND) application with the U.S. Food and Drug Administration (FDA). The FDA does not make information public about IND applications or approvals;

this information can be made public only by the applicants. In the last decade, at least two U.S. investigators were given approval to conduct clinical trials of mistletoe as a treatment for people with cancer. These clinical trials are now closed.

In 2002, the National Center for Complementary and Integrative Health (NCCIH), in cooperation with the National Cancer Institute (NCI), began enrolling patients for a phase I clinical trial of a mistletoe extract (Helixor A) and gemcitabine in patients with advanced solid tumors. This combination showed low toxicity and no botanical-drug interactions were reported.

Reviews of Many Clinical Trials Combined

Findings from over 50 clinical trials using mistletoe extracts in patients with cancer have been published. Reviews of many studies taken together have looked at the effects of mistletoe on quality of life, survival, and symptom relief in different types of cancer:

- Quality of life was measured in a review that included 26 randomized clinical trials. Of these, 22 trials showed patients had improved quality of life. All 10 nonrandomized, controlled clinical trials reviewed also reported the same benefits. Chemotherapy-related fatigue, nausea and vomiting, depression, emotional well-being, and concentration improved. Some of the studies were well designed, while others had weaknesses.
- Tumor response, quality of life, and psychological distress were measured in a review of 21 randomized clinical trials in patients with different types of cancer. A variety of mistletoe extracts were used either alone, with chemotherapy, or with radiation therapy. Most of the studies reported benefits for patients, although this review had weaknesses in design and size.
- Quality of life and survival were measured in a review of 10 randomized clinical trials which used a variety of mistletoe extracts in patients with different types of cancer. There was no difference in survival or quality of life measures in patients who received mistletoe compared to those who did not.

Have Any Side Effects or Risks Been Reported from Mistletoe?

Very few serious side effects have been reported from the use of mistletoe extract products. Common side effects include soreness and inflammation at injection sites, headache, fever, and chills.

One review surveyed many animal and human studies that used European mistletoe and mistletoe lectins. Different doses and ways to give mistletoe were used. Treatment was not found to lessen immune system responses. High doses of mistletoe lectins damaged the liver in some cases; this damage was correctable. Another review of clinical trials reported adverse effects that included increased circulatory problems, thrombophlebitis, swelling of lymph nodes, and allergic reactions.

A few cases of severe allergic reactions, including anaphylactic shock, have been reported.

Is Mistletoe Approved by the FDA for Use as a Cancer Treatment in the United States?

The FDA has not approved the use of mistletoe as a treatment for cancer or any other medical condition. The FDA does not allow injectable mistletoe extracts to be imported or used except for clinical research.

Part Four

Recurrent and Advanced Cancer

Chapter 70

Recurrent Cancer

When cancer comes back after treatment, doctors call it a recurrence or recurrent cancer. Finding out that cancer has come back can cause feelings of shock, anger, sadness, and fear. But you have something now that you didn't have before—experience. You've lived through cancer already and you know what to expect. Also, remember that treatments may have improved since you were first diagnosed. New drugs or methods may help with your treatment or in managing side effects. In some cases, improved treatments have helped turn cancer into a chronic disease that people can manage for many years.

Why Cancer Comes Back

Recurrent cancer starts with cancer cells that the first treatment didn't fully remove or destroy. This doesn't mean that the treatment you received was wrong. It just means that a small number of cancer cells survived the treatment and were too small to show up in follow-up tests. Over time, these cells grew into tumors or cancer that your doctor can now detect. Sometimes, a new type of cancer will occur in people who have a history of cancer. When this happens, the new cancer is

---

This chapter contains text excerpted from the following sources: Text in this chapter begins with excerpts from "Recurrent Cancer: When Cancer Comes Back," National Cancer Institute (NCI), January 18, 2016; Text beginning with the heading "Your Feelings" is excerpted from "Support for People With Cancer—When Cancer Returns," National Cancer Institute (NCI), September 2014. Reviewed March 2018.

known as a second primary cancer. Second primary cancer is different from recurrent cancer.

Types of Recurrent Cancer

Doctors describe recurrent cancer by where it develops and how far it has spread. The following are the different types of recurrence:

- **Local recurrence** means that the cancer is in the same place as the original cancer or very close to it.
- **Regional recurrence** means that the tumor has grown into lymph nodes or tissues near the original cancer.
- **Distant recurrence** means the cancer has spread to organs or tissues far from the original cancer. When cancer spreads to a distant place in the body, it is called metastasis or metastatic cancer. When cancer spreads, it is still the same type of cancer. For example, if you had colon cancer, it may come back in your liver. But, the cancer is still called colon cancer.

Staging Recurrent Cancer

To figure out the type of recurrence you have, you will have many of the same tests you had when your cancer was first diagnosed, such as lab tests and imaging procedures. These tests help determine where the cancer has returned in your body, if it has spread, and how far. Your doctor may refer to this new assessment of your cancer as "restaging." After these tests, the doctor may assign a new stage to the cancer. An "r" will be added to the beginning of the new stage to reflect the restaging. The original stage at diagnosis does not change.

Treatment for Recurrent Cancer

The type of treatment that you have for recurrent cancer will depend on your type of cancer and how far it has spread.

Your Feelings

People feel so many emotions when they find out that their cancer has come back. Shock, fear, anger, and denial are just a few. The new diagnosis hits them as hard as it did the first time, or even harder. Regardless of your first reaction, starting cancer treatment again can place even more demands on your mind and spirit. You'll have good days and bad days. So just remember that it's okay to feel a lot of different emotions. Some of these emotions may be ones you have had at other times in your life. But you may be feeling them more intensely.

If you have dealt with them in the past, you may be able to cope with them now, too. If some of the feelings are new, or are so strong that it is hard to get through everyday activities, you may want to ask for help. There are many people who may be able to help you. These include health psychologists, oncology social workers, other mental health experts, and leaders in your faith or spiritual community. They know many ways to help you cope with your feelings.

Stress

Stress is a normal reaction to cancer. After all, you're dealing with a lot: treatment, family, your job, money, and day-to-day living. Sometimes, you may not even notice that you are stressed. But your family and friends probably see a change. Anything that makes you feel calm or relaxed may help. So try to think of things that relax you and that you enjoy doing. Some people try deep breathing, listening to tapes that have nature sounds, or listening to music.

Hope

While you may be sad or depressed about your cancer recurrence, you do have reasons to feel hopeful. Science has advanced and cancer treatments have improved. So more people are surviving cancer than ever before. Nearly 10 million people who have a history of cancer are alive today. In other words, cancer is becoming a disease that doctors can manage. To help build your sense of hope:

- Plan your days as you have always done.
- Don't limit the things you like to do just because you have cancer.
- Look for your own reasons to have hope.

Gratitude

Some people see their cancer coming back as a "wake-up call." They may realize the importance of enjoying the little things in life. They go places they've never been. They finish projects they had started but put aside. They spend more time with friends and family. They mend broken relationships.

It may be hard at first, but you can find joy in your life. Take note of what makes you smile. Pay attention to the things you do each day that you enjoy. They can be as simple as drinking your morning coffee, sitting with a pet, or talking to a friend. These small, day-to-day activities can give you comfort and pleasure.

You can also do things that are more meaningful to you. Everyone has special things, both large and small, that bring meaning to their life. For you, it may be visiting a garden in your city or town. It may be praying in a certain chapel. Or it could be playing golf or some other sport that you love. Whatever you choose, embrace the things that bring you joy when you can.

Anxiety

Cancer takes a toll on both your body and your mind. You are coping with so much now. You may feel overwhelmed. Pain and medicines for pain can also make you feel anxious or depressed. And you may be more likely to feel this way if you have had these feelings before. The following are some signs of anxiety:

- Feeling very tense and nervous
- Racing heartbeat
- Sweating a lot
- Trouble breathing or catching your breath
- Having a lump in your throat or a knot in your stomach
- Feeling fear

Feeling anxious can be normal. But if it begins to disrupt your daily life, tell a member of your healthcare team. They can suggest someone for you to talk to. Or they can give you medicines that will help. Some of the nondrug choices for pain may work for your anxiety as well.

Fear

It's normal to feel scared and worried. You may be afraid of pain or other side effects, either from the cancer or the treatment. You may worry about looking different as a result of your treatment. You may worry about taking care of your family, paying your bills, and keeping your job. You may be afraid of dying.

It's hard to deal with the fear of so many unknowns. Some people say it helps if you know what to expect in the future. Ask your healthcare team questions, so you can understand more about your cancer and treatment choices. Also, update your will and other legal papers, if you haven't already done so. Then you won't have to worry about them. Fear can be overwhelming. Remember that others have felt this way, too. It's okay to ask for help.

Sadness and Depression

Sadness is a normal response to any serious illness. You may feel sad that you have to go through treatment again. You may feel sad that life won't be quite the same from now on. It's okay to feel blue. You don't need to be upbeat all the time or pretend to be cheerful. Many people say that they want the freedom to just give in to their feelings sometimes. But others say that it helps to look for what is good in life, even in the bad times.

Depression can happen when sadness or despair seems to take over your life. Some of the signs listed on the next page are normal at a time like this. But if they last more than two weeks, talk to your doctor. Some symptoms could be due to physical problems. This is why it's important to let your doctor know about them.

Anger

You may also feel angry or frustrated. It's normal to ask, "Why me?" You may be mad at the cancer, your doctors, or your loved ones. If you are religious, you might even be angry with God. If you feel angry, it's helpful to remember that you don't have to pretend that everything is okay. Try to figure out why you are angry. Anger sometimes comes from feelings that are hard to show. These might be fear, panic, frustration, worry, or helplessness. It's not always easy to look at what is causing your anger. But it's healthy to try. Being open and dealing with your anger may help you let go of it. It's also good to know that anger is a form of energy. You can express this energy through exercise, art, or even just hitting the bed with a pillow.

Guilt

It's normal for some people to wonder whether they did things that caused their cancer to recur. People feel guilty for a number of reasons:

- They worry about how their family and friends feel.
- They envy other people's good health and are ashamed of this feeling.

- They blame themselves for certain lifestyle choices.
- They feel guilty that their first treatment didn't work.
- They wonder if they waited too long to go back to the doctor. Or they fear that they didn't follow the doctor's instructions the right way.

But it's important to remember that the treatment failed you. You didn't fail the treatment. It's not known why cancer returns in some people and not others. So, it's important for you to try to:

- Focus on things worthy of your time and energy.
- Let go of any mistakes you think you may have made.
- Forgive yourself.

You may want to share these feelings with your loved ones. Some people blame themselves for upsetting the people they love or worry that they'll be a burden to others. If you feel this way, take comfort knowing that many family members say that it is an honor and a privilege to care for their loved one.

Many consider it a time when they can share experiences and become closer to one another. Others say that caring for someone else makes them take life more seriously and causes them to reevaluate their priorities. If you don't feel that you can talk openly about these things with your loved ones, getting counseling or joining a support group may also help. Let your healthcare team know if you would like to talk with someone about your feelings.

Loneliness

You may feel lonely, even when lots of people support and care for you. The following are some common feelings:

- You feel like no one else understands what you're going through, even those you love and care about.
- You feel distant from others. Or you find that your family and friends have a hard time dealing with your cancer.
- You realize that you aren't able to take part in as many events and activities as you used to.

Although it may be harder some days than others, remember that you aren't alone. Continue to do the things you've always done as best you can. If you want to, tell people that you don't want to be alone and that you welcome their visits. More than likely, your loved ones have feelings like yours. They may feel isolated from you and lonely if they are unable to talk with you.

Denial

You may feel that this is not happening to you. It's tough to accept that the cancer has come back. Feeling that you need more time to absorb everything is natural. You may need more time to adjust to the news. But this can become a serious problem if it lasts longer than it should. It can keep you from getting the treatment you need or talking about your treatment choices. As time passes, try to keep an open mind. Listen to what others around you suggest for your care.

Ways You Can Cope

Your feelings will come and go, just like they always have. If you have some strategies to deal with them, you have already taken a step in the right direction. Know that many other people have been where you are. Some do better when they join a support group. It helps them to talk with others who are facing the same challenges. You may prefer to join an online support group. That way you can chat with people from home. Be sure to check the privacy issues before you join. If support groups don't appeal to you, there are many experts who are trained to give cancer support. These include oncology social workers, psychologists or health psychologists, counselors, or members of your faith or spiritual community.

Chapter 71

Metastatic Cancer

What Is Metastatic Cancer?

The main reason that cancer is so serious is its ability to spread in the body. Cancer cells can spread locally by moving into nearby normal tissue. Cancer can also spread regionally, to nearby lymph nodes, tissues, or organs. And it can spread to distant parts of the body. When this happens, it is called metastatic cancer. For many types of cancer, it is also called stage IV (four) cancer. The process by which cancer cells spread to other parts of the body is called metastasis.

When observed under a microscope and tested in other ways, metastatic cancer cells have features like that of the primary cancer and not like the cells in the place where the cancer is found. This is how doctors can tell that it is cancer that has spread from another part of the body. Metastatic cancer has the same name as the primary cancer. For example, breast cancer that spreads to the lung is called metastatic breast cancer, not lung cancer. It is treated as stage IV breast cancer, not as lung cancer.

Sometimes when people are diagnosed with metastatic cancer, doctors cannot tell where it started. This type of cancer is called cancer of unknown primary origin, or carcinoma of unknown primary (CUP). When a new primary cancer occurs in a person with a history of cancer, it is known as a second primary cancer. Second primary cancers are

---

This chapter includes text excerpted from "Metastatic Cancer," National Cancer Institute (NCI), February 6, 2017.

rare. Most of the time, when someone who has had cancer has cancer again, it means the first primary cancer has returned.

How Cancer Spreads

Cancer cells spread through the body in a series of steps.

1. Growing into, or invading, nearby normal tissue
2. Moving through the walls of nearby lymph nodes or blood vessels
3. Traveling through the lymphatic system and bloodstream to other parts of the body
4. Stopping in small blood vessels at a distant location, invading the blood vessel walls, and moving into the surrounding tissue
5. Growing in this tissue until a tiny tumor forms
6. Causing new blood vessels to grow, which creates a blood supply that allows the tumor to continue growing

Most of the time, spreading cancer cells die at some point in this process. But, as long as conditions are favorable for the cancer cells at every step, some of them are able to form new tumors in other parts of the body. Metastatic cancer cells can also remain inactive at a distant site for many years before they begin to grow again, if at all.

Where Cancer Spreads

Cancer can spread to most any part of the body, although different types of cancer are more likely to spread to certain areas than others. The most common sites where cancer spreads are the bone, liver, and lung. The following list shows the most common sites of metastasis, not including the lymph nodes, for some common cancers:

Table 71.1. Common Sites of Metastasis

Cancer Type	Main Sites of Metastasis
Bladder	Bone, liver, lung
Breast	Bone, brain, liver, lung
Colon	Liver, lung, peritoneum
Kidney	Adrenal gland, bone, brain, liver, lung
Lung	Adrenal gland, bone, brain, liver, other lung

Table 71.1. Continued

Cancer Type	Main Sites of Metastasis
Melanoma	Bone, brain, liver, lung, skin, muscle
Ovary	Liver, lung, peritoneum
Pancreas	Liver, lung, peritoneum
Prostate	Adrenal gland, bone, liver, lung
Rectal	Liver, lung, peritoneum
Stomach	Liver, lung, peritoneum
Thyroid	Bone, liver, lung
Uterus	Bone, liver, lung, peritoneum, vagina

Symptoms of Metastatic Cancer

Metastatic cancer does not always cause symptoms. When symptoms do occur, their nature and frequency will depend on the size and location of the metastatic tumors. The following are some common signs of metastatic cancer:

- Pain and fractures, when cancer has spread to the bone
- Headache, seizures, or dizziness, when cancer has spread to the brain
- Shortness of breath, when cancer has spread to the lung
- Jaundice or swelling in the belly, when cancer has spread to the liver

Treatment for Metastatic Cancer

Once cancer spreads, it can be hard to control. Although some types of metastatic cancer can be cured with current treatments, most cannot. Even so, there are treatments for all patients with metastatic cancer. The goal of these treatments is to stop or slow the growth of the cancer or to relieve symptoms caused by it. In some cases, treatments for metastatic cancer may help prolong life. The treatment that you may have depends on your type of primary cancer, where it has spread, treatments you've had in the past, and your general health.

When Metastatic Cancer Can No Longer Be Controlled

If you have been told you have metastatic cancer that can no longer be controlled, you and your loved ones may want to discuss end-of-life care. Even if you choose to continue receiving treatment to try to shrink the cancer or control its growth, you can always receive palliative care to control the symptoms of cancer and the side effects of treatment.

Chapter 72

Advanced Cancer

You may have just been diagnosed with advanced cancer. Or perhaps you're struggling with the recurrence of cancer. This news may be hard to believe or accept at first. Many people say they felt like they were in shock and couldn't hear anything else. Having advanced cancer can bring anxiety and uncertainty to your life. Remember that you're still in control of your choices and actions. You get to choose how to move forward with your care. Having advanced cancer may also bring times of reflection. Many people say they started to see life in new ways as they made these new decisions. They learned the importance of making the most of each day.

Talking about Your Advanced Cancer

Once you are diagnosed with advanced cancer, or your disease has progressed to this point, you will have a number of issues to talk about with your loved ones and your healthcare team. You'll need to discuss future steps and what to expect. Having these talks may not be easy. But knowing your options and sharing them with others will make it easier for you to move forward with your care.

Talking with Your Healthcare Team

Your healthcare team needs to know what you want to know. Many people have a team of healthcare providers who work together

---

This chapter includes text excerpted from "Advanced Cancer," National Cancer Institute (NCI), November 6, 2017.

to help them. This team may include doctors, nurses, oncology social workers, dietitians, and other specialists. They need to know your goals for care at this stage of your cancer and how you would like to proceed. Tell them what is most important to you now. For example is it:

- Controlling symptoms and feeling comfortable?
- Receiving care at home?
- Being open to experimental treatments?

It's important to have good communication and an understanding of your goals with those who will be caring for you. Here are some topics you may want to discuss with your doctor or other members of your healthcare team:

- **Decision-making.** Some people want to know all the details about their care. Others prefer to know as little as possible. Some patients want to make all the decisions, while others want family members to make most of their decisions. What would you prefer? Decide what you want to know, how much you want to know, and when you've heard enough. Choose the amount of information that is most comfortable for you, and tell your doctor and family members. Ask that they follow your wishes.
- **Pain or other symptoms.** Some people assume that there will always be severe pain with advanced cancer. This does not have to be the case. Pain can be managed throughout the course of the disease. People whose pain is managed are able to focus on enjoying life. They can sleep better, enjoy friends and family, and focus on the daily activities they enjoy. It's important to be honest and open about your pain. Tell your doctors if and where you have pain.
- **Know your family's wishes.** Some family members may have trouble coping with your cancer prognosis. They may not want to know how far the disease has advanced or how much time doctors think you have. If you feel comfortable, ask your family members how much they want to know about your condition. Then let your healthcare team know their wishes. Do this as soon as possible. It will help avoid conflicts or distress among your loved ones. If you haven't done so already, it is important to fill out advance directives.

Talking with Family and Friends

Your loved ones may need time to adjust to the advanced stage of your illness. They need to come to terms with their own feelings. These may include:

- confusion
- shock
- helplessness
- anger
- sadness

Knowing that everyone copes with bad news in their own way will help you and your loved ones deal with their feelings. Let them know that the best thing they can do for you is to be themselves and feel at ease with you. Ask them to listen when you need it, rather than try to solve every problem. Many people are comforted by sharing feelings and taking the time to say what they need to say.

Keep in mind that not everyone can handle the thought that they might lose you. Or some people may not know what to say or do for you. As a result, relationships may change. This isn't because of you, but because others have trouble coping with their own painful feelings.

Some things you could do:

- Tell them that you're still the same person you always were.
- Let them know if it's alright to ask questions or tell you how they feel.
- Remind them that often just being there for you is enough.

It's also okay if you don't feel comfortable talking about these issues. Sometimes certain topics are hard to discuss with others. If this is the case, you may want to talk with a member of your medical team or a trained counselor. You could also go to a support group where patients meet to share common concerns.

Talking with Your Spouse or Partner

Some relationships grow stronger during cancer treatment, but others are weakened. It's very common for patients and their partners to feel more stress than usual as a couple. There is often stress about:

- Knowing how to give and get support
- Coping with new feelings that have come up
- Figuring out how to communicate
- Having money problems
- Making decisions
- Changing roles in the family
- Having changes in social life
- Coping with changes in daily routines

Some people feel more comfortable talking about serious issues than others. Only you and your loved one know how you communicate. Some suggestions:

- **Talk things over.** This may be hard for you or your partner. If so, ask a counselor or social worker to talk to both of you together.
- **Be realistic about demands.** Your spouse or partner may feel guilty about your illness. They may feel guilty about any time spent away from you. They could also be under stress due to changing family roles. Try to be aware of how they're feeling.
- **Spend some time apart.** Your partner needs time to address his or her own needs. If these needs are neglected, your loved one may have less energy and support to give to you and others. Remember, you didn't spend 24 hours a day together before you got sick.

Talking with Your Kids

Children of all ages can sense when things are wrong. Keeping your children's and grandchildren's trust is still very important at this time. It's best to be as open as you can about your cancer. They may worry that they did something to cause you to get sick. They may be afraid that no one will take care of them. They may also feel that you are not spending as much time with them as you used to.

Some children become very clingy. Others get into trouble in school or at home. Let the child's teacher or guidance counselor know what is going on. It helps to keep all the lines of communication open, both with your kids and with the other people in their lives.

Although you can't protect them from what they may feel, you can prepare them. If they ask if you are going to die, you can tell them the truth with comfort and understanding. What you tell them and how they take it will depend on their age and what they have gone through already in life. While you can't protect them from pain and loss, you can help them cope with it and understand it as part of life. Try to:

- **Be honest.** Tell them you are sick and that the doctors are working to help you feel comfortable.
- **Let them know that nothing they did or said caused the cancer.** And make sure they know that they can't catch it from you or others.
- **Tell them you love them.** Tell them it's okay to be upset, angry, or scared. Encourage them to talk.
- **Be clear and simple.** Children do not have the focus of adults. Use words they can understand.
- **Let them know that they will always be taken care of and loved.**
- **Let them know that it's okay to ask questions.** Tell them you will answer them as honestly as you can. In fact, children who aren't told the truth about an illness can become even more scared. They often use their imagination and fears to explain the changes around them.

Talking with Your Teenagers

Many of the things listed above also apply to teenagers. They need to hear the truth about an illness. This helps keep them from feeling guilt and stress. But be aware that they may try to avoid the subject. They may become angry, act out, or get into trouble as a way of coping. Others simply withdraw. Try to:

- **Give teenagers the space they need.** This is especially important if you have to rely on them more than before to help with family needs.
- **Give them time to deal with their feelings, alone or with their friends.**

- **Let your teenager know that they should still go to school.** Tell them they should keep taking part in sports and other fun activities.

If you have trouble talking with your teen about cancer, you might want to ask for help. Try asking a close friend, relative, or healthcare provider for advice. You could also go to a trusted coach, teacher, or youth minister. Your social worker or doctor can help you as well.

Talking with Your Adult Children

Your relationship with your adult children may change now that you have advanced cancer. You may have to rely on them differently than you have in the past. It's a normal reaction if you find that this is hard for you. Many people find this difficult. After all, you may be used to giving support rather than getting it. Or it may be hard for other reasons. Perhaps your relationship with your children has been a more formal or distant one.

Adult children have their concerns, too. They may become fearful of their own mortality. They may feel guilty because they're overwhelmed by the many demands of their lives as parents, children, and employees and unable to be there with you as much as they want.

As your illness progresses, it helps to:

- Share decision making with your children.
- Involve them in issues that are important to you. These may include treatment choices, plans for the future, or types of activities you want to continue.

Reaching out to your adult children and openly sharing your feelings and wishes may help them cope with your cancer. It could bring you closer to them as well. It may also help lessen any fears or conflicts that may arise between siblings when important decisions need to be made.

Family Disagreements

Any problems your family may have had before the cancer diagnosis are likely to be more intense now. And relatives that you or your family members don't know very well or who live far away may be around more often, which may complicate things.

It's common for families to argue over things such as:

- Treatment options or whether to continue treatment at all
- When to use hospice care
- Feelings that some family members are helping more than others

Although everyone may be trying to do what's best, some family members may disagree as to what this means. Everyone brings their own set of beliefs and values to the table, which makes these decisions hard. It's common for families to ask their healthcare team to hold a family meeting or to help with communication in some way.

Ask for Help or a Family Meeting

Often, talking with the people closest to you is harder than talking with anyone else. Some families are good at communicating with each other. And others have trouble expressing their needs to each other, even if they get along very well. Or sometimes families simply don't get along.

If you don't feel comfortable talking with family members, ask a member of your healthcare team to help start a conversation. You could also ask a social worker or other professional to hold a family meeting. This may help family members feel more comfortable to openly express their feelings. It can also be a time for you and your family to meet with your team to solve problems that may have arisen and set goals. It can be very hard to talk about the goals for care when someone has advanced cancer. But studies show that cancer care goes more smoothly when everyone stays open and talks about the issues.

Chapter 73

End-of-Life Care

When you learn you have advanced cancer, you're faced with many decisions about your end-of-life care. Talking about these decisions early can make it easier on you and your family later. The following are some questions you may want to think about:

- What's important to you during this time?
- Is it most important that you be as comfortable and alert as possible during the last stages of cancer?
- Is it most important to continue with treatments that may help you live longer but make you uncomfortable?

Some patients choose to receive all possible treatments. Others choose to receive only some treatments or no treatment at all. Some choose to receive only care that will keep them comfortable. Having information about your options will help you make these choices. Together, you, your family, and your doctor can decide on a plan for your care during the advanced stages of cancer.

Quality Care at the End of Life

You decide what quality care at the end of life means for you.

This chapter includes text excerpted from "Planning the Transition to End-of-Life Care in Advanced Cancer (PDQ®)—Patient Version," National Cancer Institute (NCI), November 24, 2015.

Your care continues even after all treatments have stopped. End-of-life care is more than what happens moments before dying. Care is needed in the days, weeks, and sometimes even months before death. During this time, many patients feel it's important to:

- Have their pain and symptoms controlled.
- Avoid a long process of dying.
- Feel a sense of control over what is happening to them.
- Cause less emotional and financial burden on the family.
- Become closer with loved ones.

Your doctors and family need to know the kind of end-of-life care you want.

Make end-of-life care decisions early. You may be able to think about your options more clearly if you talk about them before the decisions need to be made. It's a good idea to let your doctors, family, and caregivers know your wishes before there is an emergency.

End-of-Life Care Decisions to Be Made

Care decisions for the last stages of cancer can be about treatments and procedures, pain control, place of care, and spiritual issues.

Chemotherapy

Some patients choose to begin new chemotherapy treatment in the end stages of cancer. Others wish to let the disease take its course when a cure is not expected. In the end stages of cancer, chemotherapy usually doesn't help you live longer and it may lower the quality of the time that remains. Each person and each cancer is different. Talking with your doctor about the effects of treatment and your quality of life can help you make a decision. You can ask if the treatment will make you comfortable or if it will help you live longer.

Pain and Symptom Control

Controlling pain and other symptoms can help you have a better quality of life in the end stages of cancer. Pain and symptom control can be part of your care in any place of care, such as the hospital, home, and hospice.

Cardiopulmonary Resuscitation (CPR)

It's important to decide if you will want to have cardiopulmonary resuscitation (CPR). CPR is a procedure used to try to restart the heart and breathing when it stops. In advanced cancer, the heart, lungs, and other organs begin to fail and it's harder to restart them with CPR. Your doctor can help you understand how CPR works and talk with you about whether CPR is likely to work for you.

People who are near the end of life may choose not to have CPR done. Your decision about having CPR is personal. Your own spiritual or religious views about death and dying may help you decide. If you decide you don't want CPR, you can ask your doctor to write a do-not-resuscitate (DNR) order. This tells other healthcare professionals not to perform CPR if your heart or breathing stops. You can remove the DNR order at any time.

Talk with your doctors and other caregivers about CPR as early as possible (for example, when being admitted to the hospital), in case you're not able to make the decision later. If you do choose to have your doctor write a DNR, it's important to tell all your family members and caregivers about it.

In the United States, if there is no DNR order, you will be given CPR to keep you alive.

Ventilator Use

A ventilator is a machine used to help you breathe and keep you alive after normal breathing stops. It doesn't treat a disease or condition. It's used only for life support. You can tell doctors whether you would want to be put on a ventilator if your lungs stop working or if you cannot breathe on your own after CPR. If your goal of care is to live longer, you may choose to have a ventilator used. Or you may choose to have a ventilator for only a certain length of time. It's important to tell your family and healthcare providers what you want before you have trouble breathing.

Religious and Spiritual Support

Your religious or spiritual beliefs may help you with end-of-life decisions. Clergy and chaplains can give counseling. You can also talk with a member of your church, a social worker, or even other people who have cancer.

Talking with Your Doctor about End-of-Life Care

You may need to start the conversation. Some doctors don't ask patients about end-of-life issues. If you want to make choices about these issues, talk with your doctors so that your wishes can be carried out. Open communication can help you and your doctors make decisions together and create a plan of care that meets your goals and wishes. If your doctor is not comfortable talking about end-of-life plans, you can talk to other specialists for help.

Prognosis, treatment goals, and making decisions are some of the end-of-life issues to discuss with your doctor.

Understand Your Prognosis

Having a good understanding of your prognosis is important when making decisions about your care and treatment during advanced cancer. You will probably want to know how long you have to live. That's a hard question for doctors to answer. It can be different for each person and depends on the type of cancer, where it has spread, and whether you have other illnesses. Treatments can work differently for each person. Your doctor can talk about the treatment options with you and your family and explain the effects they may have on your cancer and your quality of life. Knowing the benefits and risks of available treatments can help you decide on your goals of care for the last stages of cancer.

Decide on Your Care Goals

Your care goals for advanced cancer depend in part on whether quality of life or length of life is more important to you. Your goals of care may change as your condition changes or if new treatments become available. Tell your doctor what your goals of care are, even if you aren't asked. It's important that you and your doctor are working toward the same goals.

Take Part in Making Decisions

Do you want to take part in making the decisions about your care? Or would you rather have your family and your doctors make those decisions? This is a personal choice and your family and doctors need to know what you want.

Early communication with your doctors can help you feel more prepared for end-of-life issues. Many patients who start talking with their doctors early about end-of-life issues report feeling better prepared. Better communication with your doctors may make it easier to deal with concerns about being older, living alone, relieving symptoms, spiritual well-being, and how your family will cope in the future.

There are ways to improve communication with your doctors. Tell your doctor how you and your family wish to receive information and the type of information you want. Also ask how you can get information at times when you can't meet face-to-face.

Remembering what your doctor said and even remembering what you want to ask can be hard to do. Some of the following may help communication and help you remember what was said:

- Have a family member go with you when you meet with your doctor.
- Make a list of the questions you want to ask the doctor during your visit.
- Get the information in writing.
- Record the discussion with tape recorders, smartphones, or on video.
- Ask if your doctor or clinic offers any of the following:
    - A cancer consultation preparation package, which includes aids such as a question idea sheet, booklets on decision making and patient rights, and information about the clinic
    - A talk with a psychologist about advance planning and end-of-life issues
    - An end-of-life preference interview, which includes a list of questions that can help you explain your wishes about the end of life

Supportive Care, Palliative Care, and Hospice

Even when treatments can no longer cure the cancer, medical care is still needed. Some of the end-of-life care options are supportive care, palliative care, and hospice.

Supportive Care

Supportive care is given to prevent or treat, as early as possible, the symptoms of the cancer, side effects caused by treatments, and psychological, social, and spiritual problems related to the cancer or its treatment. During active treatment to cure the cancer, supportive care helps you stay healthy and comfortable enough to continue receiving the cancer treatments. In the last stages of cancer, when a cure is no longer the goal, supportive care is used for side effects that continue.

Palliative Care

Palliative care is specialized medical care for people with serious or life-threatening illnesses. The focus of palliative care is relief from pain and other symptoms, both during active treatment and when treatment has been stopped. Palliative care is offered in some hospitals, outpatient centers, and in the home.

Palliative care helps to improve your quality of life by preventing and relieving suffering. When you're more comfortable, your family's quality of life may also be better. Palliative care includes treating physical symptoms such as pain, and helping you and your family with emotional, social, and spiritual concerns. When palliative treatment is given at the end of life, the focus is on relieving symptoms and distress caused by the process of dying and to make sure your goals of care are followed.

Hospice Care

When treatment is no longer helping, you may choose hospice. Hospice is a program that gives care to people who are near the end of life and have stopped treatment to cure or control their cancer. Hospice care focuses on quality of life rather than length of life. The hospice team offers physical, emotional, and spiritual support for patients who are expected to live no longer than six months. The goal of hospice is to help patients live each day to the fullest by making them comfortable and relieving their symptoms. This may include supportive and palliative care to control pain and other symptoms so you can be as alert and comfortable as possible. Services to help with the emotional, social, and spiritual needs of you and your family are also an important part of hospice care.

Hospice programs are designed to keep the patient at home with family and friends, but hospice care may also be given in hospice centers and in some hospitals and nursing homes. The hospice team includes doctors, nurses, spiritual advisors, social workers, nutritionists, and volunteers. Team members are specially trained on issues that occur at the end of life. The hospice program continues to give help, including grief counseling, to the family after their loved one dies. Ask your doctor for information if you wish to receive hospice care.

Advance Planning

Making end-of-life care decisions early can ease your mind and decrease stress on your family. There may come a time when you can't tell the healthcare team what you want. When that happens, would you prefer to have your doctor and family make decisions? Or would you rather make decisions early, so your wishes will be known and can be followed when the time comes? If not planned far ahead of time, the end-of-life decisions must be made by someone other than you.

Planning ahead for end-of-life care helps with the following:

- Makes sure your doctors and family know what your wishes are
- Allows you to refuse the use of treatments
- Decreases the emotional stress on your family, who would have to make decisions if you aren't able to
- Reduces the cost of care, if you choose not to receive life-saving procedures
- Eases your mind to have these decisions already made

You can make your wishes known with an advance directive.

Advance directives are documents that state what your wishes are for certain medical treatments when you can no longer communicate those wishes. Advance directive is the general term for different types of documents that state what your wishes are for certain medical treatments when you can no longer tell those wishes to your caregivers. In addition to decisions about relieving symptoms at the end of life, it is also helpful to decide if and when you want certain treatments to stop. Advance directives make sure your wishes about treatments and life-saving procedures to keep you alive are known ahead of time. Without knowing your wishes, doctors will do everything medically possible to keep you alive, such as cardiopulmonary resuscitation (CPR) and the use of a ventilator (breathing machine).

Each state has its own laws for advance directives. Make sure your advance directives follow the laws of the state where you live and are being treated.

The following are types of documents that communicate your wishes in advance:

- **Living will:** A legal document that states whether you want certain life-saving medical treatments to be used or not used under certain circumstances. Some of the treatments covered by a living will include CPR, use of a ventilator (breathing machine), and tube-feeding.

- **Healthcare proxy (HCP):** A document in which you choose a person (called a proxy) to make medical decisions if you become unable to do so. It's important that your proxy knows your values and wishes, so that he or she can make the decisions you would make if you were able. You do not have to state specific decisions about individual treatments in the document, just state that the proxy will make medical decisions for you. HCP is also known as durable power of attorney for healthcare (DPOAHC) or medical power of attorney (MPOA).
- **Do-Not-Resuscitate (DNR) order:** A document that tells medical staff in the hospital not to do cardiopulmonary resuscitation (CPR) if your heart or breathing stops. A DNR order is a decision only about CPR. It does not affect other treatments that may be used to keep you alive, such as medicine or food.
- **Out-of-hospital DNR order:** A document that tells emergency medical workers outside of a hospital that you do not wish to have CPR or other types of resuscitation. Each state has its own rules for a legal out-of-hospital DNR order, but it is usually signed by the patient, a witness, and the doctor. It's best to have several copies so one can quickly be given to emergency medical workers when needed.
- **Do-Not-Intubate (DNI) order:** A document that tells medical staff in a hospital or nursing facility that you do not wish to have a breathing tube inserted and to be put on a ventilator (breathing machine).
- **Physician Orders for Life-Sustaining Treatment (POLST):** A form that states what kind of medical treatment you want toward the end of your life. It is signed by you and your doctor.
- **Medical Orders for Life-Sustaining Treatment (MOLST):** A form that states the care you would like to receive if you are not able to communicate. This care includes CPR, intubation (breathing tubes), and other life-saving procedures. Under current law, the information in a MOLST form must be followed both in the home and hospital by all medical staff, including emergency medical workers.

All your caregivers need to have copies of your advance directives. Give copies of your advance directives to your doctors, caregivers, and family members. Advance directives need to move with you. If your doctors or your place of care changes, copies of your advance directives need to be given to your new caregivers. This will make sure that your wishes are known through all cancer stages and places of care. You can change or cancel an advance directive at any time.

Part Five

Clinical Trials and Cancer Research

Chapter 74

Clinical Trials

Chapter Contents

Section 74.1

What Are Clinical Trials?

This section includes text excerpted from "NIH Clinical Research Trials and You—The Basics," National Institutes of Health (NIH), October 20, 2017.

Clinical Research and Its Types

Clinical research is medical research that involves people like you. When you volunteer to take part in clinical research, you help doctors and researchers learn more about disease and improve healthcare for people in the future. Clinical research includes all research that involves people. Types of clinical research include the following:

- Epidemiology, which improves the understanding of a disease by studying patterns, causes, and effects of health and disease in specific groups
- Behavioral, which improves the understanding of human behavior and how it relates to health and disease
- Health services, which looks at how people access healthcare providers and healthcare services, how much care costs, and what happens to patients as a result of this care
- Clinical trials, which evaluate the effects of an intervention on health outcomes

What Are Clinical Trials and Why Would I Want to Take Part?

Clinical trials are part of clinical research and at the heart of all medical advances. Clinical trials look at new ways to prevent, detect, or treat disease. Clinical trials can study the following:

- New drugs or new combinations of drugs
- New ways of doing surgery
- New medical devices

- New ways to use existing treatments
- New ways to change behaviors to improve health
- New ways to improve the quality of life for people with acute or chronic illnesses

The goal of clinical trials is to determine if these treatment, prevention, and behavior approaches are safe and effective. People take part in clinical trials for many reasons. Healthy volunteers say they take part to help others and to contribute to moving science forward. People with an illness or disease also take part to help others, but also to possibly receive the newest treatment and to have added (or extra) care and attention from the clinical trial staff. Clinical trials offer hope for many people and a chance to help researchers find better treatments for others in the future.

How Does the Research Process Work?

The idea for a clinical trial often starts in the lab. After researchers test new treatments or procedures in the lab and in animals, the most promising treatments are moved into clinical trials. As new treatments move through a series of steps called phases, more information is gained about the treatment, its risks, and its effectiveness.

What Are Clinical Trial Protocols?

Clinical trials follow a plan known as a protocol. The protocol is carefully designed to balance the potential benefits and risks to participants, and answer specific research questions. A protocol describes the following:

- The goal of the study
- Who is eligible to take part in the trial
- Protections against risks to participants
- Details about tests, procedures, and treatments
- How long the trial is expected to last
- What information will be gathered

A clinical trial is led by a principal investigator (PI). Members of the research team regularly monitor the participants' health to determine the study's safety and effectiveness.

What Are the Types of Clinical Trials?

There are different types of clinical trials.

- Prevention trials look for better ways to prevent a disease in people who have never had the disease or to prevent the disease from returning. Approaches may include medicines, vaccines, or lifestyle changes.
- Screening trials test new ways for detecting diseases or health conditions.
- Diagnostic trials study or compare tests or procedures for diagnosing a particular disease or condition.
- Treatment trials test new treatments, new combinations of drugs, or new approaches to surgery or radiation therapy.
- Behavioral trials evaluate or compare ways to promote behavioral changes designed to improve health.
- Quality of life trials (or supportive care trials) explore and measure ways to improve the comfort and quality of life of people with conditions or illnesses.

Section 74.2

How to Find a Cancer Treatment Trial

This section includes text excerpted from "Steps to Find a Clinical Trial," National Cancer Institute (NCI), June 23, 2016.

If you are thinking about joining a clinical trial as a treatment option, the best place to start is to talk with your doctor or another member of your healthcare team. Often, your doctor may know about a clinical trial that could be a good option for you. He or she may also be able to search for a trial for you, provide information, and answer questions to help you decide about joining a clinical trial.

Some doctors may not be aware of or recommend clinical trials that could be appropriate for you. If so, you may want to get a second opinion about your treatment options, including taking part in a clinical trial. If you decide to look for trials on your own, the following steps can guide you in your search. This information should not be used in place of advice from your doctor or other members of your healthcare team. This section takes you through the following steps:

Step One: Gather Details about Your Cancer

If you decide to look for a clinical trial, you must know certain details about your cancer diagnosis. You will need to compare these details with the eligibility criteria of any trial that interests you. Eligibility criteria are the guidelines for who can and cannot take part in a certain clinical trial. To help you gather details about your cancer, complete as much of the cancer details checklist (www.cancer.gov/about-cancer/treatment/clinical-trials/search/trial-guide/detailschecklist.pdf) as possible. Refer to the form during your search for a clinical trial. If you need help filling out the form, talk with your doctor, a nurse, or social worker at your doctor's office. The more information you can gather, the easier it will be to find a clinical trial to fit your situation.

Step Two: Find Clinical Trials

There are many lists of cancer clinical trials taking place in the United States. Some trials are funded by nonprofit organizations, including the U.S. government. Others are funded by for-profit groups, such as drug companies. Hospitals and academic medical centers also sponsor trials conducted by their own researchers. Because of the many types of sponsors, no single list contains every clinical trial.

Helpful Tip: Whichever website you use to search for clinical trials, be sure to bookmark or print a copy of the protocol summary for every trial that interests you.

A protocol summary should explain the goal of the trial and describe which treatments will be tested. It should also list the locations where the trial is taking place.

Keep in mind that protocol summaries are written for healthcare providers and use medical language to describe the trial that may be difficult to understand. For help understanding the protocol summary, call, email, or chat with a trained information specialist at the National Cancer Institute (NCI) Contact Center.

NCI-Supported Clinical Trials

NCI's website helps you find NCI-supported clinical trials that are taking place across the United States, Canada, and internationally. The list includes the following:

- All NCI network trials, including trials supported through the:
    - National Clinical Trials Network (NCTN)
    - NCI Community Oncology Research Program (NCORP)
    - Experimental Therapeutics Clinical Trials Network (ETCTN)
- Trials that are funded in full or in part by NCI, including trials taking place at NCI-Designated Cancer Centers
- Trials at the National Institutes of Health (NIH) Clinical Center (CC) in Bethesda, Maryland

If you need help with your search, you can call, email, or chat with a trained information specialist at the NCI Contact Center. They will need to know details about your cancer, so have your cancer details checklist ready.

Other Lists of Trials

In addition to NCI's list of cancer clinical trials, you may want to check a few other trial lists.

Other places to look for lists of cancer clinical trials include:

ClinicalTrials.gov

ClinicalTrials.gov, which is part of the U.S. National Library of Medicine (NLM), lists clinical trials for cancer and many other diseases and conditions. It contains trials that are in NCI's list of cancer trials as well as trials sponsored by pharmaceutical or biotech companies that may not be on NCI's list.

Cancer Centers and Clinics that Conduct Cancer Clinical Trials

Many cancer centers across the United States, including NCI-Designated Cancer Centers, sponsor or take part in cancer clinical trials. The websites of these centers usually have a list of the clinical trials taking place at their institutions. Some of the trials included in these lists may not be on NCI's list.

Keep in mind that the amount of information about clinical trials on these websites can vary. You may have to contact a cancer center clinical trials office to get more information about the trials that interest you.

Drug and Biotechnology Companies

Many companies provide lists of the clinical trials that they sponsor on their websites. Sometimes, a company's website may refer you to the website of another organization that helps the company find patients for its trials. The other organization may be paid fees for this service.

The website of the Pharmaceutical Research and Manufacturers of America (PhRMA) includes a list of its member companies, many of which sponsor cancer clinical trials. PhRMA is a trade organization that represents drug and biotechnology companies in the United States.

Clinical Trial Listing Services

Some organizations provide lists of clinical trials as a part of their business. These organizations generally do not sponsor or take part in clinical trials. Some of them may receive fees from drug or biotechnology companies for listing their trials or helping find patients for their trials.

Keep the following points in mind about clinical trial listing services:

- The lists of trials provided by these organizations often draw from the trial lists that are available from the U.S. government (NCI and ClinicalTrials.gov).
- The websites of these organizations may not be updated regularly.
- The websites of these organizations may require you to register to search for clinical trials or to obtain trial contact information for trials that interest you.

Cancer Advocacy Groups

Cancer advocacy groups provide education, support, financial assistance, and advocacy to help patients and families who are dealing with cancer, its treatment, and survivorship. These organizations recognize that clinical trials are important to improving cancer care. They work to educate and empower people to find information and obtain access to appropriate treatment.

Advocacy groups work hard to know about the latest advances in cancer research. Some will have information about clinical trials that are enrolling patients.

To find trials, search the websites of advocacy groups for specific types of cancer. Many of these websites have lists of clinical trials or refer you to the websites of organizations that match patients to trials. Or, you can contact an advocacy group directly for help finding clinical trials.

Step Three: Take a Closer Look at the Trials That Interest You

Once you have completed the cancer details checklist and found some trials that interest you, you should now:

- Take a closer look at the protocol summary for each trial and
- Use the questions below to narrow your list to include only those trials for which you would like to get more information.

Helpful Tip: Don't worry if you can't answer all of the questions below just yet. The idea is to narrow your list of potential trials, if possible. However, don't give up on trials you're not sure about. You may want to talk with your doctor or another healthcare team member during this process, especially if you find the protocol summaries hard to understand.

Key Questions to Ask about Each Trial

Trial Objective

What is the main purpose of the trial? Is it to cure your cancer? To slow its growth or spread? To lessen the severity of cancer symptoms or the side effects of treatment? To determine whether a new treatment is safe and well-tolerated? Read this information carefully to learn whether the trial's main objective matches your goals for treatment.

Eligibility Criteria

Do the details of your cancer diagnosis and your current overall state of health match the trial's eligibility criteria? Some treatment trials will not accept people who have already been treated for their cancer. Other treatment trials are looking for people who have already been treated for their cancer.

Helpful Hint: If you have just found out that you have cancer, the time to think about joining a trial is before you have any treatment. Talk with your doctor about how quickly you need to make a treatment decision.

Trial Location

Is the location of the trial manageable for you? Some trials take place at more than one location. Look carefully at how often you will need to receive treatment during the course of the trial. Decide how far and how often you are willing to travel. You will also need to ask whether the sponsoring organization will pay for some or all of your travel costs.

Study Length

How long will the trial run? Not all protocol summaries provide this information. If they do, consider the time involved and whether it will work for you and your family.

After thinking about these questions, if you are still interested in a clinical trial, then you are ready to contact the team running the trial.

Step Four: Contact the Team Running the Trial

There are a few ways to reach the clinical trial team.

- **Contact the trial team directly.** The protocol summary should include the phone number of a person or an office that you can contact for more information. You do not need to talk to the lead researcher (called the "protocol chair" or "principal investigator") at this time, even if his or her name is given along with the telephone number. Instead, call the number and ask to speak with the "trial coordinator." This person can answer questions from patients and their doctors. It is also the trial coordinator's job to decide whether you are likely to be eligible to join the trial. However, a final decision will probably not be made until you have met with a doctor who is part of the trial team.

You will need to refer to the cancer details checklist during this conversation, so keep it handy.

- **Ask your doctor or another healthcare team member to contact the trial team for you.** The clinical trial coordinator will ask questions about your cancer diagnosis and your current general health that you may not be sure how to answer. So, you may want to ask your doctor or someone else on your healthcare team to contact the trial coordinator for you.
- **The trial team may contact you.** If you have registered to use the website of a clinical trial listing service and found a trial that interests you, the clinical trial team may contact you directly by using the phone number and email address you provide when you register.

Step Five: Ask Questions

Whether you or someone from your healthcare team speaks with the clinical trial team, this is the time to get answers to questions that will help you decide whether or not to take part in this particular clinical trial. Remember to keep your cancer details checklist handy to help you answer some of the questions that may be asked.

Talk with Your Doctor

To make a final decision, you will want to know the potential risks and benefits of all treatment options available to you. If you have any remaining questions or concerns, you should discuss them with your doctor. Ask your doctor some of the same questions that you asked the trial coordinator. You should also ask your doctor about the risks and benefits of standard treatment for your cancer. Then, you and your doctor can compare the risks and benefits of standard treatment with those of treatment in a clinical trial. You may decide that joining a trial is your best option, or you may decide not to join a trial. It's your choice.

Step Six: Make an Appointment

If you decide to join a clinical trial for which you are eligible, schedule a visit with the team running the trial.

Chapter 75

Cancer Biology Research

Research on Cancer Biology Is Critical to Progress against the Disease

Research on the biology of cancer starts with the simplest of questions: What is—and isn't—normal?

To understand how cancer develops and progresses, researchers first need to investigate the biological differences between normal cells and cancer cells. This work focuses on the mechanisms that underlie fundamental processes such as cell growth, the transformation of normal cells to cancer cells, and the spread, or metastasis, of cancer cells.

Knowledge gained from such studies deepens our understanding of cancer and produces insights that could lead to the development of new clinical interventions. For example, studies of cell signaling pathways in normal cells and cancer cells have contributed greatly to our knowledge about the disease, revealing molecular alterations that are shared among different types of cancer and pointing to possible strategies for treatment.

The last few decades of basic research in cancer biology have created a broad base of knowledge that has been critical to progress against the disease. In fact, many advances in the prevention, diagnosis, and treatment of cancer would not have occurred without the knowledge that has come from investigating basic questions about the biology of cancer.

This chapter includes text excerpted from "Research Areas—Cancer Biology Research," National Cancer Institute (NCI), November 30, 2016.

Opportunities in Cancer Biology Research

Scientists today have a growing understanding of the biology of a vast array of cancers driven by various mutations and across many body sites. New data and research approaches have created opportunities for researchers to study in detail many aspects of cancer biology, including how the normal biological programs of cell proliferation and death are altered during cancer and how the immune system responds to tumors.

The discovery of tumor stem cells in a range of cancers has created opportunities for researchers to identify these rare cells in both solid tumors and hematologic cancers, as well as to investigate the role of these cells at different stages of the disease.

The recognition that the cancer cell is in a symbiotic relationship with the tumor microenvironment has created opportunities to study the interactions of cancer cells within the tumor or the host microenvironment. Researchers are now studying the molecular mechanisms and signaling pathways of cancer cell development, proliferation, and metastasis.

Growing interest in the microbiome, the community of microorganisms and viruses that inhabit the human body, has led researchers to investigate the role of the human microbiome in the initiation and progression of tumors.

New genetic technologies developed over the past decade have helped researchers examine the functional effects of genetic alterations that underlie the development of cancer. These tools have also been used to study epigenetic changes associated with cancer, mechanisms of deoxyribonucleic acid (DNA) damage and repair, and gene regulation in cancer cells.

The introduction of increasingly powerful structural biology approaches has allowed researchers to characterize the structures of mutant proteins involved in cancer, such as renin-angiotensin system (RAS), and other molecules in greater detail than had been possible previously. And through approaches that allow the characterization of the entire proteome, researchers are integrating genomic analysis with the analysis of the proteins in tumor cells to learn, in detail, how cancer-associated mutant proteins affect other proteins.

There are also opportunities to explore cancer biology through systems biology approaches. Researchers use a variety of information and tools, such as mathematical modeling, to describe the complex interactions among components of a biological system and make predictions that help guide and further refine experimental science.

Challenges in Cancer Biology Research

Basic research in cancer biology is often viewed as "high risk," in part because the clinical applications of a given research project might not be clear at the outset. However, knowledge gained from studying cancer cell biology not only improves our understanding of the disease but is essential for the development of clinical advances that benefit patients, as recent progress in the areas of immunotherapy and cancer vaccines illustrates.

Nonetheless, because of the uncertainty about the outcomes of basic research in cancer biology, this area of research receives relatively little funding from sources that are driven by profit. For this reason, federal funding for cancer biology research is critical.

Collaboration across disciplines is increasingly necessary to better understand key mechanisms in cancer. Therefore, some investigators may need to develop tools and strategies for sharing and communicating research results.

NCI's Role in Cancer Biology Research

National Cancer Institute (NCI) supports and directs research on the biological differences between normal cells and cancer cells through a variety of programs and approaches. For example, the Division of Cancer Biology (DCB) supports extramural researchers who are using a variety of methods to study cancer biology.

In addition to many of the topics mentioned above, DCB supports research on:

- the metabolism of cancer cells, the responses of cancer cells to stress, and mechanisms involved in control of the cell cycle
- biological agents (such as viruses and bacteria), host factors (such as obesity, comorbid conditions, and age), and behaviors (such as dietary intake) that may cause or contribute to the development of cancer
- immune regulation of the development and spread of tumors and approaches to improve immune targeting and destruction of cancer cells
- genomic instability and related molecular, cytogenetic, and chromosomal effects during induction and progression to malignancy
- the role of the microenvironment created by inflammation and the inflammatory signaling molecules in the formation and progression of tumors

- processes and molecular targets where there is potential for therapeutic or preventive intervention
- the effects of hypoxia on tumor cell invasion and metastasis
- the role of somatic stem cells in determining tumor progression and metastatic behavior, and control of the stem cell niche by tumor microenvironment

NCI-supported research programs in cancer biology include the:

- Physical Sciences in Oncology Network (PS-ON)

  The goal of this initiative is to promote and foster the convergence of physical science and cancer research. Small transdisciplinary teams of physical scientists (engineers, physicists, mathematicians, chemists, and computer scientists) and cancer researchers (cancer biologists, oncologists, and pathologists) collaborate on solving problems such as determining which cell is the cell of origin for brain and hematopoietic tumors and exploring the use of three-dimensional images of single cells as cancer signatures.

- Cancer Systems Biology Consortium (CSBC)

  The CSBC focuses on combining advanced experimental approaches with mathematical and computational methodologies to build and test predictive models of cancer. The initiative takes an integrative approach to cancer research to complement and expand our current understanding of tumor development and progression across many physical and timescales, with the ultimate goal of improving the lives of cancer patients.

- Barrett's Esophagus Translational Research Network (BETRNet)

  This multidisciplinary, multi-institutional collaboration was established to better understand Barrett esophagus and to prevent esophageal adenocarcinoma. BETRNet aims to better understand esophageal adenocarcinoma (EA) biology; examine research opportunities associated with its precursor lesion, Barrett Esophagus; improve EA risk stratification and prediction; and provide strategies for EA prevention. The overriding goal is to decrease the incidence, morbidity, and mortality of this cancer.

- Alliance of Glycobiologists for Detection of Cancer

    This consortium of tumor glycomics laboratories and their research partners study the cancer-related dynamics of complex carbohydrates. This program, which NCI sponsors with the National Institute of General Medical Sciences (NIGMS) and the National Heart, Lung, and Blood Institute (NHLBI), aims to study the structure and function of glycans in relation to cancer.

- Molecular and Cellular Characterization of Screen-Detected Lesions Initiative

    The goal of this program is to undertake a comprehensive molecular and cellular characterization of tumor tissue, cell, and microenvironment components to distinguish screen-detected early lesions from interval and symptom-detected cancers. Researchers use various technologies and approaches to determine both the cellular and molecular phenotypes of early lesions, with the goal of better predicting the fate of early lesions.

- Clinical Proteomic Tumor Analysis Consortium (CPTAC)

    CPTAC was launched by NCI's Office of Cancer Clinical Proteomics Research (OCCPR) to systematically identify proteins that result from genetic alterations in cancer cells, study how they affect biological processes, and provide this data with accompanying assays and protocols to the public.

- Applied Proteogenomics Organizational Learning and Outcomes Network (APOLLO)

    A collaboration between the U.S. Department of Defense (DoD), U.S. Department of Veterans Affairs (VA), and NCI using the latest genomic and proteomic research methods to more rapidly and accurately identify effective drugs to treat cancer based on the proteogenomic profile of a patient's tumor. Initial collaborative efforts will focus on a cohort of 8,000 patients with lung cancer and will make data broadly available to the research community. Eventually, the effort will be expanded to additional cancer types.

NCI's Centers of Excellence bring together intramural researchers from NCI's Center for Cancer Research and Division of Cancer

Epidemiology and Genetics (DCEG) to develop new projects and initiatives in various areas of cancer biology, including:

- Chromosome Biology

  The experts affiliated with this center study the mechanisms involved in chromosome function through diverse research that includes mapping the dynamic changes of the genome and transcriptome during the development of cancer and translational research for the early diagnosis of cancer.

- Integrative Cancer Biology and Genomics

  This center's goal is to use advanced analytic technologies to define homogenous clusters of patients, who can then be treated with appropriate therapies. The researchers in this center build upon the immense amount of basic research data available in an effort to shorten the time between discovery and patient benefit by bringing together expertise in five areas: biomarkers and molecular targets, genomic approaches, human genomics and genetics, cancer inflammation, and integrative/systems biology and bioinformatics.

Chapter 76

Cancer Genomics Research

Genomics Research Is Critical to Progress against Cancer

The study of cancer genomes has revealed abnormalities in genes that drive the development and growth of many types of cancer. This knowledge has improved our understanding of the biology of cancer and led to new methods of diagnosing and treating the disease.

For example, the discovery of cancer-causing genetic and epigenetic changes in tumors has enabled the development of therapies that target these changes as well as diagnostic tests that identify patients who may benefit from these therapies. One such targeted drug is vemurafenib (Zelboraf®), which was approved by the U.S. Food and Drug Administration (FDA) in 2011 for the treatment of some patients with melanoma who have a specific mutation in the *BRAF* gene as detected by an FDA-approved test.

Over the past decade, large-scale research projects have begun to survey and catalog the genomic changes associated with a number of types of cancer. These efforts have revealed unexpected genetic similarities across different types of tumors. For instance, mutations in the *HER2* gene (distinct from amplifications of this gene, for which therapies have been developed for breast, esophageal, and gastric cancers) have been found in a number of cancers, including breast, bladder, pancreatic, and ovarian.

This chapter includes text excerpted from "Research Areas—Cancer Genomics Research," National Cancer Institute (NCI), August 4, 2017.

Researchers have also shown that a given type of cancer, such as breast, lung, and stomach, may have several molecular subtypes. For some types of cancer, the existence of certain subtypes had not been known until researchers began to profile the genomes of tumor cells.

The results of these projects illustrate the diverse landscape of genetic alterations in cancer and provide a foundation for understanding the molecular basis of this group of diseases.

Opportunities in Cancer Genomics Research

Although a large number of genetic alterations that drive the development and progression of many types of cancer have been identified through large-scale research studies, some tumor types have not been deeply characterized. New technologies and the knowledge gained from previous genomic studies could be used to define the full set of driver mutations and other alterations to deoxyribonucleic acid (DNA) and ribonucleic acid (RNA) in many cancers. Studies that compare genomic information from tumors and normal tissue from the same patient allow researchers to discover genomic changes that may drive cancer.

Another opportunity is to expand the current use of genomic methods to investigate the molecular basis of clinical phenotypes. This approach could help researchers identify genetic changes that may distinguish aggressive cancers from indolent ones, for example. Similar approaches could be used to study the molecular basis of response to a given therapy, as well as mechanisms of resistance to treatment.

The wealth of data emerging from cancer genome studies increasingly will be integrated with patients' medical histories and clinical data. These integrated results could be used to develop more tailored approaches to cancer diagnosis and treatment, as well as to improve methods of predicting cancer risk, prognosis, and response to treatment.

Challenges in Cancer Genomics Research

Comprehensive analysis of cancer genomes has revealed a great deal of diversity in the genetic abnormalities found within cancers of a single type. Moreover, recurrent genetic alterations within these cancers are often involved in only a small percentage of cases. Identifying which genetic changes initiate cancer development and discovering rare genetic alterations that drive cancers are therefore challenges for the field.

Another challenge is acquiring high-quality biological samples needed for genomic studies, particularly for tumor types that are uncommon or rare, or those not treated primarily by surgery.

Developing cell lines and animal models that capture the diversity of human cancer is also an unmet need. Models of rare cancer subtypes may be nonexistent or underrepresented, and there are no models for many recurrent genetic lesions in human cancer.

Managing and analyzing the vast amounts of data involved in genomic studies are additional challenges for the field. This area of research requires an efficient bioinformatics infrastructure and increasingly involves contributions of data and expertise from cross-disciplinary teams.

NCI's Role in Cancer Genomics Research

Pursuing the genetic foundations of cancer is a vital part of National Cancer Institute's (NCI) research efforts. In 2012, NCI established a new Center for Cancer Genomics (CCG) to focus on the study of how altered genes promote cancer. CCG uses high-throughput techniques to identify and study mutations, large rearrangements of the genome, increases and decreases in DNA copy number, chemical modifications to DNA, and changes in the expression of RNA and proteins. NCI supports diverse cancer genomics research and related efforts to translate these findings into clinical advances for patients.

Characterizing Cancer Genomes

NCI investigators analyze the DNA and RNA of cancer cells using advanced technologies such as next-generation DNA sequencing to map the landscape of the cancer genome and discover new changes linked to disease. NCI studies commonly use multiple genomic techniques. Integrating the results from several analyses helps scientists gain a better understanding of cancer, much like combining magenta, cyan, and yellow inks can generate vibrant color prints.

- The Cancer Genome Atlas (TCGA), a collaboration between NCI and the National Human Genome Research Institute (NHGRI) and Therapeutically Applicable Research to Generate Effective Treatments (TARGET) have characterized thousands of genomes and matched normal samples. This large number is important for discovering DNA, RNA, and protein abnormalities that are responsible for cancers in small numbers of patients.

- The Cancer Genome Characterization Initiative (CGCI) also studies cancer genomes, including cancers associated with human immunodeficiency virus (HIV) infection.
- CCG characterizes cancer genomes through its Genome Characterization Pipeline, which converts tissue samples donated by patients into high quality, publicly available genomic data.
- TCGA and TARGET taught the research community the importance of combining patients' medical data with cancer genomics data, leading to NCI programs that integrate rich genomic and clinical datasets.

Analyzing Standard of Care and Novel Treatments at a Molecular Level

Collaborative programs within and outside of NCI are collecting genomic data from patients receiving standard cancer treatments and patients receiving investigational treatments in clinical trials. These research collaborations have the power to answer questions critical to improving cancer outcomes, such as how tumors develop drug resistance, and what treatments are most effective against particular genomic traits.

- The Clinical Trials Sequencing Project (CTSP), a collaboration between CCG and NCI's Division of Cancer Treatment and Diagnosis, and the Cancer Driver Discovery Program (CDDP), characterize tissue samples from patients who have undergone standard-of-care or investigational treatments. These programs seek to understand the genomic basis of cancer development, metastasis, and drug resistance.
- The Exceptional Responders (ER) Initiative analyzes the genetic basis of exceptional responses to therapy. In some cases, a trial of a new drug fails to help most patients, but one or two people treated with the drug benefit. ER investigates the reason for exceptional responses to help assign the right treatments to the right patients in the future.
- Adjuvant Lung Cancer Enrichment Marker Identification and Sequencing Trial (ALCHEMIST), a set of precision medicine lung cancer trials, screens participants' genomes for molecular targets of currently available targeted therapies. By analyzing patients' tumors over the course of their treatment, ALCHEMIST aims to uncover how different cancers respond to targeted drugs and how tumors evolve during treatment.

Modeling the Activity of Cancer Genes

To translate genomic insights to the clinic, the activity of potential cancer genes that have been identified must be tested in models of cancer. These models can be cancer cell lines, organoid tissues, mice, or other model organisms. NCI supports research that helps bridge the gap between initial genomic discoveries and translation.

- The Cancer Treatment Discovery and Development Program (CTD2) is a network of scientific laboratories devoted to translating genomics into clinical benefit. CTD2 researchers study how genes linked to cancer work in cells and explore opportunities to target vulnerabilities with new therapies.
- The Human Models Cancer Initiative (HCMI) is generating new cancer models using cutting-edge technologies. These models will provide researchers with more accurate representations of a wide variety of cancers, and genomic characterization of the models may reveal links between genomic traits and how cells behave.

Relating Inherited Risk Factors to Cancer Genomics

Researchers in NCI's Division of Cancer Epidemiology and Genetics (DCEG) integrate tissue profiling into studies examining the causes of cancer to better understand the process by which normal cells are transformed into cancer cells (carcinogenesis) and to pinpoint factors associated with risk for developing specific molecular or genomic subtypes. DCEG investigators are also working to identify novel molecular and genomic signatures in tumors that are linked to germline genetic variants and environmental exposures, such as cigarette smoking and ionizing radiation. This approach will help identify new risk factors and yield novel insights into biological mechanisms of carcinogenesis.

- The DCEG Cancer Genomics Research Laboratory supports epidemiologic research by processing, characterizing, and analyzing tissue collections and other samples using genome-wide association studies, DNA sequencing, and candidate gene studies.

Data Sharing

NCI has spearheaded genomic data sharing practices since the inception of TCGA. NCI's support for cancer genomic data sharing continues by making all the data as open and accessible as possible while protecting patient privacy.

- The NCI Genomic Data Commons (GDC) is a data sharing platform that harmonizes diverse datasets and provides streamlined access for the research community. The GDC contains NCI-generated genomic datasets such as TCGA and TARGET, and continually expands its catalog by incorporating data submissions from research organizations, advocacy foundations, and industry. By standardizing patient medical information and raw genomic data using the latest bioinformatics pipelines, the GDC provides high quality processed data.
- The Cancer Genomics Cloud (CGC) Pilots facilitate large-scale computing on NCI genomic data by making them accessible through commercial cloud providers. The Cloud Pilots can reduce costs and increase efficiency for big data analyses.

Chapter 77

Cancer Diagnosis Research

Research on Diagnosis Is Critical to Progress against Cancer

Advances in the diagnosis of cancer have the potential to improve outcomes for many patients with the disease. Doctors and patients depend on accurate information derived from diagnostic tools, such as clinical laboratory tests, imaging studies, and genomic analysis, to make decisions at all stages of cancer care. Diagnostic tools can:

- help determine the impending risk of cancer
- help determine the extent of cancer within the body (staging)
- classify groups of patients with tumors that share certain genetic changes
- inform decisions about treatment, such as identifying the treatment that is most likely to be effective for a given patient
- assess a patient's response to treatment
- monitor a patient for a recurrence of cancer

Opportunities in Cancer Diagnosis Research

Cancer diagnosis has long relied on the microscopic examination of cells to see if they have the appearance of cancer cells. Diagnosis often

---

This chapter includes text excerpted from "Research Areas—Cancer Diagnosis Research," National Cancer Institute (NCI), March 13, 2015.

includes the use of molecular and cytogenetic markers to collect additional information about the tumor. The development of new technologies for analyzing deoxyribonucleic acid (DNA) and other molecules in tumors has created opportunities to develop additional biomarkers for cancer diagnosis.

Recognizing this opportunity, as well as the challenges involved in developing new tools and methods, researchers at National Cancer Institute (NCI) and elsewhere developed a checklist of criteria that can be used to determine the readiness of new omics-based tests for guiding patient care in clinical trials.

Omics tests include those based on such disciplines as genomics, epigenomics, transcriptomics, proteomics, and metabolomics, which is the study of small-molecule metabolites in cells and tissues that are present in bodily fluids, such as blood and urine.

Advances in technology have also created opportunities to develop and test new imaging methods in cancer diagnosis. For instance, a study by NCI researchers showed that an image-guided biopsy for the detection of prostate cancer did a better job of identifying men with a high-risk disease than standard biopsy, while also reducing the detection of low-risk disease that may not need treatment.

Other opportunities in imaging include the development of better tools for imaging tumors and for reading and interpreting scans.

Diagnostic tools that identify specific molecular abnormalities in tumors are also important in the context of precision medicine. With this information, doctors can determine whether a patient has the target for a particular targeted therapy or does not and should avoid taking the drug. In recent years, the U.S. Food and Drug Administration (FDA) has approved tests called companion diagnostics to help identify candidates for certain treatments. Patients may be required to undergo one of these tests prior to starting treatment with a targeted therapy.

Challenges in Cancer Diagnosis Research

To be useful in the clinic, diagnostic test results must be reliable and should be returned to patients and doctors within a relatively short time frame.

Establishing the predictive value of diagnostic tools is a challenge, particularly given the heterogeneity of cancers and variation in clinical courses, even for patients with the same type of cancer. In a diagnostic setting, the sensitivity of a test is important. For example, although many potential omics-based tests have shown promise in preclinical studies, few have been translated into clinically useful tests due to poor sensitivity.

More than 20 tumor markers are currently in use, but there are some limitations to the use of these diagnostic tools. Not everyone with a particular type of cancer will have a higher level of a tumor marker associated with that cancer, for example. Moreover, tumor markers have not been identified for every type of cancer.

Another research challenge is to develop ways to monitor, in real time, molecular changes within tumors over the course of treatment and beyond, particularly for tumors that are poorly accessible.

There is also a need to give patients information about the likelihood that a given tumor will be life threatening. Indeed, as the technology for identifying tumors has improved, the number of over-diagnosed cancers that are not likely to cause harm or death has risen. Therefore, there is an even greater need for tools to accurately assess the risks these tumors pose to patients.

NCI's Role in Cancer Diagnosis Research

NCI supports research on novel tools and methods for diagnosing cancer. This work includes the development of tests and imaging technologies that can provide specific information about an individual's cancer. Other priorities include the development of diagnostic tools that can be used in laboratory research.

Cancer Diagnosis Program (CDP)

One of eight major programs managed by NCI's Division of Cancer Treatment and Diagnosis (DCTD), the CDP aims to improve the diagnosis and assessment of cancer. Investigators supported by CDP work on a range of projects, including the development of diagnostic tests to better characterize cancers and provide information that can help doctors and patients make clinical decisions. The program supports research at medical centers, hospitals, businesses, and universities throughout the United States. Two CDP initiatives are the:

- Program for the Assessment of Clinical Cancer Tests (PACCT), which focuses, in part, on barriers that affect the development of improved tests for cancer diagnosis. PACCT helped facilitate a workshop on criteria for the use of "omics"-based predictors (such as genomic and proteomic test results) in NCI-supported clinical trials.

PACCT also played a role in developing the Trial Assigning Individualized Options for Treatment (TAILORx) clinical trial. This NCI-sponsored study is using a gene-based test to see if a panel of genes that are frequently associated with risk of recurrence in women with early-stage breast cancer can be used to assign patients to the most appropriate and effective treatment. Specifically, the test helps to assess the likely benefit from certain types of chemotherapy.

- Strategic Partnering to Evaluate Cancer Signatures (SPECS) program, which supports research groups that are exploring how information from molecular analyses can affect the care of patients and ultimately improve outcomes. The SPECS II program includes researchers who are studying lung, colon, and prostate cancers; acute leukemia; and non-Hodgkin lymphoma.

Cancer Imaging Program (CIP)

DCTD's CIP supports research on the use of imaging techniques to noninvasively diagnose cancer and the identification of disease subsets in patients, among other research areas. An area of focus for CIP researchers is functional or molecular imaging, which visualizes physiological, cellular, or molecular processes in living tissues as they occur. Molecular imaging is critical for fundamental improvements in the care of patients with cancer. CIP supports the:

- *In Vivo* Cellular and Molecular Imaging Centers (ICMIC), where scientists from a variety of fields conduct multidisciplinary research on cellular and molecular imaging related to cancer. Pre-ICMIC planning grants provide time and funds for investigators and institutions to prepare themselves, organizationally and scientifically, to establish ICMICs.

Early Detection Research Network (EDRN)

EDRN, managed by NCI's Division of Cancer Prevention (DCP), focuses on the development and testing of promising biomarkers or technologies to improve risk assessment and the early detection of cancer. A goal of the EDRN is to make molecular diagnostics a reality. EDRN is a consortium of more than 300 investigators who represent diverse scientific disciplines, including genomics, informatics, and public health.

Molecular and Cellular Screening of Screen-Detected Lesions (MCSSL) Initiative

MCSSL aims to reduce the number of over-diagnosed tumors by studying the biology of indolent tumors, those lesions that tend to grow slowly, to understand their progression from benign to invasive cancer. This program is managed jointly by DCP and NCI's Division of Cancer Biology (DCB).

NCI's Intramural Cancer Diagnosis Research

NCI's Center for Cancer Research (CCR) and Division of Cancer Epidemiology and Genetics (DCEG) have scientists in a number of programs that conduct studies related to cancer diagnosis research.

- CCR researchers in the Center for Advanced Preclinical Research (CAPR) have expertise in preclinical imaging studies and biomarker development.
- CCR's Clinical Molecular Profiling Core uses genomic technologies to analyze biospecimens obtained from NCI clinical trials.
- NCI's Center of Excellence in Integrative Cancer Biology and Genomics (CEICBG), which is sponsored by CCR and DCEG, promotes research efforts to identify, develop, and validate biomarkers for the early detection and diagnosis of cancer, among many other activities.

Chapter 78

Cancer Prevention Research

Research on Prevention Is Critical to Progress against Cancer

By 2025, an estimated 2.1 million people in the United States will be diagnosed with cancer every year. This is a 31-percent increase from 2012 that is due in part to the aging of the U.S. population and the greater use of cancer screening. The estimated number of annual cancer-related deaths is expected to increase even faster, by 37 percent, from 620,000 to 850,000 by 2025.

These increases make a compelling case for improvements in cancer prevention, and greater progress is possible. It has been estimated, for example, that between 1975 and 2000, tobacco control programs implemented in the United States saved nearly 800,000 lives. Continued efforts against tobacco, together with existing and emerging methods of reducing cancer risk, could pay tremendous dividends in terms of lives saved.

But there are also many obstacles to reducing cancer incidence and mortality in the United States, including socioeconomic disparities, barriers that limit access to healthcare, and widespread obesity.

Making strides in cancer prevention is not only a public health imperative, it is also an economic imperative. By 2020, the United States will spend an estimated $174 billion each year on cancer care.

This chapter includes text excerpted from "Research Areas—Cancer Prevention Research," National Cancer Institute (NCI), August 22, 2017.

Opportunities in Cancer Prevention Research

Studies that have more clearly defined how cancer develops and identified factors that can influence cancer risk are paving the way for important advances in cancer prevention.

Based on this knowledge, researchers are testing new approaches to prevent cancer. This work is informed by the following studies and programs:

- Identify the biological mechanisms by which common conditions such as obesity and diabetes are associated with cancer risk.
- Explain how the immune system recognizes and interacts with healthy, precancerous, and tumor cells and test ways to strengthen the immune system's ability to disrupt cancer development.
- Reveal how drugs used to treat other conditions affect cancer incidence and mortality and test whether they may have a role in cancer prevention.
- Develop and test ways to address the socioeconomic, biological, and other factors that contribute to higher cancer rates in specific population groups.
- Analyze the impact of different environmental exposures on cancer risk and develop interventions, including policies, that help to limit those exposures.
- Identify and test interventions that may prevent the development of cancer in those at increased risk.

Challenges in Cancer Prevention Research

Studying cancer prevention and risk reduction has its challenges. Some are related to time. It can take years or decades to determine whether an intervention—such as a new preventive therapy or policies that encourage behavioral changes that can decrease cancer risk—reduces the number of cases or deaths from cancer.

Studies used to identify environmental and behavioral risk factors also require a significant time investment. And conducting these studies comes with the cumbersome logistical hurdles inherent in studying large populations, such as developing and validating tools that accurately measure potential environmental and behavioral risk factors (such as exposure to certain toxins or dietary components and level of physical activity) and, in many cases, monitoring people over time.

Currently, there are genetic tests and risk assessment tools designed to identify people at substantially increased risk of only a few types of cancer. But researchers have struggled to develop tests that can identify people at risk for most types of cancer, due in part to the immense complexity of cancer.

Developing preventive therapies has many challenges. Even as researchers begin to better understand the events in cells that initiate cancer, developing interventions that specifically block or interfere with these events is a complicated and lengthy process.

In addition, prevention research often involves studying a population of people who, although they may be at increased risk of disease, are often otherwise healthy. Consequently, potential preventive therapies must meet a higher bar for safety than therapies used to treat cancer.

And, perhaps with the exception of developing vaccines, the private sector traditionally has had limited interest in spending resources on prevention and risk reduction.

NCI's Role in Cancer Prevention Research

National Cancer Institute (NCI) supports and conducts a broad range of cancer prevention research focused on developing and testing preventive interventions, expanding our understanding of the biological processes through which cancer develops, studying ways to reduce cancer risk, and disseminating preventive interventions. The Division of Cancer Prevention (DCP) leads NCI's cancer prevention research efforts and provides funding and administrative support to extramural researchers who conduct cancer prevention research.

New Cancer Prevention Approaches

NCI supports programs and studies that identify and develop interventions designed to reduce cancer risk in people with no history of the disease and to prevent recurrences or second primary malignancies in patients who have already been treated for cancer.

The Pre-Cancer Atlas (PCA), an initiative that is currently under development, will provide a comprehensive analysis of precancerous tissue and its surrounding microenvironment. The goal of PCA is to understand how precancers change to invasive cancer over time. The data generated through this initiative will help develop models for cancer researchers that can both predict and inform new or improved methods to prevent cancer.

The NCI Community Oncology Research Program (NCORP) is a national network that brings clinical trials and studies, including cancer prevention trials, to people in their own communities. NCORP is generating a broadly applicable evidence base that contributes to improving patient outcomes and to reducing cancer disparities.

The PREVENT Cancer Preclinical Drug Development Program helps bring new cancer prevention agents and biomarkers through the early stages of research. The program is currently supporting the development of a number of new agents, as well as the evaluation of several drugs already in use for other diseases and conditions, including aspirin and the diabetes drug metformin.

Through the Phase 0/I/II Cancer Prevention Clinical Trials Program, NCI conducts early-stage trials of new therapies for patients at increased cancer risk. One such trial tested whether sulindac, a nonsteroidal anti-inflammatory drug, reduces the risk of several different cancers in people at increased risk.

Research led by two scientists in NCI's Center for Cancer Research (CCR) directly contributed to the development of U.S. Food and Drug Administration (FDA)-approved human papillomavirus (HPV) vaccines—work for which they were awarded the National Medal of Technology and Innovation in 2014. CCR scientists are collaborating with other researchers to develop next-generation HPV vaccines designed to have a greater capacity to halt HPV infections, which can lead to cervical, oral, anal, and several other cancers.

Researchers from NCI's Division of Cancer Epidemiology and Genetics (DCEG) led a large clinical trial of the bivalent HPV vaccine that established its safety and efficacy with regard to cervical cancer and HPV-associated cancer at other anatomic sites. The trial has transitioned to an epidemiologic cohort study involving long-term follow-up to evaluate the vaccine's durability. DCEG scientists continue to analyze data from this trial and other HPV vaccine trials to evaluate the impact of different dosing regimens.

Enhancing Cancer Risk Reduction

Encouraging healthy behaviors that reduce cancer risk underpins NCI's involvement in the public-private National Collaborative on Childhood Obesity Research (NCCOR). Through NCCOR, researchers in NCI's Division of Cancer Control and Population Sciences are leading the Family Life, Activity, Sun, Health, and Eating Study to better understand what factors in the lives of children and their families, such as diet, physical activity, tobacco use, and sun exposure, affect their cancer risk.

One of the landmark public health achievements of the past 30 years has been the reduction in tobacco use. NCI's Tobacco Control Research Branch (TCRB) supports studies to monitor tobacco use patterns, identify factors that influence tobacco use rates (such as smoking in movies, advertising at sporting events), and develop and test ways to help tobacco users quit or prevent them from starting in the first place.

DCEG research has helped to identify numerous environmental, biological, and behavioral risk factors that increase cancer risk. A study co-led by DCEG researchers, for example, was the first to definitively link exposure to radiation from computed tomography (CT) scans and cancer risk in children—increasing awareness about the potential risks of medical radiation and emphasizing the need to keep radiation doses during CT procedures on children as low as possible.

The NCI Cohort Consortium conducts numerous studies using cohorts that include more than 4 million people in the United States and abroad. These studies seek to identify factors (including environmental, lifestyle, and genetic) that may influence cancer risk.

NCI investigators have also been among the leaders in genome-wide association studies (GWAS). By identifying genetic variations that are more common in people with a disease than those without the disease, GWAS are helping researchers better understand the mechanisms of disease initiation and development. Often using data from NCI-supported cohort and case-control studies, NCI-led GWAS have identified hundreds of genetic variants associated with cancer risk. For example, a DCEG study implicated single-nucleotide polymorphisms that play a role in the clearance of the hepatitis C virus (HCV), either spontaneously or in response to treatment.

Prevention and Cancer Disparities

Prevention is an important component in reducing cancer health disparities, including the higher incidence and mortality rates in some population groups.

NCI's Center to Reduce Cancer Health Disparities (CRCHD) supports programs that increase access to and use of preventive measures, such as smoking cessation, in communities in which marked disparities have been documented.

Disparities are also a focus of NCI's NCORP, which supports prevention-focused clinical studies at the community level. Currently, 12 of NCORP's 34 sites are Minority/Underserved Community Sites, with patient populations comprised of at least 30 percent racial/ethnic minorities or rural residents.

Chapter 79

Cancer Treatment Research

Cancer Treatment Research Is Critical to Progress against the Disease

Research on the treatment of cancer is fundamental to improving outcomes for patients affected by the disease. These efforts include the development of more effective and less toxic treatments, such as targeted therapies, immunotherapies, and cancer vaccines, as well as the improvement of therapies that have existed for decades, such as chemotherapy, radiation therapy, and surgery. And some studies address better management of a treatment's toxic effects, thereby improving a patient's ability to receive effective cancer treatment. Still, other studies test whether less intensive therapy or no therapy at all will result in the same outcome.

Opportunities in Cancer Treatment Research

Decades of research on the biology of cancer have revealed insights into the mechanisms that drive the disease. Data from molecular and other studies indicate that, even within a given cancer, there are differences in how the cancer behaves and how it responds to treatment. In addition to identifying genetic, epigenetic, and other molecular changes that may promote the development and growth of tumors,

---

This chapter includes text excerpted from "Cancer Treatment Research," National Cancer Institute (NCI), May 22, 2017.

researchers have learned about the ways that tumors can survive and thrive in the body.

For example, tumors have the ability to develop their own blood supplies, manipulate the immune system to tamp down immune responses, and recruit normal cells to help them grow. Just as important, tumor cells can ignore signals that normally tell old or damaged cells to die.

This new understanding has created opportunities to develop targeted therapies—cancer treatments that target the specific changes, most often in proteins, that underlie the growth and development of cancer. Surgery, radiation therapy, and standard chemotherapy will continue to play an important role in treating cancer, but the emergence in recent years of targeted therapies and of immunotherapies, which harness the power of the immune system to fight cancer, have expanded the treatment options available to patients with certain types of cancer.

Another important opportunity comes from the finding that similar molecular changes are shared among cancers that arise at different sites in the body. For example, The Cancer Genome Atlas (TCGA) Research Network recently identified genomic similarities between endometrial and other types of cancer, including breast, ovarian, and colorectal cancers. Therefore, treatments that target specific molecular changes may work not only against the cancer for which they were developed, but also against tumors from other sites that happen to carry the same alterations.

Challenges in Cancer Treatment Research

Although many advances in cancer treatment have been made in recent decades, numerous challenges remain before the goal of providing the best possible outcome for all patients diagnosed with cancer can be achieved.

For example, developing targeted therapies requires the identification of good molecular targets—that is, targets that play a key role in cancer cell growth and survival—and the design and development of drugs that effectively "hit," or bind to, those targets. However, some potential targets that have been identified appear to lack places to which an anticancer drug can bind and, therefore, have been called "undruggable." Finding ways to design drugs that effectively hit these targets is a major challenge.

Drug resistance—either to traditional chemotherapy drugs or to newer targeted therapies—is another challenge in cancer treatment.

More research is needed to uncover the mechanisms of drug resistance and identify ways to overcome it.

The genomic characterization of tumors has provided both new opportunities for cancer treatment and new challenges. The discovery that each individual's cancer has a unique constellation of gene mutations and other alterations increases the complexity of identifying treatments that are likely to work best for a given person's cancer. However, even within a single patient, different parts of a single tumor, or different metastatic tumor nodules in the same patient, may not be identical in terms of the molecular changes that are present. This raises the possibility that a drug might be effective in one part of a person's tumor but not in another.

Moreover, although recent advances in immunotherapy have been dramatic, this approach to treating cancer is still in its infancy. Many challenges remain, including how to optimize the immune response to eradicate cancer while avoiding runaway responses that cause autoimmune damage to normal tissues. An additional challenge is determining why current immunotherapies work in some patients but not in others.

Many challenges also remain in optimizing cancer treatment with conventional chemotherapy drugs, radiation therapy, and surgery. Research on the identification and development of additional chemotherapeutic agents is needed, as is research to refine the delivery of lethal doses of radiation therapy to tumors while sparing the surrounding normal tissues from harm. Another challenge is the development of ever more effective treatments to alleviate the side effects of all forms of cancer therapy.

NCI's Role in Cancer Treatment Research

For more than 50 years, National Cancer Institute (NCI) has played an active role in the cancer drug development process—from conducting preclinical studies in the laboratory to testing potential therapies in humans. NCI's influence is reflected in the fact that approximately half of the chemotherapeutic drugs currently used by oncologists to treat cancer were discovered and/or developed by NCI-funded researchers.

The institute sponsors treatment clinical trials that are conducted by NCI researchers at the National Institutes of Health (NIH) in Bethesda, MD, and at cancer centers, hospitals, and community practices around the country. The Cancer Therapy Evaluation Program (CTEP) in NCI's Division of Cancer Treatment and Diagnosis (DCTD) functions as the institute's primary clinical evaluator of new anticancer agents, radiation treatments, and surgical methods. For details, see NCI's Clinical Trials Programs and Initiatives.

NCI is also leading efforts on several fronts to determine the most efficient and effective ways to evaluate new anticancer therapies, such as developing new clinical trial designs that are more appropriate for precision medicine and immunotherapies.

Drug Discovery and Development

National Cancer Institute's (NCI) Developmental Therapeutics Program (DTP), which is also part of DCTD, has a repository of more than 400,000 compounds that have gone through some kind of screening process. About 80,000 compounds have been screened since 1990. DTP participates in all stages of preclinical drug discovery and development.

A compound is first screened against a variety of human tumor cell lines, growing in tissue culture dishes, to test its ability to prevent the growth of specific kinds of cancer cells. If the drug shows some evidence of anticancer activity, extensive testing in animals will determine whether it is effective enough for testing in humans.

NCI's Center for Advanced Preclinical Research (CAPR), a component of NCI's Center for Cancer Research (CCR), conducts comprehensive preclinical testing of early-stage candidate drugs. Candidate compounds are assessed for antitumor efficacy and selectivity in genetically engineered animal models. Other projects at CAPR include the development of imaging technologies to monitor disease and treatment.

Of all the compounds screened by NCI, about 40 percent come from industry, and the rest primarily come from academic collaborators. Another source of novel compounds is the Natural Products Branch, a part of the DCTD DTP that collaborates with agencies throughout the world to collect thousands of plant and marine organisms to screen for potential anticancer compounds.

To expedite drug discovery, NCI provides sample sets of more than 140,000 synthetic chemicals, 80,000 natural products extracted from plants and marine organisms, and other biological materials to investigators who might have discovered potential cancer-associated molecular targets.

The NCI Formulary, a public-private partnership between NCI and pharmaceutical and biotechnology companies, will give investigators at NCI-Designated Cancer Centers quicker access to approved and investigational agents for use in cancer clinical trials. Eligible investigators will be able to apply for access to agents from the available formulary list and test them in new preclinical or clinical studies, including combination studies of formulary agents from different companies.

Academic and private industry laboratories engaged in drug discovery may face financial and technical burdens that keep promising therapeutic agents from reaching patients. DTP has helped and will continue to help the academic and private sectors overcome various therapeutic development barriers, in particular by supporting high-risk projects and the development of therapies for rare cancers.

Human Tumor Cell Lines and Models

A unique resource in DTP's anticancer drug discovery program is a collection of 60 human tumor cell lines that can be used to evaluate compounds for anticancer activity. The NCI-60 Human Tumor Cell Lines Screen represents nine different types of cancer: breast, ovary, prostate, colon, lung, kidney, brain, leukemia, and melanoma. These are the most frequently studied human tumor cell lines in cancer research, molecular pharmacology, and drug discovery.

The *In Vitro* Cell Line Screening Project (IVCLSP) supports the DTP anticancer drug discovery program. This project is designed to screen up to 3,000 compounds per year for potential anticancer activity using the NCI-60 human tumor cell lines. The aim is to prioritize, for further evaluation, promising synthetic compounds or natural product samples with anticancer properties.

NCI has developed the Patient-Derived Models Repository (PDMR) to serve as a resource for public-private partnerships and for academic drug discovery efforts. The patient-derived models (PDMs) being developed for the repository are derived from tumor tissue or circulating tumor cells (CTCs) and are propagated both *in vitro* using 2D or 3D cell culture systems and *in vivo* passaging in mice as patient-derived xenografts (PDXs). These PDMs are early-passage, molecularly characterized, and clinically annotated and will be made available to the research community at a minimal cost. All associated metadata will be available for review through the publicly accessible website without the need to acquire a model beforehand.

The international Human Cancer Model Initiative (HCMI) is generating novel human tumor-derived culture models with the goal of creating cancer models that recapitulate patients' tumors as faithfully as possible. The models are annotated with genomic and clinical data and are available to the wider research community to define cancer pathways, determine mechanisms of drug resistance, and assess responses to small molecules. NCI contributes to the initiative by providing funding and support to two Cancer Model Development Centers.

Radiation Therapy, Cancer Vaccines, and Immunotherapies

Finding new ways to more specifically target radiation therapy to tumors and spare as much normal tissue as possible is paramount for maintaining patients' quality of life and improving cure rates. NCI's Radiation Research Program (RRP), which is part of DCTD, provides expertise to investigators who perform radiotherapy research and assists in establishing future radiation research directions.

Cancer treatment vaccines are designed to boost the body's natural ability to protect itself, through the immune system, from dangers posed by damaged or abnormal cells, such as cancer cells. Researchers are developing treatment vaccines against many types of cancer and testing them in clinical trials.

Developing effective cancer treatment vaccines requires a detailed understanding of how immune system cells and cancer cells interact. CCR's Vaccine Branch studies basic mechanisms of immune response and molecular virology. These findings are applied to the development of vaccines and immunotherapy for the prevention and treatment of cancer and acquired immune deficiency syndrome (AIDS), as well as viruses that cause cancer.

Immunotherapies are treatments that stimulate the activities of specific components of the immune system or counteract signals produced by cancer cells that suppress immune responses. CCR researchers conducted pioneering research that has led to the first effective immunotherapies for selected patients with advanced cancer. These studies of cell transfer immunotherapy have resulted in durable complete remissions in patients with metastatic melanoma.

Translational Research

DCTD's Translational Research Program (TRP) supports efforts through the Specialized Programs of Excellence (SPOREs) to translate novel scientific discoveries from the laboratory to the clinic for testing in humans and to determine the biological basis for observations made in cancer patients or in populations at risk for cancer. Recent projects have included a study to define the importance of immunity to an antigen in melanoma therapy and targeted therapies for childhood acute lymphoblastic leukemia.

CCR's Developmental Therapeutics Branch (DTB) integrates both basic science and translational clinical programs. The basic science program focuses on cancer-specific genomic and epigenomic alterations, oxidative signaling, molecular pharmacology, and drug resistance. The translational clinical program focuses on novel therapeutic agents across a spectrum of diseases and disease mechanisms.

Within DTB, the Genomics and Bioinformatics Group explores the relationships between genomic alterations in malignant cells and their response to chemotherapeutic agents using molecular databases at the deoxyribonucleic acid (DNA), ribonucleic acid (RNA), and protein levels.

The PREVENT Cancer Preclinical Drug Development Program helps bring new cancer preventing interventions and biomarkers through the early stages of research required before testing in human clinical trials. The program, which is part of NCI's Division of Cancer Prevention (DCP), currently supports the development of a number of new agents and several drugs already in use for other diseases and conditions, including aspirin and the diabetes drug metformin. Clinical evaluation of these and other promising new agents and strategies to prevent cancer is performed by the Phase 0/I/II Cancer Prevention Clinical Trials Program.

Exceptional Responders Initiative and NExT

Exceptional responders are patients who respond to treatments that are not effective for most other patients. NCI launched the Exceptional Responders Initiative to determine whether certain molecular features of the malignant tissue in patients who respond exceptionally well can predict the responses of future patients to the same or similar drugs. In the study, investigators will study the molecular characteristics of tumors from patients who had an exceptional response to a systemic cancer therapy. Where possible, nontumor specimens (or "normal" tissue) from the patients will also be examined, as these help in determining which mutations are present only in the tumor, rather than in normal cells and tissue.

NCI's Experimental Therapeutics Program (NExT) focuses on advancing breakthrough discoveries in basic and clinical research into new therapies to treat cancer patients. This translational research effort unites the drug development expertise of DCTD with CCR's dynamic research programs and the facilities at the NIH Clinical Center (CC) to advance new therapeutic interventions from both the private and public sectors.

Supportive and Palliative Care

Supportive and palliative care studies focus on the prevention and treatment of acute and chronic symptoms and side effects related to cancer and its treatment. Research is also done to study the effect of treatment on cancer patients' quality of life and the psychosocial issues and strategies for care at the end of life. The NCI Community Oncology Research Program (NCORP) network supports studies on the molecular determinants of treatment toxicities and cancer-related symptoms and on the management of treatment-related effects like fatigue, musculoskeletal pain, nerve damage, and ovarian failure.

Chapter 80

Oncolytic Virus Therapy

For more than a century, doctors have been interested in using viruses to treat cancer, and in recent years a small but growing number of patients have begun to benefit from this approach.

Some viruses tend to infect and kill tumor cells. Known as oncolytic viruses, this group includes viruses found in nature as well as viruses modified in the laboratory to reproduce efficiently in cancer cells without harming healthy cells.

To date, only one oncolytic virus—a genetically modified form of a herpesvirus for treating melanoma—has been approved by the U.S. Food and Drug Administration (FDA), though a number of viruses are being evaluated as potential treatments for cancer in clinical trials.

Oncolytic viruses have long been viewed as tools for directly killing cancer cells. But a growing body of research suggests that some oncolytic viruses may work—at least in part—by triggering an immune response in the body against the cancer.

When a virus infects a tumor cell, the virus makes copies of itself until the cell bursts. The dying cancer cell releases materials, such as tumor antigens, that allow the cancer to be recognized, or "seen," by the immune system.

"Oncolytic viruses are alerting the immune system that something's wrong," said Jason Chesney, M.D., Ph.D., director of the University of Louisville's (UofL) James Graham Brown Cancer Center. This can lead

---

This chapter includes text excerpted from "Oncolytic Virus Therapy: Using Tumor-Targeting Viruses to Treat Cancer," National Cancer Institute (NCI), February 9, 2018.

to an immune response against nearby tumor cells (a local response) or tumor cells in other parts of the body (a systemic response).

For this reason, some researchers consider oncolytic viruses to be a form of immunotherapy—a treatment that harnesses the immune system against cancer. But many in the field would agree that more studies are needed to learn how different oncolytic viruses work against cancer.

A Modern Approach to an Old Idea

Since the late 1800s, doctors have observed that some patients with cancer go into remission, if only temporarily, after a viral infection. At present, several dozen viruses—and a few strains of bacteria—are being studied as potential cancer treatments, according to research presented at an National Cancer Institute (NCI)-sponsored conference on using microbes as cancer therapies in 2017.

"Oncolytic virus therapy is of growing interest to researchers for one reason: It's working," said Juan Fueyo, M.D., of the University of Texas MD Anderson Cancer Center, who codeveloped a type of oncolytic virus being tested in patients with brain tumors.

Although the notion of using viruses in cancer therapy is old, the science only began to move forward in the 1990s with advances in genetic engineering technology, noted Matthias Gromeier, M.D., of the Duke Cancer Institute (DCI), who has led clinical trials of a genetically modified form of poliovirus.

"There was another shift—around 2005—as people began to realize that the true value of viruses in cancer therapy is in immunotherapy," Dr. Gromeier continued. "At present, viruses are firmly established as a potential option to enhance and mediate immunotherapy."

He added: "These are still early days for oncolytic viruses, but it's now getting interesting."

The First FDA-Approved Oncolytic Virus Therapy

The first oncolytic virus to receive FDA approval was a treatment for melanoma known as talimogene laherparepvec (Imlygic®) or T-VEC. The treatment, which is injected into tumors, was engineered to produce a protein that stimulates the production of immune cells in the body and to reduce the risk of causing herpes.

In some patients receiving the therapy, tumors that could not be injected have shrunk, suggesting that T-VEC can generate a systemic immune response, noted Howard Kaufman, M.D., of the Rutgers Cancer Institute of New Jersey.

"The oncolytic virus kills tumor cells and causes the release of danger signals, which help to generate an immune response," explained Dr. Kaufman, who co-led the clinical trial that led to the approval of T-VEC.

Investigating Interactions with the Immune System

At the NCI meeting about using microbes as cancer therapies last year, more than 350 investigators discussed many topics, including the need to better understand how infectious agents interact with tumors and with components of the immune system.

The biological mechanisms used by viruses to kill tumors depend on various factors, including the virus, the target tissue or cell, and which biological pathways are targeted, according to Phillip Daschner of NCI's Division of Cancer Biology (DCB), who helped organize the NCI conference.

Some viruses work primarily by killing tumor cells, whereas others work by directing local or systemic immune responses, he explained. Nonetheless, "there was a consensus at the meeting that even for directly oncolytic therapies, there probably is an important immune component to the response," he added.

Dr. Kaufman noted that T-VEC, when given alone or in combination with other therapies, generally has been well tolerated by patients in clinical trials.

"We continue to be impressed by the safety profile of these approaches," he said. "The quality of life for many of these patients is barely affected by these agents."

Using Viruses to Enhance the Body's Immune Response

One of the challenges for researchers now is to try to enhance the immune response to the tumor through a variety of strategies, including by combining oncolytic virus therapy and immunotherapy.

The promise of this approach has been demonstrated in two early-phase clinical trials. Patients with melanoma who received T-VEC plus a type of immunotherapy known as a checkpoint inhibitor had higher response rates than those who received a checkpoint inhibitor alone.

In one trial, nearly 200 patients received T-VEC with or without ipilimumab (Yervoy®). The results suggested to the researchers that the combination therapy could induce an immune response. "To me, that's the big finding of this study," said Dr. Chesney, who co-led the clinical trial with Dr. Kaufman.

In the second trial, which included 21 patients, T-VEC was combined with pembrolizumab (Keytruda®). The oncolytic virus induced the infiltration of immune cells known as T cells into tumors that had low levels of these cells prior to treatment, the researchers found.

The study suggests that the viral therapy can change the local microenvironment to make an immunologically "cold" tumor—that is, a tumor lacking T cells—into an inflamed, or "hot," tumor, noted John B.A.G. Haanen, Ph.D., of the Netherlands Cancer Institute (NKI) in a commentary accompanying the study results.

"The injection [of T-VEC] is like lighting a match—it's the spark that starts a fire," said Antoni Ribas, M.D., Ph.D., of the UCLA Jonsson Comprehensive Cancer Center (JCCC), who led the trial. The therapy was generally well tolerated, he noted, and the most common side effects were fatigue, fever, and chills.

A phase 3 clinical trial involving 600 patients with melanoma who will receive T-VEC with or without pembrolizumab is underway to assess the combination therapy in a large, randomized study.

The same combination—T-VEC plus pembrolizumab—is also being evaluated in a clinical trial for patients with advanced melanoma that has progressed despite treatment with a checkpoint inhibitor such as pembrolizumab or nivolumab (Opdivo®).

This NCI-sponsored trial is testing the idea that injections of T-VEC into accessible melanoma tumors will increase the infiltration of immune cells into these and potentially other tumors, making them susceptible to treatment with pembrolizumab.

A New Way of Delivering Viruses

Most oncolytic virus therapies have been tested in patients with melanoma or brain tumors, and most treatments have been given as injections into tumors. Two new studies highlight efforts to expand the number of cancer types treated with oncolytic virus therapies as well as the methods of delivery.

One of the studies found that an oncolytic virus delivered intravenously could cross the blood-brain barrier and enter brain tumors, killing tumor cells. The treatment uses a type of virus known as a reovirus, which causes mild symptoms of a cold or stomach bug in children.

In the second study, researchers tested the Maraba virus, which was originally isolated from a species of sand fly in Brazil, as a way to sensitize tumors to immunotherapy in a mouse model of triple-negative breast cancer.

In both studies, the researchers found that giving oncolytic virus therapy prior to surgery may alter the body's immune response and enhance the effects of subsequent treatment with a checkpoint inhibitor.

"Combination immunotherapies like these may be most effective when used early in treatment when tumor burden is less and immune systems are intact," noted Marie-Claude Bourgeois-Daigneault, Ph.D., of the University of Ottawa, an investigator on the Maraba virus study.

Testing a Modified Form of Poliovirus against Brain Tumors

At the DCI, Dr. Gromeier and his colleagues have been testing an engineered poliovirus, called PVS-RIPO, in patients with glioblastoma.

When the research began in the mid-1990s, Dr. Gromeier viewed oncolytic viruses primarily as agents for killing cancer cells. His thinking changed, however, as PVS-RIPO was tested in patients, and his team noticed clinical changes associated with immune responses in the patients.

"From the first patients, we observed very clear signs that the virus elicited antitumor immune responses," Dr. Gromeier recalled. Some patients had swelling in the brain and "profound changes in the tumor that took months to develop, which is consistent with an immune event," he explained.

Based on the results of the clinical studies, FDA in 2016 granted "breakthrough status" to Duke's poliovirus therapy, which allows officials at FDA to accelerate the agency's review of the therapy for approval.

"We are interested in exploring what we can combine with PVS-RIPO," said Dr. Gromeier. "Everyone seems to agree that no single mode of treatment will do the trick in treating cancer."

A phase 2 trial testing PVS-RIPO with or without the chemotherapy drug lomustine (Gleostine®) is underway in patients with glioblastoma.

Investigating the Mechanisms of Oncolytic Virus Therapy

To learn more about the mechanisms by which poliovirus therapy attacks tumor cells, the Duke researchers recently conducted experiments in cancer cell lines and in mice.

They found that cancer cells infected with PVS-RIPO released tumor antigens and other material that activated immune cells called dendritic cells and induced an immune response against the cancer cells.

"In the mouse model, we showed that a poliovirus could induce a T-cell response that recognizes the tumor," said Smita Nair, Ph.D., of the Duke University School of Medicine. The finding provides further support for testing the oncolytic virus in combination with other types of immunotherapies, including checkpoint inhibitors, she added.

The Duke team is planning a clinical trial to test PVS-RIPO in six patients with triple-negative breast cancer. Two weeks before undergoing surgery, the patients will receive injections of the treatment into their tumors and will be followed to determine whether the poliovirus triggers any changes in immune system molecules or in the tumor.

Future Research Questions and Priorities for the Field

As oncolytic viruses are tested in clinical trials, researchers will try to learn which patients are likely to respond. "We need biomarkers to help develop effective combination therapies and to select patients who are most likely to benefit from certain combinations," said Dr. Nair.

Another challenge for the field will be to use the knowledge gained from the melanoma clinical trials to develop treatments for patients with other types of tumors, Dr. Chesney noted.

For researchers, it will also be important to understand "how much tumor infection and killing is required to treat cancer," said Dr. Gromeier. "These are critical questions that we need to answer, and we're working on it."

Oncolytic Viruses May Also Reveal Insights into Immunotherapy

Research on oncolytic viruses may yield insights into the use of current immunotherapies.

"Viruses are great tools for helping us to understand how the antitumor immune response works," said Dr. Fueyo of MD Anderson. "What we learn from viruses will help us move the field of immunotherapy forward."

The evolution in thinking about oncolytic viruses since Dr. Fueyo began working in the field two decades ago represents an important shift that has implications for future research.

"We used to think only about making viruses better—more powerful—at killing tumor cells," said Dr. Fueyo. "Now we need to find ways to help viruses enhance the immune response."

Chapter 81

Gene Therapy for Cancer

The U.S. Food and Drug Administration (FDA) approved Yescarta (axicabtagene ciloleucel), a cell-based gene therapy, to treat adult patients with certain types of large B-cell lymphoma who have not responded to or who have relapsed after at least two other kinds of treatment. Yescarta, a chimeric antigen receptor (CAR) T cell therapy, is the second gene therapy approved by the FDA and the first for certain types of non-Hodgkin lymphoma (NHL).

"This day marks another milestone in the development of a whole new scientific paradigm for the treatment of serious diseases. In just several decades, gene therapy has gone from being a promising concept to a practical solution to deadly and largely untreatable forms of cancer," said FDA Commissioner Scott Gottlieb, M.D. "This approval demonstrates the continued momentum of this promising area of medicine and we're committed to supporting and helping expedite the development of these products. We will soon release a comprehensive policy to address how we plan to support the development of cell-based regenerative medicine. That policy will also clarify how we will apply our expedited programs to breakthrough products that use CAR-T cells and other gene therapies. We remain committed to supporting the efficient development of safe and effective treatments that leverage these scientific platforms."

This chapter includes text excerpted from "FDA Approves CAR-T Cell Therapy to Treat Adults with Certain Types of Large B-Cell Lymphoma," U.S. Food and Drug Administration (FDA), October 18, 2017.

Diffuse large B-cell lymphoma (DLBCL) is the most common type of NHL in adults. NHLs are cancers that begin in certain cells of the immune system and can be either fast growing (aggressive) or slow growing. Approximately 72,000 cases of NHL are diagnosed in the United States each year, and DLBCL represents approximately one in three newly diagnosed cases. Yescarta is approved for use in adult patients with large B-cell lymphoma after at least two other kinds of treatment failed, including DLBCL, primary mediastinal large B-cell lymphoma (PMBCL), high-grade B-cell lymphoma (HGBL), and DLBCL arising from follicular lymphoma. Yescarta is not indicated for the treatment of patients with primary central nervous system lymphoma.

Each dose of Yescarta is a customized treatment created using a patient's own immune system to help fight the lymphoma. The patient's T cells, a type of white blood cell, are collected and genetically modified to include a new gene that targets and kills the lymphoma cells. Once the cells are modified, they are infused back into the patient.

"The approval of Yescarta brings this innovative class of CAR-T cell therapies to an additional group of cancer patients with few other options—those adults with certain types of lymphoma that have not responded to previous treatments," said Peter Marks, M.D., Ph.D., director of the FDA's Center for Biologics Evaluation and Research (CBER).

The safety and efficacy of Yescarta were established in a multicenter clinical trial of more than 100 adults with refractory or relapsed large B-cell lymphoma. The complete remission rate after treatment with Yescarta was 51 percent.

Treatment with Yescarta has the potential to cause severe side effects. It carries a boxed warning for cytokine release syndrome (CRS), which is a systemic response to the activation and proliferation of CAR-T cells causing high fever and flu-like symptoms, and for neurologic toxicities. Both CRS and neurologic toxicities can be fatal or life threatening. Other side effects include serious infections, low blood cell counts, and a weakened immune system. Side effects from treatment with Yescarta usually appear within the first 1–2 weeks, but some side effects may occur later.

Because of the risk of CRS and neurologic toxicities, Yescarta is being approved with a risk evaluation and mitigation strategy (REMS), which includes elements to assure safe use (ETASU). The FDA is requiring that hospitals and their associated clinics that dispense Yescarta be specially certified. As part of that certification, staff involved in the prescribing, dispensing or administering of Yescarta are required to be trained to recognize and manage CRS and nervous system toxicities. Also, patients must be informed of the potentially serious side effects and of the importance of promptly returning to the treatment site if side effects develop. To further evaluate the long-term safety, the FDA is also requiring the manufacturer to conduct a post-marketing observational study involving patients treated with Yescarta.

The FDA granted Yescarta Priority Review and Breakthrough Therapy designations. Yescarta also received Orphan Drug designation, which provides incentives to assist and encourage the development of drugs for rare diseases. The Yescarta application was reviewed using a coordinated, cross-agency approach. The clinical review was conducted by the FDA's Oncology Center of Excellence (OCE), while CBER conducted all other aspects of review and made the final product approval determination.

The FDA granted approval of Yescarta to Kite Pharma, Inc. The FDA, an agency within the U.S. Department of Health and Human Services (HHS), protects the public health by assuring the safety, effectiveness, and security of human and veterinary drugs, vaccines, and other biological products for human use, and medical devices. The agency also is responsible for the safety and security of our nation's food supply, cosmetics, dietary supplements, products that give off electronic radiation, and for regulating tobacco products.

Chapter 82

Liquid Biopsy: Using DNA in Blood to Detect, Track, and Treat Cancer

When a patient has a suspicious lump or symptoms, one of the first things a doctor may do is perform a tissue biopsy—a procedure to collect cells for closer examination.

Examining the appearance of the cells under the microscope can determine if cancer is present, show what type of cancer it is, and give clues about the patient's prognosis. In addition, molecular analysis of a tissue biopsy sample can also reveal information that may help guide a personalized treatment strategy.

Although they are important for patient care, tissue biopsies—which may involve a large needle, an endoscope, or open surgery—can be invasive, risky, costly, and painful. And some patients may not be able to have a tissue biopsy due to the inaccessibility of their tumors or because they have other health conditions that prevent them from undergoing the procedure.

Because these factors make it difficult to perform repeated biopsies on a patient, these tests can be an impractical method to track tumors as they develop and change over time. Nevertheless, they remain the gold standard for detecting and obtaining information about cancer.

This chapter includes text excerpted from "Liquid Biopsy: Using DNA in Blood to Detect, Track, and Treat Cancer," National Cancer Institute (NCI), November 8, 2017.

But researchers have been exploring a new approach that could potentially complement or, in some cases, serve as an alternative to tissue biopsies. The approach, often called a liquid biopsy, relies on analyzing bits of tumor material—molecules as well as whole cells—that are found in bodily fluids such as blood or urine.

Although there is a widespread belief that liquid biopsies could eventually have a significant impact on patient care, most researchers in the field agree that the science around the approach is still evolving and important questions remain unanswered.

"I think the major stumbling block for moving these liquid biopsy tests forward is there is not enough clinical verification and validation to know and feel comfortable that what we're detecting with them is clinically meaningful," said Lynn Sorbara, Ph.D., of National Cancer Institute's (NCI) Division of Cancer Prevention (DCP).

Different Tests for Different Tumor Molecules

More than 100 years ago, scientists discovered that tumors shed molecules and cells into bodily fluids. Much more recently, researchers have shown that analyzing these molecules and cells can reveal some of the same information that tissue biopsies provide.

Liquid biopsy research has recently expanded, generating an entirely new field of study. Both academic and industry researchers from diverse areas of expertise are working on many fronts to develop, refine, and establish clinical uses for liquid biopsy tests.

Different liquid biopsy tests analyze different kinds of tumor material, such as deoxyribonucleic acid (DNA), ribonucleic acid (RNA), proteins, tiny vesicles called exosomes, and whole cells. The tests detect these molecules or cells in various bodily fluids, including blood, urine, cerebrospinal fluid, or saliva. These body fluids are usually readily accessible, and in most cases the procedure for collecting a sample is less invasive and more easily repeatable than a tissue biopsy.

This feature gives liquid biopsies the potential to be used for several important applications for which tissue biopsies are not well suited, explained Miguel Ossandon, M.S., program manager for the Cancer Diagnosis Program (CDP) in NCI's Division of Cancer Treatment and Diagnosis (DCTD).

For example, liquid biopsies could be used to monitor cancer development, track a patient's response to treatment, or as a "surveillance" method for people who have completed treatment but are at high risk of their disease returning, he said.

"The variety of technologies emerging to enable more precise and robust analysis of circulating molecules, cells, and everything in-between, certainly suggests that the exciting clinical potential for liquid biopsy approaches is more a question of 'when' rather than 'if'," said Tony Dickherber, Ph.D., director of NCI's Innovative Molecular Analysis Technologies (IMAT) program.

There has been a recent surge of research related to liquid biopsy tests that analyze tumor DNA in blood, called circulating tumor DNA (ctDNA), and several ctDNA-based liquid biopsy tests are in clinical development.

Using Tumor DNA to Detect Cancer Early

One potential application of ctDNA-based liquid biopsies is for detecting cancer at an early stage, when treatment may be most successful. In several studies, for example, liquid biopsy tests detected ctDNA in blood samples collected from patients months before they were diagnosed with cancer by traditional methods, such as imaging tests.

But, in these studies, the tests sometimes produced false-positive test results—that is, they detected cancerous DNA when no cancer actually developed.

Another concern is that these tests will detect early-stage tumors that will not grow much or will grow so slowly that they would never actually harm the patient.

Treating these slow-growing tumors could actually do more harm than good, and "the risk of overtreatment is a major concern with early cancer detection," Dr. Sorbara noted. "The idea of diagnosing somebody using liquid biopsy alone has not been validated yet. We're still at the early stages and have a long way to go," she continued.

Prospective cohort studies are needed to truly determine if the presence of ctDNA in a patient's blood can be used as an accurate marker for early-stage cancer, she added. For example, studies are needed to determine if the detection of ctDNA warrants treatment and if that treatment improves patient outcomes.

NCI is supporting an initiative to advance the development and validation of liquid biopsy technologies that can detect early-stage cancers, distinguish cancer from benign conditions, and identify fast- and slow-growing cancers. A major aim of the initiative is to create a public-private partnership that brings engineering and clinical experts together to accomplish these goals.

Looking forward, Dr. Sorbara envisions that liquid biopsy tests may be used to screen for early-stage cancer in high-risk individuals, such as those with hereditary cancer syndromes.

Or, she continued, they could be used in tandem with other tests, such as an magnetic resonance imaging (MRI). For example, a liquid biopsy test could be used as a routine prescreening method in healthy individuals to identify those who may have early-stage cancer and are candidates for other (possibly more costly or invasive) screening tests.

Tumor DNA May Aid Precision Cancer Treatment

There is also hope that ctDNA-based liquid biopsies may guide precision medicine treatment by identifying unique molecular characteristics of an individual's cancer. In several research studies, liquid biopsies have pinpointed ctDNA mutations that could potentially be used to determine the optimal treatment.

For example, researchers at University of California, San Diego (UCSD) Moores Cancer Center (MCC) analyzed blood samples from 168 patients with different types of cancer, including brain, lung, and breast cancer. For 58 percent of the participants, the researchers identified at least one cancer-related ctDNA mutation. For most of these patients, a U.S. Food and Drug Administration (FDA)–approved drug was available to treat cancers with that particular mutation.

Other studies have demonstrated the feasibility of using ctDNA-based liquid biopsies on a large scale to identify DNA mutations in patients' cancers. For instance, investigators used Guardant360—a commercially available test that analyzes 70 cancer-related genes in a blood sample—to identify mutations in the ctDNA of more than 15,000 patients. The investigators found that, for most patients, the genetic mutations identified by the liquid biopsy test were consistent with those identified by a tissue biopsy test.

In 2016, FDA approved a liquid biopsy test, called the cobas® EGFR Mutation Test for the detection of *EGFR* gene mutations in ctDNA of patients with lung cancer. The purpose of the test is to identify patients who may be candidates for treatment with erlotinib (Tarceva®) and osimeritinib (Tagrisso®)—targeted therapies that attack cancer cells with EGFR mutations. Because the test may produce a false-negative test result, FDA recommends a tissue biopsy if the liquid biopsy is negative (meaning it does not detect an EGFR mutation).

Many other liquid biopsy tests are commercially available but have not been rigorously tested by scientists. Clinicians and researchers are still determining the limitations of these tests and, more importantly, whether they provide clinical benefit to patients. For example, it is unknown whether using a liquid biopsy test to help select treatment improves patient outcomes.

Monitoring Treatment Response with Tumor DNA

Because they are noninvasive and easily repeated, ctDNA-based liquid biopsies may be useful for monitoring patients' responses to therapy both during treatment and after it is completed. Clinicians are hopeful that tracking a patient's response to treatment may allow adjustments to be made in real time. In other words, the treatment could be stopped or adjusted if the test indicates it is not working.

Imaging techniques such as computed tomography (CT) scans are currently used to track treatment response for patients with certain cancer types, but they are not sensitive enough to detect small changes in tumor size and they tend to be costly, explained Mark Roschewski, M.D., of NCI's Center for Cancer Research (CCR).

As a potential alternative, Dr. Roschewski and his colleagues tested the ability of a liquid biopsy test to track treatment responses in patients with lymphoma. They showed that changes in ctDNA correlated with positive responses to chemotherapy. Furthermore, they were able to use ctDNA patterns to detect when some patients' disease was coming back—months before it was possible to do so via CT scan.

"In our study, the liquid biopsy test was much more sensitive than imaging techniques," said Dr. Roschewski.

Likewise, other NCI researchers correlated changes in ctDNA levels with patients' responses to immunotherapy treatment. They found that they could detect these changes within 2 weeks of the start of treatment. Having an early indicator of the treatment's efficacy could be very helpful because only a small proportion of patients typically respond to immunotherapy treatment, they explained.

"Liquid biopsy tests have the added advantage of providing molecular information about the cancer, which can change during and after treatment," said Brian Sorg, Ph.D., also of NCI's DCTD. This additional information could potentially help doctors track the development of drug resistance and make more personalized treatment decisions.

For example, although most patients with lung cancer initially respond to treatment with a class of drugs called tyrosine kinase inhibitors, the majority develop drug resistance within 1 or 2 years of starting treatment.

In one study, a team of researchers analyzed mutations in ctDNA from patients with lung cancer that had become resistant to certain tyrosine kinase inhibitors. They detected a genetic mutation causing the drug resistance in ctDNA from 80 percent of participants.

A separate study will be needed to determine if the liquid biopsy test can identify patients whose tumors have this mutation and who are most likely to benefit from a different treatment, the researchers noted.

According to an expert review released by the American Society of Clinical Oncology (ASCO) and College of American Pathologists (CAP), most liquid biopsy tests are not yet ready for routine use in clinical cancer care. Based on an analysis of 77 liquid biopsy studies, the organizations concluded that most liquid biopsy tests designed to track treatment responses need more evidence to confirm that the tests correctly identify patients for whom a particular treatment is likely to be effective. The evidence on the validity of these tests is "still emerging," they wrote.

Limitations of ctDNA-Based Liquid Biopsies

While there are many potential applications for ctDNA-based liquid biopsies, there are also several limitations.

Most cancer types lack well-established biomarkers (such as a specific DNA mutation) that allow scientists to identify and track the disease via ctDNA. For example, a biomarker commonly used to track advanced pancreatic cancer is considered unreliable for early detection of the disease.

"While the technology for detecting ctDNA in body fluids has improved dramatically, the knowledge required to identify appropriate biomarkers for many cancer types has not," said Dr. Dickherber.

And DNA mutations vary even among patients with the same cancer type, so although a particular mutation may be common for one type of cancer, many patients with that cancer type may not have it. This adds a layer of complexity to the challenge of identifying ctDNA biomarkers for every cancer type and stage.

One possible solution could involve combining tissue and liquid biopsies, said Ossandon. First, a tissue biopsy could be used to identify unique biomarkers for an individual's tumor, he explained, and then liquid biopsy tests could be used to track those biomarkers.

Another limitation is that ctDNA in the blood may not be truly representative of DNA in the actual tumor, and, therefore, may not be the best source of information for guiding clinical decisions. Tumors are heterogeneous—meaning DNA mutations vary between cancer cells in a single tumor—and it is not known whether ctDNA is released from the whole tumor or only certain parts of it, explained Dr. Sorg.

It is also unknown whether the mutations found in ctDNA are "driver" mutations—those that play an important role in the cancer's biology—said Dr. Sorbara. They may instead be "passenger" mutations, that is, changes that accompany the development of cancer but do not control its growth.

The ASCO and CAP review also found that the results of most liquid biopsy tests don't completely match results from tissue biopsies, calling into question the accuracy of these new tests. This discordance could be the result of biological differences (between blood and tissue samples, for example) or limitations of the tests, the experts noted.

"Possibly the biggest unanswered question is whether liquid biopsy tests can improve patient survival," Dr. Roschewski said. Meaning, does using liquid biopsy tests to detect early-stage cancer, select treatment, or track disease progression ultimately extend patient survival or improve quality of life?

Many researchers, including the ASCO and CAP experts, agree that studies that prospectively analyze the effect of liquid biopsy tests on clinical outcome are needed.

For example, Stanford University and NCI are leading a clinical trial to evaluate the clinical response and overall survival of patients who receive targeted therapy based on molecular information identified via a tissue or liquid biopsy test. As of October 2017, the trial is currently recruiting adults with metastatic solid tumors.

Chapter 83

Technologies in Tumor Surgery

For surgeons, removing a tumor is a balancing act. Cut out too much and you risk removing healthy tissues that have important functions. Remove too little and you may leave behind cancer cells that could grow back into a tumor over time. National Institutes of Health (NIH)-funded researchers are developing new technologies to help surgeons determine exactly where tumors end and healthy tissue begins. Their ultimate goal is to make surgery for cancer patients safer and more effective.

"Currently, surgeons view magnetic resonance imaging (MRI) and computed tomography (CT) scans taken prior to an operation to establish where a tumor is located and to plan a surgical approach that will minimize damage to healthy tissues," says Dr. Steven Krosnick, an NIH expert in image-guided surgery. "But once the operation has begun, surgeons generally rely only on their eyes and sense of touch to distinguish tumor from healthy tissue."

Surgeons go through many years of training to understand the subtle cues that can distinguish tumor from normal surroundings. Sometimes the tumor is a slightly different color than healthy tissue, or it feels different. It might also bleed more readily or could contain calcium deposits. Even with these cues, however, surgeons don't always get it right.

This chapter includes text excerpted from "Technologies Enhance Tumor Surgery—Helping Surgeons Spot and Remove Cancer," *NIH News in Health,* National Institutes of Health (NIH), February 2016.

"In a lot of cases, we leave tumor behind that could be safely removed if only we were able to better visualize it," says Dr. Daniel Orringer, a neurosurgeon at the University of Michigan.

In today's operating rooms, pathologists can often help surgeons determine if all of a tumor has been taken out. A pathologist may view the edges of the tissue under a microscope and look for cancer cells. If they're found, the surgeon will remove more tissue from the patient and send these again to the pathologist for review. This process can occur repeatedly while the patient remains on the operating table and continue until no cancer cells are detected.

"Each time a pathologist analyzes tissue during an operation, it can take up to 30 minutes because the tissue has to be frozen, thinly sliced, and stained so it can be viewed under the microscope," Krosnick says. "If multiple rounds of tissue are taken, it can greatly increase the length of the surgery."

In the days following an operation, the pathologist conducts a more thorough review of the tissue. If cancer cells are found at the margins, the patient may undergo a second surgery to remove cancer that was left behind.

Orringer is part of a research team that's testing a new technology that could help surgeons tell the difference between a tumor and healthy brain tissue during surgery. The team developed a special microscope with NIH support that shoots a pair of low-energy lasers at the tissue. That causes the chemical bonds in the tissue's molecules to vibrate. The vibrations are then analyzed by a computer and used to create detailed images of the tissue.

From a molecular point of view, the components of a tumor differ from those in healthy tissue. This specialized microscope can reveal differences between the tissues that can't be seen with the naked eye.

"Our technology enables us to get a microscopic view of human tissues without taking them out of the body," Orringer says. "We can see cells, blood vessels, the connections between brain cells...all of the microscopic components that make up the brain."

Orringer and colleagues developed a computer program that can quickly analyze the images and assess whether or not cancer cells are present. This type of analysis could help surgeons decide whether all of a tumor has been cut out. To date, Orringer has used the specialized microscope to help remove cancer tissue in nearly 100 patients with brain tumors.

Other researchers are taking different approaches. For example, Dr. Quyen Nguyen—a head and neck surgeon at the University of California, San Diego—has developed a fluorescent molecule that's currently being tested in clinical trials. The patient receives an injection of the molecules before surgery. When exposed to certain types of light, these molecules cause cancer cells to glow, making them easier to spot and remove. The surgeon then uses a near-infrared camera to visualize the glowing tumor cells while operating.

Nguyen is also developing a fluorescent molecule to light up nerves. Accidental nerve injury during surgery can leave patients with loss of movement or feeling. In some cases, sexual function may be impaired.

"Nerves are really, really small, and they're often buried in soft tissue or encased within bone. When we have to do cancer surgery, they can be encased in the cancer itself," Nguyen says. The fluorescent molecule could help surgeons detect hard-to-spot nerves, so they can be protected. The nerve-tagging molecule is now being tested in animal studies.

Other NIH-funded researchers are focusing on ways to speed up cancer surgeries. Dr. Milind Rajadhyaksha, a researcher at Memorial Sloan Kettering Cancer Center (MSKCC), has developed a microscope technique to reduce the amount of time it takes to perform a common surgery for removing nonmelanoma skin cancers.

Each year about 2 million people in the United States undergo Mohs surgery, in which a doctor successively removes suspicious areas until the surrounding skin tissue is free of cancer. The procedure can take several hours, because each time more tissue is removed, it has to be prepared and reviewed under a microscope to determine if cancer cells remain. This step can take up to 30 minutes.

The technique developed by Rajadhyaksha shortens the time for assessing removed tissue to less than 5 minutes, which greatly reduces the overall length of the procedure. Tissue is mounted in a specialized microscope that uses a focused laser line to do multiple scans of the tissue. The resulting image "strips" are then combined, like a mosaic, into a complete microscopic image of the tissue.

About 1,000 specialized skin surgeries have already been performed guided by this technique. Rajadhyaksha is currently developing an approach that would allow doctors to use the technology directly on a patient's skin, before any tissue has been removed. This would allow doctors to identify the edges of tumors before the start of surgery and reduce the need for several presurgical "margin-mapping" biopsies. There are many types of cancer surgeries, and researchers continue to work hard to develop better techniques.

Chapter 84

Treatment of Prostate Cancer with Apalutamide

On February 14, 2018, the U.S. Food and Drug Administration (FDA) approved apalutamide (Erleada) for men with prostate cancer that has not spread (nonmetastatic) and is resistant to standard hormone therapy, also called androgen deprivation therapy (ADT).

Treatment with apalutamide decreased the risk of metastasis or death by more than 70 percent compared with placebo, the trial that led to the approval showed.

"These are very dramatic results and, in many ways, exceeded our expectations," said lead investigator Matthew Smith, M.D., Ph.D., of Massachusetts General Hospital Cancer Center. The treatment "will be an important option" for men with prostate cancer in this setting, he added.

"We're learning that using hormone therapy earlier in men with prostate cancer can delay metastasis and probably improve survival. But the balance of benefits and potential side effects will need to be evaluated on a patient-by-patient basis," said William Dahut, M.D., head of the Prostate Cancer Clinical Research Section of National Cancer Institute's (NCI) Center for Cancer Research (CCR).

This chapter includes text excerpted from "FDA Approves Apalutamide for Some Men with Prostate Cancer," National Cancer Institute (NCI), March 8, 2018.

A New Option after Hormone Therapy Resistance

Men with prostate cancer that has not spread may be treated with ADT. These treatments block the body's production and use of male sex hormones (known as androgens) that drive prostate cancer growth. But most prostate cancers eventually become castration-resistant, meaning the tumor begins to grow again despite androgen deprivation.

In the past, men with nonmetastatic castration-resistant prostate cancer (NM-CRPC) continued ADT and were carefully observed for signs that the cancer had spread, at which point they could receive therapies for metastatic prostate cancer.

"The prevention of metastases represents an important unmet medical need," trial co-investigator Eric Small, M.D., of the University of California, San Francisco (UCSF), said at the 2018 Genitourinary Cancers Symposium.

In an earlier phase 2 trial funded by NCI, Dr. Smith and his colleagues found that apalutamide had anticancer activity against castration-resistant prostate cancer. Apalutamide prevents androgens from binding to androgen receptors on cells and triggering cell growth.

In the phase 3 trial (dubbed (Selective Prostate Androgen Receptor Targeting with ARN-509 (SPARTAN) trial) that led to the FDA approval, men with castration-resistant prostate cancer and no metastatic disease detectable by standard imaging tests were randomly assigned to receive apalutamide or placebo in addition to ongoing ADT. All participants were at high risk of metastasis based on rapidly rising prostate-specific antigen (PSA) levels. The study was sponsored by Janssen Pharmaceutical Companies, the manufacturer of apalutamide.

The median length of time from the start of treatment to when tumors spread or the patient died (metastasis-free survival) was 16 months in the placebo group and 40 months in the apalutamide group. Men treated with apalutamide also went longer without worsening symptoms of cancer progression. Even when their cancer progressed on apalutamide and they went on to receive another therapy, these men had longer time to progression with the subsequent treatment than men in the placebo group.

The median length of time patients were alive after the start of treatment (overall survival) was 39 months for those who received placebo and had not been reached at the time of the study analysis for those who received apalutamide. An early analysis suggests that apalutamide may reduce the risk of death from prostate cancer, but longer patient follow-up is needed before the researchers can confirm this.

More patients in the apalutamide group than the placebo group had weight loss, fatigue, rash, falls, and bone fractures. In the apalutamide group, approximately 11 percent of patients discontinued treatment due to side effects, compared with 7 percent in the placebo group. Serious side effects were associated with the death of 1 subject in the placebo group and 10 subjects in the apalutamide group.

The researchers found no differences in quality-of-life scores reported by participants between the groups, and the scores did not get worse during treatment.

Apalutamide is the first drug to be approved by FDA based on an improvement in metastasis-free survival. Traditionally, most approvals are based on an improvement in progression-free survival or overall survival.

"This new precedent for FDA approval may permit drugs to reach the clinic more quickly," Dr. Dahut explained.

Another Potential Option for Prostate Cancer

Results from a separate clinical trial that was also reported at the 2018 Genitourinary Cancers Symposium suggest that there may soon be another potential treatment option for men with NM-CRPC.

The Prospective Study of Pravastatin in the Elderly at Risk (PROSPER) trial showed that enzalutamide (Xtandi), a hormone therapy that also counteracts castration resistance, reduced the risk of metastasis or death by 71 percent compared with placebo. Compared with placebo, enzalutamide delayed the median time before study subjects needed a different treatment because their cancer had gotten worse (18 months versus 40 months). At the time of analysis, patients were not followed long enough for the investigators to determine the median overall survival.

Enzalutamide caused side effects in a greater percentage of patients than did placebo (87% versus 77%). The most common serious side effects of enzalutamide were high blood pressure, fatigue, and blood in the urine. After the study treatment was completed, 32 patients who received enzalutamide died of unknown causes, compared with 4 patients who received placebo.

Enzalutamide is FDA-approved to treat metastatic castration-resistant prostate cancer (mCRPC) but it is not currently approved to treat men with NM-CRPC.

Considering results from the SPARTAN and PROSPER trials, it is evident that "using these more intense hormonal therapies earlier can definitely prevent the development of metastasis," Dr. Dahut said.

"But treating asymptomatic patients carries a certain burden of proof wherein benefit must clearly outweigh risk," Philip Kantoff, M.D., of Memorial Sloan Kettering Cancer Center (MSKCC), noted in a discussion of the two trials at the symposium.

It is not clear whether longer metastasis-free survival translates to benefits such as fewer symptoms or longer overall survival in these men, Dr. Kantoff explained. While it seems that both apalutamide and enzalutamide may ultimately prolong overall survival, there is not yet enough data to know for sure. "To me, the clinical benefit is not yet fully determined in both studies," he concluded.

New Imaging Techniques May Change Diagnoses

While apalutamide—and, potentially, enzalutamide—gives men with nonmetastatic castration-resistant disease a new treatment option, this patient population may decrease in the future, Dr. Dahut noted. That's because traditional imaging techniques such as a computed axial tomography (CAT) scan may not be able to detect tiny metastatic tumors, he explained. But a technique being used in research studies called molecular imaging can catch smaller tumors. If molecular imaging tests become part of clinical care, more men with prostate cancer might be classified as having metastatic disease.

"It's highly likely that apalutamide would be active" in men with mCRPC, Dr. Dahut speculated. Trials to evaluate apalutamide in this patient population are already underway, Dr. Smith noted.

Part Six

Additional Help and Information

Chapter 85

A Glossary of Cancer-Related Terms

ablation: In medicine, the removal or destruction of a body part or tissue or its function. Ablation may be performed by surgery, hormones, drugs, radio frequency, heat, or other methods.

abnormal: Not normal. An abnormal lesion or growth may be cancer, premalignant (likely to become cancer), or benign (not cancer).

acute: Symptoms or signs that begin and worsen quickly; not chronic.

adenocarcinoma: Cancer that begins in cells that line certain internal organs and that have gland-like (secretory) properties.

adenoma: A tumor that is not cancer. It starts in gland-like cells of the epithelial tissue (thin layer of tissue that covers organs, glands, and other structures within the body).

advance directive: A legal document that states the treatment or care a person wishes to receive or not receive if he or she becomes unable to make medical decisions (for example, due to being unconscious or in a coma). Some types of advance directives are living wills and do-not-resuscitate (DNR) orders.

advanced cancer: Cancer that has spread to other places in the body and usually cannot be cured or controlled with treatment.

This glossary contains terms excerpted from documents produced by several sources deemed reliable.

aggressive: In medicine, describes a tumor or disease that forms, grows, or spreads quickly. It may also describe treatment that is more severe or intense than usual.

anal cancer: Cancer that forms in tissues of the anus. The anus is the opening of the rectum (last part of the large intestine) to the outside of the body.

anaplastic: A term used to describe cancer cells that divide rapidly and have little or no resemblance to normal cells.

astrocytoma: A tumor that begins in the brain or spinal cord in small, star-shaped cells called astrocytes.

axillary: Pertaining to the armpit area, including the lymph nodes that are located there.

axillary lymph node: A lymph node in the armpit region that drains lymph from the breast and nearby areas.

basal cell: A small, round cell found in the lower part (or base) of the epidermis, the outer layer of the skin.

basal cell carcinoma: Cancer that begins in the lower part of the epidermis (the outer layer of the skin). It may appear as a small white or flesh-colored bump that grows slowly and may bleed. Basal cell carcinomas are usually found on areas of the body exposed to the sun. Basal cell carcinomas rarely metastasize (spread) to other parts of the body. They are the most common form of skin cancer.

benign: Not cancerous. Benign tumors may grow larger but do not spread to other parts of the body. Also called nonmalignant.

bile duct cancer: Cancer that forms in a bile duct. A bile duct is a tube that carries bile (fluid made by the liver that helps digest fat) between the liver and gallbladder and the intestine. Bile ducts include the common hepatic, cystic, and common bile ducts. Bile duct cancer may be found inside the liver (intrahepatic) or outside the liver (extrahepatic).

biliary: Having to do with the liver, bile ducts, and/or gallbladder.

bladder cancer: Cancer that forms in tissues of the bladder (the organ that stores urine). Most bladder cancers are transitional cell carcinomas (cancer that begins in cells that normally make up the inner lining of the bladder). Other types include squamous cell carcinoma (cancer that begins in thin, flat cells) and adenocarcinoma (cancer that begins in cells that make and release mucus and other fluids). The cells that form squamous cell carcinoma and adenocarcinoma develop in the inner lining of the bladder as a result of chronic irritation and inflammation.

bone cancer: Primary bone cancer is cancer that forms in cells of the bone. Some types of primary bone cancer are osteosarcoma, Ewing sarcoma, malignant fibrous histiocytoma, and chondrosarcoma. Secondary bone cancer is cancer that spreads to the bone from another part of the body (such as the prostate, breast, or lung).

brachytherapy: A type of radiation therapy in which radioactive material sealed in needles, seeds, wires, or catheters is placed directly into or near a tumor. Also called implant radiation therapy, internal radiation therapy, and radiation brachytherapy.

brain tumor: The growth of abnormal cells in the tissues of the brain. Brain tumors can be benign (not cancer) or malignant (cancer).

***BRCA1*:** A gene on chromosome 17 that normally helps to suppress cell growth. A person who inherits certain mutations (changes) in a *BRCA1* gene has a higher risk of getting breast, ovarian, prostate, and other types of cancer.

***BRCA2*:** A gene on chromosome 13 that normally helps to suppress cell growth. A person who inherits certain mutations (changes) in a *BRCA2* gene has a higher risk of getting breast, ovarian, prostate, and other types of cancer.

breast cancer: Cancer that forms in tissues of the breast, usually the ducts (tubes that carry milk to the nipple) and lobules (glands that make milk). It occurs in both men and women, although male breast cancer is rare.

bronchus: A large airway that leads from the trachea (windpipe) to a lung. The plural of bronchus is bronchi.

cancer: A term for diseases in which abnormal cells divide without control and can invade nearby tissues. Cancer cells can also spread to other parts of the body through the blood and lymph systems. There are several main types of cancer. Carcinoma is a cancer that begins in the skin or in tissues that line or cover internal organs. Sarcoma is a cancer that begins in bone, cartilage, fat, muscle, blood vessels, or other connective or supportive tissue. Leukemia is a cancer that starts in blood-forming tissue such as the bone marrow, and causes large numbers of abnormal blood cells to be produced and enter the blood. Lymphoma and multiple myeloma are cancers that begin in the cells of the immune system. Central nervous system cancers are cancers that begin in the tissues of the brain and spinal cord. Also called malignancy.

carcinoembryonic antigen (CEA): A substance that is sometimes found in an increased amount in the blood of people who have certain cancers, other diseases, or who smoke. It is used as a tumor marker for colorectal cancer. Also called CEA.

carcinogen: Any substance that causes cancer.

carcinoid: A slow-growing type of tumor usually found in the gastro-intestinal system (most often in the appendix), and sometimes in the lungs or other sites. Carcinoid tumors may spread to the liver or other sites in the body, and they may secrete substances such as serotonin or prostaglandins, causing carcinoid syndrome.

carcinoma: Cancer that begins in the skin or in tissues that line or cover internal organs.

carcinoma in situ: A group of abnormal cells that remain in the place where they first formed. They have not spread. These abnormal cells may become cancer and spread into nearby normal tissue. Also called stage 0 disease.

cervical cancer: Cancer that forms in tissues of the cervix (the organ connecting the uterus and vagina). It is usually a slow-growing cancer that may not have symptoms but can be found with regular Pap tests (a procedure in which cells are scraped from the cervix and looked at under a microscope). Cervical cancer is almost always caused by human papillomavirus (HPV) infection.

chemotherapy: Treatment with drugs that kill cancer cells.

chondrosarcoma: A type of cancer that forms in bone cartilage. It usually starts in the pelvis (between the hip bones), the shoulder, the ribs, or at the ends of the long bones of the arms and legs. A rare type of chondrosarcoma called extraskeletal chondrosarcoma does not form in bone cartilage. Instead, it forms in the soft tissues of the upper part of the arms and legs. Chondrosarcoma can occur at any age but is more common in people older than 40 years. It is a type of bone cancer.

chronic: A disease or condition that persists or progresses over a long period of time.

colon cancer: Cancer that forms in the tissues of the colon (the longest part of the large intestine). Most colon cancers are adenocarcinomas (cancers that begin in cells that make and release mucus and other fluids).

colonoscopy: Examination of the inside of the colon using a colonoscope, inserted into the rectum. A colonoscope is a thin, tube-like instrument with a light and a lens for viewing. It may also have a tool to remove tissue to be checked under a microscope for signs of disease.

colorectal cancer: Cancer that develops in the colon (the longest part of the large intestine) and/or the rectum (the last several inches of the large intestine before the anus).

colostomy: An opening into the colon from the outside of the body. A colostomy provides a new path for waste material to leave the body after part of the colon has been removed.

cyst: A sac or capsule in the body. It may be filled with fluid or other material.

endometrial cancer: Cancer that forms in the tissue lining the uterus (the small, hollow, pear-shaped organ in a woman's pelvis in which a fetus develops). Most endometrial cancers are adenocarcinomas (cancers that begin in cells that make and release mucus and other fluids).

endoscopy: A procedure that uses an endoscope to examine the inside of the body. An endoscope is a thin, tube-like instrument with a light and a lens for viewing. It may also have a tool to remove tissue to be checked under a microscope for signs of disease.

ependymoma: A type of brain tumor that begins in cells lining the spinal cord central canal (fluid-filled space down the center) or the ventricles (fluid-filled spaces of the brain). Ependymomas may also form in the choroid plexus (tissue in the ventricles that makes cerebrospinal fluid). Also called ependymal tumor.

esophageal cancer: Cancer that forms in tissues lining the esophagus (the muscular tube through which food passes from the throat to the stomach). Two types of esophageal cancer are squamous cell carcinoma (cancer that begins in flat cells lining the esophagus) and adenocarcinoma (cancer that begins in cells that make and release mucus and other fluids).

gallbladder cancer: Cancer that forms in tissues of the gallbladder. The gallbladder is a pear-shaped organ below the liver that collects and stores bile (a fluid made by the liver to digest fat). Gallbladder cancer begins in the innermost layer of tissue and spreads through the outer layers as it grows.

gastric cancer: Cancer that forms in tissues lining the stomach. Also called stomach cancer.

gastrinoma: A tumor that causes overproduction of gastric acid. It usually begins in the duodenum (first part of the small intestine that connects to the stomach) or the islet cells of the pancreas. Rarely, it may also begin in other organs, including the stomach, liver, jejunum (the middle part of the small intestine), biliary tract (organs and ducts that make and store bile), mesentery, or heart. It is a type of neuroendocrine tumor, and it may metastasize (spread) to the liver and the lymph nodes.

gastrointestinal stromal tumor (GIST): A type of tumor that usually begins in cells in the wall of the gastrointestinal tract. It can be benign or malignant.

gene therapy: Treatment that alters a gene. In studies of gene therapy for cancer, researchers are trying to improve the body's natural ability to fight the disease or to make the cancer cells more sensitive to other kinds of therapy.

germ cell tumor: A type of tumor that begins in the cells that give rise to sperm or eggs. Germ cell tumors can occur almost anywhere in the body and can be either benign or malignant.

glioblastoma: A fast-growing type of central nervous system tumor that forms from glial (supportive) tissue of the brain and spinal cord and has cells that look very different from normal cells. Glioblastoma usually occurs in adults and affects the brain more often than the spinal cord. Also called GBM, glioblastoma multiforme, and grade IV astrocytoma.

***Helicobacter pylori (H. pylori)*:** A type of bacterium that causes inflammation and ulcers in the stomach or small intestine. People with *H. pylori* infections may be more likely to develop cancer in the stomach, including MALT (mucosa-associated lymphoid tissue) lymphoma.

HER2/neu: A protein involved in normal cell growth. It is found on some types of cancer cells, including breast and ovarian. Cancer cells removed from the body may be tested for the presence of HER2/neu to help decide the best type of treatment. HER2/neu is a type of receptor tyrosine kinase. Also called c-erbB-2, human EGF receptor 2, and human epidermal growth factor receptor 2.

high-dose chemotherapy: An intensive drug treatment to kill cancer cells, but that also destroys the bone marrow and can cause other severe side effects. High-dose chemotherapy is usually followed by bone marrow or stem cell transplantation to rebuild the bone marrow.

Hodgkin lymphoma: A cancer of the immune system that is marked by the presence of a type of cell called the Reed-Sternberg cell. The two major types of Hodgkin lymphoma are classical Hodgkin lymphoma and nodular lymphocyte-predominant Hodgkin lymphoma. Symptoms include the painless enlargement of lymph nodes, spleen, or other immune tissue. Other symptoms include fever, weight loss, fatigue, or night sweats. Also called Hodgkin disease.

hormone: One of many chemicals made by glands in the body. Hormones circulate in the bloodstream and control the actions of certain cells or organs. Some hormones can also be made in the laboratory.

hormone receptor: A cell protein that binds a specific hormone. The hormone receptor may be on the surface of the cell or inside the cell. Many changes take place in a cell after a hormone binds to its receptor.

hospice: A program that provides special care for people who are near the end of life and for their families, either at home, in freestanding facilities, or within hospitals.

hysterectomy: Surgery to remove the uterus and, sometimes, the cervix. When the uterus and the cervix are removed, it is called a total hysterectomy. When only the uterus is removed, it is called a partial hysterectomy.

imaging: In medicine, a process that makes pictures of areas inside the body. Imaging uses methods such as X-rays (high-energy radiation), ultrasound (high-energy sound waves), and radio waves.

immunotherapy: Treatment to boost or restore the ability of the immune system to fight cancer, infections, and other diseases. Also used to lessen certain side effects that may be caused by some cancer treatments. Agents used in immunotherapy include monoclonal antibodies, growth factors, and vaccines. These agents may also have a direct antitumor effect. Also called biological response modifier therapy, biological therapy, biotherapy, and BRM therapy.

in situ: In its original place. For example, in carcinoma in situ, abnormal cells are found only in the place where they first formed. They have not spread.

indolent: A type of cancer that grows slowly.

inflammatory breast cancer: A type of breast cancer in which the breast looks red and swollen and feels warm. The skin of the breast may also show the pitted appearance called peau d'orange (like the skin of an orange). The redness and warmth occur because the cancer cells block the lymph vessels in the skin.

interferon: A biological response modifier (a substance that can improve the body's natural response to infections and other diseases). Interferons interfere with the division of cancer cells and can slow tumor growth. There are several types of interferons, including interferon-alpha, -beta, and -gamma. The body normally produces these substances. They are also made in the laboratory to treat cancer and other diseases.

interleukin: One of a group of related proteins made by leukocytes (white blood cells) and other cells in the body. Interleukins regulate immune responses. Interleukins made in the laboratory are used as biological response modifiers to boost the immune system in cancer therapy. Also called IL.

jaundice: A condition in which the skin and the whites of the eyes become yellow, urine darkens, and the color of stool becomes lighter than normal. Jaundice occurs when the liver is not working properly or when a bile duct is blocked.

Kaposi sarcoma: A type of cancer characterized by the abnormal growth of blood vessels that develop into skin lesions or occur internally.

kidney cancer: Cancer that forms in tissues of the kidneys. Kidney cancer includes renal cell carcinoma (cancer that forms in the lining of very small tubes in the kidney that filter the blood and remove waste products) and renal pelvis carcinoma (cancer that forms in the center of the kidney where urine collects). It also includes Wilms tumor, which is a type of kidney cancer that usually develops in children under the age of five.

laryngeal cancer: Cancer that forms in tissues of the larynx (area of the throat that contains the vocal cords and is used for breathing, swallowing, and talking). Most laryngeal cancers are squamous cell carcinomas (cancer that begins in flat cells lining the larynx).

laryngectomy: An operation to remove all or part of the larynx (voicebox).

laser therapy: Treatment that uses intense, narrow beams of light to cut and destroy tissue, such as cancer tissue. Laser therapy may also be used to reduce lymphedema (swelling caused by a buildup of lymph fluid in tissue) after breast cancer surgery.

late effects: Side effects of cancer treatment that appear months or years after treatment has ended. Late effects include physical and mental problems and second cancers.

leukemia: Cancer that starts in blood-forming tissue such as the bone marrow and causes large numbers of blood cells to be produced and enter the bloodstream.

liver cancer: Primary liver cancer is cancer that forms in the tissues of the liver. Secondary liver cancer is cancer that spreads to the liver from another part of the body.

lobe: A portion of an organ, such as the liver, lung, breast, thyroid, or brain.

localized: Restricted to the site of origin, without evidence of spread.

lung cancer: Cancer that forms in tissues of the lung, usually in the cells lining air passages. The two main types are small cell lung cancer and nonsmall cell lung cancer. These types are diagnosed based on how the cells look under a microscope.

lymph node: A rounded mass of lymphatic tissue that is surrounded by a capsule of connective tissue. Lymph nodes filter lymph (lymphatic fluid), and they store lymphocytes (white blood cells). They are located along lymphatic vessels. Also called lymph gland.

lymphedema: A condition in which extra lymph fluid builds up in tissues and causes swelling. It may occur in an arm or leg if lymph vessels are blocked, damaged, or removed by surgery.

lymphoma: Cancer that begins in cells of the immune system. There are two basic categories of lymphomas. One kind is Hodgkin lymphoma, which is marked by the presence of a type of cell called the Reed-Sternberg cell. The other category is non-Hodgkin lymphomas, which includes a large, diverse group of cancers of immune system cells. Non-Hodgkin lymphomas can be further divided into cancers that have an indolent (slow growing) course and those that have an aggressive (fast growing) course. These subtypes behave and respond to treatment differently. Both Hodgkin and non-Hodgkin lymphomas can occur in children and adults, and prognosis and treatment depend on the stage and the type of cancer.

magnetic resonance imaging (MRI): A procedure in which radio waves and a powerful magnet linked to a computer are used to create detailed pictures of areas inside the body. These pictures can show the difference between normal and diseased tissue. Magnetic resonance imaging makes better images of organs and soft tissue than other scanning techniques, such as computed tomography (CT) or X-ray. Magnetic resonance imaging is especially useful for imaging the brain, the spine, the soft tissue of joints, and the inside of bones. Also called MRI, NMRI, and nuclear magnetic resonance imaging.

mammography: The use of film or a computer to create a picture of the breast.

mass: In medicine, a lump in the body. It may be caused by the abnormal growth of cells, a cyst, hormonal changes, or an immune reaction. A mass may be benign (not cancer) or malignant (cancer).

mastectomy: Surgery to remove the breast (or as much of the breast tissue as possible).

medullary thyroid cancer: Cancer that develops in C cells of the thyroid. The C cells make a hormone (calcitonin) that helps maintain a healthy level of calcium in the blood.

melanoma: A form of cancer that begins in melanocytes (cells that make the pigment melanin). It may begin in a mole (skin melanoma), but can also begin in other pigmented tissues, such as in the eye or in the intestines.

meningioma: A type of slow-growing tumor that forms in the meninges (thin layers of tissue that cover and protect the brain and spinal cord). Meningiomas usually occur in adults.

Merkel cell carcinoma: A rare type of cancer that forms on or just beneath the skin, usually in parts of the body that have been exposed to the sun. It is most common in older people and in people with weakened immune systems. Also called Merkel cell cancer, neuroendocrine carcinoma of the skin, and trabecular cancer.

mesothelioma: A benign (not cancer) or malignant (cancer) tumor affecting the lining of the chest or abdomen. Exposure to asbestos particles in the air increases the risk of developing malignant mesothelioma.

metastasis: The spread of cancer from one part of the body to another. A tumor formed by cells that have spread is called a "metastatic tumor" or a "metastasis." The metastatic tumor contains cells that are like those in the original (primary) tumor. The plural form of metastasis is metastases.

mole: A benign (not cancer) growth on the skin that is formed by a cluster of melanocytes (cells that make a substance called melanin, which gives color to skin and eyes). A mole is usually dark and may be raised from the skin. Also called nevus.

monoclonal antibody: A type of protein made in the laboratory that can bind to substances in the body, including tumor cells. There are many kinds of monoclonal antibodies. Each monoclonal antibody is made to find one substance. Monoclonal antibodies are being used to treat some types of cancer and are being studied in the treatment of other types. They can be used alone or to carry drugs, toxins, or radioactive materials directly to a tumor.

multiple myeloma: A type of cancer that begins in plasma cells (white blood cells that produce antibodies). Also called Kahler disease, myelomatosis, and plasma cell myeloma.

mutation: Any change in the DNA of a cell. Mutations may be caused by mistakes during cell division, or they may be caused by exposure to DNA-damaging agents in the environment. Mutations can be harmful, beneficial, or have no effect. If they occur in cells that make eggs or sperm, they can be inherited; if mutations occur in other types of cells, they are not inherited. Certain mutations may lead to cancer or other diseases.

myelogenous: Having to do with, produced by, or resembling the bone marrow. Sometimes used as a synonym for myeloid; for example, acute myeloid leukemia and acute myelogenous leukemia are the same disease.

myeloid: Having to do with or resembling the bone marrow. May also refer to certain types of hematopoietic (blood forming) cells found in the bone marrow. Sometimes used as a synonym for myelogenous.

myeloma: Cancer that arises in plasma cells, a type of white blood cell.

neoplasm: An abnormal mass of tissue that results when cells divide more than they should or do not die when they should. Neoplasms may be benign (not cancer), or malignant (cancer). Also called tumor.

neuroblastoma: Cancer that arises in immature nerve cells and affects mostly infants and children.

neuroendocrine tumor: A tumor that forms from cells that release hormones in response to a signal from the nervous system. Some examples of neuroendocrine tumors are carcinoid tumors, islet cell tumors, medullary thyroid carcinomas, pheochromocytomas, and neuroendocrine carcinomas of the skin (Merkel cell cancer). These tumors may secrete higher-than-normal amounts of hormones, which can cause many different symptoms.

nevus: A benign (not cancer) growth on the skin that is formed by a cluster of melanocytes (cells that make a substance called melanin, which gives color to skin and eyes). A nevus is usually dark and may be raised from the skin. Also called mole.

nodule: A growth or lump that may be malignant (cancer) or benign (not cancer).

non-Hodgkin lymphoma (NHL): Any of a large group of cancers of lymphocytes (white blood cells). Non-Hodgkin lymphomas can occur at any age and are often marked by lymph nodes that are larger than normal, fever, and weight loss. There are many different types of non-Hodgkin lymphoma. These types can be divided into aggressive (fast growing) and indolent (slow growing) types, and they can be formed from either B-cells or T-cells. B-cell non-Hodgkin lymphomas include Burkitt lymphoma, chronic lymphocytic leukemia/small lymphocytic lymphoma (CLL/SLL), diffuse large B-cell lymphoma, follicular lymphoma, immunoblastic large cell lymphoma, precursor B-lymphoblastic lymphoma, and mantle cell lymphoma. T-cell non-Hodgkin lymphomas include mycosis fungoides, anaplastic large cell lymphoma, and precursor T-lymphoblastic lymphoma. Lymphomas that occur after bone marrow or stem cell transplantation are usually B-cell non-Hodgkin lymphomas. Prognosis and treatment depend on the stage and type of disease. Also called NHL.

noninvasive: In medicine, it describes a procedure that does not require inserting an instrument through the skin or into a body opening. In cancer, it describes disease that has not spread outside the tissue in which it began.

nonmelanoma skin cancer: Skin cancer that forms in the lower part of the epidermis (the outer layer of the skin) or in squamous cells, but not in melanocytes (skin cells that make pigment).

nonseminoma: A group of testicular cancers that begin in the germ cells (cells that give rise to sperm). Nonseminomas are identified by the type of cell in which they begin and include embryonal carcinoma, teratoma, choriocarcinoma, and yolk sac carcinoma.

oncologist: A doctor who specializes in treating cancer. Some oncologists specialize in a particular type of cancer treatment. For example, a radiation oncologist specializes in treating cancer with radiation.

oral cavity cancer: Cancer that forms in tissues of the oral cavity (the mouth). The tissues of the oral cavity include the lips, the lining inside the cheeks and lips, the front two-thirds of the tongue, the upper and lower gums, the floor of the mouth under the tongue, the bony roof of the mouth, and the small area behind the wisdom teeth.

oropharyngeal cancer: Cancer that forms in tissues of the oropharynx (the part of the throat at the back of the mouth, including the soft palate, the base of the tongue, and the tonsils). Most oropharyngeal cancers are squamous cell carcinomas (cancer that begins in flat cells lining the oropharynx).

osteosarcoma: A cancer of the bone that usually affects the large bones of the arm or leg. It occurs most commonly in young people and affects more males than females. Also called osteogenic sarcoma.

ovarian cancer: Cancer that forms in tissues of the ovary (one of a pair of female reproductive glands in which the ova, or eggs, are formed). Most ovarian cancers are either ovarian epithelial carcinomas (cancer that begins in the cells on the surface of the ovary) or malignant germ cell tumors (cancer that begins in egg cells).

palliative care: Care given to improve the quality of life of patients who have a serious or life-threatening disease. The goal of palliative care is to prevent or treat as early as possible the symptoms of a disease, side effects caused by treatment of a disease, and psychological, social, and spiritual problems related to a disease or its treatment. Also called comfort care, supportive care, and symptom management.

palliative therapy: Treatment given to relieve the symptoms and reduce the suffering caused by cancer and other life-threatening diseases. Palliative cancer therapies are given together with other cancer treatments, from the time of diagnosis, through treatment, survivorship, recurrent, or advanced disease, and at the end of life.

pancreatic cancer: A disease in which malignant (cancer) cells are found in the tissues of the pancreas. Also called exocrine cancer.

pathologist: A doctor who identifies diseases by studying cells and tissues under a microscope.

penile cancer: A rare cancer that forms in the penis (an external male reproductive organ). Most penile cancers are squamous cell carcinomas (cancer that begins in flat cells lining the penis).

peritoneal cancer: Cancer of the tissue that lines the abdominal wall and covers organs in the abdomen.

pituitary tumor: A tumor that forms in the pituitary gland. The pituitary is a pea-sized organ in the center of the brain above the back of the nose. It makes hormones that affect other glands and many body functions, especially growth. Most pituitary tumors are benign (not cancer).

placebo: An inactive substance or treatment that looks the same as, and is given the same way as, an active drug or treatment being tested. The effects of the active drug or treatment are compared to the effects of the placebo.

plasmacytoma: A type of cancer that begins in plasma cells (white blood cells that produce antibodies). A plasmacytoma may turn into multiple myeloma.

primary tumor: The original tumor.

radiation therapy: The use of high-energy radiation from X-rays, gamma rays, neutrons, protons, and other sources to kill cancer cells and shrink tumors. Radiation may come from a machine outside the body (external-beam radiation therapy), or it may come from radioactive material placed in the body near cancer cells (internal radiation therapy). Systemic radiation therapy uses a radioactive substance, such as a radiolabeled monoclonal antibody, that travels in the blood to tissues throughout the body. Also called irradiation and radiotherapy.

radioactive iodine: A radioactive form of iodine, often used for imaging tests or to treat an overactive thyroid, thyroid cancer, and certain other cancers. For imaging tests, the patient takes a small dose of radioactive iodine that collects in thyroid cells and certain kinds of tumors and can be detected by a scanner. To treat thyroid cancer, the patient takes a large dose of radioactive iodine, which kills thyroid cells. Radioactive iodine is also used in internal radiation therapy for prostate cancer, intraocular (eye) melanoma, and carcinoid tumors. Radioactive iodine is given by mouth as a liquid or in capsules, by infusion, or sealed in seeds, which are placed in or near the tumor to kill cancer cells.

radiosurgery: A type of external radiation therapy that uses special equipment to position the patient and precisely give a single large dose of radiation to a tumor. It is used to treat brain tumors and other brain disorders that cannot be treated by regular surgery. It is also being studied in the treatment of other types of cancer. Also called radiation surgery, stereotactic radiosurgery, and stereotaxic radiosurgery.

randomized clinical trial: A study in which the participants are assigned by chance to separate groups that compare different treatments; neither the researchers nor the participants can choose which group. Using chance to assign people to groups means that the groups will be similar and that the treatments they receive can be compared objectively. At the time of the trial, it is not known which treatment is best. It is the patients choice to be in a randomized trial.

recurrent cancer: Cancer that has recurred (come back), usually after a period of time during which the cancer could not be detected. The cancer may come back to the same place as the original (primary) tumor or to another place in the body. Also called recurrence.

remission: A decrease in or disappearance of signs and symptoms of cancer. In partial remission, some, but not all, signs and symptoms of cancer have disappeared. In complete remission, all signs and symptoms of cancer have disappeared, although cancer still may be in the body.

resection: Surgery to remove tissue or part or all of an organ.

retinoblastoma: Cancer that forms in the tissues of the retina (the light-sensitive layers of nerve tissue at the back of the eye). Retinoblastoma usually occurs in children younger than five years. It may be hereditary or nonhereditary (sporadic).

risk factor: Something that increases the chance of developing a disease. Some examples of risk factors for cancer are age, a family history of certain cancers, use of tobacco products, being exposed to radiation or certain chemicals, infection with certain viruses or bacteria, and certain genetic changes.

salpingo-oophorectomy: Surgical removal of the fallopian tubes and ovaries.

sarcoma: A cancer of the bone, cartilage, fat, muscle, blood vessels, or other connective or supportive tissue.

seminoma: A type of cancer of the testicles. Seminomas may spread to the lung, bone, liver, or brain.

sentinel lymph node biopsy: Removal and examination of the sentinel node(s) (the first lymph node(s) to which cancer cells are likely to spread from a primary tumor). To identify the sentinel lymph node(s), the surgeon injects a radioactive substance, blue dye, or both near the tumor. The surgeon then uses a probe to find the sentinel lymph node(s) containing the radioactive substance or looks for the lymph node(s) stained with dye. The surgeon then removes the sentinel node(s) to check for the presence of cancer cells.

skin cancer: Cancer that forms in the tissues of the skin. There are several types of skin cancer. Skin cancer that forms in melanocytes (skin cells that make pigment) is called melanoma. Skin cancer that forms in the lower part of the epidermis (the outer layer of the skin) is called basal cell carcinoma. Skin cancer that forms in squamous cells (flat cells that form the surface of the skin) is called squamous cell carcinoma. Skin cancer that forms in neuroendocrine cells (cells that release hormones in response to signals from the nervous system) is called neuroendocrine carcinoma of the skin. Most skin cancers form in older people on parts of the body exposed to the sun or in people who have weakened immune systems.

small cell lung cancer: An aggressive (fast-growing) cancer that forms in tissues of the lung and can spread to other parts of the body. The cancer cells look small and oval-shaped when looked at under a microscope.

small intestine cancer: A rare cancer that forms in tissues of the small intestine (the part of the digestive tract between the stomach and the large intestine). The most common type is adenocarcinoma (cancer that begins in cells that make and release mucus and other fluids). Other types of small intestine cancer include sarcoma (cancer that begins in connective or supportive tissue), carcinoid tumor (a slow-growing type of cancer), gastrointestinal stromal tumor (a type of soft tissue sarcoma), and lymphoma (cancer that begins in immune system cells).

soft tissue sarcoma: A cancer that begins in the muscle, fat, fibrous tissue, blood vessels, or other supporting tissue of the body.

solid tumor: An abnormal mass of tissue that usually does not contain cysts or liquid areas. Solid tumors may be benign (not cancer), or malignant (cancer). Different types of solid tumors are named for the type of cells that form them. Examples of solid tumors are sarcomas, carcinomas, and lymphomas. Leukemias (cancers of the blood) generally do not form solid tumors.

squamous cell carcinoma: Cancer that begins in squamous cells, which are thin, flat cells that look like fish scales. Squamous cells are found in the tissue that forms the surface of the skin, the lining of the hollow organs of the body, and the passages of the respiratory and digestive tracts. Also called epidermoid carcinoma.

stage: The extent of a cancer in the body. Staging is usually based on the size of the tumor, whether lymph nodes contain cancer, and whether the cancer has spread from the original site to other parts of the body.

staging: Performing exams and tests to learn the extent of the cancer within the body, especially whether the disease has spread from the original site to other parts of the body. It is important to know the stage of the disease in order to plan the best treatment.

stem cell transplant: A method of replacing immature blood-forming cells in the bone marrow that have been destroyed by drugs, radiation, or disease. Stem cells are injected into the patient and make healthy blood cells. A stem cell transplant may be autologous (using a patient's own stem cells that were saved before treatment), allogeneic (using stem cells donated by someone who is not an identical twin), or syngeneic (using stem cells donated by an identical twin).

stereotactic biopsy: A biopsy procedure that uses a computer and a three-dimensional scanning device to find a tumor site and guide the removal of tissue for examination under a microscope.

stoma: A surgically created opening from an area inside the body to the outside.

stomach cancer: Cancer that forms in tissues lining the stomach. Also called gastric cancer.

supportive care: Care given to improve the quality of life of patients who have a serious or life-threatening disease. The goal of supportive care is to prevent or treat as early as possible the symptoms of a disease, side effects caused by treatment of a disease, and psychological, social, and spiritual problems related to a disease or its treatment. Also called comfort care, palliative care, and symptom management.

survivorship: In cancer, survivorship covers the physical, psychosocial, and economic issues of cancer, from diagnosis until the end of life. It focuses on the health and life of a person with cancer beyond the diagnosis and treatment phases. Survivorship includes issues related to the ability to get healthcare and follow-up treatment, late effects of treatment, second cancers, and quality of life. Family members, friends, and caregivers are also part of the survivorship experience.

systemic chemotherapy: Treatment with anticancer drugs that travel through the blood to cells all over the body.

targeted therapy: A type of treatment that uses drugs or other substances, such as monoclonal antibodies, to identify and attack specific cancer cells. Targeted therapy may have fewer side effects than other types of cancer treatments.

teratoma: A type of germ cell tumor that may contain several different types of tissue, such as hair, muscle, and bone. Teratomas occur most often in the ovaries in women, the testicles in men, and the tailbone in children. Not all teratomas are malignant.

testicular cancer: Cancer that forms in tissues of the testis (one of two egg-shaped glands inside the scrotum that make sperm and male hormones). Testicular cancer usually occurs in young or middle-aged men. Two main types of testicular cancer are seminomas (cancers that grow slowly and are sensitive to radiation therapy) and nonseminomas (different cell types that grow more quickly than seminomas).

thymic carcinoma: A rare type of thymus gland cancer. It usually spreads, has a high risk of recurrence, and has a poor survival rate. Thymic carcinoma is divided into subtypes, depending on the types of cells in which the cancer began. Also called type C thymoma.

thymoma: A tumor of the thymus, an organ that is part of the system and is located in the chest, behind the breastbone.

thyroid cancer: Cancer that forms in the thyroid gland (an organ at the base of the throat that makes hormones that help control heart rate, blood pressure, body temperature, and weight). Four main types of thyroid cancer are papillary, follicular, medullary, and anaplastic thyroid cancer. The four types are based on how the cancer cells look under a microscope.

tumor: An abnormal mass of tissue that results when cells divide more than they should or do not die when they should. Tumors may be benign (not cancer), or malignant (cancer). Also called neoplasm.

tumor marker: A substance that may be found in tumor tissue or released from a tumor into the blood or other body fluids. A high level of a tumor marker may mean that a certain type of cancer is in the body. Examples of tumor markers include CA 125 (in ovarian cancer), CA 15-3 (in breast cancer), CEA (in ovarian, lung, breast, pancreas, and gastrointestinal tract cancers), and PSA (in prostate cancer).

unresectable: Unable to be removed with surgery.

upper GI series: A series of X-ray pictures of the esophagus, stomach, and duodenum (the first part of the small intestine). The X-ray pictures are taken after the patient drinks a liquid containing barium sulfate (a form of the silver-white metallic element barium). The barium sulfate coats and outlines the inner walls of the upper gastrointestinal tract so that they can be seen on the X-ray pictures. Also called upper gastrointestinal series.

urethral cancer: A rare cancer that forms in tissues of the urethra (the tube through which urine empties the bladder and leaves the body). Types of urethral cancer include transitional cell carcinoma (cancer that begins in cells that can change shape and stretch without breaking apart), squamous cell carcinoma (cancer that begins in flat cells lining the urethra), and adenocarcinoma (cancer that begins in cells that make and release mucus and other fluids).

vaginal cancer: Cancer that forms in the tissues of the vagina (birth canal). The vagina leads from the cervix (the opening of the uterus) to the outside of the body. The most common type of vaginal cancer is squamous cell carcinoma, which starts in the thin, flat cells lining the vagina. Another type of vaginal cancer is adenocarcinoma, cancer that begins in glandular cells in the lining of the vagina.

virtual colonoscopy: A method to examine the inside of the colon by taking a series of X-rays. A computer is used to make two-dimensional (2-D) and three-dimensional (3-D) pictures of the colon from these X-rays. The pictures can be saved, changed to give better viewing angles, and reviewed after the procedure, even years later. Also called computed tomographic colonography, computed tomography colonography, CT colonography, and CTC.

vulvar cancer: Cancer of the vulva (the external female genital organs, including the clitoris, vaginal lips, and the opening to the vagina).

wound: A break in the skin or other body tissues caused by injury or surgical incision (cut).

X-ray: A type of high-energy radiation. In low doses, X-rays are used to diagnose diseases by making pictures of the inside of the body. In high doses, X-rays are used to treat cancer.

Chapter 86

National Organizations Offering Cancer-Related Services

Government Agencies That Provide Information about Cancer

Benefits.gov
U.S. Department of Labor (DOL)
200 Constitution Ave. N.W.
Washington, DC 20210
Toll-Free: 866-4-USA-DOL
(866-487-2365)
Website: www.benefits.gov

Colorectal Cancer Control Program (CCCP)
Centers for Disease Control and Prevention (CDC)
1600 Clifton Rd.
Atlanta, GA 30329-4027
Toll-Free: 800-CDC-INFO
(800-232-4636)
Toll-Free TTY: 888-232-6348
Website: www.cdc.gov/cancer/crccp
E-mail: cdcinfo@cdc.gov

Resources in this chapter were compiled from several sources deemed reliable; all contact information was verified and updated in March 2018.

Eldercare Locator
Administration on Aging (AOA)
330 C St. S.W.
Washington, DC 20201
Toll-Free: 800-677-1116
Website: www.eldercare.gov
E-mail: eldercarelocator@n4a.org

Health Resources & Services Administration (HRSA)
U.S. Department of Health and Human Services (HHS)
5600 Fishers Ln.
Rockville, MD 20857
Toll-Free: 877-464-4772
Phone: 301-443-3376
Toll-Free TTY: 877-897-9910
Website: www.hrsa.gov

Healthcare.gov
Centers for Medicare and Medicaid Services (CMS)
7500 Security Blvd.
Baltimore, MD 21244
Toll-Free TTY: 855-889-4325
Website: www.healthcare.gov

Medicaid.gov
Centers for Medicare and Medicaid Services (CMS)
7500 Security Blvd.
Baltimore, MD 21244-1850
Toll-Free: 877-267-2323
Phone: 410-786-3000
Toll-Free TTY: 866-226-1819
TTY: 410-786-0727
Website: www.cms.gov/MedicaidGenInfo

National Breast and Cervical Cancer Early Detection Program (NBCCEDP)
Centers for Disease Control and Prevention (CDC)
1600 Clifton Rd.
Atlanta, GA 30329-4027
Toll-Free: 800-CDC-INFO (800-232-4636)
Toll-Free TTY: 888-232-6348
Website: www.cdc.gov/cancer/nbccedp
E-mail: cdcinfo@cdc.gov

National Cancer Institute (NCI)
9609 Medical Center Dr.
BG 9609 MSC 9760
Bethesda, MD 20892-9760
Toll-Free: 800-4-CANCER (800-422-6237)
Website: www.cancer.gov

National Women's Health Information Center (NWHIC)
8270 Willow Oaks Corporate Dr.
Fairfax, VA 22031
Toll-Free: 800-994-9662
Toll-Free TTY: 888-220-5446
Website: www.womenshealth.gov

U.S. Department of Housing and Urban Development (HUD)
451 Seventh St. S.W.
Washington, DC 20410
Toll-Free: 800-569-4287
Phone: 202-708-1112
TTY: 202-708-1455
Website: www.hud.gov

U.S. Social Security Administration (SSA)
1100 W. High Rise
6401 Security Blvd.
Baltimore, MD 21235
Toll-Free: 800-772-1213
Toll-Free TTY: 800-325-0778
Website: www.ssa.gov

Private Agencies That Provide Information about Cancer

Air Charity Network (ACN)
Toll-Free: 877-621-7177
Website: www.
aircharitynetwork.org

American Cancer Society (ACS)
250 Williams St. N.W.
Ste. 600
Atlanta, GA 30303
Toll-Free: 800-227-2345
Website: www.cancer.org

American Childhood Cancer Organization (ACCO)
6868 Distribution Dr.
Beltsville, MD 20705
Toll-Free: 855-858-2226
Phone: 301-962-3520
Fax: 301-962-3521
Website: www.acco.org
E-mail: staff@acco.org

Be the Match
National Marrow Donor
Program (NMDP)
500 N. Fifth St.
Minneapolis, MN 55401-1206
Toll-Free: 800-MARROW2
(800-627-7692)
Website: www.bethematch.org
E-mail: patientinfo@nmdp.org

Camp Kesem
P.O. Box 452
Culver City, CA 90232
Phone: 260-22-KESEM
(260-225-3736)
Website: www.campkesem.org
E-mail: magic@campkesem.org

Cancer Hope Network (CHN)
2 North Rd., Ste. A
Chester, NJ 07930
Toll-Free: 877-HOPENET
(877-467-3638)
Phone: 908-879-4039
Fax: 908-879-6518
Website: www.
cancerhopenetwork.org
E-mail: info@
cancerhopenetwork.org

Cancer Support Community (CSC)
734 15th St. N.W.
Ste. 300
Washington, DC 20005
Toll-Free: 888-793-9355
Phone: 202-659-9709
Website: www.cancersupportcommunity.org
E-mail: help@cancersupportcommunity.org

***Cancer*Care**
275 Seventh Ave.
22nd Fl.
New York, NY 10001
Toll-Free: 800-813-HOPE (800-813-4673)
Phone: 212-712-8495
Website: www.cancercare.org
E-mail: info@cancercare.org

Caritas Internationalis
777 United Nations Plaza
S.10G
New York, NY 10017-3521
Website: www.caritas.org

Catholic Charities USA
2050 Ballenger Ave.
Ste. 400
Alexandria, VA 22314
Toll-Free: 800-919-9338
Phone: 703-549-1390
Fax: 703-549-1656
Website: www.catholiccharitiesusa.org
E-mail: info@catholiccharitiesusa.org

Children's Brain Tumor Foundation (CBTF)
1460 Bdwy.
New York, NY 10036
Toll-Free: 866-228-4673
Phone: 212-448-9494
Website: www.cbtf.org
E-mail: info@cbtf.org

Cleaning for a Reason Foundation (CRF)
211 S. Stemmons
Ste. G
Lewisville, TX 75067
Toll-Free: 877-337-3348
Fax: 972-316-4138
Website: www.cleaningforareason.org

Colorectal Care Line (CCCL)
421 Butler Farm Rd.
Hampton, VA 23666
Toll-Free: 866-657-8634
Website: www.colorectalcareline.org

Corporate Angel Network (CAN)
One Loop Rd.
White Plains, NY 10604-1215
Phone: 914-328-1313
Fax: 914-328-3938
Website: www.corpangelnetwork.org
E-mail: info@corpangelnetwork.org

Cure Search for Children's Cancer (CSCC)
4600 East West Hwy
Ste. 600
Bethesda, MD 20814
Toll-Free: 800-458-6223
Phone: 301-718-0047
Website: www.curesearch.org
E-mail: info@curesearch.org

Facing Our Risk of Cancer Empowered (FORCE)
16057 Tampa Palms Blvd. W
PMB 373
Tampa, FL 33647
Toll-Free: 866-288-RISK (866-288-7475)
Fax: 954-827-2200
Website: www.facingourrisk.org
E-mail: info@facingourrisk.org

Good Days
6900 N. Dallas Pkwy
Ste. 200
Plano, TX 75024
Toll-Free: 877-968-7233
Phone: 972-608-7141
Fax: 214-570-3621
Website: www.mygooddays.org

HealthWell Foundation
20440 Century Blvd.
Ste. 250
Germantown, MD 20874
Toll-Free: 800-675-8416
Toll-Free Fax: 800-282-7692
Website: www.healthwellfoundation.org
E-mail: grants@healthwellfoundation.org

Intercultural Cancer Council (ICC)
Baylor College of Medicine (BCM)
1720 Dryden Rd.
Ste. 1025
Houston, TX 77030
Phone: 713-798-4614
Website: iccnetwork.org
E-mail: info@iccnetwork.org

International Cancer Information Service Group (ICISG)
Website: www.icisg.org
E-mail: info@icisg.org

Joe's House
505 E. 79th St.
Ste. 17E
New York, NY 10075
Toll-Free: 877-563-7468
Website: www.joeshouse.org
E-mail: info@joeshouse.org

Leukemia and Lymphoma Society (LLS)
3 International Dr.
Ste. 200
Rye Brook, NY 10573
Toll-Free: 888-557-7177
Website: www.lls.org

Livestrong
2201 E. Sixth St.
Austin, TX 78702
Toll-Free: 877-236-8820
Website: www.livestrong.org
E-mail: livestrong@livestrong.org

Look Good Feel Better (LGFB)
Toll-Free: 800-395-LOOK (800-395-5665)
Website: www.lookgoodfeelbetter.org

M.D. Anderson Cancer Center
1515 Holcombe Blvd.
Houston, TX 77030
Toll-Free: 844-854-4601
Website: www.mdanderson.org

Melanoma International Foundation (MIF)
250 Mapleflower Rd.
Glenmoore, PA 19343
Toll-Free: 866-463-6663
Phone: 610-942-3432
Website: melanomainternational.org
E-mail: contact@melanomainternational.org

Memorial Sloan-Kettering Cancer Center (MSKCC)
1275 York Ave.
New York, NY 10065
Toll-Free: 800-525-2225
Phone: 212-639-2000
Website: www.mskcc.org

Mesothelioma Applied Research Foundation (MARF)
c/o WeWork
641 S. St. N.W.
Washington, DC 20001
Toll-Free: 877-363-6376
Fax: 571-363-2784
Website: www.curemeso.org
E-mail: info@curemeso.org

National Association of Insurance Commissioners (NAIC)
1100 Walnut St.
Ste. 1500
Kansas City, MO 64106-2197
Phone: 816-842-3600
Fax: 816-783-8175
Website: www.naic.org
E-mail: help@naic.org

The National Children's Cancer Society (NCCS)
500 N. Bdwy.
Ste. 1850
St. Louis, MO 63102
Toll-Free: 800-532-6459
Phone: 314-241-1600
Fax: 314-241-1996
Website: www.thenccs.org

National Coalition for Cancer Survivorship (NCCS)
8455 Colesville Rd.
Ste. 930
Silver Spring, MD 20910
Toll-Free: 877-NCCS-YES (877-622-7937)
Website: www.canceradvocacy.org
E-mail: info@canceradvocacy.org

National Lymphedema Network (NLN)
411 Lafayette St.
Sixth Fl.
New York, NY 10003
Toll-Free: 800-541-3259
Phone: 646-772-7410
Website: www.lymphnet.org
E-mail: nln@lymphnet.org

NeedyMeds
P.O. Box 219
Gloucester, MA 01931
Toll-Free: 800-503-6897
Fax: 206-260-8850
Website: www.needymeds.org
E-mail: info@needymeds.org

Patient Advocate Foundation (PAF)
421 Butler Farm Rd.
Hampton, VA 23666
Toll-Free: 800-532-5274
Fax: 757-873-8999
Website: www.patientadvocate.org
E-mail: help@patientadvocate.org

Physicians Committee
5100 Wisconsin Ave.
Ste. 400
Washington, DC 20016
Phone: 202-244-5038
Website: www.pcrm.org
E-mail: pcrm@pcrm.org

R.A. Bloch Cancer Foundation
One H&R Block Way
Kansas City, MO 64105
Toll-Free: 800-433-0464
Phone: 816-854-5050
Fax: 816-854-8024
Website: www.blochcancer.org
E-mail: hotline@blochcancer.org

Ronald McDonald House Charities (RMHC)
One Kroc Dr.
Oak Brook, IL 60523
Website: www.rmhc.org
E-mail: info@rmhc.org

The Salvation Army National Headquarters
615 Slaters Ln.
P.O. Box 269
Alexandria, VA 22313
Toll-Free: 800-SA-TRUCK (800-728-7825)
Website: www.salvationarmyusa.org

The Samfund
89 South St.
Ste. LL02
Boston, MA 02111
Toll-Free: 866-439-9365
Phone: 617-938-3484
Toll-Free Fax: 866-496-8070
Website: www.thesamfund.org

Sarcoma Alliance
775 Blithedale Ave.
Ste. 334
Mill Valley, CA 94941
Phone: 415-381-7236
Fax: 415-381-7235
Website: www.sarcomaalliance.org
E-mail: info@sarcomaalliance.org

Sisters Network, Inc.
2922 Rosedale St.
Houston, TX 77004
Toll-Free: 866-781-1808
Phone: 713-781-0255
Fax: 713-780-8998
Website: www.sistersnetworkinc.org
E-mail: infonet@sistersnetworkinc.org

Stupid Cancer
40 worth st.
Ste. 808
New York, NY 10013
Toll-Free: 877-735-4673
Website: www.stupidcancer.org
E-mail: contact@stupidcancer.org

Susan G. Komen
5005 LBJ Fwy
Ste. 526
Dallas, TX 75244
Toll-Free: 877-GO-KOMEN
(877-465-6636)
Website: ww5.komen.org
E-mail: helpline@komen.org

Teens Living with Cancer
1000 Elmood Ave.
Rochester, NY 14620
Phone: 585-563-6221
Website: www.
teenslivingwithcancer.org

13thirty Cancer Connect
1000 Elmwood Ave.
Rochester, NY 14620
Phone: 585-563-6221
Website: 13thirty.org
E-mail: staff@13thirty.org

The Ulman Cancer Fund for Young Adults
1215 E. Fort Ave.
Ste. 104
Baltimore, MD 21230
Toll-Free: 888-393-FUND
(888-393-3863)
Phone: 410-964-0202
Toll-Free Fax: 888-964-0402
Website: www.ulmanfund.org
E-mail: info@ulmanfund.org

United Healthcare Children's Foundation (UHCCF)
9700 Health Care Ln.
MN017-W400
Minneapolis, MN 55343
Toll-Free: 855-MY-UHCCF
(855-698-4223)
Website: www.uhccf.org
E-mail: customerservice@uhccf.
org

United Way Worldwide
701 N. Fairfax St.
Alexandria, VA 22314
Phone: 703-836-7112
Website: www.unitedway.org

Us TOO International, Inc.
2720 S. River Rd.
Ste. 112
Des Plaines, IL 60018
Toll-Free: 800-808-7866
Phone: 630-795-1002
Fax: 630-795-1602
Website: www.ustoo.org
E-mail: ustoo@ustoo.org

Young Survival Coalition (YSC)
80 Broad St.
Ste. 1700
New York, NY 10004
Toll-Free: 877-972-1011
Fax: 646-257-3030
Website: www.youngsurvival.org
E-mail: info@youngsurvival.org

Chapter 87

Using Trusted Resources

Health information, whether in print or online, should come from a trusted, credible source. Government agencies, hospitals, universities, and medical journals and books that provide evidence-based information are sources you can trust. Too often, other sources can provide misleading or incorrect information. If a source makes claims that are too good to be true, remember—they usually are.

There are many websites, books, and magazines that provide health information to the public, but not all of them are trustworthy. Use the resources provided below to safeguard yourself when reviewing sources of health information.

Websites

Online sources of health information should make it easy for people to learn who is responsible for posting the information. They should make clear the original source of the information, along with the medical credentials of the people who prepare or review the posted material.

Use the following questions to determine the credibility of health information published online.

- **Who manages this information?**

  The person or group that has published health information online should be easy to find somewhere on the page.

This chapter includes text excerpted from "Using Trusted Resources," National Cancer Institute (NCI), May 3, 2017.

- **What are the letters at the end of the web address?**

  Government websites end in ".gov" and those ending with ".edu" are run by a university or other educational institution. These are sources that you can usually trust. If you see ".org" or ".com" at the end of a web address, it may also be a trusted site. However, check it closely to make sure.

- **Who is paying for the project, and what is their purpose?**

  You should be able to find this information in the "About Us" section.

- **What is the original source of the information that they have posted?**

  If the information was originally published in a research journal or a book, they should say which one(s) so that you can find it.

- **How is information reviewed before it gets posted?**

  Most health information publications have someone with medical or research credentials (e.g., someone who has earned an M.D., D.O., or Ph.D.) review the information before it gets posted, to make sure it is correct.

- **How current is the information?**

  Online health information sources should show you when the information was posted or last reviewed.

- **If they are asking for personal information, how will they use that information and how will they protect your privacy?**

  This is very important. Do not share personal information until you understand the policies under which it will be used and you are comfortable with any risk involved in sharing your information online.

Social Media

Social media sites (such as Facebook, Twitter) are good ways to stay connected. However, when you're seeking medical information, only follow social media from reputable sources. Many trusted organizations have social media accounts that link to their websites. For example, the National Cancer Institute (NCI) has an official Facebook pages (www.cancer.gov/social-media#facebook) and many Twitter accounts (www.cancer.gov/social-media#twitter) from its offices and departments.

When it comes to personal social media accounts, it's common for users to post their experiences with illness. This may include:

- How they're feeling physically
- Treatments they're going through
- Complementary therapies they're using, such as a type of diet or supplements
- What feelings they're having

But remember that everyone is different. Even someone with the exact same kind of cancer has a different body and health history from you. And never take recommendations for treatment or medicines from someone other than your doctor. You don't know where or how the user got their information. You also don't know if the information is current, or what the user's knowledge of cancer is.

Books

A number of books have been written about cancer, cancer treatment, and complementary and alternative medicine (CAM). Some books contain trustworthy content, while others do not.

It's important to know that information is always changing and that new research results are reported every day. Be aware that if a book is written by only one person, you may only be getting that one person's view.

If you go to the library, ask the staff for suggestions. Or if you live near a college or university, there may be a medical library available. Local bookstores may also have people on staff who can help you. If you find a book online, look very carefully at the author's credentials, background, and expertise. Questions you may want to ask yourself are:

- Is the author an expert on this subject?
- Do you know anyone else who has read the book?
- Has the book been reviewed by other experts?
- Was it published in the past 5 years?
- Does the book offer different points of view, or does it seem to hold one opinion?

- Has the author researched the topic in full?
- Are the references listed in the back?

Magazines

If you want to look for articles you can trust, search online medical journal databases or ask your librarian to help you look for medical journals, books, and other research that has been done by experts.

Articles in popular magazines are usually not written by experts. Rather, the authors speak with experts, gather information, and then write the article. If claims are made in a magazine, remember:

- The authors may not have expert knowledge in this area.
- They may not say where they found their information.
- The articles have not been reviewed by experts.
- The publisher may have ties to advertisers or other organizations. Therefore, the article may be one-sided in the information or view(s) it presents.

When you read these articles, you can use the same process that the magazine writer uses:

- Speak with experts
- Ask lots of questions
- Then decide if the therapy is right for you

Where to Get More Help

Cancer Treatment Scams

A page (www.consumer.ftc.gov/articles/0104-cancer-treatment-scams) from the Federal Trade Commission (FTC) that advises people to ask their healthcare provider about products that claim to cure or treat cancer and offers tips for spotting treatment scams.

For Consumers: Protecting Yourself

A page (www.fda.gov/ForConsumers/ProtectYourself/default.htm) from the U.S. Food and Drug Administration (FDA) that includes links to several resources that have tips about buying medicines and other products online.

Evaluating Cancer Information on the Internet

Developed by the American Society of Clinical Oncology (ASCO), Cancer.Net provides information, including common misconceptions about cancer and tips to evaluate the credibility of online cancer information.

Chapter 88

Beware of Online Cancer Fraud

Products Claiming to "Cure" Cancer Are a Cruel Deception

Beware of products claiming to cure cancer on websites or social media platforms, such as Facebook and Instagram. According to Nicole Kornspan, M.P.H., a consumer safety officer at the U.S. Food and Drug Administration (FDA), they're rampant these days.

"Anyone who suffers from cancer, or knows someone who does, understands the fear and desperation that can set in," says Kornspan. "There can be a great temptation to jump at anything that appears to offer a chance for a cure."

Legitimate medical products such as drugs and devices intended to treat cancer must gain FDA approval or clearance before they are marketed and sold. The agency's review process helps ensure that these products are safe and effective for their intended uses.

Nevertheless, it's always possible to find someone or some company hawking bogus cancer "treatments," which come in many forms, including pills, capsules, powders, creams, teas, oils, and treatment kits. Frequently advertised as "natural" treatments and often falsely

---

This chapter includes text excerpted from "Products Claiming to "Cure" Cancer Are a Cruel Deception," U.S. Food and Drug Administration (FDA), January 8, 2018.

labeled as dietary supplements, such products may appear harmless, but may cause harm by delaying or interfering with proven, beneficial treatments. Absent FDA approval or clearance for safety, they could also contain dangerous ingredients.

That holds true for treatments intended for humans and those intended for pets. "Increasingly, bogus remedies claiming to cure cancer in cats and dogs are showing up online," Kornspan says. "People who cannot afford to spend large sums at the animal hospital to treat cancer in their beloved dogs and cats are searching for less expensive remedies."

The FDA urges consumers to steer clear of these potentially unsafe and unproven products and to always discuss cancer treatment options with their licensed healthcare provider.

FDA Takes Action

In April 2017, the FDA sent out warning letters to 14 companies, advising them to change or remove the fraudulent claims on their websites. If the companies don't comply, the FDA may take further legal action to prevent their products from reaching consumers.

Red Flags

While some fraudulent products claim to cure a variety of diseases and conditions, fraudulent cancer products often use a particular vocabulary, Kornspan says. Consumers should recognize certain phrases as red flags, including:

- Treats all forms of cancer
- Miraculously kills cancer cells and tumors
- Shrinks malignant tumors
- Selectively kills cancer cells
- More effective than chemotherapy
- Attacks cancer cells, leaving healthy cells intact
- Cures cancer

Moreover, whether products claim to cure cancer or another disease, there are a number of catchphrases that can tip you off that they're bogus.

"There are legal ways for patients to access investigational drugs, for example taking part in clinical trials," says Kornspan. Patients looking to try an experimental cancer treatment should talk to their doctor about treatment options.

Index

Index

Page numbers followed by 'n' indicate a footnote. Page numbers in *italics* indicate a table or illustration.

D

E

F

G

H

I

M

N

O

P

S

T

U

V